A Clinician's Guide to Autism

A Clinician's Guide to Autism

Editor: Paul Hiddleston

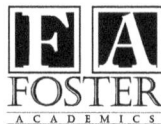

FA
FOSTER
ACADEMICS

www.fosteracademics.com

www.fosteracademics.com

FA FOSTER
ACADEMICS

Cataloging-in-Publication Data

A clinician's guide to autism / edited by Paul Hiddleston.
    p. cm.
Includes bibliographical references and index.
ISBN 978-1-63242-785-4
1. Autism. 2. Autism--Diagnosis. 3. Hyperlexia. 4. Autism spectrum disorders.
I. Hiddleston, Paul.
RC553.A88 C55 2019
616.858 82--dc23

Foster Academics,
118-35 Queens Blvd., Suite 400,
Forest Hills, NY 11375, USA

ISBN 978-1-63242-785-4 (Hardback)

Contents

Preface..VII

Chapter 1 **Alterations in the inferior longitudinal fasciculus in autism and associations with visual processing: a diffusion-weighted MRI study**..1
Bart Boets, Lien Van Eylen, Kevin Sitek, Pieter Moors, Ilse Noens,
Jean Steyaert, Stefan Sunaer and Johan Wagemans

Chapter 2 **Autism spectrum disorder: prospects for treatment using gene therapy**.................15
Matthew Benger, Maria Kinali and Nicholas D. Mazarakis

Chapter 3 **CRISPR/Cas9-induced *shank3b* mutant zebrafish display autism-like behaviors**..................25
Chun-xue Liu, Chun-yang Li, Chun-chun Hu, Yi Wang, Jia Lin,
Yong-hui Jiang, Qiang Li and Xiu Xu

Chapter 4 **Operationalizing atypical gaze in toddlers with autism spectrum disorders: a cohesion-based approach**..................38
Quan Wang, Daniel J. Campbell, Suzanne L. Macari, Katarzyna Chawarska and
Frederick Shic

Chapter 5 **Prenatal mercury exposure and features of autism**..................47
Jean Golding, Dheeraj Rai, Steven Gregory, Genette Ellis, Alan Emond,
Yasmin Iles-Caven, Joseph Hibbeln and Caroline Taylor

Chapter 6 **Impairment of social behaviors in *Arhgef10* knockout mice**..................56
Dai-Hua Lu, Hsiao-Mei Liao, Chia-Hsiang Chen, Huang-Ju Tu,
Houng-Chi Liou, Susan Shur-Fen Gau and Wen-Mei Fu

Chapter 7 **Risk markers for suicidality in autistic adults**..................69
Sarah Cassidy, Louise Bradley, Rebecca Shaw and Simon Baron-Cohen

Chapter 8 **Abnormal coherence and sleep composition in children with Angelman syndrome**..................83
Hanna den Bakker, Michael S. Sidorov, Zheng Fan, David J. Lee,
Lynne M. Bird, Catherine J. Chu and Benjamin D. Philpot

Chapter 9 **The impact of robotic intervention on joint attention in children with autism spectrum disorders**..................95
Hirokazu Kumazaki, Yuichiro Yoshikawa, Yuko Yoshimura, Takashi Ikeda,
Chiaki Hasegawa, Daisuke N. Saito, Sara Tomiyama, Kyung-min An, Jiro Shimaya,
Hiroshi Ishiguro, Yoshio Matsumoto, Yoshio Minabe and Mitsuru Kikuchi

Chapter 10 **Sleep disturbances are associated with specific sensory sensitivities in children with autism**..................105
Orna Tzischinsky, Gal Meiri, Liora Manelis, Asif Bar-Sinai, Hagit Flusser,
Analya Michaelovski, Orit Zivan, Michal Ilan, Michal Faroy,
Idan Menashe and Ilan Dinstein

Chapter 11   **Oscillatory rhythm of reward: anticipation and processing of rewards in children with and without autism** 115
Katherine Kuhl-Meltzoff Stavropoulos and Leslie J. Carver

Chapter 12   **The effect of age on vertex-based measures of the grey-white matter tissue contrast in autism spectrum disorder** 130
Caroline Mann, Anke Bletsch, Derek Andrews, Eileen Daly, Clodagh Murphy, Declan Murphy and Christine Ecker

Chapter 13   **Analysis of neuroanatomical differences in mice with genetically modified serotonin transporters assessed by structural magnetic resonance imaging** 143
Jacob Ellegood, Yohan Yee, Travis M. Kerr, Christopher L. Muller, Randy D. Blakely, R. Mark Henkelman, Jeremy Veenstra-VanderWeele and Jason P. Lerch

Chapter 14   **17-β estradiol increases parvalbumin levels in *Pvalb* heterozygous mice and attenuates behavioral phenotypes with relevance to autism core symptoms** 155
Federica Filice, Emanuel Lauber, Karl Jakob Vörckel, Markus Wöhr and Beat Schwaller

Chapter 15   **Self-reported sex differences in high-functioning adults with autism** 168
R. L. Moseley, R. Hitchiner and J. A. Kirkby

Chapter 16   **Practice patterns and determinants of wait time for autism spectrum disorder diagnosis** 180
Melanie Penner, Evdokia Anagnostou and Wendy J. Ungar

Chapter 17   **Does stereopsis account for the link between motor and social skills in adults?** 193
Danielle Smith, Danielle Ropar and Harriet A Allen

Chapter 18   **Intranasal administration of exosomes derived from mesenchymal stem cells ameliorates autistic-like behaviors of BTBR mice** 208
Nisim Perets, Stav Hertz, Michael London and Daniel Offen

Chapter 19   **Savant syndrome has a distinct psychological profile in autism** 220
James E A Hughes, Jamie Ward, Elin Gruffydd, Simon Baron-Cohen, Paula Smith, Carrie Allison and Julia Simner

                Permissions

                List of Contributors

                Index

Preface

Autism is a developmental disorder. It is identified by the problems associated with social interaction, and restricted and repetitive behavior. These signs can generally be detected in the first two or three years of a child's life. Some of the common characteristics of autistic children are avoidance of eye contact and turn-taking, preference of loneliness, and difficulty in maintaining friendships. Echolalia and use of reverse pronouns are commonly witnessed in an autistic child. Rubella, alcohol, pesticides, cocaine, air pollution and valproic acid are some common risk factors during pregnancy, which may cause autism in the unborn child. Different approaches, evaluations, methodologies and advanced studies on autism have been included in this book. It brings forth some of the most innovative concepts and elucidates the unexplored aspects of autism. Students, doctors, and experts actively engaged in this field will find this book full of crucial and unexplored concepts.

After months of intensive research and writing, this book is the end result of all who devoted their time and efforts in the initiation and progress of this book. It will surely be a source of reference in enhancing the required knowledge of the new developments in the area. During the course of developing this book, certain measures such as accuracy, authenticity and research focused analytical studies were given preference in order to produce a comprehensive book in the area of study.

This book would not have been possible without the efforts of the authors and the publisher. I extend my sincere thanks to them. Secondly, I express my gratitude to my family and well-wishers. And most importantly, I thank my students for constantly expressing their willingness and curiosity in enhancing their knowledge in the field, which encourages me to take up further research projects for the advancement of the area.

Editor

Alterations in the inferior longitudinal fasciculus in autism and associations with visual processing: a diffusion-weighted MRI study

Bart Boets[1,2,3*], Lien Van Eylen[1,2], Kevin Sitek[3,4], Pieter Moors[5], Ilse Noens[6], Jean Steyaert[1,2], Stefan Sunaert[7] and Johan Wagemans[2,5]

Abstract

Background: One of the most reported neural features of autism spectrum disorder (ASD) is the alteration of multiple long-range white matter fiber tracts, as assessed by diffusion-weighted imaging and indexed by reduced fractional anisotropy (FA). Recent methodological advances, however, have shown that this same pattern of reduced FA may be an artifact resulting from excessive head motion and poorer data quality and that aberrant structural connectivity in children with ASD is confined to the right inferior longitudinal fasciculus (ILF). This study aimed at replicating the observation of reduced FA along the right ILF in ASD, while controlling for group differences in head motion and data quality. In addition, we explored associations between reduced FA in the right ILF and quantitative ASD characteristics, and the involvement of the right ILF in visual processing, which is known to be altered in ASD.

Method: Global probabilistic tractography was performed on diffusion-weighted imaging data of 17 adolescent boys with ASD and 17 typically developing boys, matched for age, performance IQ, handedness, and data quality. Four tasks were administered to measure various aspects of visual information processing, together with questionnaires assessing ASD characteristics. Group differences were examined and the neural data were integrated with previously published findings using Bayesian statistics to quantify evidence for replication and to pool data and thus increase statistical power. (Partial) correlations were calculated to investigate associations between measures.

Results: The ASD group showed consistently reduced FA only in the right ILF and slower performance on the visual search task. Bayesian statistics pooling data across studies confirmed that group differences in FA were confined to the right ILF only, with the evidence for altered FA in the left ILF being indecisive. Lower FA in the right ILF tended to covary with slower visual search and a more fragmented part-oriented processing style. Individual differences in FA of the right ILF were not reliably associated with the severity of ASD traits after controlling for clinical status.

Conclusion: Our findings support the growing evidence for reduced FA along a specific fiber tract in ASD, the right ILF.

Keywords: Autism spectrum disorder, Structural connectivity, Diffusion-weighted imaging, Visual processing, Inferior longitudinal fasciculus

* Correspondence: bart.boets@kuleuven.be
Bart Boets and Lien Van Eylen are joint first author.
Bart Boets and Lien Van Eylen contributed equally to this work.
[1]Center for Developmental Psychiatry, Department of Neurosciences, KU Leuven, Kapucijnenvoer 7h, PB 7001, 3000 Leuven, Belgium
[2]Leuven Autism Research (LAuRes), KU Leuven, 3000 Leuven, Belgium
Full list of author information is available at the end of the article

Background

Autism spectrum disorder (ASD) is a neurodevelopmental disorder characterized by impairments in social reciprocity and communication, combined with restricted, repetitive and stereotyped patterns of behavior, interests or activities (RRBIs) [1]. Atypical sensory processing is also often reported and has been included in the new diagnostic RRBI criteria of ASD in DSM-5 [1]. Although the etiology of the disorder remains largely unknown, advanced genetic and neuroimaging studies point towards the involvement of altered brain connectivity [2], and the core behavioral and cognitive atypicalities have been related to reduced integration of information between different brain regions [3–5]. Reduced long-range connectivity has often been investigated in ASD, but there are many inconsistencies regarding the existence, the direction, and the specific anatomical location of this aberrant brain connectivity [6–10].

Here, we investigated structural brain connectivity in ASD using diffusion-weighted imaging (DWI). This noninvasive magnetic resonance imaging (MRI) technique indirectly assesses the structural properties and orientation of white matter tracts based on the diffusion of water molecules [11]. Typically, reduced diffusivity along the principal axis (i.e., axial diffusivity or AD) and increased diffusivity perpendicular to it (i.e., radial diffusivity or RD), resulting in a reduced directionality of diffusion (i.e., lower fractional anisotropy or FA), are considered indicative of reduced white matter integrity and thus reduced structural connectivity [11]. However, this interpretation might be misleading as the exact microstructural and macrostructural substrates of reduced FA are only partly understood (e.g., axonal density, axonal diameter, degree of myelination, homogeneity of axon orientation) [12, 13]. Therefore, in the present report, we will refer to the observed diffusion properties per se, without making inferences about white matter integrity.

Previous studies have observed widespread reductions of FA in individuals with ASD and have interpreted these findings as indicative of generally reduced white matter connectivity in ASD [8, 9]. A meta-analysis of diffusion imaging studies revealed four clusters with consistently lower FA in individuals with ASD [8]. The largest cluster was located in the right occipito-temporal region and extended from the inferior occipital and lingual gyrus into the fusiform and inferior temporal gyrus. Fiber tracking through this cluster pinpointed aberrant connectivity along the right inferior longitudinal fasciculus (ILF) in ASD [8].

Recent findings, however, revealed that differences in diffusion properties may be an artifact resulting from excessive head motion and poorer DWI data quality [14, 15]. Individuals with ASD may be more prone to greater head motion and the resulting DWI artifacts, as shown by Koldewyn and colleagues [16]. These authors applied diffusion-weighted imaging combined with global probabilistic tractography in school-aged children with ASD versus typically developing (TD) children and showed reduced FA in ASD along multiple white matter tracts. However, after carefully matching data quality and head motion parameters between both groups, all these effects disappeared, except for consistently reduced FA in one single tract, the right ILF [16]. This study thus challenged the hypothesis of widespread changes in FA-related structural connectivity in ASD and highlighted the importance of matching for data quality.

The ILF is a white matter association tract, extending from the occipital cortex into the anterior temporal lobe [17]. The right ILF connects several brain regions that are crucially involved in face processing (e.g., the occipital face area, the fusiform face area, the superior temporal sulcus, and the amygdala) [6], and lesions of the right ILF have been associated with face processing impairments [18]. Given the characteristic difficulties of individuals with ASD with processing faces [19–21], Koldewyn and colleagues [16] a priori hypothesized to observe structural abnormalities in the right ILF in individuals with ASD. Yet, as the ILF (both right and left) carries information from many extrastriate visual areas throughout the ventral visual stream, it is also implicated in visual perceptual organization and object recognition in general [17, 22]. Therefore, alterations in the ILF may (at least partially) underlie the known visual processing anomalies of individuals with ASD. Although these perceptual atypicalities are often subtle and dependent on particular task and sample characteristics [23], it has been shown that individuals with ASD have problems with global integrative processing and are more inclined to process and attend to parts and details [24–26], as postulated by the Weak Central Coherence (WCC) account [24].

The overall aim of this study was threefold. First of all, we aimed to replicate the findings of Koldewyn and colleagues [16], obtained in children, in an independent sample of adolescents with ASD and TD controls, using an identical methodological approach. In particular, we expected individuals with ASD to show selectively reduced FA of the right ILF. Therefore, the right ILF constituted the main anatomical target, along with 17 other major white matter tracts that were also included in the study of Koldewyn and colleagues [16]. Second, we explored whether reduced FA of the right ILF is associated with increased ASD symptom severity, both regarding the social and the non-social (i.e., RRBI) domains. Given its involvement in face processing, which is crucial for efficient social communication and interaction, we mainly expected an association of ILF properties with the social symptom domain. Yet, the ILF also plays a role in visual perception [17, 22], and given that the perceptual peculiarities of individuals with ASD are proposed to underlie (at least some of) their RRBIs [27], it is warranted to also explore the association between ILF properties and general RRBI symptomatology. Third, given the involvement of the ILF in ventral visual stream processing, we examined the association between ILF diffusion properties and performance on several visual processing measures. Although both left and right ILF play a role in visual processing, within the context of studying an ASD sample and in line with our previous hypothesis, we mainly focused on the association between individual differences in FA of the right ILF and visual processing measures. Four tasks that are often used in ASD research and that each target visual information integration in a different manner were administered: a Fragmented Object Outlines task, a Coherent Motion task, a visual search task, and the Rey-Osterrieth Complex Figure task (ROCF) (for a detailed conceptual and technical description of these tasks, see Van Eylen et al. [23]). Both the Fragmented Object Outlines task and the Coherent Motion task require visual information integration. However, the Fragmented Object Outlines task relies more on ventral visual stream functioning, as it requires form integration [28, 29], whereas the Coherent Motion task relies on dorsal visual stream functioning, since it requires the integration of motion signals [30]. Therefore, it is expected that only performance on the Fragmented Object Outlines task is associated with ILF properties. The visual search task is more controversial in terms of the implicated visual processes. While it has traditionally been conceptualized to measure local processing abilities, it also requires various types of grouping and feature integration [31, 32] and may therefore also be associated with ventral stream ILF diffusion properties. Finally, the ROCF task does not provide an indication of processing abilities but provides an indication

of processing style, with a higher score indicating a more fragmented, locally oriented processing style, and a lower score reflecting a more global integrative processing style [23]. For this task, we expect that a more integrative processing style is related to higher FA in the ILF.

Methods

Participants

Nineteen boys with ASD and 19 TD boys participated in the study. All participants were aged between 11 and 18 years, had a full-scale IQ (FSIQ) above 80 and had normal or corrected-to-normal vision (with glasses or lenses). Data on pubertal development were not collected. Participants were excluded if they had a history of epilepsy, traumatic brain injury, and attention deficit/hyperactivity disorder or if ASD was associated with a genetic syndrome. One individual with ASD had dyslexia and one had a developmental coordination disorder. None of the participants took psychotropic medication. Inclusion criteria for the ASD group were (1) a diagnosis of ASD made by the multidisciplinary Expertise Center for Autism (University Hospitals KU Leuven) in a standardized way according to DSM-IV-TR criteria [33]; (2) confirmation of their diagnosis with the Developmental, Dimensional, and Diagnostic interview (3di) [34] and (3) T-scores above 65 on the Social Responsiveness Scale (SRS) [35, 36]. None of the TD participants, nor their first degree relatives, had a history of neurological or psychiatric conditions, nor a current medical, developmental or psychiatric diagnosis. Parents of the control children completed the SRS questionnaire [35, 36] to exclude the presence of substantial ASD characteristics.

Application of a strict DWI data quality criterion (cf. supra) resulted in the selection of 17 adolescents with ASD (two left-handed) and 17 TD adolescents (two left-handed), matched for age, performance IQ, sex, handedness, and MRI data quality (see Tables 1 and 2). Both groups differed (marginally) significantly with regard to

Table 1 Participant characteristics

	ASD (n = 17)		TD (n = 17)		
	M	SD	M	SD	p value
Age (years)	13.8	1.3	14.4	2.0	.27
Performance IQ[a]	104	15	112	15	.14
Verbal IQ[a]	105	18	116	13	.05
Total IQ[a]	105	14	114	10	.03
Social Responsiveness Scale (Total T)[b]	90	10	44	8	< .0001
SRS Social Communication and Interaction	78	15	14	10	< .0001
SRS RRBI	16	5	1.3	1.6	< .0001
Repetitive Behavior Scale—Revised	21	11	0.5	1.3	< .0001

[a]Standardized scores with population average M = 100 and SD = 15
[b]Standardized scores with population average M = 50 and SD = 10

Table 2 Between-group differences for DWI data quality measures and for FA per tract

	ASD (n = 17)		TD (n = 17)		F	p value
	M	SD	M	SD		
DWI data quality measures						
Average translation	1.4279	0.3591	1.4271	0.3597	0.00	0.995
Average rotation	0.0130	0.0047	0.0114	0.0041	1.16	0.290
Percentage of slices with drop-out	0.2781	0.4457	0.1903	0.6030	0.23	0.633
Average signal drop-out score	1.0381	0.0437	1.0187	0.0332	2.12	0.155
Fractional anisotropy (FA) per tract						
R inferior longitudinal fasciculus [*,°]	0.4395	0.0259	0.4622	0.0293	5.74	0.023
L inferior longitudinal fasciculus [*]	0.4561	0.0319	0.4779	0.0286	4.43	0.043
R anterior thalamic radiations	0.3900	0.0261	0.4012	0.0208	1.94	0.173
L anterior thalamic radiations	0.3928	0.0248	0.4033	0.0295	1.26	0.269
R cingulum-angular bundle	0.3131	0.0351	0.2983	0.0215	2.21	0.147
L cingulum-angular bundle	0.2953	0.0379	0.2880	0.0303	0.38	0.541
R cingulum-cingulate gyrus bundle	0.4161	0.0373	0.4302	0.0527	0.81	0.374
L cingulum-cingulate gyrys bundle	0.4492	0.0468	0.4725	0.0596	1.61	0.214
R corticospinal tract	0.5243	0.0196	0.5228	0.0397	0.02	0.888
L corticospinal tract	0.5352	0.0230	0.5197	0.0307	2.79	0.105
R superior longitudinal fasciculus—parietal	0.4037	0.0253	0.4103	0.0263	0.56	0.461
L superior longitudinal fasciculus—parietal	0.4234	0.0485	0.4300	0.0381	0.19	0.662
R superior longitudinal fasciculus—temporal	0.4711	0.0271	0.4816	0.0270	1.30	0.263
L superior longitudinal fasciculus—temporal	0.4642	0.0304	0.4714	0.0274	0.52	0.477
R uncinate fasciculus	0.4002	0.0247	0.4018	0.0276	0.03	0.862
L uncinate fasciculus	0.3810	0.0247	0.3855	0.0244	0.28	0.603
Forceps major (corpus callosum)	0.5252	0.0866	0.5326	0.0759	0.07	0.793
Forceps minor (corpus callosum)	0.4976	0.0329	0.4938	0.0329	0.11	0.737

Note. [*] $p < .05$, [°] group difference that survives Bonferroni correction ($\alpha = 0.05/18 = 0.0028$), after outlier exclusion ($F(1,30) = 12.40$, $p = .0014$)

verbal and total IQ. However, as we aimed to replicate the study of Koldewyn and colleagues [16] as closely as possible, we ensured to control for the same participant characteristics as these authors (i.e., age, performance IQ, sex, and data quality measures).

The study was approved by the local Ethical Board and informed consent was obtained from all parents/guardians according to the Declaration of Helsinki, with additional assent from all participating children.

DWI data acquisition

After familiarization in a mock scanner, scanning was performed with a 32 head coil 3T Philips Achieva system at the University Hospitals Leuven. DWI data covering the entire brain and brainstem were acquired using an optimized single-shot spin-echo, echo planar imaging sequence with the following parameters: 58 contiguous saggital slices, slice thickness = 2.5 mm, repetition time (TR) = 7600 ms, echo time (TE) = 65 ms, field-of-view (FOV) = $240 \times 200 \times 145$ mm^2, matrix size = 96 × 94, in-plane pixel size = 2.12×2.5 mm^2, acquisition time = 10 min 33 s. Diffusion gradients were applied in 60 non-collinear directions ($b = 1300$ s/mm^2) and one image without diffusion-weighting was acquired. Additionally, a high-resolution T_1-weighted anatomical scan was collected (182 contiguous coronal slices, TR = 9.6 ms, TE = 4.6 ms, FOV = $250 \times 250 \times 218$ mm^3, acquisition matrix = 256 × 256, voxel size = $0.98 \times 0.98 \times 1.2$ mm^3, acquisition time = 6 min 23 s).

DWI data processing

DWI data were analyzed using anatomically constrained global probabilistic tractography combined with an extensive data quality control, identical to the approach pursued by Koldewyn and colleagues [16]. Tractography was carried out using the Tracts Constrained by Underlying Anatomy (TRACULA) tool within FreeSurfer [37] (Fig. 1a). TRACULA is a tool for automatic reconstruction of 18 major white matter pathways in native subject-space from diffusion-weighted MR images. It uses global probabilistic tractography with anatomical

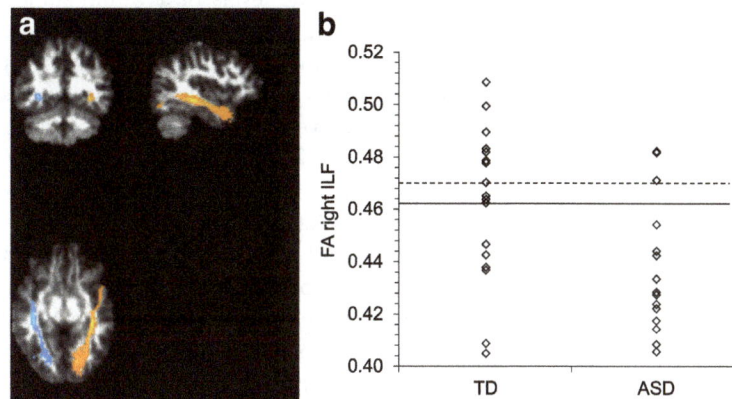

Fig. 1 a Illustrative result of the left (in blue) and right (in orange) ILF pathway reconstructed by TRACULA for one representative subject, plotted on its DWI FA map. **b** Individual FA scores for the right ILF for TD and ASD participants. The solid line indicates the mean of the TD group. The dotted line indicates the mean of the TD group after exclusion of the two outliers

priors. Prior distributions on the neighboring anatomical structures of each pathway are derived from an atlas and combined with the FreeSurfer cortical parcellation and subcortical segmentation of each subject's T1 structural image [38] to constrain the tractography solutions. The posterior distribution of each of the white matter pathways is modeled as the product of (1) a data likelihood term, which uses the ball-and-stick model of diffusion and (2) a pathway prior term, which incorporates prior anatomical knowledge about the pathway trajectory from a set of training subjects. There is no assumption that the pathways have the same shape in the study subjects as in the training subjects, and thus, TRACULA does not rely on perfect alignment between study and training subjects.

Automated parcellation of the T_1-weighted images was performed with FreeSurfer 5.3.0 to identify gray and white matter volumes and to define specific cortical and subcortical regions in each participant [39]. All preprocessing of the diffusion-weighted images (image corrections, image quality assessment, intra-subject and inter-subject-registration, mask creation, tensor fitting, estimation of pathway priors), ball-and-stick model fitting, pathway reconstruction, and extraction of DWI statistics were done using standard TRACULA settings. For each of the reconstructed tracts, mean values for FA, mean diffusivity (MD), RD, and AD were calculated by averaging the voxel values along the entire tract. In addition, supplementary analyses were performed where we calculated the DWI statistics only for the center of each tract (i.e., the single-voxel wide path with the highest probability, along the entire tract) or where we calculated a weighted tract average by weighting each DWI measure at each voxel in the tract by the pathway probability at that voxel.

DWI data quality measures comprised the average volume-by-volume translation, the average volume-by-volume rotation, the percentage of slices with excessive intensity drop-out, and the average drop-out score for slices with excessive intensity drop-out [40]. Subjects exceeding an average translation of 2.5 mm and/or rotation of 1.5° were discarded from the sample. This head motion criterion resulted in the removal of two ASD and two TD participants, and resulted in two participant groups that were well matched in terms of the four motion characteristics (see Table 2).

Visual processing measures and behavioral questionnaires

Prior to scanning, all participants performed four visual processing tasks, as part of a study of Van Eylen and colleagues [23]. In the *Fragmented Object Outlines* task, the outline of an object was gradually built up in ten steps, from the most fragmented image (showing 10% of the contour) to the completely closed contour, and participants had to correctly identify the object as soon as possible. The main outcome measure was the correct identification latency (in ms), with a higher score reflecting slower performance. This task requires bottom-up contour integration, as well as top-down matching of the perceptual input with object representations stored in memory, and semantically labeling it. In the *Coherent Motion* task, participants were presented with a random dot kinematogram and had to detect the direction of coherently moving dots by integrating the motion stimuli. A coherent motion threshold was estimated by varying the percentage of coherently moving dots. This threshold reflects the smallest proportion of coherently moving dots that is necessary to reliably perceive the global direction of motion, with higher scores reflecting reduced performance. In the *visual search* task, participants

6   A Clinician's Guide to Autism

watched a stimulus display containing a pre-specified target hidden among distractors, and participants had to touch the target as soon as possible on a touch screen. Two within-subject factors were manipulated: the number of distractors (14 vs. 24) and the target-distractor similarity (low vs. high). The target detection latency (in ms) was registered, which is the time needed to touch the correct target. Finally, the *Rey-Osterrieth Complex Figure* (ROCF) task provided an indication of the visual processing style. Participants had to copy the ROCF, and the degree of continuity or coherence in the drawing process was evaluated by calculating a fragmentation score. This score ranged from 0 to 9, with a higher score indicating a more fragmented, locally oriented processing style, and a lower score reflecting a more global integrative processing style. A more detailed description of each of these tasks and their analysis approach is provided by Van Eylen and colleagues [23].

In addition to the experimental tasks, two questionnaires were administered to assess ASD characteristics. The *Social Responsiveness Scale* (SRS) assesses a wide range of behaviors characteristic of ASD and covers subscales for "social communication and interaction" and for "restricted and repetitive patterns of behavior and interests" (RRBIs) [36]. Likewise, the *Repetitive Behavior Scale—Revised* (RBS-R) assesses the RRBIs observed in individuals with ASD [41].

Statistical analysis

Distribution analyses were performed and measures were $\log_{10}$ or square root transformed to obtain normal distributions. For the DWI data, two outliers were identified in the FA data of the right ILF in the TD group (cf. Fig. 1b). All analyses were performed with these outliers included as well as excluded, and we report the more valid analysis, i.e., including the outliers for the group comparison and excluding the outliers for the correlation analyses (since the correlation analyses were disturbed by these outliers). Concerning the group comparisons, standard ANOVAs were performed for the DWI measures, the SRS and RBS-R questionnaires, the Coherent Motion test, and the ROCF fragmentation score. For the Fragmented Objects Outline task, a repeated measures mixed model analysis was carried out with group (ASD vs. TD) as between-subject variable and stimulus type (curved vs. straight) and stimulus homogeneity (low vs. high) as within-subject variables. For the visual search task, a repeated measures mixed model analysis was carried out with group (ASD vs. TD) as between-subject variable and target-distractor similarity (low vs. high) and number of distractors (14 vs. 24) as within-subject variables. For the repeated measures analyses, the Kenward-Roger method was used to calculate the degrees of freedom, and group contrasts for

specific levels of a within-subject factor were corrected using the Tukey-Kramer procedure. Regarding the correlation analyses, whole-sample (partial) Pearson correlations were calculated to investigate the association between FA values of the white matter tracts, ASD characteristics, and visual processing measures. All analyses were conducted using the general statistical software package SAS Version 9.4 [42].

All reported *p* values are uncorrected for multiple comparisons, except for a Tukey-Kramer correction for the post-hoc group contrasts in the repeated measures analyses (i.e., when comparing both groups on the low and high similarity condition of the visual search task). A Bonferroni correction for multiple comparisons was applied by dividing the significance level ($\alpha = 0.05$) by the number of comparisons per type of analysis. For each type of analysis, we also report the Bonferroni corrected significance level (α) in the "Results" section. Note, however, that within the context of this replication study, we had a clear a priori hypothesis in which tract to observe group differences in diffusion properties, thus reducing the need to correct for multiple comparisons. Moreover, in a study with a relatively small sample and a large number of measures, correction for multiple comparisons would not only reduce the chance of making a type I error (i.e., incorrectly rejecting a null hypothesis, which results in false positives) but also dramatically enhance the chance of making a type II error (i.e., incorrectly accepting the null hypothesis, which results in false negatives) [43]. As studies in smaller samples are less sensitive to trivial effects and type I errors, correction for multiple comparisons is less relevant and scientific importance is better reflected by effect sizes and their confidence intervals [44]. Accordingly, Cohen's *d* group effect sizes (and confidence intervals) were calculated by dividing the estimated group difference by the pooled standard deviation. To calculate the pooled standard deviation, a simplified formula could be used ($\sqrt{[(\sigma 1^2 + \sigma 2^2)/2]}$), because our samples have equal size. An effect size ranging from 0.2 to 0.3 is considered small, values around 0.5 are medium, and values of 0.8 or above are considered large effects [45].

Finally, to quantify the success or failure of our attempt to replicate the findings of Koldewyn and colleagues [16] concerning group differences in FA values for the 18 tracts, we performed three Bayes factor tests [46] (for the applied R-script, see Additional file 1). All these Bayes factors express the weighted likelihood ratio between a null hypothesis and an alternative hypothesis. Firstly, the *equality-of-effect-size Bayes factor* quantifies the evidence for the null hypothesis that the effect sizes in our study equal the effect sizes in the study of Koldewyn and colleagues [16], versus the alternative hypothesis that the effect sizes in both studies are not equal. For this

Bayes factor, values higher than 1 indicate support for the null hypothesis (suggesting successful replication), whereas values lower than 1 indicate support for the alternative hypothesis. Secondly, the *replication Bayes factor* quantifies the evidence that the data provide for the hypothesis that the effect that we found in our replication attempt is consistent with the effect found in the original study of Koldewyn and colleagues [16], versus the null hypothesis that the effect is zero. Values higher than 1 indicate support for the replication hypothesis, whereas values lower than 1 indicate support for the null hypothesis. However, values between 3 and 1/3 are considered anecdotal and indicate that the outcome is indecisive [47]. This is the case when the difference between the postulated effect in the null hypothesis and the replication hypothesis is small, so when the effect found in the original study is non-significant and the effect size is close to zero. Therefore, this test is mainly relevant to evaluate the replication success of the significantly lower FA value in the right ILF for the ASD group, as reported by Koldewyn and colleagues [16]. Thirdly, we calculated the *fixed-effect meta-analysis Bayes factor*, in which we pooled the data from our study and the study of Koldewyn and colleagues [16]. This factor quantifies the evidence that the pooled data provide for the hypothesis that the true effect is present (i.e., the alternative hypothesis) versus absent (i.e., the null hypothesis), with values higher than 1 providing support for the alternative hypothesis. By pooling the data from both studies, we overcome the power problem of our current study. More specifically, with a sample size of 17 included participants per group, the population effect size

needs to be 0.99 or higher, to achieve a power of 80%. Furthermore, only effect sizes of 0.69 or higher achieve a power of 50% and can thus result in a significant group difference ($p < 0.05$). We therefore lack power to detect more subtle group differences with an effect size smaller than 0.69. However, by pooling the data from both studies and by calculating the fixed-effect meta-analysis Bayes factor, we can quantify the combined evidence for the presence or absence of an effect for each of the 18 fiber tracts. For all Bayes factors (BFs), values in between 3 and 1/3 indicate that the data are ambiguous, making the outcome indecisive.

Results

Statistics for the DWI data quality measures average volume-by-volume translation, average volume-by-volume rotation, percentage of slices with signal drop-out, and average signal drop-out severity are displayed in Table 2 and indicate that groups were well matched in terms of DWI data quality.

Given our aim to replicate the findings of Koldewyn and colleagues [16], we primarily focused on the FA values of the white matter tracts, especially of the right ILF. A one-way ANOVA comparing ASD vs. TD on each of the 18 tracts revealed similar FA values for both groups on every tract, with the exception of significantly reduced FA in ASD for the right and left ILF (see Table 2, and Figs. 1b and 2). To quantify the evidence that our data provide for replicating the findings from the study of Koldewyn and colleagues [16], we calculated three Bayes Factors (see Table 3). Firstly, the equality-of-effect-

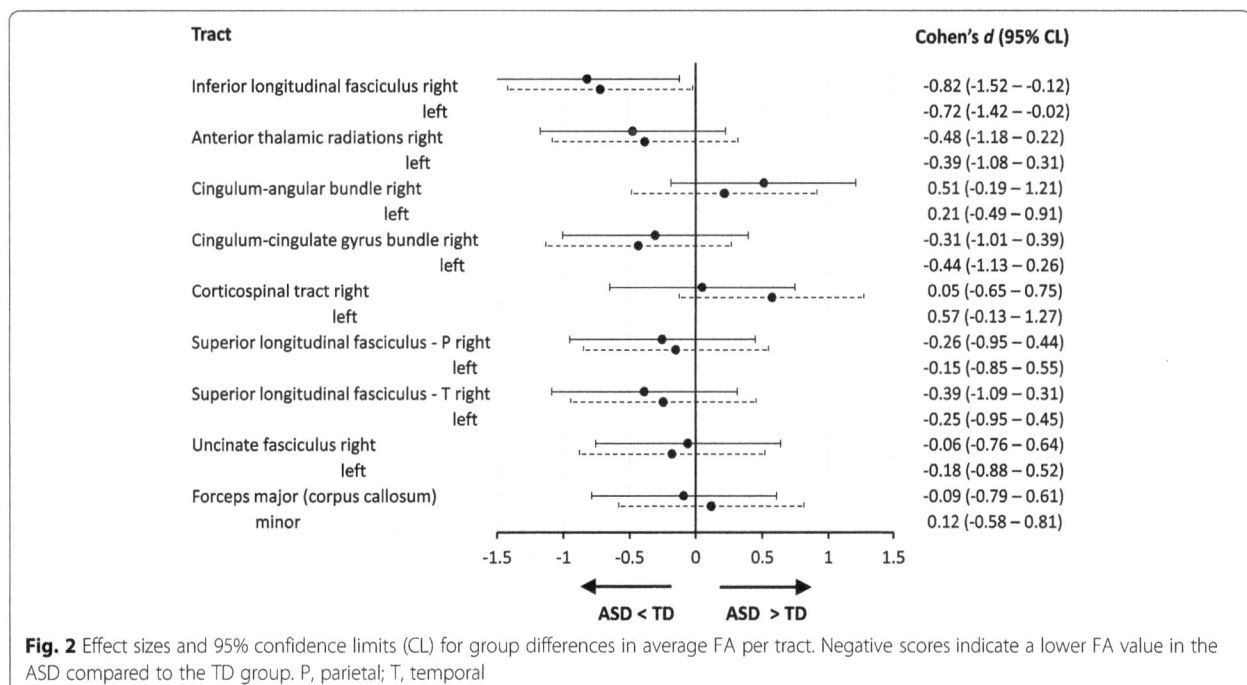

Fig. 2 Effect sizes and 95% confidence limits (CL) for group differences in average FA per tract. Negative scores indicate a lower FA value in the ASD compared to the TD group. P, parietal; T, temporal

Table 3 An overview of the Bayes factors (BF) per tract to quantify the replication results [46]. For an explanation of each of these BFs, see the "Statistical analysis" section

	Equality-of-effect-size BF	Replication BF	Fixed-effect meta-analysis BF
R inferior longitudinal fasciculus	3.89	11.56	124.67
L inferior longitudinal fasciculus	2.69	4.45	2.00
R anterior thalamic radiations	1.93	0.95	0.05
L anterior thalamic radiations	2.77	1.00	0.05
R cingulum-angular bundle	0.54	0.26	0.12
L cingulum-angular bundle	4.08	1.00	0.16
R cingulum-cingulate gyrus bundle	3.33	0.97	0.12
L cingulum-cingulate gyrys bundle	2.58	1.11	0.14
R corticospinal tract	4.11	0.83	0.08
L corticospinal tract	1.56	1.15	0.04
R superior longitudinal fasciculus—parietal	3.32	0.89	0.06
L superior longitudinal fasciculus—parietal	3.42	0.73	0.09
R superior longitudinal fasciculus—temporal	2.85	1.07	0.13
L superior longitudinal fasciculus—temporal	3.97	1.02	0.15
R uncinate fasciculus	3.89	0.78	0.10
L uncinate fasciculus	3.81	0.86	0.06
Forceps major (corpus callosum)	4.18	0.87	0.10
Forceps minor (corpus callosum)	3.35	0.69	0.11

size Bayes factor was higher than 1 for all of the tracts, except for the right CAB, indicating that for all those tracts, there is more evidence that the effect sizes of both studies are equal. However, for several tracts, this Bayes factor was between 3 and 1/3 (i.e., for the left and right ATR, for the left CCG, CST and ILF, and for the right SLFT and CAB), indicating that the evidence for those tracts is indecisive (see Table 3). Secondly, the replication Bayes factor for the right ILF showed that it is 11.6 times more likely that the observed reduction in FA in the ASD group is a replication of the effect found in the study of Koldewyn and colleagues [16] than that this effect is truly zero. Interestingly, for the left ILF, the replication Bayes factor was also larger than 3 (i.e., 4.5). In line with our expectations, the replication Bayes factor was inconclusive ($1/3 < BF < 3$) for almost all other tracts (see Table 3), since the postulated effect under the replication hypothesis was close to that predicted under the null hypothesis. For the right CAB, however, this Bayes factor indicates that it is 3.8 times more likely that the difference in FA is truly zero than that we replicated the effect described by Koldewyn and colleagues [16]. Thirdly, the fixed-effect meta-analysis Bayes factor also provided strong evidence that the observed lower FA value in the right ILF for the pooled ASD group is a true effect (BF = 125). For the left ILF, the evidence is indecisive (BF = 2), but for all other tracts, this factor indicated that it is 6 to 23 times more likely that the effect is truly zero than that there is a group difference in FA ($1/23.3 < BF < 1/6.3$).

Concerning AD, RD, and MD, a one-way ANOVA comparing ASD vs. TD revealed similar values for both groups on each of the 18 tracts (all $p > .10$), with the exception of significantly increased RD in ASD in the right ILF ($F(1,32) = 4.54$, $p = .041$, $d = .73$).

Four supplementary analyses were performed on the DWI statistics. First, we calculated the DWI statistics only for the center of each tract, revealing reduced FA in ASD in right ILF ($F(1,32) = 5.09$, $p = .031$, $d = -0.77$), marginally significantly reduced FA in ASD in left ILF ($F(1,32) = 4.07$, $p = .052$, $d = -0.69$), and increased RD in ASD in right ILF ($F(1,32) = 6.61$, $p = .015$, $d = 0.88$), with all other measures similar for both groups ($p > .10$). Second, we calculated weighted DWI averages by weighting each DWI measure at each voxel in the tract by the pathway probability at that voxel. This analysis revealed reduced FA in ASD in right ILF ($F(1,32) = .4.58$, $p = .040$, $d = -0.73$) and increased RD in ASD in right ILF ($F(1,32) = 4.49$, $p = .042$, $d = 0.72$), with all other measures similar for both groups ($p > .098$). Third, we reanalyzed the data of FA of right ILF after excluding two outlying TD subjects (as evidenced in Fig. 1b). This analysis revealed significantly reduced FA of the right ILF in ASD ($F(1,30) = 12.40$, $p = .0014$, $d = -1.25$), which survives Bonferroni multiple comparison correction for the 18 assessed tracts ($\alpha = .05/18$). Fourth, we reanalyzed the data of FA of the right ILF after excluding the four left-handed subjects, as handedness may reflect lateralization of language, which in turn may impact upon lateralization of face-sensitive areas [48]. This analysis again revealed significantly reduced FA of the right ILF in ASD ($F(1,28) = 6.11$, $p = .019$, $d = - 0.90$).

As expected, individuals with ASD scored significantly higher on each of the questionnaires assessing ASD characteristics, both for impairments in social communication and interaction and for RRBIs (cf. SRS, RBS-R; see Table 1). These results survive Bonferroni correction, since the p value is smaller than 0.0125 ($\alpha = 0.05/4$).

Pertaining to the visual measures, individuals with ASD were slower to detect the target in the visual search task, particularly in the high-similarity condition with highly similar target-distractor items (see Table 4). When applying a stringent Bonferroni correction, this last group difference became marginally significant ($\alpha = 0.05/4 = 0.0125$), although the effect size was medium to large ($d = 0.72$). No significant group differences were found on the other visual processing measures (i.e., the Fragmented Object Outlines task, the Coherent Motion task, and the ROCF task) (see Table 4).

Next, we calculated whole-group Pearson correlations between FA of the right ILF and ASD characteristics and between FA of the right ILF and visual processing measures (see Additional files 2 and 3). As both groups were preselected to differ in terms of ASD symptoms, group membership was partialed out from all correlations involving ASD characteristics. While lower FA in the right ILF showed a slight association with the presence of more ASD characteristics (SRS total score: *partial* $r(29) = - 0.27$, $p = .15$; SRS Social Communication and Interaction scale: *partial* $r(29) = - 0.26$, $p = .17$; SRS RRBI scale: *partial* $r(29) = - 0.18$, $p = .34$), none of these correlations were significant, and the association only approached significance for the RBS-R questionnaire (*partial* $r(29) = - 0.37$, $p = .05$). Pertaining to the visual measures, lower FA in the right ILF showed a marginally significant association with slower visual search ($r(29) = - 0.34$, $p = .059$) and a more part-oriented processing

style as indexed by the fragmentation score on the ROCF ($r(30) = - 0.34$, $p = .05$). However, these results did not survive Bonferroni correction ($\alpha = 0.006$). No association was observed with coherent motion sensitivity ($r(30) = - 0.23$, $p = .22$) or performance on the Fragmented Object Outlines task ($r(30) = - 0.23$, $p = .21$). Due to the small sample size, none of these correlations sustained in the separate participant groups, except for associations in the ASD sample between lower FA in right ILF and a more fragmented processing style (ROCF: $r(15) = - 0.50$, $p = .04$) and a trend towards more RRBIs on the RBS-R questionnaire ($r(14) = - 0.46$, $p = .07$). In the TD group, the association with ASD characteristics was substantial but not significant (SRS: $r(13) = -.42$, $p = .12$). None of the 17 other white matter tracts showed an association with quantitative ASD characteristics or visual processing measures, except for two tracts: lower FA in the left and right cingulate-cingulum gyrus (CCG) bundle was associated with slower performance on the Fragmented Objects Outline task ($r(30) = - 0.43$, $p = .01$ and $r(30) = - 0.35$, $p = .04$, respectively) and with slower visual search ($r(29) = - 0.45$, $p = .009$ and $r(29) = - 0.34$, $p = .049$, respectively) (see Additional file 3). However, none of these associations survived Bonferroni correction ($\alpha = 0.006$).

Discussion

The literature on neural processing in ASD is extensive and characterized by divergent and inconsistent findings. This partially reflects the characteristic heterogeneity of the disorder [49], but may also be due to the use of suboptimal analysis approaches and less reliable data quality assessment. A recent study applied state-of-the-art global probabilistic tractography combined with stringent DWI data quality criteria and found that aberrant structural connectivity in children with ASD may be confined to one specific white matter tract, the right inferior longitudinal fasciculus or ILF [16]. To further consolidate

Table 4 Between-group differences for the visual processing measures

	ASD ($n = 17$)		TD ($n = 17$)		Group test statistic	p value	Cohen's d
	M	SD	M	SD			
Fragmented Objects Outline Task (ms) [a]	4335	1252	4031	919	$F = 0.91$	.35	0.31
Coherent Motion Task (% coherence)	29	12	24	11	$F = 2.02$	.17	0.48
Visual search task (ms) [b]	2075	505	1825	295	$F = 2.93$	.09	0.52
Low similarity [c]	1792	421	1677	295	$t = 0.72$	.47	0.25
High similarity [c]	2360	634	1973	381	$t = 2.51$	.017	0.72
ROCF fragmentation score	5.4	2.1	4.2	2.8	$F = 1.76$	.19	0.46

Note. Since the groups were compared on four tasks, a Bonferroni correction results in a significance level (α) of 0.0125
[a]Other effects retained in the model for Fragmented Objects Outline Task: within-subject factors type ($F(1,1279) = 13.07$, $p < .001$) and homogeneity ($F(1,1279) = 54$, $p = < .001$)
[b]Other effects retained in the model for visual search: within-subject factors target-distractor similarity ($F(1,1285) = 86.07$, $p < .001$), number of distractors ($F(1,1285) = 57.67$, $p < .001$), and the interaction between group and target-distractor similarity ($F(1,1285) = 7.68$, $p = .006$)
[c]Tukey-Kramer correction was performed for group contrasts for the specific levels of a within-subject factor

this finding, we replicated the study design of Koldewyn and colleagues [16], by applying an identical analysis approach and identical head motion and DWI data quality matching, in adolescents with and without ASD.

Similar to the findings of Koldewyn and colleagues [16], we found that adolescents with ASD showed reduced FA in the ILF and not in any of the 16 other white matter tracts. In our study, significantly reduced FA in the right ILF was consistently observed across a number of different analysis approaches and the effect size was large (i.e., $d = -0.82$ in the current adolescent sample, as compared to $d = -0.68$, in the school-aged sample of Koldewyn and colleagues). Furthermore, the Bayes factor tests provided strong evidence that we replicated the findings of Koldewyn and colleagues [16] and that the observed lower FA value in the right ILF for the ASD group is a true effect. Likewise, in both studies, reduced FA in the right ILF was driven by increased RD in the ASD sample. The particular anatomical location of aberrant diffusion in ASD coincides with the major cluster of reduced FA across a series of whole-brain DWI studies (as calculated in a meta-analysis [8]) and is also supported by a number of DWI tractography studies [50–52]. Together with findings of reduced functional occipito-temporal connectivity [10], this suggests a dysfunction of the right ILF in ASD.

Contrary to previous studies and reviews [6, 8, 9, 16], we also observed significantly reduced FA in the left ILF ($d = -0.72$) in the ASD group. However, this group difference was less consistently observed across different analysis approaches, and—as it was not a priori predicted—it did not survive correction for multiple comparisons. A closer look at the data of Koldewyn and colleagues [16] shows that FA in the left ILF was also significantly reduced in ASD in their original analysis without head motion and data-quality matching. Yet, in the more stringent analysis, the group difference was no longer significant, but still substantial ($d = -0.34$). The replication Bayes factor also indicated that the observed lower FA value in the left ILF for the ASD group corresponds to the effect reported by Koldewyn and colleagues [16], rather than showing that the effect is zero. However, according to the fixed-effect meta-analysis Bayes factor, the pooled data of both studies provide indecisive evidence. Taken together, this indicates that the observation of reduced FA in the left ILF is not as robust as in the right ILF and should be interpreted with caution.

Concerning the issue of *selective* alterations in one particular white matter tract in ASD, it should be noted that our sample was too small to reliably demonstrate the *absence* of more subtle group differences in white matter properties. To overcome this limitation, we calculated the fixed-effect meta-analysis Bayes factor on the pooled data from our study and the study of Koldewyn

and colleagues [16]. This Bayes factor provided strong evidence that the observed lower FA value in the right ILF of the ASD group is indeed a true effect (in fact, based on the findings in both studies, it is 125 times more likely that this effect is truly present instead of absent). For the left ILF, the evidence was inconclusive, but for all other tracts, the meta-analysis Bayes factor clearly suggested that group differences are absent (depending on the tract it is 6 to 23 times more likely that FA values across groups are similar instead of different). Therefore, the combined findings across both studies confirm the presence of alterations in right ILF in ASD and may question the common idea of more widespread alterations in white matter in ASD (although they leave us with uncertainty regarding the left ILF).

Additionally, our findings also illustrate the heterogeneity in white matter properties within the ASD population (see Fig. 1b), indicating that results of group comparisons should be interpreted with caution. This heterogeneity implies that not every individual participant with ASD has reduced FA in the right ILF, despite the observed group difference. Likewise, for the other tracts, the absence of a group difference in FA does not imply that none of the participants with ASD may show alterations in any of these tracts. Besides heterogeneity at the brain level [49], ASD is also characterized by heterogeneity at the cognitive level [53] and at the behavioral level, as each ASD symptom has a wide range of manifestations [1]. This heterogeneity at different levels stimulates a more dimensional approach to examine the link between alterations in white mater organization and variations in cognition and ASD symptom severity.

The observed alterations in white matter organization can potentially underlie some of the cognitive characteristics of ASD. In this study, we focused on the role of the right ILF in visual processing. According to one of the dominant theories on visual processing in ASD (i.e., the Weak Central Coherence account), individuals with ASD show relatively impaired global integrative processing and are more inclined to process and attend to parts or details [24]. Nevertheless, group differences in visual processing are often subtle, and many studies yield inconsistent results with weak effect sizes comparing individuals with ASD versus TD controls [25, 26]. The adolescents of our ASD sample showed reduced performance on the visual search task, compared to the TD group. Intact performance was found on the Fragmented Object Outlines task, the Coherent Motion task, and the ROCF. This pattern of results is in line with similar findings on the same visual measures in larger samples of individuals with and without ASD [23]. Van Eylen and colleagues [23] demonstrated that group differences on visual processing measures were small and depended on the age and/or sex of the participants. More specifically, the group difference on the ROCF task was only found in girls and the group difference on the Coherent Motion task was restricted to younger children, thus corresponding to the absence of group differences in the current sample of adolescent boys. Generally, these findings challenge the claim that individuals with ASD have a general inability to integrate information [23], although the cognitive heterogeneity within ASD should be taken into account when interpreting results.

Reduced brain connectivity has been suggested as the biological mechanism underlying atypical visual processing in individuals with ASD [4]. Here, we observed reduced FA in the right ILF of boys with ASD. As the ILF connects the occipital and the temporal lobe, reduced FA along this tract may impact upon information integration along the ventral visual stream. In line with this hypothesis, we found that lower FA in the right ILF was associated with slower performance on the visual search task and a trend towards a more part/detail-oriented processing style. Ortibus and colleagues [22] previously demonstrated that reduced FA of the ILF was also associated with impaired object recognition in children with cerebral visual impairment. As expected, FA in the ILF was not associated with Coherent Motion sensitivity, a traditional measure of dorsal visual stream functioning [30]. Contrary to our expectations, no correlation was found between FA in the ILF and performance on the Fragmented Object Outlines task, and no group difference was found on this task, despite the lower FA values in the right ILF of the ASD group. A possible explanation is that the Fragmented Object Outlines task targets higher-level top-down visual processing and, thus, does not solely rely on diffusion along the ILF. Therefore, specific alterations of the ILF may only partially determine performance on this task, due to compensation by other brain mechanisms. For example, our data pointed towards a possible involvement of the cingulum-cingulate gyrus bundle (CCG), given the observed association between FA in the CCG (bilaterally) and performance on the Fragmented Object Outlines task. Low- and mid-level visual processing tasks in which the right ILF plays a more unique role are expected to show a higher correlation with FA in the right ILF and a greater impairment in individuals with ASD.

One cognitive process in which the right ILF is particularly implicated is face processing, by interconnecting several key brain regions (i.e., the occipital and the fusiform face area, the superior temporal sulcus and the amygdala) [6, 18, 54–57]. Impaired (emotional) face processing has repeatedly been described in ASD [19–21] and may impact upon social functioning and communication in general. As a result, disruption of the right ILF may be linked with ASD symptom severity via face processing impairments. However, after controlling for clinical status, we

could not observe any reliable associations between individual differences in FA of right ILF and individual differences in socio-communicative ASD characteristics. On the other hand, there was a marginally significant association between lower FA of the right ILF and the increased presence of RRBI characteristics as rated on the RBS-R questionnaire, which was entirely driven by the ASD sample. As some of these RBS-R items involve atypical sensory processing and a possible preoccupation with parts of objects, the link with altered ILF properties may be partially mediated by atypical visual processing [27].

Although this study replicated the previously observed reduction in FA in the right ILF in individuals with ASD [16], some limitations should be considered. First, as indicated above, by itself, our study was underpowered to demonstrate the selectivity of the ILF alterations in ASD, i.e., that *only* the right ILF and no other tracts may display reduced FA in ASD. Likewise, the power of our study was limited to demonstrate reliable associations with visual processing and ASD characteristics, especially at the subgroup level. Therefore, larger studies are needed to examine these associations more thoroughly, including the association with face processing abilities. Second, although both our study and the one of Koldewyn and colleagues [16] demonstrated reduced FA in right ILF in adolescents and school-aged children with ASD, respectively, it remains to be validated whether this ILF alteration is consistently present across the developmental trajectory, thus also at preschool and adult age. It may be particularly relevant to investigate how group differences in diffusion properties of association tracts evolve throughout pubertal development and how this relates to differences in hormone levels, such as testosterone. In this regards, it has been demonstrated that the development of association tracts, such as the ILF, is influenced by this hormone [58, 59] and that boys with and without ASD have different testosterone levels during puberty [60]. Third, the present study (as well as the one of Koldewyn and colleagues [16]) included a relatively selective subset of participants in terms of IQ (above 80), calling into question to what extent the findings may generalize to the whole ASD spectrum.

In this regard, future research should also investigate how heterogeneity at the behavioral level in the ASD population (in terms of IQ, age, comorbid symptoms etc.) may relate to heterogeneity at the neural level [61]. Future research is also needed to directly examine the hypothesized association between structural ILF properties and face processing abilities and to investigate (the directionality of) possible causal pathways linking lower FA in right ILF with ASD symptom severity. A longitudinal investigation of the intrinsic association between fine-grained local connectivity patterns and (atypical) functional brain activity in the fusiform face area [62] may be particularly elucidating in this regard. Finally, more fundamental research is needed to pinpoint the exact micro- and macrostructural factors underlying the reduced FA in the right ILF in individuals with ASD and the functional implications in terms of brain connectivity, neural communication, and information transmission.

Conclusion

To conclude, our results replicate the findings of Koldewyn and colleagues [16] and support the growing evidence for altered structural connectivity along the right ILF in ASD, although they leave us with uncertainty regarding alterations in the left ILF. Nevertheless, these findings need to be interpreted in the light of the known heterogeneity of the disorder. This heterogeneity calls for a more dimensional approach to examine the link between alterations in ILF properties and variations in cognition and ASD symptom severity. In that regard, this study suggests that alterations in structural ILF properties in individuals with ASD may underlie (at least some of) the visual processing atypicalities and RRBI characteristics of ASD. To move the field forward, we need large interdisciplinary, multi-dimensional studies that examine inter-individual differences at different levels and the corresponding biological pathways. This will increase our understanding of the links between the brain, cognition, and behavior and will reveal the factors that induce, or at least increase the risk for, ASD, but may also elucidate protective factors.

Additional files

Additional file 1: Supplementary R-script. The applied R-script to calculated the three Bayes factor tests, to quantify the result of our replication attempt [46]. (TXT 4 kb)

Additional file 2: Figure S1. Scatter plots displaying the association between individual differences in FA in right ILF (depicted on the X axis) and individual differences in quantitative ASD characteristics and visual processing measures (depicted on the Y axis). First row: Associations with (square root transformed) scores on the SRS questionnaire, the SRS Social and Communication subscale, the SRS RRBI subscale, and the RBS-R questionnaire. Second row: Associations with reaction time on the Fragmented Object Outlines task, (log-transformed) percentage coherence threshold on the Coherent Motion Task, (log-transformed) reaction time on the visual search task, and (square root transformed) fragmentation score on the Rey-Osterrieth Complex Figure task. ASD subjects are depicted by empty squares, TD subjects by filled diamonds. (PPTX 130 kb)

Additional file 3: Table S1. Pearson (partial) correlations between ASD characteristics, visual processing measures and fractional anisotropy (FA) in the white matter tracts. (DOCX 19 kb)

Abbreviations
AD: Axial diffusivity; ASD: Autism spectrum disorder; DFlex: Detail and flexibility questionnaire; DWI: Diffusion-weighted Imaging; FA: Fractional anisotropy; FOV: Field-of-view; ILF: Inferior longitudinal fasciculus; MD: Mean diffusivity; MRI: Magnetic resonance imaging; RBS-R: Repetitive Behavior Scale—Revised; RD: Radial diffusivity; ROCF: Rey-Osterrieth Complex Figure; RRBIs: Restricted and repetitive patterns of behavior and interests; SRS: Social Responsiveness Scale; TD: Typically developing; TE: Echo time; TR: Repetition time; TRACULA: Tracts Constrained by Underlying Anatomy

Acknowledgements
We thank all participating children and their families for their time and effort. We also acknowledge S. Ghosh at the McGovern Institute for Brain Research (MIT), for assistance with the implementation of the FreeSurfer and TRACULA analysis pipelines as well as Claudia Dillen and the master students Karen Van Bouwel and Evelyne Vereecke from the KU Leuven, for their assistance during scanning.

Funding
BB was supported by a postdoctoral fellowship of the Research Foundation Flanders and a visiting researcher grant of Fulbright. LVE was supported by a doctoral fellowship of the Research Foundation Flanders and a postdoctoral fellowship of the M.M. Delacroix Foundation. The research was financed by grants from the Research Council of KU Leuven (IDO/08/013 and StG/15/014BF awarded to BB) and a long-term structural funding from the Flemish Government (METH/14/02) to JW. The funding bodies in itself had no role in the design of the study nor in the collection, analysis, and interpretation of data or in writing the manuscript.

Authors' contributions
BB and LVE collected, analyzed, and interpreted the data and wrote the manuscript. BB took the lead in the conception and design of the imaging part of the study and analyzed the imaging data. LVE took the lead in the conception, design, and analyses of the visual processing measures. KS substantially contributed to the analysis of the imaging data. PM contributed to the Bayesian statistics. IN critically revised the manuscript and provided important intellectual content. JS provided feedback on the draft of the manuscript. SS provided support in the design of the imaging protocol. JW aided with the interpretation of the results and gave detailed feedback on the manuscript. All authors read and approved the final manuscript.

Competing interests
The authors declare that they have no competing interests.

Author details
[1]Center for Developmental Psychiatry, Department of Neurosciences, KU Leuven, Kapucijnenvoer 7h, PB 7001, 3000 Leuven, Belgium. [2]Leuven Autism Research (LAuRes), KU Leuven, 3000 Leuven, Belgium. [3]Department of Brain and Cognitive Sciences, Massachusetts Institute of Technology, Cambridge, MA 02139, USA. [4]Speech and Hearing Bioscience and Technology, Division of Medical Sciences, Harvard Medical School, Boston, MA 02115, USA. [5]Laboratory of Experimental Psychology, KU Leuven, 3000 Leuven, Belgium. [6]Parenting and Special Education Research Unit, KU Leuven, 3000 Leuven, Belgium. [7]Translational MRI, KU Leuven, 3000 Leuven, Belgium.

References
1. American Psychiatric Association. Diagnostic and statistical manual of mental disorders: DSM-5. 5th ed. Washington, D.C: American Psychiatric Association; 2013.

2. Ameis SH, Szatmari P. Imaging-genetics in autism spectrum disorder: advances, translational impact, and future directions. Neuroimaging Stimul. 2012;3:46.

3. Belmonte MK, Allen G, Beckel-Mitchener A, Boulanger LM, Carper RA, Webb SJ. Autism and abnormal development of brain connectivity. J Neurosci. 2004;24:9228–31.

4. Hill EL, Frith U. Understanding autism: insights from mind and brain. Philos Trans R Soc B Biol Sci. 2003;358:281–9.

5. Just MA, Cherkassky VL, Keller TA, Minshew NJ. Cortical activation and synchronization during sentence comprehension in high-functioning autism: evidence of underconnectivity. Brain. 2004;127:1811–21.

6. Ameis SH, Catani M. Altered white matter connectivity as a neural substrate for social impairment in autism spectrum disorder. Cortex. 2015;62:158–81.

7. Aoki Y, Abe O, Nippashi Y, Yamasue H. Comparison of white matter integrity between autism spectrum disorder subjects and typically developing individuals: a meta-analysis of diffusion tensor imaging tractography studies. Mol Autism. 2013;4:25.

8. Hoppenbrouwers M, Vandermosten M, Boets B. Autism as a disconnection syndrome: a qualitative and quantitative review of diffusion tensor imaging studies. Res Autism Spectr Disord. 2014;8:387–412.

9. Travers BG, Adluru N, Ennis C, DPM T, Destiche D, Doran S, et al. Diffusion tensor imaging in autism spectrum disorder: a review. Autism Res. 2012;5:289–313.

10. Vissers ME, Cohen MX, Geurts HM. Brain connectivity and high functioning autism: a promising path of research that needs refined models, methodological convergence, and stronger behavioral links. Neurosci Biobehav Rev. 2012;36:604–25.

11. Le Bihan D. Looking into the functional architecture of the brain with diffusion MRI. Nat Rev Neurosci. 2003;4:469–80.

12. Song S-K, Sun S-W, Ramsbottom MJ, Chang C, Russell J, Cross AH. Dysmyelination revealed through MRI as increased radial (but unchanged axial) diffusion of water. NeuroImage. 2002;17:1429–36.

13. Jones DK, Knösche TR, Turner R. White matter integrity, fiber count, and other fallacies: the do's and don'ts of diffusion MRI. NeuroImage. 2013;73:239–54.

14. Yendiki A, Koldewyn K, Kakunoori S, Kanwisher N, Fischl B. Spurious group differences due to head motion in a diffusion MRI study. NeuroImage. 2014;88:79–90.

15. Walker L, Gozzi M, Lenroot R, Thurm A, Behseta B, Swedo S, et al. Diffusion tensor imaging in young children with autism: biological effects and potential confounds. Biol Psychiatry. 2012;72:1043–51.

16. Koldewyn K, Yendiki A, Weigelt S, Gweon H, Julian J, Richardson H, et al. Differences in the right inferior longitudinal fasciculus but no general disruption of white matter tracts in children with autism spectrum disorder. Proc Natl Acad Sci U S A. 2014;111:1981–6.

17. Catani M, Jones DK, Donato R, Ffytche DH. Occipito-temporal connections in the human brain. Brain J Neurol. 2003;126(Pt 9):2093–107.

18. Thomas C, Avidan G, Humphreys K, Jung K, Gao F, Behrmann M. Reduced structural connectivity in ventral visual cortex in congenital prosopagnosia. Nat Neurosci. 2009;12:29–31.

19. Harms MB, Martin A, Wallace GL. Facial emotion recognition in autism spectrum disorders: a review of behavioral and neuroimaging studies. Neuropsychol Rev. 2010;20:290–322.

20. Uljarevic M, Hamilton A. Recognition of emotions in autism: a formal meta-analysis. J Autism Dev Disord. 2013;43:1517–26.

21. Weigelt S, Koldewyn K, Kanwisher N. Face identity recognition in autism spectrum disorders: a review of behavioral studies. Neurosci Biobehav Rev. 2012;36:1060–84.

22. Ortibus E, Verhoeven J, Sunaert S, Casteels I, De Cock P, Lagae L. Integrity of the inferior longitudinal fasciculus and impaired object recognition in children: a diffusion tensor imaging study. Dev Med Child Neurol. 2012;54:38–43.

23. Van Eylen L, Boets B, Steyaert J, Wagemans J, Noens I. Local and global visual processing in autism spectrum disorders: influence of task and sample characteristics and relation to symptom severity. J Autism Dev Disord. 2015; https://doi.org/10.1007/s10803-015-2526-2.

24. Happé FGE, Booth RDL. The power of the positive: revisiting weak coherence in autism spectrum disorders. Q J Exp Psychol. 2008;61:50–63.

25. Simmons DR, Robertson AE, McKay LS, Toal E, McAleer P, Pollick FE. Vision in autism spectrum disorders. Vis Res. 2009;49:2705–39.

26. Van der Hallen R, Evers K, Brewaeys K, Van den Noortgate W, Wagemans J. Global processing takes time: a meta-analysis on local-global visual processing in ASD. Psychol Bull. 2015;141:549–73.

27. Brunsdon VEA, Happé F. Exploring the 'fractionation' of autism at the cognitive level. Autism. 2014;18:17–30.

28. Altmann CF, Bülthoff HH, Kourtzi Z. Perceptual organization of local elements into global shapes in the human visual cortex. Curr Biol CB. 2003;13:342–9.

29. Grill-Spector K, Weiner KS. The functional architecture of the ventral temporal cortex and its role in categorization. Nat Rev Neurosci. 2014;15:536–48.

30. Braddick O, Atkinson J, Wattam-Bell J. Normal and anomalous development of visual motion processing: motion coherence and 'dorsal-stream vulnerability'. Neuropsychologia. 2003;41:1769–84.

31. Kaldy Z, Giserman I, Carter AS, Blaser E. The mechanisms underlying the ASD advantage in visual search. J Autism Dev Disord. 2016;46(5):1513—27.

32. Wolfe JM. Visual search. In: Pashler H, editor. Attention. Hove: Psychology Press; 1998. p. 13–73.

33. American Psychiatric Association. Diagnostic and statistical manual of mental disorders: DSM-IV-TR. 4th ed. Washington, DC: American Psychiatric Association. p. 2000.

34. Skuse D, Warrington R, Bishop D, Chowdhury U, Lau J, Mandy W, et al. The developmental, dimensional and diagnostic interview (3di): a novel computerized assessment for autism spectrum disorders. J Am Acad Child Adolesc Psychiatry. 2004;43:548–58.

35. Roeyers H, Thys M, Druart C, De Schryver M, Schittekatte M. Screeningslijst voor autismespectrumstoornissen: SRS. Amsterdan: Hogrefe; 2011.

36. Roeyers H, Thys M, Druart C, De Schryver M, Schittekatte M. Screeningslijst voor autismespectrumstoornissen: SRS-2. Amsterdan: Hogrefe; 2013.

37. Yendiki A, Panneck P, Srinivasan P, Stevens A, Zöllei L, Augustinack J, et al. Automated probabilistic reconstruction of white-matter pathways in health and disease using an atlas of the underlying anatomy. Front Neuroinform. 2011;5:23.

38. Fischl B, Salat DH, Busa E, Albert M, Dieterich M, Haselgrove C, et al. Whole brain segmentation: automated labeling of neuroanatomical structures in the human brain. Neuron. 2002;33:341–55.

39. Fischl B. FreeSurfer. NeuroImage. 2012;62:774–81.

40. Benner T, van der Kouwe AJW, Sorensen AG. Diffusion imaging with prospective motion correction and reacquisition. Magn Reson Med. 2011;66:154–67.

41. Bodfish JW, Symons FJ, Parker DE, Lewis MH. Varieties of repetitive behavior in autism: comparisons to mental retardation. J Autism Dev Disord. 2000;30:237–43.

42. SAS Institute Inc. SAS University edition, version 9.4. Cary: SAS Institute Inc.; 2013.

43. Nakagawa S. A farewell to Bonferroni: the problems of low statistical power and publication bias. Behav Ecol. 2004;15:1044–5.

44. Friston K. Ten ironic rules for non-statistical reviewers. NeuroImage. 2012;61:1300–10.

45. Cohen J. Statistical power analysis for the behavioral sciences. 2nd ed. Hillsdale: Lawrence Erlbaum Associates; 1988.

46. Verhagen J, Wagenmakers E-J. Bayesian tests to quantify the result of a replication attempt. J Exp Psychol Gen. 2014;143:1457.

47. Jeffreys H. Theory of probability. 3rd ed. Oxford: Oxford University Press; 1961.

48. Behrmann M, Plaut DC. Distributed circuits, not circumscribed centers, mediate visual recognition. Trends Cogn Sci. 2013;17:210–9.

49. Lenroot RK, Yeung PK. Heterogeneity within autism spectrum disorders: what have we learned from neuroimaging studies? Front Hum Neurosci. 2013;7:733.

50. Ameis SH, Fan J, Rockel C, Voineskos AN, Lobaugh NJ, Soorya L, et al. Impaired structural connectivity of socio-emotional circuits in autism spectrum disorders: a diffusion tensor imaging study. PLoS One. 2011;6:e28044.

51. Cheon K-A, Kim Y-S, Oh S-H, Park S-Y, Yoon H-W, Herrington J, et al. Involvement of the anterior thalamic radiation in boys with high functioning autism spectrum disorders: a diffusion tensor imaging study. Brain Res. 2011;1417:77–86.

52. Pugliese L, Catani M, Ameis S, Dell'Acqua F, Thiebaut de Schotten M, Murphy C, et al. The anatomy of extended limbic pathways in Asperger syndrome: a preliminary diffusion tensor imaging tractography study. NeuroImage. 2009;47:427–34.

53. Geurts H, Sinzig J, Booth R, Happ F. Neuropsychological heterogeneity in executive functioning in autism spectrum disorders. Int J Dev Disabil. 2014; 60:155–62.

54. Haxby J, Gobbini M. Distributed neural systems for face perception. In: Rhodes, G, Calder A, Johnson M, Haxby J, editors. Oxford Handbook of Face Perception. Oxford: Oxford University Press; 2011.

55. Fox CJ, Iaria G, Barton JJS. Disconnection in prosopagnosia and face processing. Cortex J Devoted Study Nerv Syst Behav. 2008;44:996–1009.

56. Kleinhans NM, Richards T, Sterling L, Stegbauer KC, Mahurin R, Johnson LC, et al. Abnormal functional connectivity in autism spectrum disorders during face processing. Brain J Neurol. 2008;131(Pt 4):1000–12.

57. Rudrauf D, David O, Lachaux J-P, Kovach CK, Martinerie J, Renault B, et al. Rapid interactions between the ventral visual stream and emotion-related structures rely on a two-pathway architecture. J Neurosci. 2008;28:2793–803.

58. Herting MM, Maxwell EC, Irvine C, Nagel BJ. The impact of sex, puberty, and hormones on white matter microstructure in adolescents. Cereb Cortex. 2012;22:1979–92.

59. Menzies L, Goddings A-L, Whitaker KJ, Blakemore S-J, Viner RM. The effects of puberty on white matter development in boys. Dev Cogn Neurosci. 2015;11:116–28.

60. Croonenberghs J, Van Grieken S, Wauters A, Van West D, Brouw L, Maes M, et al. Serum testosterone concentration in male autistic youngsters. Neuro Endocrinol Lett. 2010;31:483–8.

61. Happé F, Ronald A, Plomin R. Time to give up on a single explanation for autism. Nat Neurosci. 2006;9:1218–20.

62. Saygin ZM, Osher DE, Koldewyn K, Reynolds G, JDE G, Saxe RR. Anatomical connectivity patterns predict face selectivity in the fusiform gyrus. Nat Neurosci. 2012;15:321–7.

Autism spectrum disorder: prospects for treatment using gene therapy

Matthew Benger[1], Maria Kinali[2] and Nicholas D. Mazarakis[1]* (iD)

Abstract

Autism spectrum disorder (ASD) is characterised by the concomitant occurrence of impaired social interaction; restricted, perseverative and stereotypical behaviour; and abnormal communication skills. Recent epidemiological studies have reported a dramatic increase in the prevalence of ASD with as many as 1 in every 59 children being diagnosed with ASD. The fact that ASD appears to be principally genetically driven, and may be reversible postnatally, has raised the exciting possibility of using gene therapy as a disease-modifying treatment. Such therapies have already started to seriously impact on human disease and particularly monogenic disorders (e.g. metachromatic leukodystrophy, SMA type 1). In regard to ASD, technical advances in both our capacity to model the disorder in animals and also our ability to deliver genes to the central nervous system (CNS) have led to the first preclinical studies in monogenic ASD, involving both gene replacement and silencing. Furthermore, our increasing awareness and understanding of common dysregulated pathways in ASD have broadened gene therapy's potential scope to include various polygenic ASDs. As this review highlights, despite a number of outstanding challenges, gene therapy has excellent potential to address cognitive dysfunction in ASD.

Keywords: Autistic spectrum disorder, Synaptic dysfunction, ASD models, Gene therapy, Viral vector

Background

"Between stimulus and response there is a space. In that space is our power to choose our response. In our response lies our growth and our freedom"—Viktor E Frankl.

In autism spectrum disorder (ASD), a neurodevelopmental disorder affecting ~ 1.5% of the population [1], aetiologically diverse deficits in cognitive plasticity lead to broad impairments in communication and restricted, repetitive behaviours [2]. Comorbidities are common (~ 70% of cases) and include epilepsy; attention, mood and language disorders; sleep disturbance; gastrointestinal problems; and intellectual disability [3].

Despite the great personal and sociological cost of ASD (estimated to be $2 million/patient/year [4]), only the antipsychotics risperidone and aripiprazole are currently FDA-approved to treat ASD, indicated solely in the treatment of irritability symptoms [5]. A fundamental reason for this lack of disease-modifying therapies may relate to ASD's pathogenesis, which appears to be principally driven by heterogeneous genetic mutations and variants and modulated by diverse gene × environment interactions, to include pregnancy-related factors (e.g. maternal immune activation, maternal toxins) and perinatal trauma [2, 6–10]. Many of the encoded proteins implicated in ASD pathogenesis—such as cytoskeletal proteins, cell adhesion molecules and DNA-binding proteins—may be 'undruggable' using conventional small molecule drugs, which principally only modulate the function of receptors and enzymes [11].

In contrast, gene therapy—broadly defined as the delivery of nucleic acid polymers into cells to treat disease—may be used to repair, replace, augment or silence essentially any gene of interest in a target cell, opening up new areas of the proteome for drug targeting [12]. Other advantages of gene therapy versus small molecules include the ability to effect long-lasting clinical benefit with a single treatment and the potential to control cellular targeting via vector modifications [13].

Indeed, gene therapy is already making a clinical impact in the field of neurology, with Nusinersen, an

* Correspondence: n.mazarakis@imperial.ac.uk
[1]Gene Therapy, Centre for Neuroinflammation and Neurodegeneration, Division of Brain Sciences, Faculty of Medicine, Imperial College London, Hammersmith Hospital Campus, W12 0NN, London, UK
Full list of author information is available at the end of the article

antisense oligonucleotide therapy approved in Spinal muscular atrophy (SMA), and more recently Luxturna, a viral-based gene replacement strategy approved in Leber's congenital amaurosis, acting as the first disease-modifying therapies in both of these diseases [14, 15]. In addition, a clinical trial in SMA by AveXis using systemic delivery of recombinant adeno-associated virus 9 (rAAV9) carrying a replacement SMN1 gene recently proved safe and efficacious in neonates [16]. On the other hand, gene therapies are clearly expensive in the short-term, with current therapies costing at least $500,000 per treatment, and thus remaining unaffordable in many healthcare systems (see ref [17] for a thorough economic analysis).

This review will highlight key targets for ASD gene therapy, the utility of ASD models, and recent advances in our ability to deliver such therapies to the central nervous system (CNS). It will then move on to discuss recent gene therapy strategies in ASD, concentrating on conditions with available preclinical data, and the roadblocks facing their clinical translation.

Genetic targets in ASD

ASD may be divided into conditions driven by a single genetic defect (monogenic ASD) and conditions driven by multiple genetic defects (polygenic ASD). Monogenic ASD conditions often contain a variable cluster of phenotypes which include autism as part of a syndrome [18]. Whilst only accounting for ~ 5% of ASD cases [18], such disorders are prime candidates for gene therapy for two major reasons: firstly, they lend themselves to developing genetic models of ASD, which enable elucidation of the genotype to phenotype pathway, the potential for disease reversibility postnatally, and the efficacy/toxicity of novel therapeutics; secondly,

correction of a single causative protein defect has the potential to arrest and possibly reverse disease pathology. Indeed, a basis for preclinical gene therapy studies in ASD was founded by identification of the nature and function of causative genes for a number of monogenic conditions with autistic features, including Rett syndrome (RS), fragile X syndrome (FXS), Angelman syndrome (AS) and tuberous sclerosis (TSC) [19–23] (Table 1).

More recently, our understanding of the genetic landscape of ASD has been revolutionised by several whole-exome and whole-genome sequencing studies, identifying hundreds of de novo and rare inherited variants influencing sporadic ASD risk [24–32]. Many of these genes appear to be involved, either directly or indirectly, in synaptic morphology and activity, leading to the concept of ASD as a 'synaptopathy' [33, 34] (Fig. 1). Certainly, the idea of using gene therapy to increase or decrease the expression of target proteins within this network and 'retune' the synapse is a powerful one, which may be applicable to certain ASD cases.

However, in such a heterogeneous condition as ASD, it is important not to become evangelical about a single causative mechanism, especially given recent insights into the apparently critical roles of immune dysfunction and epigenetics in at least certain ASD cases [35, 36]. Furthermore, recent phase II clinical trials which looked to regulate synaptic function via GABA and glutamate receptor modulation failed to demonstrate significant overall benefit, despite strongly positive responses in certain patients [37, 38]. Thus, it is important to consider whether targeting the synapse using gene therapy may be most appropriate for correcting particular ASD endophenotypes in specific patient subsets, rather than seeing it as a panacea for ASD, a topic that is returned to later in this article.

Table 1 Genotypic and phenotypic characteristics of monogenic conditions with ASD features

Monogenic ASD	Mutated gene	Chromosome	Protein function	Autism prevalence	Other characteristics
Fragile X syndrome	FMR1 (encodes FMRP)	X	Binds and transports specific mRNAs from the nucleus to the ribosome [123]	~ 30% [124]	Long/narrow face, macroorchidism, long ears and p hiltrum, mild to moderate intellectual disability, hyperactivity, intellectual disability (ID), seizures
Rett syndrome	MECP2	X	Chromatin modification [125]	~ 60% [124]	Microcephaly, breathing irregularities, language deficits, repetitive/stereotyped hand movements, epilepsy, ID
MECP2 duplication syndrome	MECP2	X	Chromatin modification [125]	~ 100% [126]	Brachycephaly, spasticity, recurrent respiratory infections, gastrointestinal hypermotility, genitourinary abnormalities, epilepsy, ID
Tuberous sclerosis	TSC1 TSC2	9 16	Inhibition of translation via mTORC1 inhibition [127]	~ 50% [124]	Benign tumours in multiple organs, epilepsy
Angelman syndrome	UBE3A	15	Targeting of proteins for destruction via ubiquitin-tagging [41]	~ 30% [124]	Cheerful demeanour, microcephaly, epilepsy, speech deficits, sleep disturbance, epilepsy, ID

Abbreviations: *FMR1* fragile X mental retardation 1, *FMRP* fragile X mental retardation protein, *MECP2* methyl-CpG-binding protein 2, *TSC1* tuberous sclerosis 1, *TSC2* tuberous sclerosis 2, *UBE3A* ubiquitin-protein ligase E3A

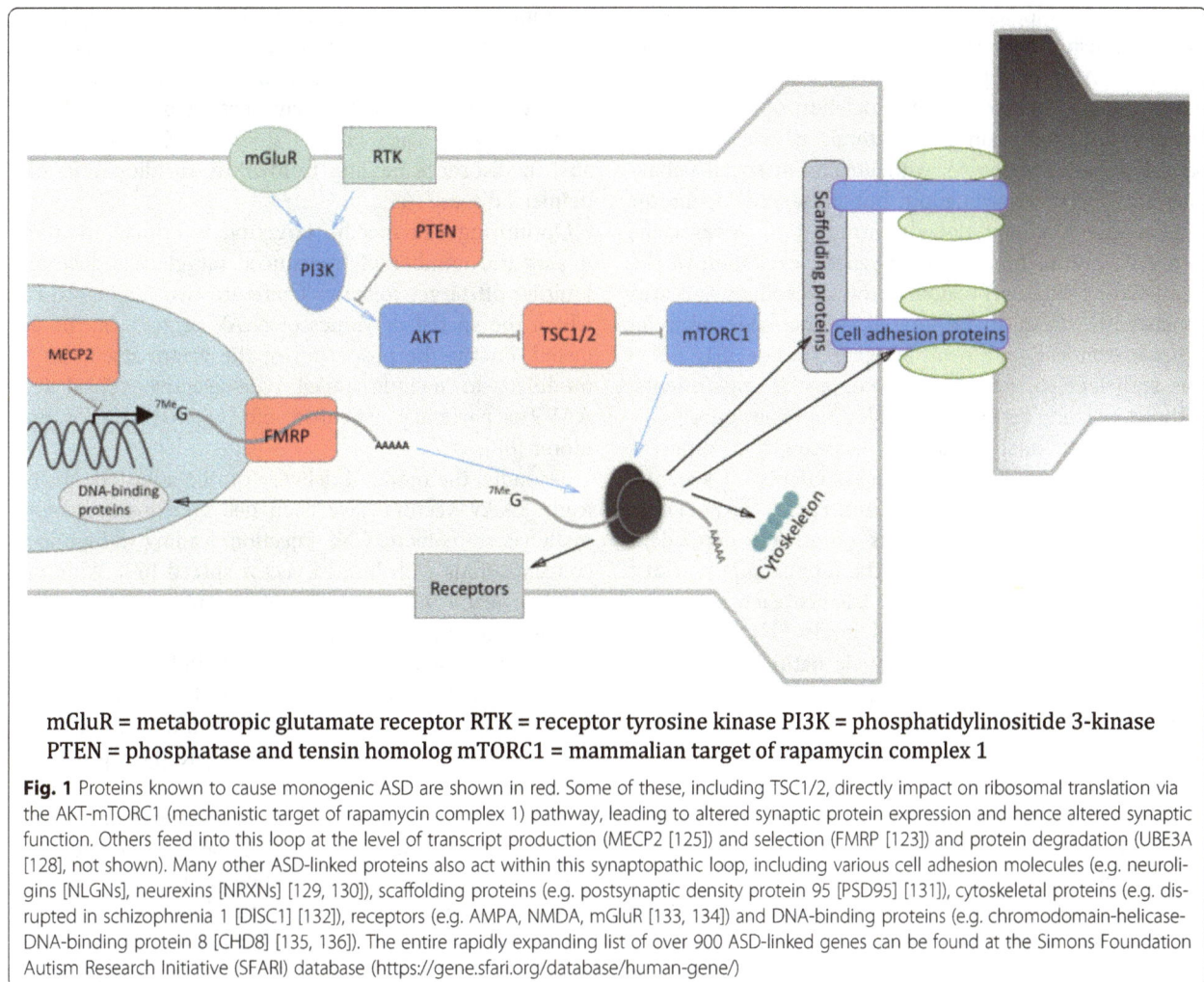

mGluR = metabotropic glutamate receptor RTK = receptor tyrosine kinase PI3K = phosphatidylinositide 3-kinase PTEN = phosphatase and tensin homolog mTORC1 = mammalian target of rapamycin complex 1

Fig. 1 Proteins known to cause monogenic ASD are shown in red. Some of these, including TSC1/2, directly impact on ribosomal translation via the AKT-mTORC1 (mechanistic target of rapamycin complex 1) pathway, leading to altered synaptic protein expression and hence altered synaptic function. Others feed into this loop at the level of transcript production (MECP2 [125]) and selection (FMRP [123]) and protein degradation (UBE3A [128], not shown). Many other ASD-linked proteins also act within this synaptopathic loop, including various cell adhesion molecules (e.g. neuroligins [NLGNs], neurexins [NRXNs] [129, 130]), scaffolding proteins (e.g. postsynaptic density protein 95 [PSD95] [131]), cytoskeletal proteins (e.g. disrupted in schizophrenia 1 [DISC1] [132]), receptors (e.g. AMPA, NMDA, mGluR [133, 134]) and DNA-binding proteins (e.g. chromodomain-helicase-DNA-binding protein 8 [CHD8] [135, 136]). The entire rapidly expanding list of over 900 ASD-linked genes can be found at the Simons Foundation Autism Research Initiative (SFARI) database (https://gene.sfari.org/database/human-gene/)

Modelling ASD in rodents: a platform for proof-of-principle studies

The field of gene therapy is littered with examples of therapies which failed to translate from their preclinical promise. In many cases, blame can be attributed to the predictive validity of the animal model used, which is itself related to its construct validity (i.e. how well the model mimics disease aetiology) and face validity (i.e. how closely the model's phenotype represents the human disorder) [39].

Given the challenges clinicians have faced in developing diagnostic criteria for ASD [40], and how various social traits often appear to be inherently 'human' qualities (although this is itself highly contested [41]), it is little wonder that generating ASD animal models with good face validity has been challenging. Nevertheless, whilst caution should always be taken when ascribing behavioural outcomes in animals to autism, various monogenic ASD rodent models have capably demonstrated quantifiable social and communicative behavioural traits [42–44], laying the ground for preclinical therapeutic studies.

As a caveat, it must be noted that a major limitation of ASD animal models relates to their inability to reflect heterogeneous environmental influences on the ASD phenotype, with various toxic, inflammatory and psychosocial factors difficult to incorporate in robust, reproducible animal models. This deficit in construct validity is especially relevant in modelling polygenic ASD, in which the gene × environment interaction plays a more fundamental role [45], and which therefore bears a particular risk for future translational work.

Locating and reversing ASD pathophysiology

Identifying specific cells and circuits dysregulated in ASD is crucial in gene therapy design, as vectors may be targeted to specific brain regions or cell types (discussed in detail later). In particular, nascent data suggest the hippocampus, cerebellum and corpus callosum contain key pathogenic circuits [34, 46–48], whilst influential cell types include pyramidal cells, Purkinje cells and glial cells [34, 49].

Recent technological advances have begun to elucidate the relationship between cell type-specific function and particular ASD endophenotypes. For example, in a RS mouse model, cre/lox-mediated deletion of MECP2 specifically from forebrain glutamatergic neurons led to a partial disease phenotype, with deficits in social behaviour and motor coordination, but preserved locomotor activity and fear-conditioned learning [50]. Meanwhile, in a TSC mouse model, chemogenetic excitation of the Right Crus I (RCrusI) region of the cerebellum—an area consistently noted to be altered in the ASD brain in neuroanatomical and neuroimaging studies [51, 52]—was sufficient to specifically rescue social impairments, without rescuing repetitive or inflexible behaviours [53].

Within individual circuits, it appears that different ASD mutations may have opposing effects on synaptic function. For example, $TSC2^{+/-}$ and $FMR1^{-/y}$ knockouts appear to have opposite effects on mGluR-dependent long-term depression (LTD) in the hippocampus, whilst mice bred with both mutations balance each other out at the synaptic and behavioural levels [54]. Such data not only exemplify the heterogeneic nature of ASD but also highlight the necessity of optimal synaptic control, and are the first hint that a successful gene therapy must walk a narrow therapeutic tightrope between over- and under-stimulating synaptic transmissions.

A crucial further question is whether autistic phenotypes can be reversed or are neurodevelopmentally fixed. Remarkably, an array of studies in different monogenic ASD animal models have consistently demonstrated the potential for reversal of established neuronal dysfunction, either after pharmacological intervention or genetic reactivation of silenced alleles [55–60]. These findings imply that postnatally, indeed post-symptomatically, the genetic horse may not yet have bolted, and genetic correction via a delivered vector might be useful in treating cognitive dysfunction.

Delivering gene therapies to the CNS

If the ASD phenotype is reversible rather than neurodevelopmentally fixed, as implied by studies in monogenic animal models, then it follows that continuous genetic correction will be necessary for a sustained therapeutic effect. Currently, only viral packaging systems have combined efficient transduction with long-term gene expression in vivo [61] (although, as will be discussed later, certain ASD conditions may be amenable to non-virally delivered antisense nucleic acid therapies).

Of the viruses which can transduce post-mitotic cells, rAAVs have emerged as the principal CNS delivery candidate [62]. This is based upon their relatively low immunogenicity (compared to adenovirus and herpes simplex virus), limiting the likelihood of an encephalitic

immune response, their ability to persist in episomal form, reducing their oncogenic potential (compared to retroviruses [63, 64]), and their high production titres [12]. Indeed, rAAV vectors have already been used safely in a number of early clinical studies in CNS gene therapy, in disorders ranging from SMA to idiopathic Alzheimer's disease [65].

Optimising cell-specific targeting is critical in maximising the number of transduced target cells/dose and limiting off-target toxicity. There are two major ways in which the spatial dynamics of rAAV vectors can be adjusted. Firstly, the properties of the vector itself can be modified, to include a cell type-selective capsid (e.g. AAV9 is particularly neurotropic [66, 67]) and/or promoter [68].

Secondly, the mode of delivery can be adjusted. Historically, rAAV vectors have been delivered intraparenchymally via stereotactic CNS injection, leading to high local concentrations with limited vector spread [69]. Although invasive (each injection requiring a craniotomy), such a localising method of delivery might have utility in correcting specific dysregulated ASD circuits linked to particular clinical endophenotypes, analogous to the recent improvement in motor scores seen after lentiviral vector delivery of a dopamine-producing gene therapy to the nigrostriatal pathway in Parkinson's disease [70].

However, ASD appears to involve global synaptic dysregulation and thus will require global CNS gene correction to fully reverse cognitive phenotypes [71, 72]. The discovery that rAAV9 crosses the blood-brain barrier (BBB) and globally transduces CNS neurons and glial cells [73], and the recent derivation of more efficient BBB-traversing rAAVs by targeted evolution [74], has opened up the possibility of using intravenous injection in ASD gene therapy.

It remains to be seen, however, whether side effects relating to peripheral tissue transduction, as well as the presence of neutralising circulating antibodies (anti-AAV9 antibodies are present in 47% of humans), will preclude intravenous administration in various ASDs [75–77]. Changes to the viral vector nucleic acid sequence outside of the transgene—such as the inclusion of 'detargeting' sequences recognised by micro RNAs (miRNAs) expressed specifically in off-target cells [78]—might circumvent the former issue, but use up highly limited space (rAAV's packaging capacity is limited to ~ 5 kb [79]). The latter issue may be negotiated by the use of engineered rAAV capsids, which may have lower neutralising antibody seropravalences [80].

An alternative to systemic delivery is intrathecal administration, which potentially combines (relatively) safe administration and global CNS transduction with fewer peripheral complications, and a higher spatial resolution limiting the dose requirements. However, there are conflicting data regarding the ability of intrathecally delivered rAAV to efficiently transduce areas outside the spinal cord [81], as well its own ability to avoid both peripheral leakage [82] and a neutralising antibody response [83, 84]. Of note, an intrathecal AAV9 approach has been corrective in a model of giant axonal neuropathy [85] and has progressed to a clinical trial.

Gene therapy strategies in monogenic ASD
Gene replacement

In ASD disorders defined by loss of function mutations (e.g. RS, FXS, TSC), simple gene replacement may restore synaptic function [12]. Given the limitations imposed by imperfect gene delivery strategies, a key question is whether sufficient transduction of target cell types can be attained to exert phenotypic benefit.

Encouragingly, a number of studies using monogenic animal models have demonstrated behavioural improvements after rAAV-delivered gene replacement. In a RS mouse model, systemic delivery of a rAAV9-MECP2 vector sufficient for ~ 10% CNS transduction (of principally neuronal cells) led to moderate behavioural improvements [86, 87]. Meanwhile, at an ~ 6-fold higher vector dose, ~ 25% CNS transduction resulted in marked behavioural and phenotypic improvements [88]. Finally, it was recently demonstrated that rAAV-mediated delivery of even a fragment of the MECP2 gene (lacking N- and C- terminal regions along with a central domain) led to phenotypic improvement in RS mice, potentially allowing extra room for construct modifications to aid target cell transduction and expression [89]. Similarly, substantial phenotypic improvements were seen in studies using FXS and TSC models after intra-CNS delivery of replacement genes, although none of these studies quantified CNS transduction [90–92].

Although a cause for optimism, none of the above studies evidenced total phenotypic reversal after gene replacement. Such incomplete phenotypic reversal may be secondary to insufficient CNS transduction. In RS for example, ~ 80% gene reactivation in neuronal cells appears to be sufficient and necessary for total phenotypic reversal [56, 93]. However, increasing the vector dose in order to increase transduction must be balanced against the risk of dose-related toxicity. This may occur secondary to off-target cell transgene expression: for example, transgene-specific liver toxicity was seen at high doses of rAAV9-MECP2 [86, 94], possibly due to MECP2's role in liver metabolism [95].

Toxicity may also occur secondary to supraphysiological expression in target cells. For example, after rAAV-mediated delivery of FMRP in FXS, toxicity developed at 2.5-fold expression above wild type [96], whilst duplication of MECP2 leads to MECP2 duplication syndrome in males [97–99]. Such toxicity may occur even at low transduction percentages due to uneven vector

distribution within the CNS or, in the case of X-linked disorders in females, due to a mosaic pattern of CNS expression caused by random X-inactivation [100]. Reassuringly, a fragmented version of the MECP2 promoter appeared to limit MECP2 expression to physiological levels in both wild type and $MECP2^{null/x}$ female mice, even at vector doses leading to ~ 25% CNS transduction [88].

Nonetheless, further studies are required to pinpoint the optimum balance between CNS transduction and on-target toxicity in various ASD syndromes. Additionally, future gene replacement studies must better characterise the relationship between gene dose and dendritic function (which was not assessed in any of the above studies).

RNA knockdown

Gene expression can be silenced by sequence-specific knockdown of mRNA transcripts using techniques such as antisense oligonucleotides (ASOs) and short interfering RNAs (siRNAs), which use the exquisite specificity conferred by Watson-Crick base pairing to bind particular mRNA transcripts and prevent their translation (for a detailed mechanism see ref [101]). These nucleic acids are typically relatively easy to manufacture, can be modified to limit degradation and inflammation, and do not require a viral vector (although long-term expression of ASOs is possible using viral delivery of short hairpin RNAs [shRNAs]) [101, 102]. Indeed, such therapies are already being used in the treatment of SMA and in clinical trials for Huntington's disease [103, 104].

These techniques are principally useful when total or partial knockdown of a particular transcript may restore synaptic function. For example in MECP2 duplication syndrome, halving MECP2 expression was shown to restore cellular function and phenotype postnatally in a conditional MECP2-overexpressing mouse model [105]. In the same study, intraventricular delivery of ASOs (delivered at a constant rate by a pump) specifically targeting MECP2 led to widespread ASO distribution in the CNS, effective knockdown of MECP2 to nearly wild type levels, and sustained phenotypic reversal (~ 10 weeks) [105].

Another strategy in which RNA silencing may be useful is in knocking down a gene which inhibits a target gene's expression, i.e. disinhibition. For example, triplication of 15q11-13 leads to a relatively common and highly penetrant type of autism linked to increased expression of UBE3A (which functions as a transcription regulator in addition to its ubiquitin ligase function) and subsequent downregulation of Cerebellin 1 Precursor (Cbln1), a synaptic organising protein, in the ventral tegmental area (VTA) [106]. Thus, knockdown of UBE3A could be used to restore sufficient Cbln1 expression in the VTA, which has already been shown to effect phenotypic change after cre/lox-mediated restoration in a UBE3A-triplicated mouse model [106].

Another application of this strategy could be in AS, where the long non-coding UBE3A antisense transcript (UBE3A-AST) causes imprinting of the paternal UBE3A allele, ensuring that a loss of maternal UBE3A allele function yields the AS phenotype (another example of how genetic defects in ASD may be bidirectional, with optimal gene expression in specific brain regions crucial). Indeed, a recent paper demonstrated that a single intracerebroventricular injection of a degradation-resistant ASO targeting UBE3A-AST in an adult AS mouse model led to specific and sustained reductions in UBE3A-AST levels, with partial restoration (~ 40%) of UBE3A levels throughout the CNS [107].

Interestingly, in the same study, whilst motor deficits were restored, other behaviours—such as anxiety and repetitive behaviours—were not. A later study, using Cre-dependent UBE3A reactivation in an AS mouse model, showed a temporal dependence for specific phenotype reversal, with anxiety and repetitive behaviours requiring gene reactivation during early development, whilst motor deficits could be restored into adulthood [108]. Such temporal factors have not been thoroughly investigated in other monogenic ASDs but are clearly critical when considering the time point of useful intervention in humans.

Finally, in a similar vein to excessive gene replacement, hyper-knockdown of target RNA may lead to rebound toxicity in both target cells and off-target cells. Furthermore, both ASOs and siRNA may cause unpredictable off-target knockdown [109]. From this perspective, the requirement for regular intra-CNS administration of ASOs is a double-edged sword in ASD: whilst on the one hand, it is clearly less convenient than a once-off injection of viral vector, on the other hand, it allows for the possibility of dose uptitration and determination of an optimal therapeutic level.

Gene editing

One of the most exciting recent developments in gene therapy is the advent of easily customised sequence-specific editing techniques, such as CRISPR (clustered regularly interspaced short palindromic repeats)-Cas9, enabling either correction of a genetic mutation via non-homologous recombination (providing there is a suitable template) or gene silencing via non-homologous end-joining [110]. Such techniques would generally enable gene expression at physiological levels in target cells, negating the problems of transgene-associated toxicity seen with both gene replacement and RNA knockdown techniques.

Unfortunately, at least in vivo, gene editing techniques still remain a distant therapeutic prospect, with a wealth of technical hurdles to overcome, including how to deliver gene editing systems to target cells, how to increase the efficiency of editing, and how to avoid off-target editing [111, 112]. Still, recent work by Doudna and colleagues provides optimism in this regard, with the demonstration of greatly improved editing of post-mitotic neurons in adult mouse brains using cell-penetrating peptides tagged onto Cas9 ribonucleoprotein complexes [113].

Prospects for gene therapy in polygenic ASD

As previously mentioned, in comparison with monogenic ASD, polygenic ASD has a greater environmental component driving its phenotype [45]. In this respect, damaging, nonsynonymous postzygotic mutations in whole-exome sequences from the largest collection of trios with ASD were recently identified, with some of these genes being particularly enriched for expression in the amygdala, a key brain region for social conditioning and learning [114]. Such factors, combined with the current paucity and constructional limitations of animal models in polygenic ASD, make it a less obvious target for gene therapy.

Nonetheless, despite the bewildering array of rare genetic mutations linked to polygenic ASD, an important focus of these mutations appears to be in the regulation of synaptic function, with diverse ASD mutations potentially connecting aberrant translational inputs and outputs (Fig. 1) [34]. For example, in mice, deletion of the translational repressor Eukaryotic translation initiation factor 4E-binding protein 2 (4E-BP2) led to overexpression of the NLGN class of cell adhesion molecules [115], mutations of which have been causally linked to ASD [46, 116, 117]. Furthermore, such deletion resulted in disruption of the ratio of excitatory to inhibitory synaptic inputs, as well as an ASD behavioural phenotype, which was corrected by NLGN1 knockdown [115].

This leads to the idea that many ASD mutations might be treated by fine-tuning the expression of influential proteins acting within dynamic translational loops. The apparently fundamental role of the PI3K-AKT-mTOR pathway in various causes of monogenic ASD [118], as well as the phenotypic reversal seen using small molecule inhibitors of mTORC1 preclinically [119], suggests that this pathway may be a critical target for gene therapy in certain cases of ASD.

However, given ASD's heterogeneity, it is once again important not to focus myopically on a single pathway. Rather, instead of embarking on a 'one size fits all' therapeutic approach, the effect of any particular ASD mutation on translational output and synaptic function should be categorised, before deciding whether and how to target a particular gene or pathway. For instance, NLGN3 knockout mice demonstrate a FXS-like disruption of mGluR-dependent synaptic plasticity [120], suggesting that either FMRP overexpression or PI3K-AKT-mTOR pathway knockdown (given the afore-mentioned opposition of these two pathways) might correct this phenotype.

Finally, recent evidence has emerged of ASD behaviours caused by amino acid deficits [121, 122]. For example, homozygous dysfunction of the BBB solute carrier transporter 7a5 (SLC7A5) and corresponding CNS loss of branched chain amino acids (BCAAs) has been linked to ASD, which is reversible in mouse models upon intra-CNS administration of BCAAs [122]. Thus, direct protein replacement therapy might provide an important additional therapeutic avenue in certain ASD cases. It is also possible to imagine using gene therapy as an adjunct here: for example, combining systemic BCAA replacement with vector-delivered SLC7A5 targeting BBB cells.

Conclusions

Given the heritable component of ASD, gene therapy offers a promising alternative to conventional small molecule therapies. Preclinical studies over the last 5 years using animal models displaying autism-like traits have demonstrated that directly altering gene expression using rAAV-delivered transgenes can reverse the behavioural phenotype, either via gene replacement or RNA knockdown. Such studies establish proof-of-concept and set up a platform for clinical translation in various monogenic ASDs, with RS being a frontrunner in this regard.

However, major hurdles remain, not least the fact that the majority of ASD disorders, even monogenic ones, show variable penetrance, with epistatic and gene × environment interactions determining phenotype. Not only is such genetic and environmental heterogeneity inherently difficult to model, hindering clinical translation, but also in clinical trials that do go ahead, ASD subgroups that benefit from a particular treatment may be lost amongst other unsuitable subgroups. Furthermore, we still do not know whether, or in which cases, epigenetic factors may preclude reversibility in humans. Cyclically, this brings us back to the question of animal models and whether these have sufficient construct validity to actually begin to answer such questions in the first place.

A number of additional questions remain: Firstly, can vector design be optimised to the extent that intravenous delivery achieves sufficient CNS transduction without peripheral toxicity? Secondly, where is the optimum balance between CNS transduction and the risk of on-target transgene-related toxicity for each ASD syndrome? Thirdly, will demonstrations of acceptable levels of CNS toxicity hold when studies commence in larger animal models? Fourthly, is there a time point beyond which some or all autistic features lose their reversibility? Answering these questions will be key to moving ASD gene therapy into clinical trials, and perhaps one day generating a genetic treatment for ASD.

Abbreviations

AS: Angelman syndrome; ASD: Autistic spectrum disorder; ASO: Antisense oligonucleotide; BBB: Blood-brain barrier; BCAA: Branched chain amino acids; Cbln1: Cerebellin 1 precursor; CHD8: Chromodomain-helicase-DNA-binding protein 8; CNS: Central nervous system; CRISPR: Clustered regularly interspaced short palindromic repeats; DISC1: Disrupted in schizophrenia 1; FMR1: Fragile X mental retardation 1; FMRP: Fragile X mental retardation protein; FXS: Fragile X syndrome; LTD: Long-term depression; MECP2: Methyl-CpG-binding protein 2; mGluR: Metabotropic glutamate receptor; miRNA: MicroRNA; mTORC1: Mammalian target of rapamycin complex 1; NLGN: Neuroligin; NRXN: Neurexin; PI3K: Phosphatidylinositide 3-kinase; PSD95: Postsynaptic density protein 95; PTEN: Phosphatase and tensin homolog; rAAV: Recombinant adeno-associated virus; RCrusI: Right Crus I; RS: Rett syndrome; RTK: Receptor tyrosine kinase; SFARI: Simons Foundation Autism Research Initiative; shRNA: Short hairpin RNA; siRNA: Short interfering RNA; SLC7A5: Solute carrier transporter 7a5; SMA: Spinal muscular atrophy; TSC: Tuberous Sclerosis; TSC1: Tuberous sclerosis 1; TSC2: Tuberous sclerosis 2; UBE3A: Ubiquitin-protein ligase E3A; VTA: Ventral tegmental area

Acknowledgements
We thank Dr. C. Proukakis for interesting discussions around the subject of this review.

Funding
NDM was supported by the ERC and CDKL5 Foundation grants during the period of this work.

Authors' contributions
NDM and MB did the literature review; MB wrote the manuscript. MK assisted with the writing of the manuscript. All authors read, corrected and approved the final manuscript.

Competing interests
The authors declare that they have no competing interests.

Author details
[1]Gene Therapy, Centre for Neuroinflammation and Neurodegeneration, Division of Brain Sciences, Faculty of Medicine, Imperial College London, Hammersmith Hospital Campus, W12 0NN, London, UK. [2]Present address: The Portland Hospital, 205-209 Great Portland Street, London W1W 5AH, UK.

References
1. Christensen DL, et al. Prevalence of autism spectrum disorder among children aged 8 years—autism and developmental disabilities monitoring network, 11 sites, United States, 2010," Morb. Mortal. Wkly. Rep. Surveill. Summ. Wash. DC 2002, vol. 63, no. 2, pp. 1–21, Mar. 2014.
2. Chahrour M, O'Roak BJ, Santini E, Samaco RC, Kleiman RJ, Manzini MC. Current perspectives in autism disorder: from genes to therapy. J. Neurosci. 2016;36(45):11402.
3. Zafeiriou DI, Ververi A, Vargiami E. Childhood autism and associated comorbidities. Brain Dev. 29(5):257–72.
4. Buescher AVS, Cidav Z, Knapp M, Mandell DS. Costs of autism spectrum disorders in the United Kingdom and the United States. JAMA Pediatr. 2014; 168(8):721–8.
5. LeClerc S, Easley D. Pharmacological therapies for autism spectrum disorder: a review. Pharm Ther. 2015;40(6):389–97.
6. Freitag CM. The genetics of autistic disorders and its clinical relevance: a review of the literature. Mol Psychiatry. 2006;12(1):2–22.
7. Geschwind DH, State MW. Gene hunting in autism spectrum disorder: on the path to precision medicine. Lancet Neurol. 2015;14(11):1109–20.

8. Careaga M, Murai T, Bauman MD. Maternal immune activation and autism spectrum disorder: from rodents to nonhuman and human primates. Biol Psychiatry. 2017;81(5):391–401.

9. Modabbernia A, Velthorst E, Reichenberg A. Environmental risk factors for autism: an evidence-based review of systematic reviews and meta-analyses. *Mol. Autism.* 2017;8(1):13.

10. Tordjman S, et al. Gene × Environment interactions in autism spectrum disorders: role of epigenetic mechanisms. Front Psychiatry. 2014;5:53.

11. Hopkins AL, Groom CR. The druggable genome. Nat Rev Drug Discov. 2002; 1(9):727–30.

12. Templeton NS. Gene and cell therapy: therapeutic mechanisms and strategies. 4th ed: CRC Press; 2015, Boca Raton, FL.

13. Naldini L. Gene therapy returns to centre stage. Nature. 2015;526(7573):351–60.

14. Hoy SM. Nusinersen: first global approval. Drugs. 2017;77(4):473–9.

15. Shaberman B. A retinal research nonprofit paves the way for commercializing gene therapies. Hum Gene Ther. 2017;28(12):1118–21.

16. Mendell JR, et al. Single-dose gene-replacement therapy for spinal muscular atrophy. N Engl J Med. 2017;377(18):1713–22.

17. Hampson G, Towse A, Pearson SD, Dreitlein WB, Henshall C. Gene therapy: evidence, value and affordability in the US health care system. J Comp Eff Res. 2018;7(1):15–28.

18. Sztainberg Y, Zoghbi HY. Lessons learned from studying syndromic autism spectrum disorders. Nat Neurosci. 2016;19(11):1408–17.

19. Amir RE, Van den Veyver IB, Wan M, Tran CQ, Francke U, Zoghbi HY. Rett syndrome is caused by mutations in X-linked MECP2, encoding methyl-CpG-binding protein 2. Nat Genet. 1999;23(2):185–8.

20. Kishino T, Lalande M, Wagstaff J. UBE3A/E6-AP mutations cause Angelman syndrome. Nat Genet. 1997;15(1):70–3.

21. Splawski I, et al. CaV1.2 calcium channel dysfunction causes a multisystem disorder including arrhythmia and autism. Cell. 119(1):19–31.

22. van Slegtenhorst M, et al. Identification of the tuberous sclerosis gene TSC1 on chromosome 9q34. Science. 1997;277(5327):805–8.

23. Verkerk AJ, et al. Identification of a gene (FMR-1) containing a CGG repeat coincident with a breakpoint cluster region exhibiting length variation in fragile X syndrome. Cell. 1991;65(5):905–14.

24. Yuen RKC, et al. Whole genome sequencing resource identifies 18 new candidate genes for autism spectrum disorder. Nat Neurosci. 2017;20(4):602–11.

25. De Rubeis S, et al. Synaptic, transcriptional and chromatin genes disrupted in autism. Nature. 2014;515(7526):209–15.

26. Iossifov I, et al. The contribution of de novo coding mutations to autism spectrum disorder. Nature. 2014;515(7526):216–21.

27. Iossifov I, et al. De novo gene disruptions in children on the autistic spectrum. Neuron. 2012;74(2):285–99.

28. Jiang Y, et al. Detection of clinically relevant genetic variants in autism spectrum disorder by whole-genome sequencing. Am J Hum Genet. 2013; 93(2):249–63.

29. Neale BM, et al. Patterns and rates of exonic de novo mutations in autism spectrum disorders. Nature. 2012;485(7397):242–5.

30. O'Roak BJ, et al. Exome sequencing in sporadic autism spectrum disorders identifies severe de novo mutations. Nat Genet. 2011;43(6):585–9.

31. Sanders SJ, et al. De novo mutations revealed by whole-exome sequencing are strongly associated with autism. Nature. 2012;485(7397):237–41.

32. Yuen RKC, et al. Whole-genome sequencing of quartet families with autism spectrum disorder. Nat Med. 2015;21(2):185–91.

33. Zoghbi HY, Bear MF. Synaptic dysfunction in neurodevelopmental disorders associated with autism and intellectual disabilities. *Cold Spring Harb. Perspect. Biol.* 2012;4(3)

34. Kleijer KTE, et al. Neurobiology of autism gene products: towards pathogenesis and drug targets. Psychopharmacology. 2014;231(6):1037–62.

35. Loke YJ, Hannan AJ, Craig JM. The role of epigenetic change in autism spectrum disorders. Front Neurol. 2015;6:107.

36. Onore C, Careaga M, Ashwood P. The role of immune dysfunction in the pathophysiology of autism. Brain Behav Immun. 2012;26(3):383–92.

37. Beversdorf DQ, MISSOURI AUTISM SUMMIT CONSORTIUM. Phenotyping, etiological factors, and biomarkers: toward precision medicine in autism spectrum disorders. J Dev Behav Pediatr. 2016;37(8):659–73.

38. Berry-Kravis EM, et al. Effects of STX209 (arbaclofen) on neurobehavioral function in children and adults with fragile X syndrome: a randomized, controlled, phase 2 trial. *Sci. Transl. Med.* 2012;4(152):152ra127.

39. Denayer T, Stöhr T, Van Roy M. Animal models in translational medicine: validation and prediction. New Horiz Transl Med. 2014;2(1):5–11.

40. Huerta M, Lord C. Diagnostic evaluation of autism spectrum disorders. Pediatr Clin N Am. 2012;59(1):103–11.

41. Bekoff M. Animal Emotions: Exploring Passionate Natures: current interdisciplinary research provides compelling evidence that many animals experience such emotions as joy, fear, love, despair, and grief—we are not alone. BioScience. 2000;50(10):861–70.

42. Stafstrom CE, Benke TA. Autism and epilepsy: exploring the relationship using experimental models. Epilepsy Curr. 2015;15(4):206–10.

43. Crawley JN. Translational animal models of autism and neurodevelopmental disorders. Dialogues Clin Neurosci. 2012;14(3):293–305.

44. Hulbert SW, Jiang Y. Monogenic mouse models of autism spectrum disorders: common mechanisms and missing links. Neuroscience. 2016;321:3–23.

45. Persico AM, Napolioni V. Autism genetics. Behav Brain Res. 2013;251:95–112.

46. Kim H, Lim C-S, Kaang B-K. Neuronal mechanisms and circuits underlying repetitive behaviors in mouse models of autism spectrum disorder. *Behav. Brain Funct.* 2016;12(1):3.

47. D'Mello AM, Stoodley CJ. Cerebro-cerebellar circuits in autism spectrum disorder. Front Neurosci. 2015;9:408.

48. Li J, et al. Integrated systems analysis reveals a molecular network underlying autism spectrum disorders. *Mol. Syst. Biol.* 2014;10(12):774.

49. Petrelli F, Pucci L, Bezzi P. Astrocytes and microglia and their potential link with autism spectrum disorders. Front Cell Neurosci. 2016;10:21.

50. Gemelli T, Berton O, Nelson ED, Perrotti LI, Jaenisch R, Monteggia LM. Postnatal loss of methyl-CpG binding protein 2 in the forebrain is sufficient to mediate behavioral aspects of Rett syndrome in mice. Biol Psychiatry. 2006;59(5):468–76.

51. Skefos J, et al. Regional alterations in purkinje ell density in patients with autism. *PLoS ONE.* 2014;9(2):e81255.

52. D'Mello AM, Crocetti D, Mostofsky SH, Stoodley CJ. Cerebellar gray matter and lobular volumes correlate with core autism symptoms. NeuroImage Clin. 2015;7:631–9.

53. Stoodley CJ, et al. Altered cerebellar connectivity in autism and cerebellar-mediated rescue of autism-related behaviors in mice. Nat Neurosci. 2017; 20(12):1744–51.

54. Auerbach BD, Osterweil EK, Bear MF. Mutations causing syndromic autism define an axis of synaptic pathophysiology. Nature. 2011;480(7375):63–8.

55. Dolen G, et al. Correction of fragile X syndrome in mice. Neuron. 2007;56(6): 955–62.

56. Guy J, Gan J, Selfridge J, Cobb S, Bird A. Reversal of neurological defects in a mouse model of Rett syndrome. Science. 2007;315(5815):1143–7.

57. Ehninger D, et al. Reversal of learning deficits in a Tsc2+/− mouse model of tuberous sclerosis. Nat Med. 2008;14(8):843–8.

58. Dolan BM, et al. Rescue of fragile X syndrome phenotypes in Fmr1 KO mice by the small-molecule PAK inhibitor FRAX486. Proc Natl Acad Sci U S A. 2013;110(14):5671–6.

59. Sztainberg Y, et al. Reversal of phenotypes in MECP2 duplication mice using genetic rescue or antisense oligonucleotides. Nature. 2015;528(7580):123–6.

60. Mei Y, et al. Adult restoration of Shank3 expression rescues selective autistic-like phenotypes. Nature. 2016;530(7591):481–4.

61. Choudhury SR, Hudry E, Maguire CA, Sena-Esteves M, Breakefield XO, Grandi P. Viral vectors for therapy of neurologic diseases. *Small Mol. Neurol. Disord.* 2017;120(Supplement C):63–80.

62. Gray SJ. Gene therapy and neurodevelopmental disorders. *Neurodev. Disord.* 2013;68(Supplement C):136–42.

63. Modlich U, et al. Insertional transformation of hematopoietic cells by self-inactivating lentiviral and gammaretroviral vectors. *Mol. Ther.* 1919–1928; 17(11)

64. Hacein-Bey-Abina S, et al. Insertional oncogenesis in 4 patients after retrovirus-mediated gene therapy of SCID-X1. J Clin Invest. 2008;118(9): 3132–42.

65. Hocquemiller M, Giersch L, Audrain M, Parker S, Cartier N. Adeno-associated virus-based gene therapy for CNS diseases. Hum Gene Ther. 2016;27(7):478–96.

66. Taymans J-M, et al. Comparative analysis of adeno-associated viral vector serotypes 1, 2, 5, 7, and 8 in mouse brain. Hum Gene Ther. 2007;18(3):195–206.

67. Aschauer DF, Kreuz S, Rumpel S. Analysis of transduction efficiency, tropism and axonal transport of AAV serotypes 1, 2, 5, 6, 8 and 9 in the mouse brain. *PLOS ONE.* 2013;8(9):e76310.

68. Powell SK, Rivera-Soto R, Gray SJ. Viral expression cassette elements to enhance transgene target specificity and expression in gene therapy. Discov Med. 2015;19(102):49–57.

69. Vite CH, Passini MA, Haskins ME, Wolfe JH. Adeno-associated virus vector-mediated transduction in the cat brain. *Gene Ther*. 2003;10(22):1874–81.

70. S. Palfi *et al.*, "Long-term safety and tolerability of ProSavin, a lentiviral vector-based gene therapy for Parkinson's disease: a dose escalation, open-label, phase 1/2 trial," *The Lancet*, 383, 9923, 1138–1146. 2014

71. Katz DM, et al. Rett syndrome: crossing the threshold to clinical translation. *Trends Neurosci*. 39(2):100–13.

72. Bruno JL, Hosseini SMH, Saggar M, Quintin E-M, Raman MM, Reiss AL. Altered brain network segregation in fragile X syndrome revealed by structural connectomics. Cereb Cortex. 2017;27(3):2249–59.

73. Dehay B, Dalkara D, Dovero S, Li Q, Bezard E. Systemic scAAV9 variant mediates brain transduction in newborn rhesus macaques. 2012;2:253.

74. Deverman BE, et al. Cre-dependent selection yields AAV variants for widespread gene transfer to the adult brain. Nat Biotech. 2016;34(2):204–9.

75. Boutin S, et al. Prevalence of serum IgG and neutralizing factors against adeno-associated virus (AAV) types 1, 2, 5, 6, 8, and 9 in the healthy population: implications for gene therapy using AAV vectors. Hum Gene Ther. 2010;21(6):704–12.

76. Gray SJ, Matagne V, Bachaboina L, Yadav S, Ojeda SR, Samulski RJ. Preclinical differences of intravascular AAV9 delivery to neurons and glia: a comparative study of adult mice and nonhuman primates. *Mol. Ther*. 19(6):1058–69.

77. Mingozzi F, High KA. Immune responses to AAV vectors: overcoming barriers to successful gene therapy. Blood. 2013;122(1):23–36.

78. Geisler A, Fechner H. MicroRNA-regulated viral vectors for gene therapy. World J Exp Med. 2016;6(2):37–54.

79. Grieger JC, Samulski RJ. Packaging capacity of adeno-associated virus serotypes: impact of larger genomes on infectivity and postentry steps. J Virol. 2005;79(15):9933–44.

80. Tse LV, et al. Structure-guided evolution of antigenically distinct adeno-associated virus variants for immune evasion. Proc Natl Acad Sci. 2017; 114(24):E4812–21.

81. Federici T, et al. Robust spinal motor neuron transduction following intrathecal delivery of AAV9 in pigs. Gene Ther. 2012;19(8):852–9.

82. Schuster DJ, et al. Biodistribution of adeno-associated virus serotype 9 (AAV9) vector after intrathecal and intravenous delivery in mouse. Front Neuroanat. 2014;8:42.

83. Samaranch L, et al. Adeno-associated virus serotype 9 transduction in the central nervous system of nonhuman primates. Hum Gene Ther. 2012;23(4):382–9.

84. Saraiva J, Nobre RJ, Pereira de Almeida L. Gene therapy for the CNS using AAVs: the impact of systemic delivery by AAV9. *J. Controlled Release*. 2016; 241(Supplement C):94–109.

85. Mussche S, et al. Restoration of cytoskeleton homeostasis after gigaxonin gene transfer for giant axonal neuropathy. Hum Gene Ther. 2013;24(2):209–19.

86. Gadalla KK, et al. Improved survival and reduced phenotypic severity following AAV9/MECP2 gene transfer to neonatal and juvenile male Mecp2 knockout mice. Mol Ther. 2013;21(1):18–30.

87. Matagne V, et al. A codon-optimized Mecp2 transgene corrects breathing deficits and improves survival in a mouse model of Rett syndrome. Neurobiol Dis. 2017;99:1–11.

88. Garg SK, et al. Systemic delivery of MeCP2 rescues behavioral and cellular deficits in female mouse models of Rett syndrome. *J. Neurosci*. 2013;33(34):13612.

89. Tillotson R, et al. Radically truncated MeCP2 rescues Rett syndrome-like neurological defects. Nature. 2017;550:398.

90. Zeier Z, Kumar A, Bodhinathan K, Feller JA, Foster TC, Bloom DC. Fragile X mental retardation protein replacement restores hippocampal synaptic function in a mouse model of fragile X syndrome. Gene Ther. 2009;16(9):1122–9.

91. Gholizadeh S, Arsenault J, Xuan ICY, Pacey LK, Hampson DR. Reduced phenotypic severity following adeno-associated virus-mediated Fmr1 gene delivery in fragile X mice. Neuropsychopharmacol Off Publ Am Coll Neuropsychopharmacol. 2014;39(13):3100–11.

92. Prabhakar S, et al. Survival benefit and phenotypic improvement by hamartin gene therapy in a tuberous sclerosis mouse brain model. Neurobiol Dis. 2015;82:22–31.

93. Robinson L, et al. Morphological and functional reversal of phenotypes in a mouse model of Rett syndrome. Brain. 2012;135(9):2699–710.

94. Gadalla KK, et al. Development of a novel AAV gene therapy cassette with improved safety features and efficacy in a mouse model of Rett syndrome. Mol Ther Methods Clin Dev. 2017;5:180–90.

95. Kyle SM, Saha PK, Brown HM, Chan LC, Justice MJ. MeCP2 co-ordinates liver lipid metabolism with the NCoR1/HDAC3 corepressor complex. Hum Mol Genet. 2016;25(14):3029–41.

96. Arsenault J, et al. FMRP expression levels in mouse central nervous system neurons determine behavioral phenotype. Hum Gene Ther. 2016;27(12):982–96.

97. Friez MJ, et al. Recurrent infections, hypotonia, and mental retardation caused by duplication of MECP2 and adjacent region in Xq28. *Pediatrics*. 2006;118(6):e1687.

98. Meins M, et al. Submicroscopic duplication in Xq28 causes increased expression of the MECP2 gene in a boy with severe mental retardation and features of Rett syndrome. J Med Genet. 2005;42(2):e12.

99. Van Esch H, et al. Duplication of the MECP2 region is a frequent cause of severe mental retardation and progressive neurological symptoms in males. Am J Hum Genet. 2005;77(3):442–53.

100. Lyon MF. X-chromosome inactivation and human genetic disease. Acta Paediatr Oslo Nor 1992 Suppl. 2002;91(439):107–12.

101. Kole R, Krainer AR, Altman S. RNA therapeutics: beyond RNA interference and antisense oligonucleotides. Nat Rev Drug Discov. 2012;11(2):125–40.

102. Wittrup A, Lieberman J. Knocking down disease: a progress report on siRNA therapeutics. Nat Rev Genet. 2015;16(9):543–52.

103. Scoto M, Finkel RS, Mercuri E, Muntoni F. Therapeutic approaches for spinal muscular atrophy (SMA). Gene Ther. 2017;24(9):514–9.

104. Wild EJ, Tabrizi SJ. Therapies targeting DNA and RNA in Huntington's disease. *Lancet Neurol*. 16, 10:837–47.

105. Sztainberg Y, et al. Reversal of phenotypes in MECP2 duplication mice using genetic rescue or antisense oligos. Nature. 2015;528(7580):123–6.

106. Krishnan V, et al. Autism gene Ube3a and seizures impair sociability by repressing VTA Cbln1. Nature. 2017;543(7646):507–12.

107. Meng L, Ward AJ, Chun S, Bennett CF, Beaudet AL, Rigo F. Towards a therapy for Angelman syndrome by reduction of a long non-coding RNA. Nature. 2015;518(7539):409–12.

108. Silva-Santos S, et al. Ube3a reinstatement identifies distinct developmental windows in a murine Angelman syndrome model. J Clin Invest. 2015;125(5):2069–76.

109. Watts JK, Corey DR. Gene silencing by siRNAs and antisense oligonucleotides in the laboratory and the clinic. J Pathol. 2012;226(2):365–79.

110. Maeder ML, Gersbach CA. Genome-editing technologies for gene and cell therapy. Mol Ther. 2016;24(3):430–46.

111. Peng R, Lin G, Li J. Potential pitfalls of CRISPR/Cas9-mediated genome editing. FEBS J. 2016;283(7):1218–31.

112. Wang L, et al. In vivo delivery systems for therapeutic genome editing. Int J Mol Sci. 2016;17(5):626.

113. Staahl BT, et al. Efficient genome editing in the mouse brain by local delivery of engineered Cas9 ribonucleoprotein complexes. Nat Biotech. 2017;35(5):431–4.

114. Lim ET, et al. Rates, distribution and implications of postzygotic mosaic mutations in autism spectrum disorder. Nat Neurosci. 2017;20:1217.

115. Gkogkas CG, et al. Autism-related deficits via dysregulated eIF4E-dependent translational control. Nature. 2013;493(7432):371–7.

116. Südhof TC. Neuroligins and neurexins link synaptic function to cognitive disease. Nature. 2008;455(7215):903–11.

117. Singh SK, Eroglu C. Neuroligins provide molecular links between syndromic and nonsyndromic autism. Sci Signal. 2013;6(283):re4.

118. Sato A. mTOR, a potential target to treat autism spectrum disorder. CNS Neurol Disord Drug Targets. 2016;15(5):533–43.

119. Sato A, et al. "Rapamycin reverses impaired social interaction in mouse models of tuberous sclerosis complex," Nat Commun. 2012;3:1292.

120. Baudouin SJ, et al. Shared synaptic pathophysiology in syndromic and nonsyndromic rodent models of autism. Science. 2012;338(6103):128–32.

121. Novarino G, et al. Mutations in BCKD-kinase lead to a potentially treatable form of autism with epilepsy. Science. 2012;338(6105):394–7.

122. Tarlungeanu DC, et al. Impaired amino acid transport at the blood brain barrier is a cause of autism spectrum disorder. Cell. 2016;167(6):1481–1494.e18.

123. Sethna F, Moon C, Wang H. From FMRP function to potential therapies for fragile X syndrome. Neurochem Res. 2014;39(6):1016–31.

124. Richards C, Jones C, Groves L, Moss J, Oliver C. Prevalence of autism spectrum disorder phenomenology in genetic disorders: a systematic review and meta-analysis. Lancet Psychiatry. 2015;2(10):909–16.

125. Guy J, Cheval H, Selfridge J, Bird A. The role of MeCP2 in the brain. Annu Rev Cell Dev Biol. 2011;27(1):631–52.

126. Ramocki MB, et al. Autism and other neuropsychiatric symptoms are prevalent in individuals with MECP2 duplication syndrome. Ann Neurol. 2009;66(6):771–82.

127. Tee AR, Fingar DC, Manning BD, Kwiatkowski DJ, Cantley LC, Blenis J. Tuberous sclerosis complex-1 and -2 gene products function together to

inhibit mammalian target of rapamycin (mTOR)-mediated downstream
signaling. Proc Natl Acad Sci. 2002;99(21):13571–6.

128. Tomaic V, Banks L. Angelman syndrome-associated ubiquitin ligase UBE3A/
E6AP mutants interfere with the proteolytic activity of the proteasome. Cell
Death Dis. 2015;6:e1625.

129. Betancur C, Sakurai T, Buxbaum JD. The emerging role of synaptic cell-
adhesion pathways in the pathogenesis of autism spectrum disorders.
Trends Neurosci. 32(7):402–12.

130. Ye H, Liu J, Wu JY. Cell adhesion molecules and their involvement in autism
spectrum disorder. Neurosignals. 2010;18(2):62–71.

131. Ting JT, Peça J, Feng G. Functional consequences of mutations in
postsynaptic scaffolding proteins and relevance to psychiatric disorders.
Annu Rev Neurosci. 2012;35(1):49–71.

132. Zheng F, et al. Evidence for association between Disrupted-in-schizophrenia
1 (DISC1) gene polymorphisms and autism in Chinese Han population: a
family-based association study. *Behav. Brain Funct*. 2011;7(1):14.

133. Chen J, Yu S, Fu Y, Li X. Synaptic proteins and receptors defects in autism
spectrum disorders. Front Cell Neurosci. 2014;8:276.

134. Rojas DC. The role of glutamate and its receptors in autism and the use of
glutamate receptor antagonists in treatment. J Neural Transm Vienna
Austria 1996. 2014;121(8):891–905.

135. Platt RJ, et al. Chd8 mutation leads to autistic-like behaviors and impaired
striatal circuits. *Cell Rep*. 19(2):335–50.

136. Breuss MW, Gleeson JG. When size matters: CHD8 in autism. Nat Neurosci.
2016;19(11):1430–2.

CRISPR/Cas9-induced *shank3b* mutant zebrafish display autism-like behaviors

Chun-xue Liu[1], Chun-yang Li[1], Chun-chun Hu[1], Yi Wang[1], Jia Lin[2], Yong-hui Jiang[3], Qiang Li[2*] and Xiu Xu[1*]

Abstract

Background: Human genetic and genomic studies have supported a strong causal role of *SHANK3* deficiency in autism spectrum disorder (ASD). However, the molecular mechanism underlying *SHANK3* deficiency resulting in ASD is not fully understood. Recently, the zebrafish has become an attractive organism to model ASD because of its high efficiency of genetic manipulation and robust behavioral phenotypes. The orthologous gene to human *SHANK3* is duplicated in the zebrafish genome and has two homologs, *shank3a* and *shank3b*. Previous studies have reported *shank3* morphants in zebrafish using the morpholino method. Here, we report the generation and characterization of *shank3b* mutant zebrafish in larval and adult stages using the CRISPR/Cas9 genome editing technique.

Methods: CRISPR/Cas9 was applied to generate a *shank3b* loss-of-function mutation ($shank3b^{-/-}$) in zebrafish. A series of morphological measurements, behavioral tests, and molecular analyses were performed to systematically characterize the behavioral and molecular changes in *shank3b* mutant zebrafish.

Results: $shank3b^{-/-}$ zebrafish exhibited abnormal morphology in early development. They showed reduced locomotor activity both as larvae and adults, reduced social interaction and time spent near conspecifics, and significant repetitive swimming behaviors. Additionally, the levels of both postsynaptic homer1 and presynaptic synaptophysin were significantly reduced in the adult brain of *shank3b*-deficient zebrafish.

Conclusions: We generated the first inheritable *shank3b* mutant zebrafish model using CRISPR/Cas9 gene editing approach. $shank3b^{-/-}$ zebrafish displayed robust autism-like behaviors and altered levels of the synaptic proteins homer1 and synaptophysin. The versatility of zebrafish as a model for studying neurodevelopment and conducting drug screening will likely have a significant contribution to future studies of human *SHANK3* function and ASD.

Keywords: shank3, CRISPR/Cas9, Zebrafish, ASD, Social behavior, Animal model

Background

SHANK3 is a master scaffolding protein enriched at the postsynaptic density of excitatory glutamatergic synapses in the brain that has critical roles in synaptogenesis and synaptic function [1–6]. *SHANK3* is the key gene implicated in the neurobehavioral features of individuals with chromosome 22q13.3 deletion syndrome or Phelan-McDermid syndrome (PMS) [7, 8]. Moreover, genetic studies have identified point mutations in the *SHANK3* gene in cases of autism spectrum disorder (ASD) that establish the causal role of *SHANK3* mutations in ~ 1% of individuals with ASD [9–11].

Animal models of ASD that mimic *SHANK3* genetic detects have facilitated a better understanding of the underlying molecular mechanisms and development of more effective treatments [2, 12]. More than a dozen different lines of *Shank3* mutant mice have been generated and characterized [4, 13–15]. Almost all *Shank3* mutant mice exhibit some of the core behavioral features of ASD [4, 13, 14]. Despite significant advantages, there are clear disadvantages associated with the use of rodent models. For example, it remains difficult to scale up for high-throughput drug screening in rodent models [12]. Compared to rodent models, zebrafish (*Danio rerio*) exhibit much more efficient reproduction, rapid external development [12, 16, 17], and optical transparency [17].

* Correspondence: liq@fudan.edu.cn; xuxiu@shmu.edu.cn
[2]Center for Translational Medicine, Institute of Pediatrics, Shanghai Key Laboratory of Birth Defect, Children's Hospital of Fudan University, 399 Wanyuan Road, Shanghai 201102, China
[1]Division of Child Health Care, Children's Hospital of Fudan University, 399 Wanyuan Road, Shanghai 201102, China
Full list of author information is available at the end of the article

Previous studies have shown that the gene orthologous to human *SHANK3* is duplicated in zebrafish as *shank3a* (in chromosome 18) and *shank3b* (in chromosome 4) [18, 19]. Transient knockdown of both *shank3a* and *shank3b* expressions by morpholino method has been reported [19, 20]. However, previously, the analysis of developmental and behavioral characteristics was only conducted within 5 days of post-fertilization (dpf), an early stage of development [19]. In the present study, we generated and characterized the first CRISPR/Cas9 engineered *shank3b* loss-of-function mutation that is stably transmitted in zebrafish. This model will enable a comprehensive study of a mechanistic link between *shank3* loss-of-function and ASD and provide a new experimental platform for high throughput drug screening in the future.

Methods

Generation of *shank3b* mutant zebrafish

The detailed procedure for CRISPR/Cas9 editing in zebrafish was described previously [21, 22]. The *shank3b* target in this study was 5′-GGGCGTGTTGTTGCCAC GGCCGG-3′ (Additional file 1: Table S1). Injection mixtures included 500 pg of Cas9 mRNA and 120 pg of gRNA. Eighty zebrafish were screened to identify a founder, and the germline mutation frequency was approximately 35%. Mutant sites were verified by comparison to the WT unaffected sequences (chimerism). Chimeric zebrafish were mated onto a Tu background for three generations to obtain *shank3b*$^{+/-}$ zebrafish. We crossed *shank3b*$^{+/-}$ males and *shank3b*$^{+/-}$ females to obtain *shank3b*$^{+/+}$, *shank3b*$^{+/-}$, and *shank3b*$^{-/-}$ littermates for all experiments of phenotypic analyses.

Tg (*HuC*: RFP) transgenic line and zebrafish maintenance

The wild-type (WT) Tu zebrafish strain was acquired from the Institute of Zebrafish, Children's Hospital of Fudan University. The zebrafish were raised and maintained in a standard laboratory environment (28.5 °C) and a 14 h light/10 h dark cycle according to a standard protocol [17, 23]. The *Tg* (*shank3b*$^{+/+}$-*HuC*: RFP$^{+/-}$) transgenic line, kindly provided by Dr. Xu Wang (Fudan University), was made via plasmid injection with tol2 mRNA at single-cell stage followed by screening for germline transmission. The vector was generated by inserting the *HuC* promoter [24] upstream of RFP cDNA followed by polyA sequence in a Tol2 destination vector, using multisite Gateway cloning [25]. In order to collect enough eggs efficiently for the RFP imaging experiments, we crossed *Tg* (*shank3b*$^{+/-}$-*HuC*: RFP$^{+/-}$) with *Tg* (*shank3b*$^{+/-}$-*HuC*: RFP$^{+/-}$) to obtain *Tg* (*shank3b*$^{-/-}$-*HuC*: RFP$^{+/+}$) for the experimental group. We crossed *Tg* (*shank3b*$^{+/+}$-*HuC*: RFP$^{+/-}$) and *Tg* (*shank3b*$^{+/+}$-*HuC*: RFP$^{+/-}$) to obtain the control group, *Tg* (*shank3b*$^{+/+}$-*HuC*: RFP$^{+/+}$).

RT-qPCR

Real-time quantitative polymerase chain reaction (RT-qPCR) was performed in triplicate, with 4–10 zebrafish per sample. Total RNA was extracted from the larval or adult brains using TRIzol reagent (Ambion, USA). Reverse transcription was performed with a Prime-Script™ RT Reagent Kit (RR037A, TaKaRa, Japan), according to the manufacturer's protocol. Oligo dT primer (25 pmol) and random 6 mers (50 pmol) were added in 10 μl mixture to efficiently obtain full-length cDNA. RT-qPCR was performed using a LightCycler® 480 apparatus (Roche, Germany) and SuperRealPreMix Plus (Tiangen, China), according to the manufacturers' instructions. Finally, we used the delta delta CT method to calculate the expression levels. The primers used in this study are described in Table S1 in Additional file 1.

Larval activity and light/dark tests

A ViewPoint setup combined with an automated computer recording system equipped with VideoTrack software was used to measure locomotor activity. The camera was a Point Grey black-and-white camera with a resolution of 1024×768. Videos were recorded for 60 min at 25 fps and were pooled into 1-min time bins. The detection threshold was set to 25. Activity was quantified using Zebralab software. The distance traveled by the larvae in the well was measured to analyze general locomotor activity. For all behavioral analyses, we used a commercial Viewpoint tracking system and custom software written in C++. All behavioral assays were analyzed by experimenters who were blinded to the genotypes. To further analyze the variances of different activity intensity scales among WT, *shank3b*$^{+/-}$, and *shank3b*$^{-/-}$ zebrafish, we divided the activity equally into five levels (10, 20, 30, 40, and 50) (Additional file 1: Figure S6). Next, we calculated the activity frequency of different activity intensity scales.

Larvae were habituated in 48-well plates, with one animal per well, in our behavioral assessment room, and videos were recorded for 60 min. The diameter of each well was 1.2 cm. After 30 min of habituation, each larva was recorded for a total of 30 min with three light/dark cycles (each consisting of 5 min of light and 5 min of dark). The light intensity for photo motor response (PMR) was 100 lx and the frame rate was 25/s.

Open-field test

Behavioral experiments were conducted between 10 a.m. and 4 p.m. Each tank was $30 \times 30 \times 30$ cm, with walls made of opaque partitions, and a video camera was suspended above the tank. Adult male zebrafish were allowed to freely swim inside the tank, and videos were recorded for 30 min. The timing of all supplementary videos began at approximately the 10th min.

The thigmotaxis test was performed in the tank divided into two equal zones, a peripheral and a central zone. Adult zebrafish swam freely in the tank. The longer the zebrafish stayed in the peripheral zone, the greater their awareness of danger [12]. The time ratio was the time the zebrafish spent in the peripheral zone divided by the total time spent in tank, and the distance ratio was the distance the zebrafish traveled in the peripheral zone divided by the total distance traveled.

Shoaling test

Adult male zebrafish were acclimated to the novel tank apparatus for 1–2 min before the test [26]. Videos were recorded for 30 min. The shoaling assessment was performed by measuring the inter-fish distance that represents the average of all distance between each zebrafish in a shoal [27, 28].

Social preference test

Social preference testing was performed in a standard mating tank (inner dimensions 21 × 10 × 7.5 cm). The tank was separated into two halves by a Plexiglas transparent barrier that allowed the zebrafish to swim freely and was provided sufficient visual information to allow the zebrafish to form a social preference. Behavioral recordings typically started after an acclimation period (1–2 min), when zebrafish usually explored the tank. Videos were recorded for 30 min. The zebrafish behaviors were quantified as a distance distribution or as presence in a zone adjacent to the group or conspecifics. The time ratio was the time spent in the conspecific sector divided by the total time. The distance ratio was the distance traveled in the conspecific sector divided by the total distance traveled. The zebrafish tested were all adult males.

Kin preference test

The specifications of the mating cylinder were the same as those in the social preference test. Two opaque separators divided the cylinder into three compartments. Videos were recorded for 30 min. Kin preference was represented by the ratio of time spent in the kin sector divided by the total time. The zebrafish tested were all adult males.

Western blot and antibodies

WT and $shank3b^{-/-}$ zebrafish brains were prepared for western blotting by dissociating the tissues in lysis buffer (RIPA, Beyotime Biotechnology, China) and 1% protease inhibitor mixture Set I (Calbiochem, San Diego, CA, USA). The lysates were then centrifuged at 12,000 rpm for 5 min, and the supernatant was collected and denatured. 20 μg of total protein were separated on an SDS-PAGE gel (12%) and were blotted onto a polyvinylidene difluoride membrane (Bio-Rad Laboratories, Hercules, CA, USA). Next, the membrane was blocked with 5% bovine serum albumin for 1–2 h at room temperature and was incubated with primary antibodies overnight at 4 °C. The membrane was rinsed and incubated with HRP-conjugated secondary antibodies for 2 h. Finally, chemiluminescent detection was performed with an ECL kit (Rockford, IL, USA). ImageJ software was used for the densitometric analysis ($N = 3$ for each group).

The synaptophysin (1:2000; ab32594) and homer1 (1:1000; ARP40181_P050) antibodies were purchased from Abcam (Cambridge, UK) and Aviva Systems Biology (San Diego, USA), respectively. The β-actin antibody was obtained from Biotech Well (1:2000; code No. WB0196, Shanghai, China).

Statistical analysis

Statistical analyses were performed using GraphPad Prism software. Simple comparisons between adult $shank3b^{+/+}$ and $shank3b^{-/-}$ zebrafish were performed with two-sided unpaired Student's t tests. Analysis of variance (ANOVA) tests were used to compare three genotypes. All the experiments were conducted in triplicate using different samples. P values < 0.05 were considered as statistically significant. Values are presented as mean ± SEM.

Results

Conservation of human SHANK family genes in zebrafish

Previous analyses have suggested that the zebrafish ortholog of human SHANK3 is duplicated in the zebrafish genome because of the presence of two highly similar copies of human SHANK3: shank3a and shank3b [19]. To further analyze the evolutionary conservation between human and zebrafish, we performed a phylogenetic analysis of the SHANK gene family (SHANK1, SHANK2, and SHANK3). As shown in Additional file 1: Table S2 and Figure S1, SHANK1 and SHANK2 each have only one homolog that is believed to be an ortholog in the zebrafish genome. Consistent with previous reports [18, 19], we identified two homologs, shank3a (1933 aa) and shank3b (1643 aa), in the zebrafish genome. shank3a and shank3b share 59 and 55% identity with human SHANK3, respectively (Additional file 1: Table S3 and Figure S2; https://blast.ncbi.nlm.nih.gov/Blast.cgi). shank3a displayed an overall 59% identity and 68% similarity with shank3b but close to 100% identity in several blocks of amino acids within the protein (Additional file 1: Table S4 and Figure S3). This observation supports that shank3a and shank3b may have evolved from the same ancestral DNA during their evolution. Although human SHANK3 was slightly more conserved in shank3a than shank3b, both of them may be relevant to understand the functions of human SHANK3 protein.

Generation of shank3b⁻/⁻ zebrafish

Zebrafish *shank3b* specific guide-RNA (gRNA) comprising a 23-base sequence was designed for the gene-specific editing of exon 2 of *shank3b*. We generated a *shank3b* mutant by co-injection of Cas9 mRNA and gRNA into zebrafish embryos (one-cell stage). DNA sequencing of target-specific PCR products confirmed that the *shank3b* targeted allele carried a deletion of 5 bases and an insertion of 13 bases, resulting in a frameshift mutation and truncated protein 90 amino acids after the mutation. The mutation disrupted all known functional domains of the shank3b protein (Fig. 1a; Additional file 1: Figure S4). Homozygous mutants for *shank3b* (*shank3b⁻/⁻*) were obtained from the heterozygotes cross (*shank3b⁺/⁻♂ × shank3b⁺/⁻♀*) after mating mutants with the original Tu strain for three generations (*shank3b⁺/⁻*). RT-qPCR analysis confirmed that the expression of *Shank3b* mRNA was significantly reduced in *shank3b⁻/⁻*

zebrafish (Fig. 1b), whereas the expression of *shank3a* mRNA was not affected (Fig. 1c). Thus, these results indicated that we have successfully generated a transgenic line of *shank3b*-deficient zebrafish.

Morphological analysis of shank3b⁻/⁻ zebrafish

We measured morphological changes in *shank3b⁻/⁻* zebrafish to examine the consequences of *shank3b* deficiency during zebrafish development. Compared with *shank3b⁺/⁺* and *shank3b⁺/⁻* zebrafish, a significantly greater proportion of *shank3b⁻/⁻* zebrafish died (*shank3b⁺/⁺*, 3%; *shank3b⁺/⁻*, 9%; *shank3b⁻/⁻*, 20%) and exhibited morphological changes at a very early stage (1 dpf). The morphological changes included neurodevelopmental delay, tail bending, and a reduction of melanin content in eye (Fig. 2a, b). However, over the course of development, these differences in the general

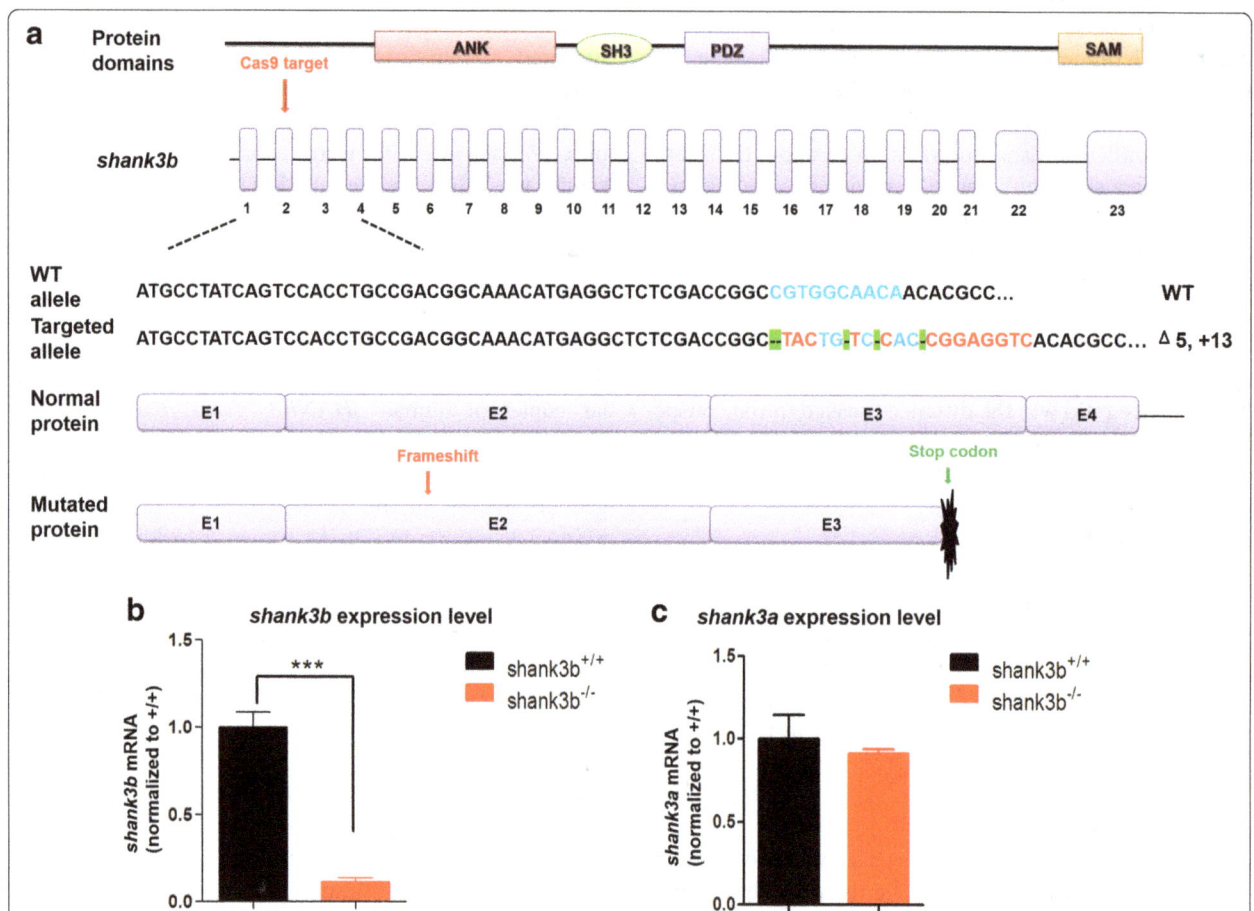

Fig. 1 Generation of *shank3b* mutation in zebrafish by CRISPR-Cas9 gene editing. **a** Structure of zebrafish *shank3b* gene and protein. The protein domains (ANK, ankyrin repeat domain; SH3, Src homology 3 domain; PDZ, PSD-95/Discs large/ZO-1 domain; SAM, sterile alpha motif domain) are aligned to the corresponding exons. Exon 2 is the target for CRISPR/Cas9 gene editing in zebrafish *shank3b*. The CRISPR/Cas9-induced mutation (5-base deletion and 13-base insertion) in *shank3b* is shown in annotated *shank3b* mutant sequences. The nucleotides in red are inserted sequences and the green highlighted "-" are deleted nucleotides. **b** Reduced expression of *shank3b* mRNA in the brain of *shank3b⁺/⁺* and *shank3b⁻/⁻* adult (6 mpf) male zebrafish analyzed by RT-qPCR. **c** The expression of *shank3a* mRNA in the brain of *shank3b⁺/⁺* and *shank3b⁻/⁻* adult (6 mpf) male zebrafish was not affected. Data are shown as mean ± SEM; ***$p < 0.001$

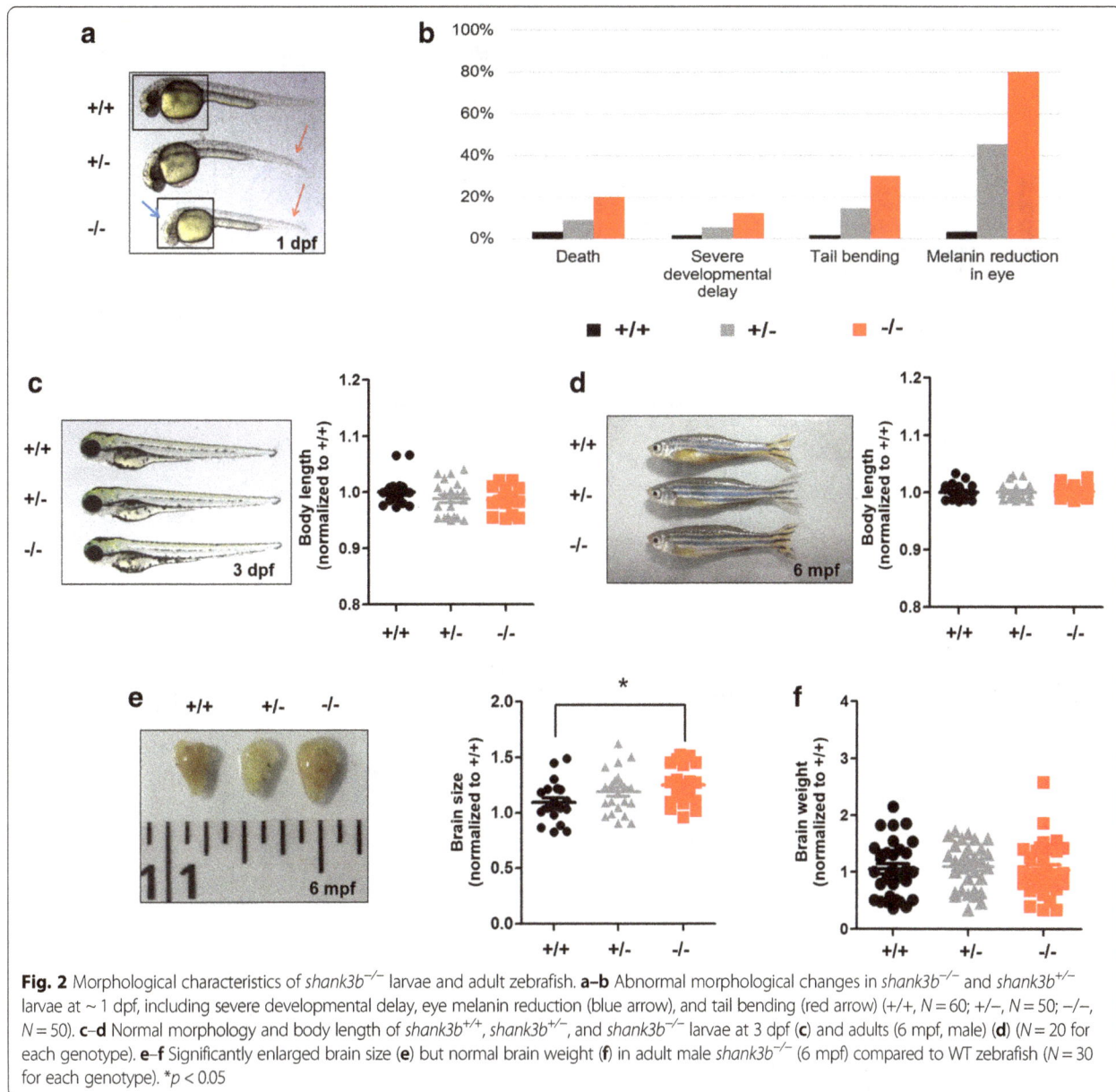

Fig. 2 Morphological characteristics of *shank3b*$^{-/-}$ larvae and adult zebrafish. **a–b** Abnormal morphological changes in *shank3b*$^{-/-}$ and *shank3b*$^{+/-}$ larvae at ~ 1 dpf, including severe developmental delay, eye melanin reduction (blue arrow), and tail bending (red arrow) (+/+, N = 60; +/−, N = 50; −/−, N = 50). **c–d** Normal morphology and body length of *shank3b*$^{+/+}$, *shank3b*$^{+/-}$, and *shank3b*$^{-/-}$ larvae at 3 dpf (**c**) and adults (6 mpf, male) (**d**) (N = 20 for each genotype). **e–f** Significantly enlarged brain size (**e**) but normal brain weight (**f**) in adult male *shank3b*$^{-/-}$ (6 mpf) compared to WT zebrafish (N = 30 for each genotype). *$p < 0.05$

phenotypes gradually become less noticeable (Fig. 2c, d). To determine whether there is a maternal or paternal origin effect on the phenotypes observed among *shank3b*$^{-/-}$ zebrafish, *shank3b*$^{-/-}$ females were crossed with WT males and *shank3b*$^{-/-}$ males were crossed with WT females, respectively. We compared the morphological phenotypes of the offspring from these two breeding schemes and did not find any significant differences (Additional file 1: Figure S5A).

The brain size of adult *shank3b*$^{-/-}$ zebrafish was significantly larger than that of *shank3b*$^{+/+}$ zebrafish ($p = 0.01$, Fig. 2e), whereas the weight of *shank3b*$^{-/-}$ brains was comparable to that of *shank3b*$^{+/+}$ and *shank3b*$^{+/-}$ brains (Fig. 2f).

shank3b$^{-/-}$ larvae exhibited impaired locomotor activity

To determine whether the loss of function of *shank3b* modulates the larval behaviors during development, the frequency was measured at five activity intensities (10, 20, 30, 40, and 50) among *shank3b*$^{+/+}$, *shank3b*$^{+/-}$, and *shank3b*$^{-/-}$ zebrafish (Additional file 1: Figure S6). The spontaneous activity of individual larva was measured for 30 min in a 48-well plate at 2, 5, and 7 dpf under light exposure (full light strength is 100 lx). Compared with *shank3b*$^{+/+}$ larvae, *shank3b*$^{-/-}$ and *shank3b*$^{+/-}$ larvae exhibited a trend of reduced activity at 2 dpf, but the differences did not reach statistically significance (Fig. 3a). *shank3b*$^{-/-}$ and *shank3b*$^{+/-}$ larvae moved significantly less than *shank3b*$^{+/+}$ larvae at higher activity

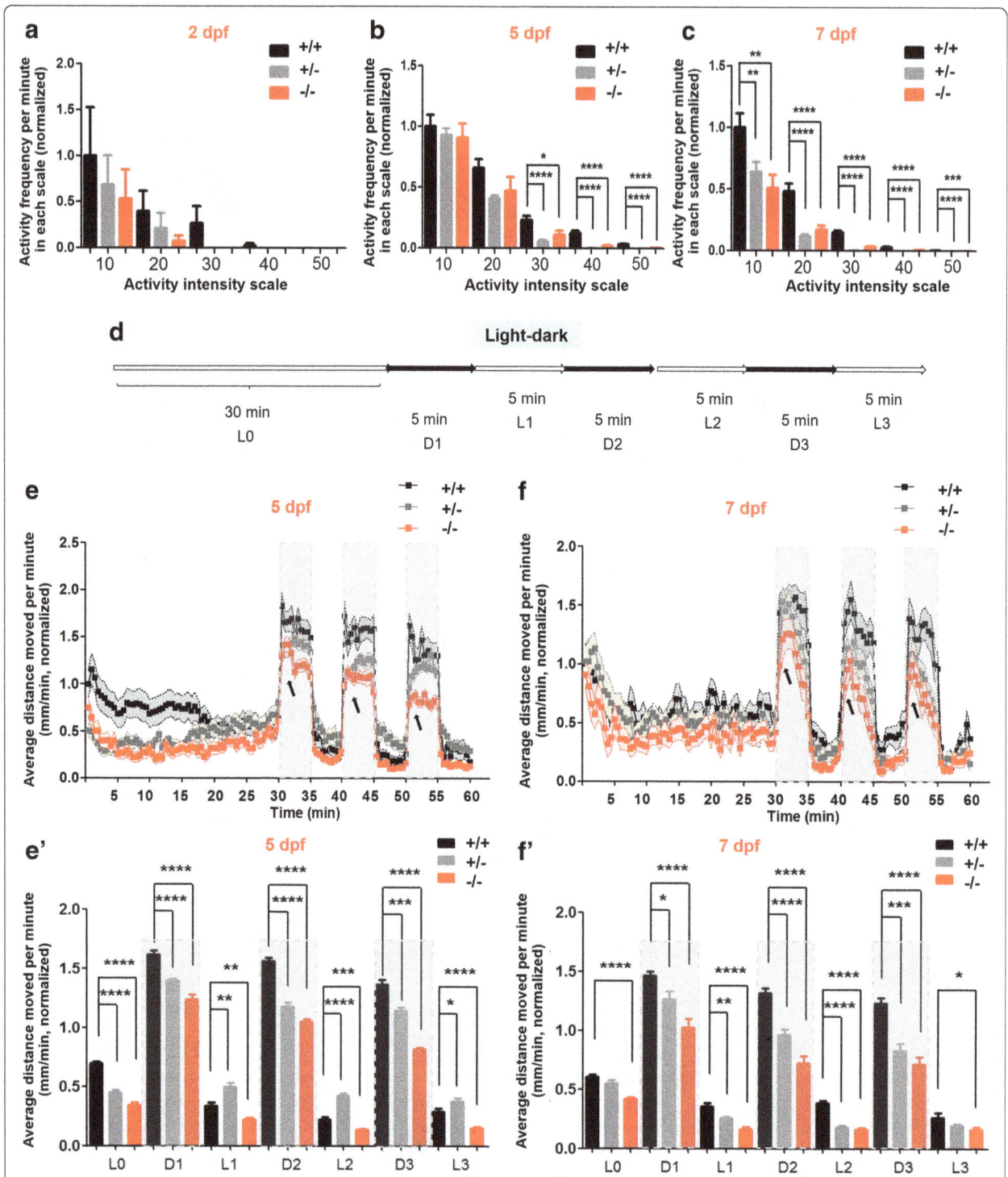

Fig. 3 *shank3b*$^{-/-}$ larvae displayed impaired locomotion activity. **a–c** Spontaneous activity of *shank3b*$^{+/+}$, *shank3b*$^{+/-}$, and *shank3b*$^{-/-}$ larvae was significantly reduced at 5 and 7 dpf, but not at 2 dpf. The *X* axis shows the intensity scale of the activity and *Y* axis shows the normalized activity frequency traveled by larvae in 1-min bin on each intensity scale (*N* = 24 for each genotype). **d–f'** Light/dark test of *shank3b*$^{+/+}$, *shank3b*$^{+/-}$, and *shank3b*$^{-/-}$ larvae at 5 and 7 dpf. The activity was recorded during 30 min of light (L0) and three 5-min light/dark intervals (D1/L1, D2/L2, and D3/L3) (**d**). The average distance moved within each 1-min bin under either light or dark conditions is plotted. Experiments were performed at 5 dpf (**e** and **e'**) and 7 dpf (**f** and **f'**). The vertical axis shows the normalized distance (millimeters) traveled by larvae in each 1-min bin. Data are shown as mean ± SEM (*N* = 24 for each genotype); *$p < 0.05$, **$p < 0.01$, ***$p < 0.001$, ****$p < 0.0001$

scales on 5 dpf (Fig. 3b), and at all activity scales on 7 dpf (Fig. 3c).

We also examined the responses evoked by light changes (light/dark switch, 100 lx for brightness and 0 lx for dark). After a 30-min habituation period, each larva displayed relatively stable activity and was recorded for 30 min over three light/dark cycles (each consisting of 5 min in light and 5 min in dark setting per cycle, Fig. 3d). Under continuous illumination, the total distance traveled was measured. Compared with shank3b$^{+/+}$ larvae, shank3b$^{-/-}$ and shank3b$^{+/-}$ larvae traveled significantly less, and shank3b$^{-/-}$ larvae performed significantly worse than shank3b$^{+/-}$ larvae. Light-to-dark transitions elicited sudden increases of total distance traveled, while dark-to-light transitions resulted in sudden decreased distance traveled (Fig. 3e, f, e', f'). However, shank3b$^{-/-}$ and shank3b$^{+/-}$ larvae showed fewer responses to changes in illumination (arrows in Fig. 3e, f).

To test whether there is a maternal or paternal origin effect on behavioral phenotypes, we compared larval activity and light/dark switch responses in the offspring of shank3b$^{-/-}$ female and shank3b$^{-/-}$ male zebrafish. However, no significant differences were observed among these two groups (Additional file 1: Figs. S5B–5F and S5B'–5F').

shank3b$^{-/-}$ adult zebrafish displayed impaired locomotor activity and abnormal repetitive movements

The locomotor activity of adult shank3b$^{-/-}$ zebrafish was also examined in an illuminated tank (Fig. 4a). Significantly reduced swimming velocity was observed in shank3b$^{-/-}$ zebrafish, compared with shank3b$^{+/+}$ zebrafish (Fig. 4b). Although shank3b$^{+/+}$ zebrafish displayed reduced velocities with increased time in the tank, shank3b$^{-/-}$ zebrafish showed steadily lower locomotor activity throughout the examination window (Fig. 4c).

To determine whether disruption of shank3b alters thigmotaxis, the two groups of adult zebrafish were assessed for the percentage of time spent and the distance traveled in the center vs. the peripheral zones in a new water tank (Fig. 4a). Compared with shank3b$^{+/+}$ zebrafish, shank3b$^{-/-}$ zebrafish spent considerably more time and traveled longer distances in the center of the tank than in the peripheral area (Fig. 4d, e).

When the trajectories of activity and pattern of swimming were analyzed in a blinded fashion, we noticed that shank3b$^{-/-}$ zebrafish exhibited a significantly higher frequency of stereotypical behaviors (Fig. 4f, g; Additional file 1: Table S5) than shank3b$^{+/+}$ zebrafish (Additional file 2: Movie S1). The repetitive behaviors include repetitive or stereotypic figure "8" swimming, circling, cornering, and walling (Additional file 3: Movie S2, Additional file 4: Movie S3, Additional file 5: Movie S4, Additional file 6: Movie S5).

shank3b$^{-/-}$ zebrafish displayed impaired social preference behaviors

It is known that wild-type zebrafish typically swim together in a school that reflects the social nature of the species. We therefore used the shoaling test to assess the social cohesion among homogeneous groups of zebrafish [26, 29]. In this assay, adult shank3b$^{+/+}$ or shank3b$^{-/-}$ zebrafish were placed in the testing tank. The average inter-fish distance was measured every 30 s for all pair combinations (Fig. 5a). As shown in Fig. 5b, shank3b$^{+/+}$ zebrafish typically swim as schools, which is characterized by a short inter-fish distance, a short average diameter of the group, and a clear polarization (Additional file 7: Movie S6), whereas shank3b$^{-/-}$ zebrafish exhibited larger and looser schools, increased average inter-fish distance, and a greater number of zebrafish swimming away from the group and spending more time outside the group (Additional file 8: Movie S7).

The social preference and interaction tests were subsequently performed using a two-sector tank, divided in the middle with clear Plexiglas to allow visualization. A group of six conspecific zebrafish was placed in the right side, and a single shank3b$^{+/+}$ or shank3b$^{-/-}$ test zebrafish was placed on the left side (Fig. 5c). shank3b$^{+/+}$ zebrafish generally contacted the group on the right side and spent more time in the conspecific sector rather than the empty sector, showing a strong group tendency (Fig. 5d; Additional file 9: Movie S8). In contrast, shank3b$^{-/-}$ zebrafish spent their time evenly throughout the region and exhibited reduced duration and frequency of social contacts with the peer group (Additional file 10: Movie S9). Quantitatively, compared with shank3b$^{+/+}$ zebrafish, shank3b$^{-/-}$ zebrafish exhibited a significantly decreased time ratio (Fig. 5e) and distance ratio (Fig. 5f) in the conspecific sector.

In the related kin recognition and preference test, the zebrafish (shank3b$^{+/+}$ or shank3b$^{-/-}$) was placed in the middle of a three-chamber apparatus with Plexiglas dividers, with kin zebrafish placed on the right and non-kin (red color) zebrafish placed on the left (Fig. 5g). shank3b$^{+/+}$ zebrafish typically spent more time near the kin group (conspecific and same color) than near the non-kin group (Additional file 11: Movie S10), indicating kin recognition and preference. In contrast, shank3b$^{-/-}$ zebrafish swam in a loose and irregular manner, and the total time spent parallel to conspecifics was much less than that found in shank3b$^{+/+}$ zebrafish (Fig. 5h; Additional file 12: Movie S11).

shank3b deficiency affected neurodevelopment in larvae

To further study neural development, the HuC-RFP transgenic line that is widely expressed in the nervous system during embryonic development was used in

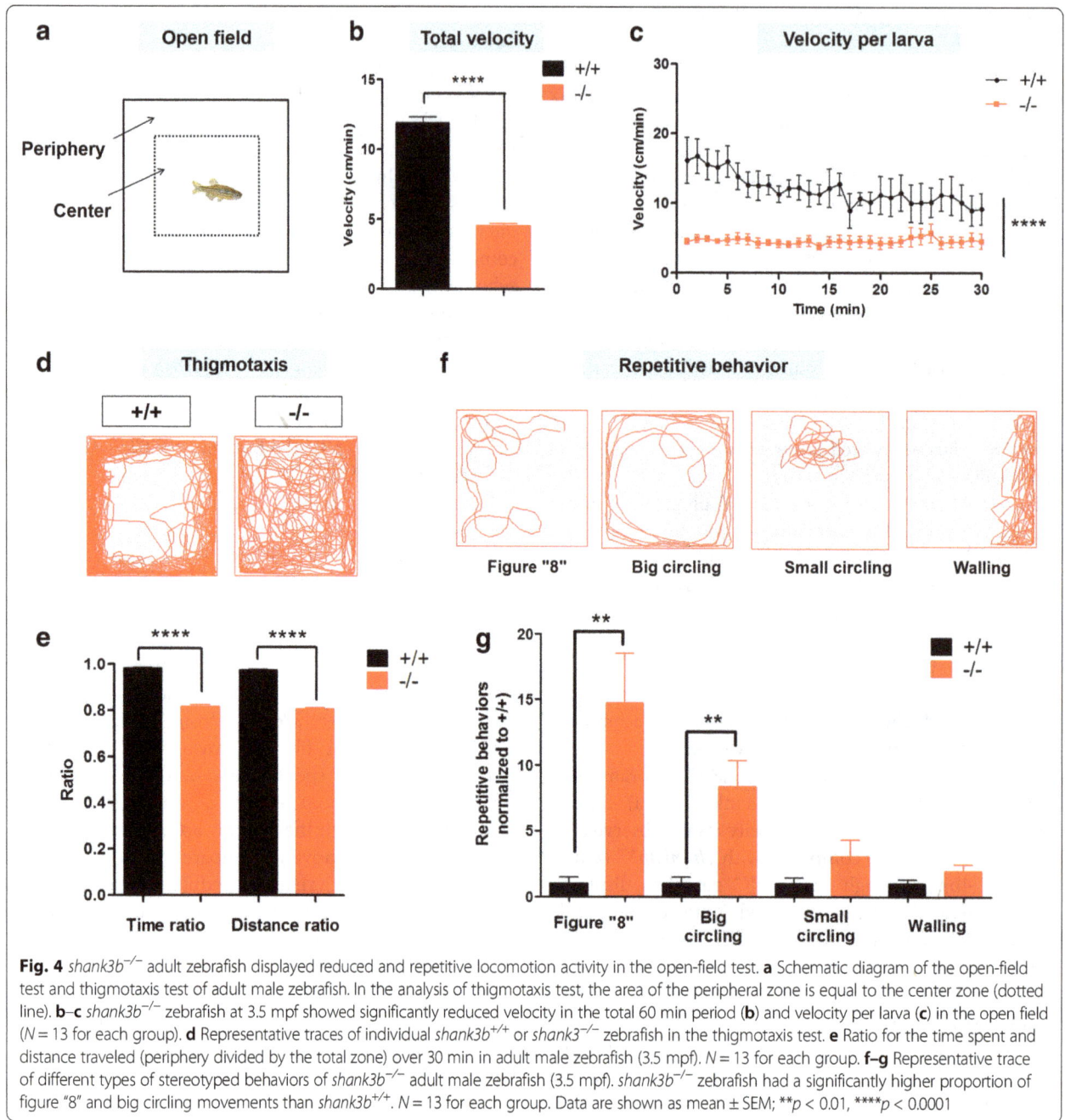

Fig. 4 shank3b$^{-/-}$ adult zebrafish displayed reduced and repetitive locomotion activity in the open-field test. **a** Schematic diagram of the open-field test and thigmotaxis test of adult male zebrafish. In the analysis of thigmotaxis test, the area of the peripheral zone is equal to the center zone (dotted line). **b–c** shank3b$^{-/-}$ zebrafish at 3.5 mpf showed significantly reduced velocity in the total 60 min period (**b**) and velocity per larva (**c**) in the open field (N = 13 for each group). **d** Representative traces of individual shank3b$^{+/+}$ or shank3$^{-/-}$ zebrafish in the thigmotaxis test. **e** Ratio for the time spent and distance traveled (periphery divided by the total zone) over 30 min in adult male zebrafish (3.5 mpf). N = 13 for each group. **f–g** Representative trace of different types of stereotyped behaviors of shank3b$^{-/-}$ adult male zebrafish (3.5 mpf). shank3b$^{-/-}$ zebrafish had a significantly higher proportion of figure "8" and big circling movements than shank3b$^{+/+}$. N = 13 for each group. Data are shown as mean ± SEM; **p < 0.01, ****p < 0.0001

this study. The *HuC*-RFP transgene, in which the *HuC* promoter drives RFP expression, enables clear and direct visualization of neurodevelopment in transparent larvae (Fig. 6a–c). Compared with *shank3b*$^{+/+}$ larvae, the expression of the RFP reporter was significantly reduced in *shank3b*$^{-/-}$ larvae from 1 to 3 dpf, indicating that the neurodevelopment of *shank3b*$^{-/-}$ larvae was altered (Fig. 6a'–c'). In addition, the differences in RFP expression at 1 dpf decreased over time, consistent with the developmental delay shown in Fig. 2.

shank3b deficiency resulted in reduced homer1 and synaptophysin protein levels in the adult zebrafish brain

Shank3 is a core scaffolding protein located at the postsynaptic density [1]. Significantly reduced Homer1, a major postsynaptic protein, is reported in *Shank3* mutant mice [4]. We therefore examined homer1 protein levels in adult *shank3b*$^{-/-}$ zebrafish brains. We found that the level of homer1 protein was significantly decreased (27% of *shank3b*$^{+/+}$) in the brain of *shank3b*$^{-/-}$ zebrafish (n = 3, mean ± SD, 0.27

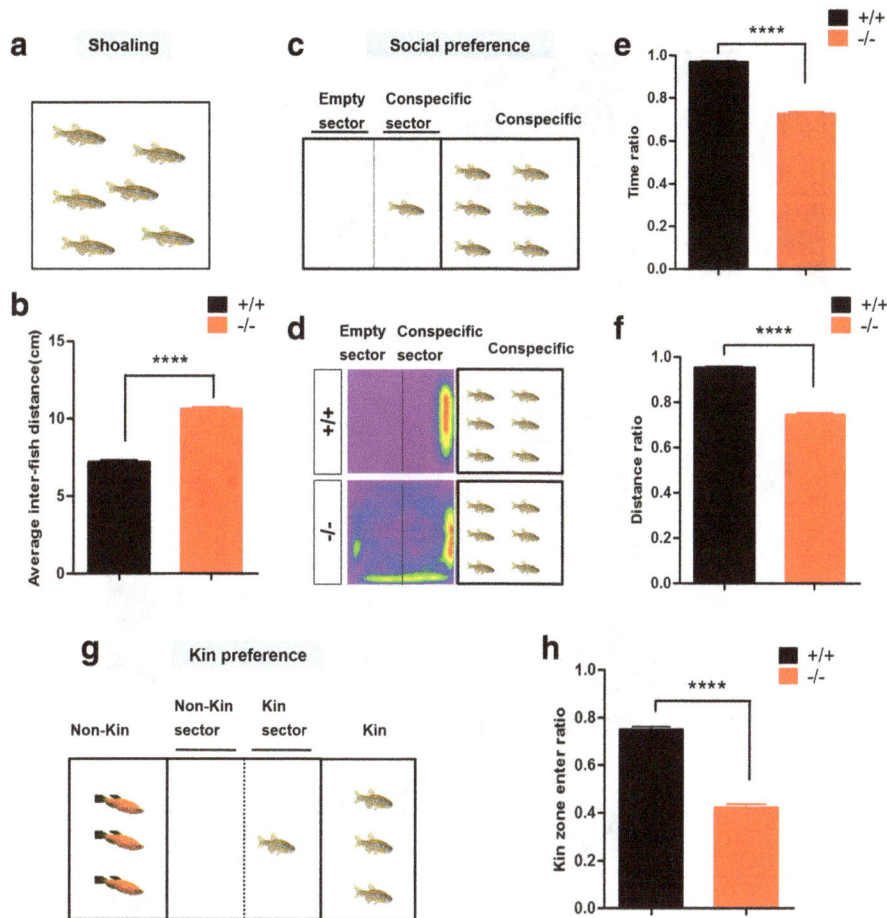

Fig. 5 *shank3b⁻/⁻* zebrafish displayed social interaction defect. **a–b** Schematic of shoaling test (**a**) and significantly increased inter-fish distance of adult male *shank3b⁻/⁻* zebrafish (3.5 mpf) (**b**). $N = 18$ for each group. **c–f** Schematic of social preference test of adult male zebrafish (3.5 mpf) (**c**). Heat map (**d**) shows that *shank3b⁺/⁺* zebrafish displayed significant higher frequency near a group of zebrafish than *shank3b⁻/⁻* zebrafish. Time ratio (**e**) and distance ratio (**f**) in the conspecific sector were significantly reduced in *shank3b⁻/⁻* zebrafish compared to *shank3b⁺/⁺* zebrafish. $N = 16$ for each group. **g–h** Schematic of kin recognition and preference test of adult male zebrafish (3.5 mpf) (**g**) and significantly reduced ratio of kin zone entering in *shank3b⁻/⁻* zebrafish compared to *shank3⁺/⁺* zebrafish (**h**). $N = 10$ for each group. Data are presented as mean ± SEM; ****$p < 0.0001$

± 0.02) compared with *shank3b⁺/⁺* zebrafish ($n = 3$, 1.00 ± 0.25; Fig. 7a).

Shank3 deletion has also been reported to impair synaptic transmission, and neurexin and neuroligin mediated trans-synaptic signaling [30]. We investigated whether presynaptic proteins were also affected in the *shank3b⁻/⁻* zebrafish brain. Synaptophysin is exclusively located in synaptic vesicles and is generally used as a marker for presynaptic terminals [31]. As shown in Fig. 7b, the levels of synaptophysin were markedly decreased in *shank3b⁻/⁻* zebrafish (49% of *shank3b⁺/⁺*; $n = 3$, 0.54 ± 0.13) compared with *shank3b⁺/⁺* zebrafish ($n = 3$, 1.10 ± 0.31).

Discussion

In this study, we generated the first *shank3b* loss-of-function mutation in zebrafish using the CRISPR/Cas9 gene editing method and reported the morphological,

behavioral and neurological characterizations of *shank3b* zebrafish mutants at both early developmental stage and adulthood. The *shank3b* deficiency caused partial lethality during early development as well as defective and delayed neurodevelopment at the larval stage. The brain volume of *shank3b⁻/⁻* zebrafish is enlarged but the brain weight is comparable to *shank3b⁺/⁺*, which may indicate the ventricles in *shank3b⁻/⁻* are larger than in WT zebrafish. This observation is reminiscent of the enlarged ventricular size frequently reported in human PMS patients [32, 33]. However, it is interesting to note that the defective and delayed neurodevelopment in *shank3b⁻/⁻* larvae becomes less noticeable later in development. The exact reason for the finding is not immediately clear but may support a different functional role of shank3b protein at different developmental stages.

shank3b⁻/⁻ zebrafish in adulthood display significantly abnormal behaviors while *shank3b⁺/⁻* zebrafish showed

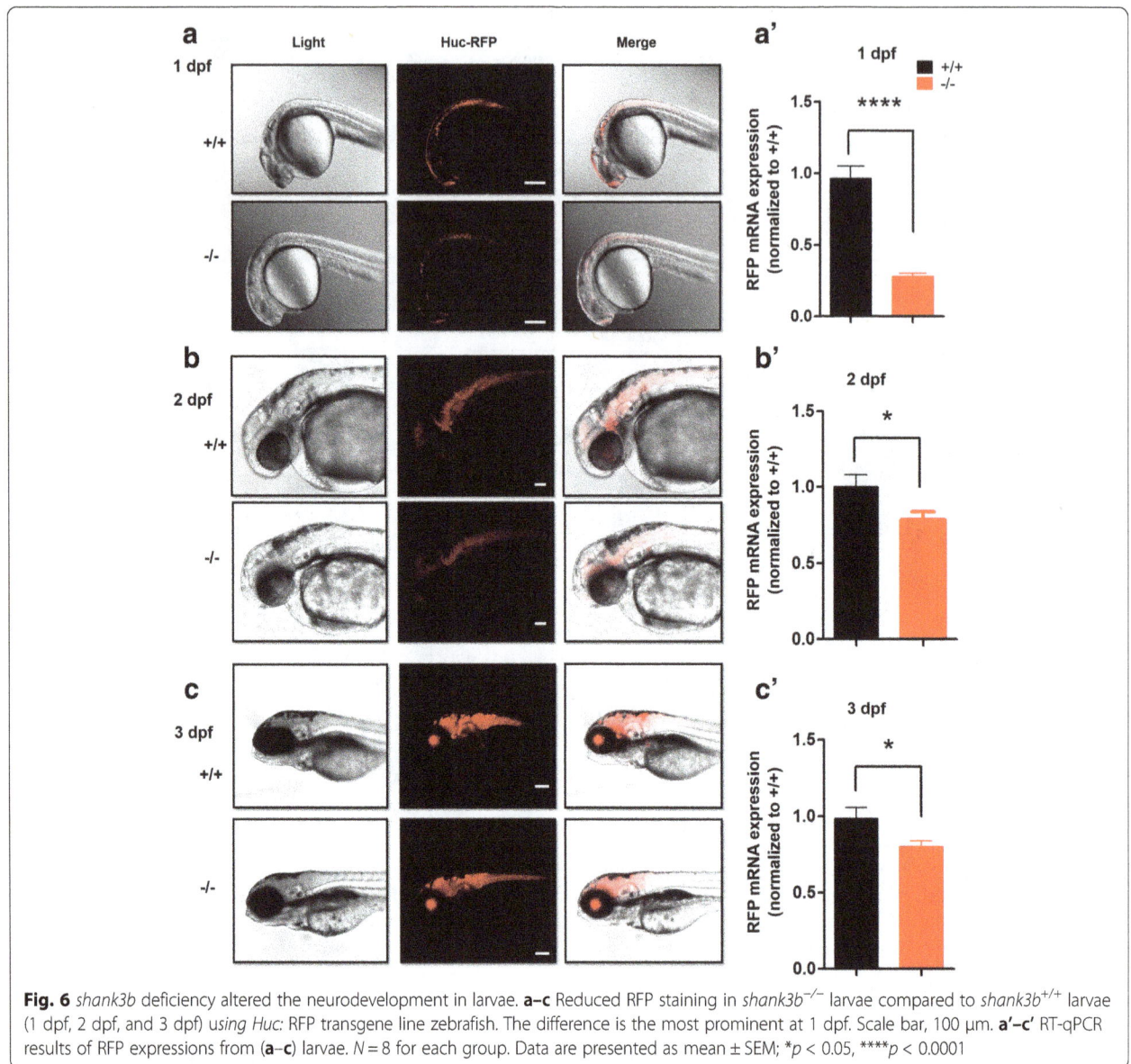

Fig. 6 *shank3b* deficiency altered the neurodevelopment in larvae. **a–c** Reduced RFP staining in *shank3b*$^{-/-}$ larvae compared to *shank3b*$^{+/+}$ larvae (1 dpf, 2 dpf, and 3 dpf) u*sing Huc:* RFP transgene line zebrafish. The difference is the most prominent at 1 dpf. Scale bar, 100 μm. **a'–c'** RT-qPCR results of RFP expressions from (**a–c**) larvae. *N* = 8 for each group. Data are presented as mean ± SEM; *p < 0.05, ****p < 0.0001

intermediate phenotypes compared to those of *shank3b*$^{-/-}$ and *shank3b*$^{+/+}$ zebrafish. The phenotypes observed in *shank3b*$^{+/-}$ zebrafish are analogous to the haploinsufficiency of *SHANK3* seen in PMS and *SHANK3*-related disorders [9, 34]. The observed early-stage developmental defects and abnormal behaviors in both *shank3b*$^{+/-}$ and *shank3b*$^{-/-}$ zebrafish larvae are different from *Shank3* rodent models, in which early developmental defects have not been reported, and phenotypes in heterozygous mutants are generally not significant [4, 35, 36]. The reason for these differences between the two species is not clear. Considering that zebrafish have both *shank3a* and *shank3b* homologs to human *SHANK3*, it is somewhat unexpected or counterintuitive that *shank3b* mutant zebrafish have more prominent phenotypes for survival and behavior. An alternative

explanation for the behavioral phenotypes is that the more significant abnormal behaviors in *shank3*$^{+/-}$ zebrafish are because behavioral assays in zebrafish are more sensitive than that in rodents.

The ortholog of human *SHANK3* is duplicated in the zebrafish genome as *shank3a* and *shank3b* during teleost evolution [12, 17]. The duplicated and conserved shank3a and shank3b share high identity at the amino acid level and are expected to have a similar function in zebrafish [17]. In a previous study, Kozol et al. reported the knock down of *shank3a* and *shank3b* by morpholino and observed embryonic defects in both morphants and impaired touch-induced startle responses in *shank3a* morphants [19]. However, abnormal ASD-like behaviors were not detected due to the limitations of morpholino technology. It would be interesting to compare the

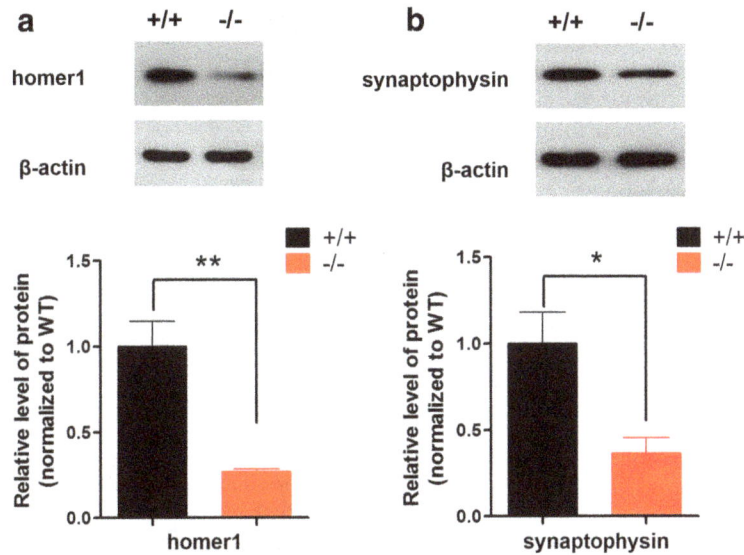

Fig. 7 *shank3b* deficiency resulted in the reduction of post- and presynaptic proteins in adult zebrafish brain. **a** Quantitative immunoblot blot analysis showed that the postsynaptic protein homer1 was significantly decreased (27% of *shank3b^(+/+)*) in the *shank3b^(-/-)* male zebrafish brain relative to *shank3b^(+/+)* zebrafish (3.5 mpf, N = 3 for each group). **b** The expression of presynaptic synaptophysin protein was markedly reduced in *shank3b^(-/-)* male zebrafish brain compared with that of *shank3b^(+/+)* zebrafish (3.5 mpf, 49% of *shank3b^(+/+)*). N = 3 for each group. Data are presented as mean ± SEM; *$p < 0.05$, **$p < 0.01$

phenotypes of *shank3a* and *shank3b* mutants engineered by CRISPR/Cas9 in parallel or even the phenotypes of *shank3a* and *shank3b* double mutants in the future.

In recent years, the zebrafish has become an attractive alternative model for ASD researchers [19, 27, 37]. Many behavioral assays have been developed in zebrafish models, including the assessment of social interaction, novelty seeking, courtship, inhibitory avoidance, fear and anxiety responses, repetitive/stereotyped behaviors, seizures, and aggression [12, 38–41]. We employed some of the behavioral assays in the analyses of *shank3b* mutant zebrafish and found striking differences in social and repetitive behavioral domains between *shank3b^(-/-)* and *shank3b^(+/+)* zebrafish. For instance, in shoaling and kin-preference assays, *shank3b^(-/-)* zebrafish preferred to swim in loose schools and showed significantly decreased preference for conspecifics. These abnormal behaviors are reminiscent of reduced social interaction in the home cage or abnormal social novelty and preference using the three chamber paradigm reported in several lines of *Shank3* mutant mice [35, 36, 42, 43]. In the open field, *shank3b^(-/-)* zebrafish displayed abnormal locomotor activity, such as figure "8" and "circling" movements that are apparently repetitive. Similarly, repetitive behavior measured by increased self-grooming has been observed in several lines of *Shank3* mutant mice [4, 42]. However, like many other behavioral findings observed in animal models, the challenge remains to determine whether the abnormal behaviors observed in *shank3b*-deficient zebrafish can be directly translated

to human *SHANK3*-related ASD. The study of the predictive validity of these abnormal behaviors to ASD may be warranted in the future, when feasible. Positive results could potentially provide further support for the translational value of these behavioral phenotypes. It also remains to be seen if these assays are universally valid and effective for ASD models caused by different genetic defects. Clinical and molecular heterogeneity have been well recognized in ASD in humans [44]. Additional behavioral assays are certainly needed to assess face validity for ASD-like behaviors, and also for common comorbidities such as seizures and cognitive impairments.

Our finding of reduced postsynaptic homer1 protein levels in *shank3b*-deficient zebrafish is consistent with the known function of SHANK3 as a scaffolding protein at the postsynaptic density from studies of *Shank3* mutant mice [4, 45]. This finding, although limited, would suggest that the molecular mechanism-associated SHANK3 deficiency may be conserved between different species. It would be interesting to examine if the same defect occurs in *shank3a*-deficient zebrafish. The finding of significantly reduced synaptophysin protein levels in the brain of *shank3b^(-/-)* zebrafish is novel, as synaptophysin is a known presynaptic protein [31]. This observation implies that *shank3b* deficiency may affect presynaptic function directly or via a trans-synaptic mechanism in zebrafish. Several recent studies have suggested that SHANK3 protein is located at the presynaptic terminus in the brain as well as in dorsal root ganglion neurons in rodents [46]. Our finding in zebrafish also potentially suggests a role of shank3 protein in the presynaptic terminus. Future studies on the presynaptic function of $shank3b^{-/-}$ are warranted and may shed additional insight in this direction.

The amenability to high-throughput drug screening is a tremendous advantage of the zebrafish model. The list of confirmed ASD-causing genes continues to grow, but the development of targeted molecular treatments significantly lags behind. A validated experimental platform that can translate the genetic discoveries to drug screening at a fast pace is urgently needed. We believe that the $shank3b^{-/-}$ model described in this study and other similar ASD zebrafish models will lay an important foundation for the development of a productive drug screening program for ASD and may ultimately lead to the discovery of an effective intervention.

Conclusions

For the first time, we successfully generated a $shank3b^{-/-}$ zebrafish model that displays robust autism-like behavioral characteristics. Reduced levels of the postsynaptic scaffolding protein homer1 in $shank3b^{-/-}$ zebrafish suggest a high conservation of the molecular mechanism underlying SHANK3 deficiency among different species. The reduced levels of synaptophysin in the brain of $shank3b^{-/-}$ zebrafish also provide further evidence supporting the potential role of shank3 in presynaptic terminus. The $shank3b$ mutant zebrafish represents a valuable model to dissect the molecular pathogenesis and conduct high-throughput drug screening for SHANK3-related disorders in the future.

Additional files

Additional file 1: Table S1. gRNA gene-target sequences, oligonucleotides for PCR knock-out validation, and RT-qPCR probes used in this study. **Table S2.** SHANK family sequences used in this study. **Table S3.** Homology analysis of zebrafish shank3a and shank3b compared with human SHANK3. **Table S4.** Homology comparison between zebrafish shank3a and shank3b. Table S5. Repetitive behaviors of shank3b⁻/⁻ adult male zebrafish (3.5 mpf). **Figure S1.** Phylogenetic tree of evolutionary relationship of SHANK family proteins. **Figure S2.** Homology comparison of zebrafish shank3a and shank3b with human SHANK3. **Figure S3.** Homology comparison between zebrafish shank3a and shank3b. **Figure S4.** shank3b target-mutation in zebrafish via CRISPR-Cas9 system. **Figure S5.** Examination of maternal or paternal origin effects on the morphological and behavioral phenotypes. **Figure S6.** Analysis of activity frequency at different activity intensity scales. (PDF 1211 kb)

Additional file 2: Movie S1. WT zebrafish swimming in the open field. (MP4 657 kb)

Additional file 3: Movie S2. shank3b⁻/⁻ zebrafish swimming in repetitive figure "8" pattern. (MP4 484 kb)

Additional file 4: Movie S3. shank3b⁻/⁻ zebrafish swimming in repetitive big circling pattern. (MP4 1193 kb)

Additional file 5: Movie S4. shank3b⁻/⁻ zebrafish swimming in repetitive small circling pattern. (MP4 380 kb)

Additional file 6: Movie S5. shank3b⁻/⁻ zebrafish swimming in repetitive walling pattern. (MP4 1535 kb)

Additional file 7: Movie S6. Performance of WT zebrafish in the shoaling test. (MPG 2510 kb)

Additional file 8: Movie S7. Performance of shank3b⁻/⁻ zebrafish in the shoaling test. (MPG 2022 kb)

Additional file 9: Movie S8. Performance of WT zebrafish in the social preference test. (MPG 2562 kb)

Additional file 10: Movie S9. Performance of shank3b⁻/⁻ zebrafish in the social preference test. (MPG 1992 kb)

Additional file 11: Movie S10. Performance of WT zebrafish in the kin recognition and preference test. (MPG 2894 kb)

Additional file 12: Movie S11. Performance of shank3b⁻/⁻ zebrafish in the kin recognition and preference test. (MPG 2044 kb)

Abbreviations

ASD: Autism spectrum disorder; dpf: Days post-fertilization; gRNA: Guide-RNA; KO: Knockout; mpf: Months post-fertilization; PCR: Polymerase chain reaction; RT-qPCR: Real-time quantitative polymerase chain reaction; SHANK3: SH3 and multiple ankyrin (ANK) repeat domain 3; WT: Wild type

Acknowledgements

We thank all members of the Division of Child Health Care and Zebrafish Core of Children's Hospital of Fudan University in China; Xiang Yu, Xiao-ming Wang, and Ning Guo for the guidance on the experiments; Xu Wang from Fudan University for providing the Tg (Huc: RFP) transgenic line; and Dong-yun Li and Samuel Hulbert for critical reading and editing of the manuscript.

Funding

This study was supported by grants from the National Natural Science Foundation of China (NSFC, no. 81371270) and the National Key Research and Development Program of China (no. 2016YFC1306205) to XX. QL is supported by grants from the NSFC (no. 8127509). YHJ is supported by grants from the National Institute of Health (MH098114, HD087795, and MH104316).

Authors' contributions

The study was conceived by XX. XX, QL and CXL designed the study. CXL performed the experiments. CXL, CYL, CCH, and YW provided homozygous identification assistance. QL and JL provided technical assistance in behavior analyses. CXL wrote the manuscript with comments from all authors. YHJ contributed to the experimental design, data analysis, and manuscript preparation. All authors read and approved the final manuscript.

Competing interests

The authors declare that they have no competing interests.

Author details

[1]Division of Child Health Care, Children's Hospital of Fudan University, 399 Wanyuan Road, Shanghai 201102, China. [2]Center for Translational Medicine, Institute of Pediatrics, Shanghai Key Laboratory of Birth Defect, Children's Hospital of Fudan University, 399 Wanyuan Road, Shanghai 201102, China. [3]Department of Pediatrics and Neurobiology, Duke University School of Medicine, Durham, NC 27614, USA.

References

1. Monteiro P, Feng G. SHANK proteins: roles at the synapse and in autism spectrum disorder. Nat Rev Neurosci. 2017;18(3):147–57.
2. Jiang YH, Ehlers MD. Modeling autism by SHANK gene mutations in mice. Neuron. 2013;78(1):8–27.
3. Grabrucker AM, Schmeisser MJ, Schoen M, et al. Postsynaptic ProSAP/Shank scaffolds in the cross-hair of synaptopathies. Trends Cell Biol. 2011;21(10): 594–603.
4. Wang X, Bey AL, Katz BM, et al. Altered mGluR5-Homer scaffolds and corticostriatal connectivity in a Shank3 complete knockout model of autism. Nat Commun. 2016;7:11459.
5. Sala C, Vicidomini C, Bigi I, et al. Shank synaptic scaffold proteins: keys to understanding the pathogenesis of autism and other synaptic disorders. J Neurochem. 2015;135(5):849–58.
6. Verpelli C, Dvoretskova E, Vicidomini C, et al. Importance of Shank3 protein in regulating metabotropic glutamate receptor 5 (mGluR5) expression and signaling at synapses. J Biol Chem. 2011;286(40):34839–50.
7. Bonaglia MC, Giorda R, Borgatti R, et al. Disruption of the ProSAP2 gene in a t(12;22)(q24.1;q13.3) is associated with the 22q13.3 deletion syndrome. Am J Hum Genet. 2001;69(2):261–8.
8. Bonaglia MC, Giorda R, Beri S, et al. Molecular mechanisms generating and stabilizing terminal 22q13 deletions in 44 subjects with Phelan/McDermid syndrome. PLoS Genet. 2011;7(7):e1002173.
9. Moessner R, Marshall CR, Sutcliffe JS, et al. Contribution of SHANK3 mutations to autism spectrum disorder. Am J Hum Genet. 2007;81(6):1289–97.
10. Betancur C, Buxbaum JD. SHANK3 haploinsufficiency: a "common" but underdiagnosed highly penetrant monogenic cause of autism spectrum disorders. Mol Autism. 2013;4(1):17.
11. Durand CM, Betancur C, Boeckers TM, et al. Mutations in the gene encoding the synaptic scaffolding protein SHANK3 are associated with autism spectrum disorders. Nat Genet. 2007;39(1):25–7.
12. Mathur P, Guo S. Use of zebrafish as a model to understand mechanisms of addiction and complex neurobehavioral phenotypes. Neurobiol Dis. 2010; 40(1):66–72.
13. Jaramillo TC, Speed HE, Xuan Z, et al. Altered striatal synaptic function and abnormal behaviour in Shank3 Exon4-9 deletion mouse model of autism. Autism Res. 2016;9(3):350–75.
14. Speed HE, Kouser M, Xuan Z, et al. Autism-associated insertion mutation (InsG) of Shank3 exon 21 causes impaired synaptic transmission and behavioral deficits. J Neurosci. 2015;35(26):9648–65.
15. Lee J, Chung C, Ha S, et al. Shank3-mutant mice lacking exon 9 show altered excitation/inhibition balance, enhanced rearing, and spatial memory deficit. Front Cell Neurosci. 2015;9:94.
16. Stewart AM, Nguyen M, Wong K, et al. Developing zebrafish models of autism spectrum disorder (ASD). Prog Neuro-Psychopharmacol Biol Psychiatry. 2014;50:27–36.
17. Kalueff AV, Stewart AM, Gerlai R. Zebrafish as an emerging model for studying complex brain disorders. Trends Pharmacol Sci. 2014;35(2):63–75.
18. Liu C, Peng X, Hu C, et al. Developmental profiling of ASD-related shank3 transcripts and their differential regulation by valproic acid in zebrafish. Dev Genes Evol. 2016;226(6):389–400.
19. Kozol RA, Cukier HN, Zou B, et al. Two knockdown models of the autism genes SYNGAP1 and SHANK3 in zebrafish produce similar behavioral phenotypes associated with embryonic disruptions of brain morphogenesis. Hum Mol Genet. 2015;24(14):4006–23.
20. Gauthier J, Champagne N, Lafrenière RG, et al. De novo mutations in the gene encoding the synaptic scaffolding protein SHANK3 in patients ascertained for schizophrenia. Proc Natl Acad Sci. 2010;107(17):7863–8.
21. Mali P, Yang L, Esvelt KM, et al. RNA-guided human genome engineering via Cas9. Science. 2013;339(6121):823–6.
22. Hwang WY, Fu Y, Reyon D, et al. Efficient genome editing in zebrafish using a CRISPR-Cas system. Nat Biotechnol. 2013;31(3):227–9.
23. Westerfield M. The zebrafish book: a guide for the laboratory use of zebrafish, Brachydanio rerio. Eugene: University of Oregon Press; 1995.
24. Park HC, Kim CH, Bae YK, et al. Analysis of upstream elements in the HuC promoter leads to the establishment of transgenic zebrafish with fluorescent neurons. Dev Biol. 2000;227(2):279–93.
25. Kwan KM, Fujimoto E, Grabher C, et al. The Tol2kit: a multisite gateway-based construction kit for Tol2 transposon transgenesis constructs. Dev Dyn. 2007; 236(11):3088–99.
26. Buske C, Gerlai R. Maturation of shoaling behavior is accompanied by changes in the dopaminergic and serotoninergic systems in zebrafish. Dev Psychobiol. 2012;54(1):28–35.
27. Meshalkina DA, N Kizlyk M, V Kysil E, et al. Zebrafish models of autism spectrum disorder. Exp Neurol. 2017;299(Pt A):207–16.
28. Kalueff AV, Gebhardt M, Stewart AM, et al. Towards a comprehensive catalog of zebrafish behavior 1.0 and beyond. Zebrafish. 2013;10(1):70–86.
29. Miller NY, Gerlai R. Shoaling in zebrafish: what we don't know. Rev Neurosci. 2011;22(1):17–25.
30. Arons MH, Thynne CJ, Grabrucker AM, et al. Autism-associated mutations in ProSAP2/Shank3 impair synaptic transmission and neurexin-neuroligin-mediated transsynaptic signaling. J Neurosci. 2012;32(43):14966–78.
31. Kwon SE, Chapman ER. Synaptophysin regulates the kinetics of synaptic vesicle endocytosis in central neurons. Neuron. 2011;70(5):847–54.
32. Sarasua SM, Dwivedi A, Boccuto L, et al. Association between deletion size and important phenotypes expands the genomic region of interest in Phelan-McDermid syndrome (22q13 deletion syndrome). J Med Genet. 2011;48(11):761–6.
33. Soorya L, Kolevzon A, Zweifach J, et al. Prospective investigation of autism and genotype-phenotype correlations in 22q13 deletion syndrome and SHANK3 deficiency. Mol. Autism. 2013;4(1):18.
34. Sarasua SM, Dwivedi A, Boccuto L, et al. 22q13.2q13.32 genomic regions associated with severity of speech delay, developmental delay, and physical features in Phelan-McDermid syndrome. Genet Med. 2014;16(4):318–28.
35. Zhou Y, Kaiser T, Monteiro P, et al. Mice with Shank3 mutations associated with ASD and schizophrenia display both shared and distinct defects. Neuron. 2016;89(1):147–62.
36. Yang M, Bozdagi O, Scattoni ML, et al. Reduced excitatory neurotransmission and mild autism-relevant phenotypes in adolescent Shank3 null mutant mice. J Neurosci. 2012;32(19):6525–41.
37. Hoffman EJ, Turner KJ, Fernandez JM, et al. Estrogens suppress a behavioral phenotype in zebrafish mutants of the autism risk gene, CNTNAP2. Neuron. 2016;89(4):725–33.
38. Dadda M, Domenichini A, Piffer L, et al. Early differences in epithalamic left-right asymmetry influence lateralization and personality of adult zebrafish. Behav Brain Res. 2010;206(2):208–15.
39. Blaser R, Gerlai R. Behavioral phenotyping in zebrafish: comparison of three behavioral quantification methods. Behav Res Methods. 2006;38(3):456–69.
40. Delaney M, Follet C, Ryan N, et al. Social interaction and distribution of female zebrafish (Danio rerio) in a large aquarium. Biol Bull. 2002;203(2):240–1.
41. D Amico D, Estivill X, Terriente J. Switching to zebrafish neurobehavioral models: the obsessive–compulsive disorder paradigm. Eur J Pharmacol. 2015;759:142–50.
42. Peca J, Feliciano C, Ting JT, et al. Shank3 mutant mice display autistic-like behaviours and striatal dysfunction. Nature. 2011;472(7344):437–42.
43. Vicidomini C, Ponzoni L, Lim D, et al. Pharmacological enhancement of mGlu5 receptors rescues behavioral deficits in SHANK3 knock-out mice. Mol Psychiatry. 2017;22(5):784.
44. Hyman SE. A glimmer of light for neuropsychiatric disorders. Nature. 2008; 455(7215):890–3.
45. Tu JC, Xiao B, Naisbitt S, et al. Coupling of mGluR/Homer and PSD-95 complexes by the Shank family of postsynaptic density proteins. Neuron. 1999; 23(3):583–92.
46. Han Q, Kim YH, Wang X, et al. SHANK3 deficiency impairs heat hyperalgesia and TRPV1 signaling in primary sensory neurons. Neuron. 2016;92(6):1279–93.

Operationalizing atypical gaze in toddlers with autism spectrum disorders: a cohesion-based approach

Quan Wang[1], Daniel J. Campbell[2], Suzanne L. Macari[1], Katarzyna Chawarska[1] and Frederick Shic[3,4]* (iD)

Abstract

Background: Multiple eye-tracking studies have highlighted the "atypical" nature of social attention in autism. However, it is unclear how "atypical" or "typical" should be quantified.

Methods: We developed a method for identifying moments when members of a group looked at similar places (High-Cohesion Time Frames; HCTFs). We defined typicality as the proximity of gaze points to typically developing (TD) gaze points during TD HCTFs. Comparing toddlers with ASD ($n = 112$) to developmentally delayed (DD, $n = 36$) and TD ($n = 163$) toddlers during a video with Dyadic Bid, Sandwich-Making, Joint Attention, and Animated Toys conditions, we examined (a) individual typicality scores, (b) the relationship between typicality and symptom severity, and (c) HCTF distributions associated with each diagnostic group.

Results: The ASD group had lower gaze typicality scores compared to the TD and DD groups in the Dyadic Bid and Sandwich-Making conditions but not during Animated Toys. The DD and TD groups did not differ in any condition. Correlational analyses indicated that higher typicality scores were associated with increased looking at pre-planned locations of the scene indexed by each experimental condition. In the ASD group, lower gaze typicality was associated with more severe autism symptoms. Examining ASD HCTFs, the gaze of toddlers with ASD was least cohesive during Dyadic Bid and most cohesive during Animated Toys.

Conclusion: In contrast to non-ASD groups, toddlers with ASD show high cohesion during salient nonsocial events, suggesting that consistency in looking strategies may depend more on perceptual features. These findings are consequential for understanding individual differences in visual attention in ASD and for the design of more sensitive biomarker tasks for stratification, between-group differentiation, and measuring response to treatment.

Keywords: Autism, ASD, Eye tracking, Cohesion, Visual attention, Attentional synchrony, Atypicality

Background

Eye tracking has been widely used to study gaze behaviors and visual attention and cognition in individuals with and without autism spectrum disorder (ASD) [1, 2]. The most prevalent approach to parsing gaze behaviors involves identifying a priori regions of interest (ROIs) in a displayed scene (e.g., faces, hands, background) and analyzing gaze behaviors as they relate to these ROIs (e.g., how looking times at ROIs differ across populations and experimental conditions). Studies employing ROI approaches have

demonstrated that, compared to controls, toddlers with ASD spend less time attending to people, their faces, and their goal-oriented activities [3–7]; for a recent meta-analysis of eye tracking in autism research see [1, 8]. These studies also highlight the differential impact of social context on attention in toddlers with ASD compared to those without autism. For instance, unlike typically developing (TD) and developmentally delayed (DD) toddlers, toddlers with ASD show decreased attention to a speaker's face only when the person looks at or speaks to the viewer and not in other conditions [3]. In addition, in children with ASD, heterogeneous gaze patterns in response to dynamic social stimuli have been linked to differences in the severity of autism symptoms and

* Correspondence: fshic@uw.edu
[3]Center for Child Health, Behavior and Development, Seattle Children's Research Institute, 2001 8th Ave Suite 400, Seattle, WA 98121, USA
[4]Department of Pediatrics, University of Washington, Seattle, WA, USA
Full list of author information is available at the end of the article

levels of developmental functioning as measured 1–2 years later [9].

These findings demonstrate how context and development affect the gaze behaviors of children with ASD, highlighting the complexities of precisely defining atypical gaze behavior. Furthermore, "atypical" can only be defined in reference to "typical," and defining "typical" behavior poses some challenges. For instance, gaze patterns vary developmentally, with attention to faces gradually increasing during the first year of life [10–13] and the significance of looking at the eyes or mouth changing as children begin to acquire language [14]. Even within normative samples studied within narrowly defined developmental periods, there is high inter-individual variability in gaze behaviors. For instance, Tenenbaum and colleagues [15] demonstrated large inter-individual variation in looking preferences for the mouth of a speaking or smiling face in young, TD infants. Similar variability has been linked to language outcomes in infant siblings of children with ASD [16]. These results illustrate that using a single norm (or simple set of ROIs) as representative of typical gaze patterns might not reflect the complex realities of intergroup or contextual gaze dynamics. These complexities are further compounded in studies of videos in which the contextual changes vary in a moment-by-moment fashion alongside corresponding ROIs. Moreover, ROI-based approaches to gaze analyses in ASD are based on top-down (investigator-defined) strategies, and differences in how ROIs are defined may introduce discrepancies when comparing results across different studies. Finally, it is not clear if ROIs, defined by experimenters who themselves are typically developing adults, fairly capture axes of variation in atypical or very young populations, especially in response to complex dynamic stimuli, in which context unfolds rapidly along multiple dimensions. These issues surrounding the multiplicity of interpretative possibilities in ROI analyses, at the core, stem from the a priori assumption of spatial points of regard characterizing constructs of interest that are more-arbitrarily defined than they are data-driven (for additional discussions, including alternative algorithms, see [17, 18] and Additional file 1: Materials 1).

Here we propose a new approach to the analysis of dynamic eye-tracking data that is based on empirically derived gaze behaviors of TD children, applicable to studies of scene looking with a priori ROI hypotheses as well as to those without. Despite the observed inter-individual variability in scanning patterns among TD children, attributable to individual neural, biological, and experiential differences, there are moments in time when the gaze behaviors of TD children converge on the same spatial location. This convergence suggests a common response to a combination of perceptual and semantic scene characteristics. We propose to use the term *cohesion* to describe this phenomenon of convergence by multiple individuals on the same area of the visual scene within a specified time frame, i.e., when the gaze points of individuals fall within close proximity to one another and those individuals participate in a consistent, unified visual experience. Each frame for each individual can be assigned a typicality score in reference to normative patterns of cohesion derived from the TD group. Using a cohesion value metric, we identified frames where the cohesion of gaze behaviors within the typical group was the highest (high-cohesion time frames, HCTFs) and argue that the analysis of HCTFs can inform studies of gaze behaviors across typical and atypical development in novel and generative ways. By identifying when and where the gaze behaviors of TD children converge in response to complex visual scenes, we can define spatial and temporal windows reflective of typical gaze behavior patterns. Subsequently, we can compute indices of similarity between TD and atypically developing samples during these windows to quantify the degree of deviation of gaze behaviors from those typically observed. Similarly, we can examine what constitutes the most "consistent" gaze behaviors *within* the notoriously heterogeneous samples of children with developmental issues by computing cohesion indices specific to these samples. That is, rather than examining deviance from a norm based on TD samples, we can also establish "norms" for specific clinical groups.

In the present study, we applied the cohesion approach to eye-tracking data derived from a large sample of toddlers with autism and developmental delays, as well as typically developing controls. We aimed to operationalize and examine gaze behaviors in clinical groups by building a data-driven normative model of gaze behavior in TD toddlers, comparing the performance of the ASD, DD, and TD groups using a gaze typicality score within the context of this normative model, and examining the relationship between gaze typicality scores and autism symptoms in the ASD group. We also aimed to investigate "normative" gaze patterns within the ASD and DD groups by examining how the proportion of HCTFs differed across conditions in ASD and DD toddlers, as compared to TD toddlers.

Methods

Participants

Participants included toddlers with ASD (age $M = 22.39$, SD = 3.02 months, $n = 112$), DD (age $M = 21.71$, SD = 3.38 months, $n = 36$), and TD (age $M = 21.89$, SD = 3.39 months, $n = 163$). ASD participants were recruited at a university-based research clinic specializing in the early differential diagnosis of autism and other developmental disorders. The study of children with ASD at this early age afforded the examination of visual gaze strategies typically at the age of first diagnosis and therefore before the potential secondary effects of interventions would likely take hold. The TD and DD toddlers had no family history of autism in first or second degree relatives. Developmental skills were evaluated using Mullen Scales of Early Learning (MSEL, 1995 [19]); (see Table 1). The MSEL captures developmental functioning in nonverbal (fine motor and visual reception) and verbal (receptive language and expressive language) domains. For this study, developmental quotients were computed for the verbal (VDQ) and nonverbal (NVDQ) scores. The severity of autism symptoms was measured using the Autism Diagnostic Observation Schedule-Generic Module 1 (ADOS-G [20, 21]); (see Table 1). The ADOS-G provides scores in the domains of social affect (SA) and restrictive and repetitive behaviors (RRB), as well as a total score reflecting the sum of SA and RRB scores. The three groups did not differ with regard to age ($F(2, 308) = 1.00$, $p = .37$). The ASD group consisted of 85.7% males, as compared to 88.9% in DD and 59.5% in TD groups ($\chi^2(2) = 28.4$, $p < .01$). The ASD and DD groups were comparable with regard to MSEL NVDQ ($p = 0.25$), and both had lower scores than the TD group ($ps < .001$). The MSEL VDQ of the ASD group ($M = 55.8$, $SD = 2.4$) was significantly lower than that of the TD ($p < .001$) and DD groups ($p < .01$). The VDQ of the DD group was also lower than that of the TD group ($p < .001$). All ASD diagnoses were based on clinical best estimate (CBE). In 79.5% ($n = 89$) of cases, CBE was conducted in a follow-up visit at 36 months (mean age at eye tracking 22.5 months; at CBE 38.7 months); in the remaining 20.5% ($n = 23$) of cases, CBE was conducted at the time of eye tracking (mean age 22.2 months). CBE was based on the direct assessment of developmental, social, communication, and adaptive skills, as well as review of developmental and medical history, by a multidisciplinary team of expert clinicians. Standard measures included the ADOS-G [20, 21], MSEL [19], PLS-5 [22], Vineland [23], and ADI-R [24]. Previous studies have indicated that CBE diagnoses of ASD in clinic-referred children are highly

stable (~ 90%) between the second and third year of life [25–27]. Given the large size of our samples, this is unlikely to significantly impact study results. The DD group included toddlers with a score less than 1.5 SDs below age-norms on one or more subscales of the MSEL and included toddlers with global developmental delays or language delays. Children in the TD group exhibited typical developmental profiles. This research was approved by the Yale University Institutional Review Board, and informed consent was obtained from the legal guardians of all participants enrolled in this study. Subsets of this data have been previously reported in [3, 9, 28].

Stimuli

The stimulus consisted of a 3-min video depicting an actress engaged in several activities in a setting shown in Fig. 1 (for a detailed description, see [3]). The video has four interleaved conditions (Dyadic Bid, Sandwich, Joint Attention, and Animated Toys), without breaks to re-engage or re-center the child's visual attention. In the Dyadic Bid condition, the actress looks directly at the camera and uses child-directed speech (e.g., "Hi, baby, how are you today?") to elicit dyadic (face-to-face) attention (11 episodes, total duration of 69 s). In the Sandwich condition, she looks down at the ingredients and tools on a table with no direct gaze or speech (2 episodes, total duration of 63 s). In the Joint Attention condition, the actress looks up briefly at the camera and then says "uh-oh" as she turns toward one of the toys and looks at it for 4 s (4 episodes, total duration of 30 s). In the Animated Toys condition, the actress looks up briefly at the camera, then a toy begins to move and make noise, followed by the actress turning to look at a toy on the opposite side of the animated toy (4 episodes, total duration of 27 s).

Apparatus

An SMI iView X RED 60 Hz eye-tracking system was used to record toddlers' eye movements. Eye-tracking data were post-processed with a custom data pipeline programmed

Table 1 Sample characterization

	ASD			DD			TD		
Male	85.7%			88.9%			59.5%		
	N	Mean	SD	N	Mean	SD	N	Mean	SD
Age (months)	112	22.39	3.02	36	21.71	3.38	163	21.89	3.39
MSEL NVDQ	110	82.70	16.67	36	85.86	11.81	161	109.96	13.00
MSEL VDQ	110	55.84	30.97	36	69.76	16.89	154	111.34	21.23
ADOS SA	109	13.35	4.66	35	5.83	3.97	–	–	–
ADOS RRB	109	4.07	2.03	35	1.37	1.52	–	–	–
ADOS TOTAL	109	17.42	5.69	35	7.20	4.52	–	–	–

ASD, autism spectrum disorder; *DD*, developmental delay; *TD*, typical development; *MSEL*, Mullen Scales of Early Learning; *NV*, non-verbal; *V*, verbal; *DQ*, developmental quotient; *ADOS*, Autism diagnostic observation schedule; *SA*, social affect; *RRB*, restricted and repetitive behaviors

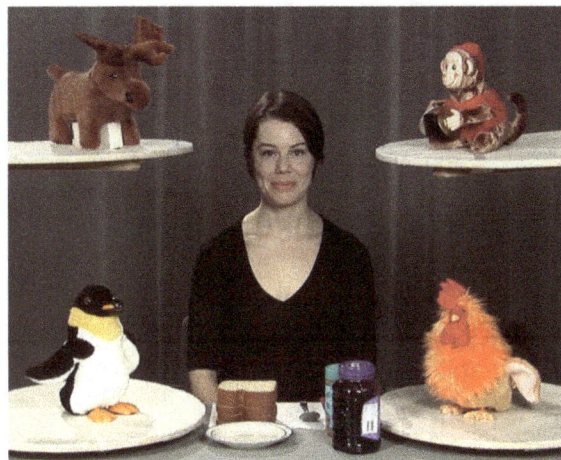

Fig. 1 The stimulus shown to participants: a 3-min video depicting an actress engaged in several activities in four interleaved conditions (Dyadic Bid, Sandwich, Joint Attention, and Animated Toys)

in MATLAB. Processing steps included calibration, recalibration, blink detection [29, 30], and cohesion analysis. Participants were included if they spent more than 30% of the video attending to the scenes (i.e., if the amount of time the eye tracker detected looking at the monitor, divided by the total stimulus presentation time, was greater than 30%) and had calibration uncertainty less than 2 degrees.

Procedure

The eye-tracking experiment was conducted in a dark and quiet room. A toddler sat in front of a 24-in. computer screen at an average distance of 75 cm. The experiment began with a child-friendly video to direct the toddler's attention to the screen, followed by a five-point calibration before the stimulus video began. Calibration targets included dynamic animations with sound (e.g., a walking cartoon tiger with a meowing sound).

Analytic strategy

Normative mode

In order to operationalize typical scanning patterns, we created a normative model using the following steps (see Additional file 1 Materials 1 for more details): step 1 aimed to define a *cohesion value* which would represent the similarity in gaze locations during a given time frame (each 200 ms) between a TD toddler and all other TD toddlers (i.e., how similar a TD participant was to other TD participants). More formally, the cohesion value was defined as being proportional to the inverse median pairwise distance between a participant and all other participants in his or her group. In step 2, we defined HCTF as the time frames when the median cohesion values of TD participants were the top 10% of all frames. Conceptually, an HCTF

represents a time interval when TD toddlers focus their attention on a similar location of the screen (i.e., when a majority of TD participants are looking at the scene content in a similar way). In step 3, we defined *typicality scores* as cohesion values during HCTFs, representing the similarity of each participant's gaze patterns to TD participants during moments when the TD group exhibited the most cohesive gaze behavior. Typicality scores were calculated for each individual, for each condition (for an example of time-varying cohesion values across conditions, see Fig. 2). We compared typicality scores between diagnostic groups (ASD, DD, and TD), across conditions, using linear mixed models (compound symmetry repeated covariance structure, type III sum of squares), and post hoc comparisons Holm-Bonferroni corrected for multiple comparisons (consistent with our prior work [31]). To clarify how typicality scores corresponded to spatial locations in each experimental condition, we isolated the HCTFs referenced to the TD sample (i.e., the normative model) and applied conventional ROI analyses to each condition. We then conducted a Pearson's r correlation analysis to examine how spatial ROI looking percentages related to typicality scores across all participants. Pearson's r correlation analysis was used to explore relationships between typicality scores and autism-related symptoms in the ASD group.

ASD and DD cohesion models

To examine cohesive behaviors within each diagnostic group, we also created *within-group cohesion models* for ASD and DD toddlers. Similar to the normative model of TD toddlers, toddlers with ASD were compared to all other toddlers with ASD, and DD toddlers to all other toddlers with DD. This aim involved computing the *proportion of HCTFs* for each condition for each within-group cohesion model. Allocation of HCTFs across conditions could deviate from chance (10%, the proportion of frames selected as HCTFs), by exceeding (greater-than-chance proportions of HCTFs within a condition) or being lower than chance (lower-than-chance proportions of HCTFs). Statistical analyses for expression levels of cohesion in different conditions across the diagnostic groups allowed us to identify commonalities in attentional salience that may be shared across members of particular groups (e.g., what draws attention most consistently in the ASD group).

Results

Normative model

Cohesion values of the TD group are presented as a line plot, with different video conditions represented by different background colors in Fig. 2. The top 10% of cohesion values in the normative model were labeled as HCTFs and are shown as red rectangles in Fig. 2. This 10% cutoff,

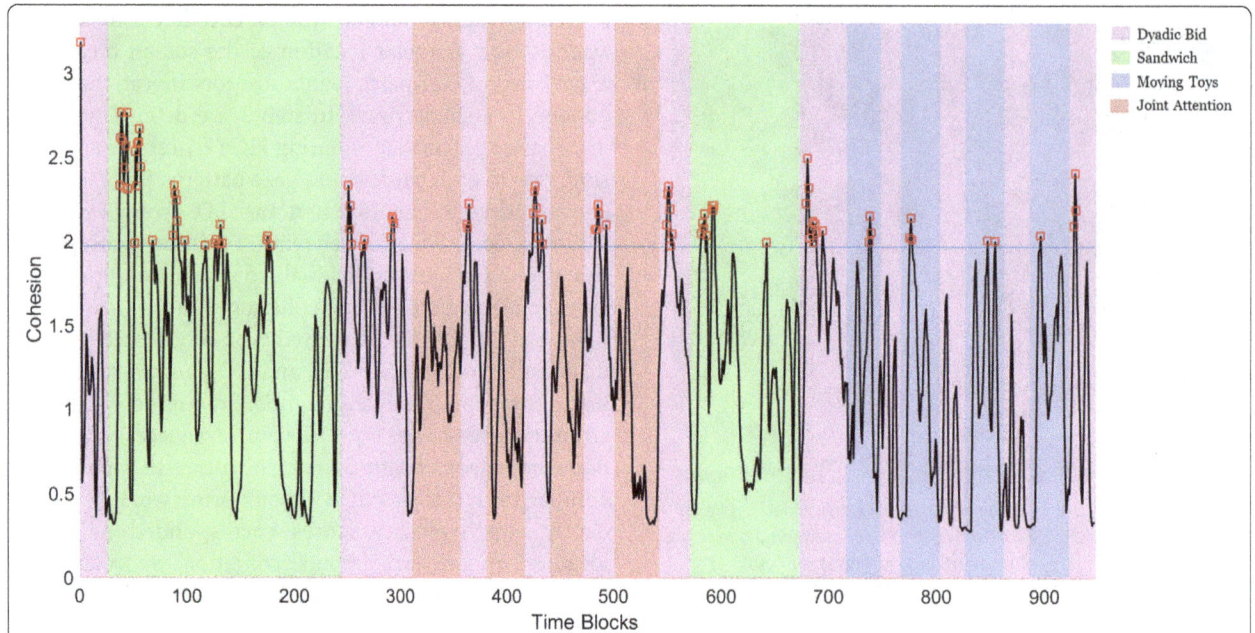

Fig. 2 High-cohesion time frames (HCTFs) in the normative model. We calculated the median cohesion value among TD toddlers for each time frame, shown as the black line plot. HCTFs included in the normative model are indicated with red boxes. Time frames belonging to one of four different conditions are identified by corresponding background colors: Purple: Dyadic Bid; light green: Sandwich; Blue: Animated Toys; Orange: Joint Attention. Typicality scores in different conditions represent the median of cohesion values within the HCTFs in the corresponding video condition

determined a priori, was found to be equivalent to a median pairwise distance between TD participants of less than 49.8 pixels on the screen (~ 1.5° of visual angle), which is correspondent to the size of foveal avascular zone, the area of highest acuity in the visual field [32, 33]. Interestingly, the algorithm identifying HCTFs within the TD group revealed no HCTFs drawn from the Joint Attention condition. For this reason, subsequent analyses do not contain the Joint Attention condition.

Typicality score group comparison (see Fig. 3 and Table 2)

To examine whether children in the DD and ASD groups showed similar gaze behaviors to the TD group during periods when TD gaze behaviors were highly convergent, we computed a diagnosis (3) × condition (3) linear mixed model on typicality scores. The analysis indicated a diagnosis effect ($F(2, 307.6) = 24.9$, $p < .001$) and a diagnosis × condition interaction ($F(4, 613.6) = 5.9$, $p < .001$), but no condition effect ($F(2, 613.4) = 2.1$, $p = .13$). The ASD group had lower typicality scores compared to the TD and DD group in Sandwich ($p < .001$, Cohen's $d = -0.64$; $p = .02$, $d = -0.41$, respectively) and Dyadic Bid ($p < .001$, $d = -0.93$; $p < .001$, $d = -0.80$) conditions but not Animated Toys ($p = .06$, $d = -0.34$; $p = .94$, $d = -0.02$). The DD group did not differ from the TD group in any conditions (Sandwich, $p = .88$; Dyadic Bid, $p = 1.00$; Animated Toys, $p = .36$). Inclusion of NVDQ, VDQ, calibration accuracy, or percentage valid as covariates

in the linear mixed model did not change these statistical results (see Additional file 1 Materials 1).

Correlation between typicality scores and ROI looking-time percentages across all groups

ROI looking-time percentages are presented in Additional file 1: Material 1, Table S1. In the Sandwich

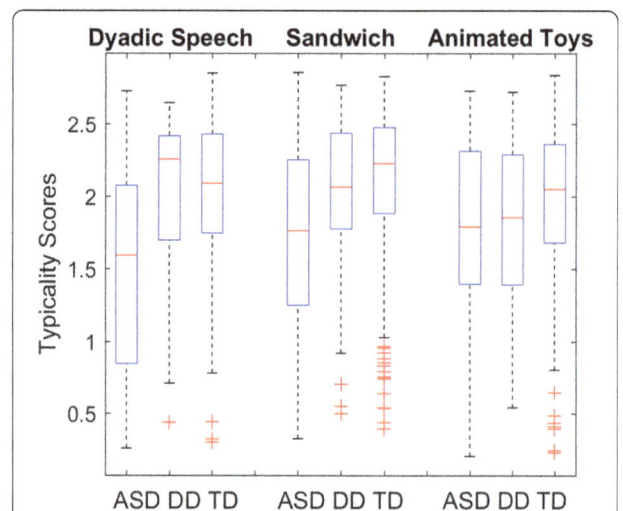

Fig. 3 Typicality score box plots for ASD, DD, and TD groups in the normative model. Comparisons are made between the diagnostic groups in the three video conditions. For Sandwich: ASD < (DD*,TD**); Dyadic Bid: ASD < (DD**,TD**); Animated Toys: no differences. *$p < .05$, **$p < .01$

Table 2 Mean and standard deviation (SD) of typicality scores of the ASD, DD, and TD groups in the Sandwich (SW), Dyadic Bid (DB), and Animated Toys (Toy) conditions. Joint Attention (JA) is not included since, in the TD normative model, no cohesive frames were allocated to the JA condition

Typicality scores	Diagnosis								
	ASD			DD			TD		
Conditions	SW	DB	TOY	SW	DB	TOY	SW	DB	TOY
Mean	1.70	1.47	1.77	1.98	2.01	1.77	2.09	2.03	1.96
SD	0.67	0.71	0.64	0.60	0.55	0.66	0.56	0.52	0.55

Table 4 Mean and standard deviation (SD) of proportion (in %) of high-cohesion time frames (HCTF) in the Sandwich (SW), Dyadic Bid (DB), and Animated Toys (TOY) conditions in the ASD, DD, and TD groups. Above 10% is greater-than-chance proportions of cohesive frames, under 10% is less-than-chance

Typicality scores	Diagnosis								
	ASD			DD			TD		
Conditions	SW	DB	TOY	SW	DB	TOY	SW	DB	TOY
Mean	14.32	6.30	14.60	9.79	14.29	3.82	13.42	12.50	6.74
SD	2.20	1.47	3.61	1.11	1.35	0.82	1.70	1.42	3.40

(SW) condition, typicality scores were positively correlated with looking at the table (the activity area of sandwich making) and negatively correlated with other ROIs. In the Dyadic Bid (DB) condition, typicality scores were positively correlated with looking at the face of the actress and negatively correlated with other ROIs. In the Toy condition, typicality scores were positively correlated with looking at the four toys and negatively correlated with other ROIs (Table 3). Similar relationships were observed when groups were considered independently (see Additional file 1: Material 1, Table S2).

Correlation between typicality score and severity of autism symptoms in the ASD group

Subsequently, we conducted Pearson's r correlation tests between typicality scores for each condition and ADOS social affect (SA) and restricted and repetitive behavior (RRB) scores, as an exploratory analysis. ADOS SA scores were negatively correlated with the typicality scores in the Sandwich ($r(109) = -0.235$, $p = .014$) and Dyadic Bid condition ($r(109) = -0.199$, $p = .038$), but not in Animated Toys ($r(109) = -0.06$, $p = 0.538$). ADOS RRB scores were not correlated with any condition ($r(109) = -0.158$, 0.003, and -0.117, all $ps > .05$, for Sandwich, Dyadic Bid, and Animated Toys conditions respectively). Statistical results were unchanged using Spearman's rank correlation.

Proportion of frames with highest cohesion scores

For ASD and the DD groups, we identified the proportion of HCTFs in each condition (Table 4). We excluded the Joint Attention condition for comparability with the TD

Table 3 Correlation between typicality score and percentage looking at predefined regions of interest (ROIs) in the cohesive frames of the normative model, stratified by experimental condition across all groups

Looking percentage on ROIs***	Face	Toys	Body	Table	BG
SW typicality score	− .47	− .46	− .43	**.75**	− .48
DB typicality score	.79	− .51	− .40	− .45	− .51
Toy typicality score	− .24	.68	− .24	− .19	− .57

Bold entries highlight positive associations

group, which had no HCTFs in the Joint Attention condition in the normative model. Similarly, for comparability, we maintained the 10% threshold for HCTF identification. Because the 10% of frames, across all conditions, with the highest cohesion were defined as HCTFs, if guided purely by random uniform chance, each condition would be expected to show a 10% composition of HCTFs. Thus, conditions with more than 10% of HCTFs were labeled as demonstrating greater-than-chance proportions of HCTFs (i.e., showing more cohesion that would be expected by chance, thus demonstrating more homogeneous group behavior) and conditions with less than 10% of HCTFs were labeled as demonstrating lower-than-chance proportions.

Within-group linear mixed models were run to examine potential differences in the proportion of HCTFs allocated to each condition within each group (Fig. 4 and Table 4). In the TD group, condition was significant ($F(2, 324) = 532.9$, $p < .001$), with post hoc comparisons indicating the highest proportion of HCTFs in the Sandwich condition (13.4%), next highest in the Dyadic Bid condition (12.5%),

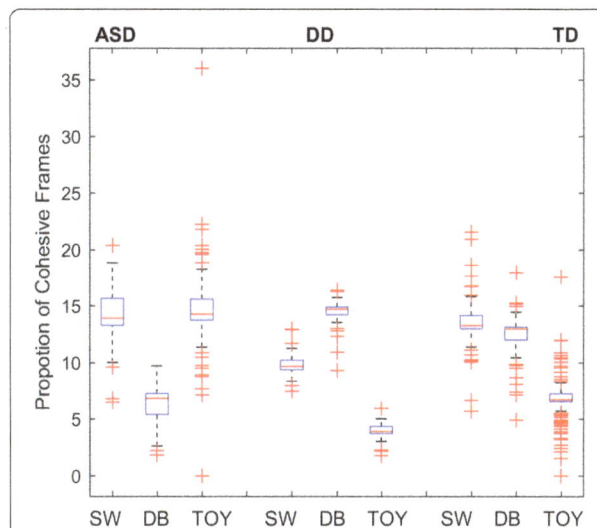

Fig. 4 Box plots illustrating proportion of HCTFs in Dyadic Bid (DB), Sandwich (SW), and Animated Toy (TOY) conditions in within-group model. For ASD: DB<SW<TOY; for DD: TOY<SW<DB; and for TD: TOY<DB<SW. All effects $p < .001$

and the lowest in the Animated Toys condition (6.7%) (all pairwise $p < .001$). In the DD group, condition was significant ($F(2, 70) = 554.8$, $p < .001$), with the highest proportion of HCTFs in the Dyadic Bid (14.3%) condition, next highest in the Sandwich (9.8%) condition, and, like the TD group, the lowest proportion in the Animated Toys condition (3.8%) (all pairwise $p < .001$). In the ASD group, condition was significant ($F(2, 222) = 272.3$, $p < .001$), but, in contrast, the highest proportion of HCTFs occurred in the Animated Toys (14.6%) and Sandwich conditions (14.3%) and the lowest in the Dyadic Bid condition (6.3%) (pairwise $p < .001$, excepting Animated Toys vs Sandwich, $p = .491$). Except for the DD group in the Sandwich condition, all proportions of HCTFs significantly differed from chance (10%) in one sample T tests. Between-condition group-specific effect sizes are provided in Additional file 1: Material 1, Table S3.

Discussion

This is the first study to apply a data-driven cohesion-based approach to the analysis of eye-tracking data collected in response to dynamic complex scenes in toddlers with and without social disability. This study provides a unique perspective on defining atypical gaze behaviors in ASD. We conducted the cohesion model analysis with a sample of over 300 well-characterized toddlers with and without autism and other developmental disabilities at the earliest age of ASD diagnosis. This cohesion approach was data-driven and free of assumptions associated with pre-defined ROIs, though results comparing correlations between typicality and standard ROI-based measures of looking suggested that typicality scores reflected the pre-planned point-of-regard manipulated and targeted by experimental conditions. Differences in patterns of looking in cohesive frames in the normative model replicated results observed in high-level between group analyses in [3] (see Supplement).

Results suggested that the gaze behaviors of toddlers with ASD were most atypical in contexts involving face-to-face interactions (Dyadic Bid) and goal-oriented activities (Sandwich condition). Despite the presence of developmental delays in the DD group, the DD and TD children did not differ in their gaze behaviors in any condition, suggesting that intellectual functioning alone cannot explain the differences observed in the ASD group. These findings are consistent with previous ROI-based findings suggesting atypical gaze behaviors in response to social bids and limited activity monitoring in children with ASD at this age [3, 5].

In the ASD group, lower typicality scores in Sandwich and Dyadic Bid conditions were associated with higher severity of social-affective symptoms. This suggests that cohesion-based metrics may be clinically meaningful and that cohesion may provide a powerful method for indexing severity of autism symptoms and understanding individual variation within the autism spectrum. Given that gaze behavior guides learning throughout development, atypical looking patterns would provide access to different experiences for children with ASD as compared to TD or DD toddlers, potentially leading to more impoverished opportunities for social learning. Our results are consistent with previous work that has suggested that gaze atypicality is associated with symptom severity [9].

There were no differences in gaze patterns during the Animated Toys condition between the ASD and DD groups. This lack of differences could be due to shared similarities in attraction to physical properties of the scene, such as motion [34–37]. It may also be the case that the non-social nature of the Animated Toys condition did not tap into ASD-DD between-group differences in as stark a fashion as the more socially oriented Dyadic Bid and Sandwich conditions. Furthermore, there were no correlations between typicality scores and autism symptoms in the ASD group within the Animated Toys condition, reinforcing the perspective that attention to non-social events may be less powerful for stratification along the autism spectrum.

However, it is important to note that typicality scores only tell us how much toddlers in the ASD or DD groups deviate from TD toddlers; they do not tell us about the inherent gaze patterns within groups, e.g., when and on what areas of the scene children with ASD or DD tend to converge compared to other children within their own group. To address this, we constructed cohesion models for each diagnostic group independently, identifying the moments of highest cohesion within each group, and then examined structural differences in cohesion points across conditions within different diagnostic groups.

In the TD group, toddlers showed greater-than-chance proportions of HCTFs in both Sandwich and Dyadic Bid conditions and lower-than-chance proportions in Animated Toys. This suggests that they were more likely to look at the same region at the same time when potent social cues for attention, such as eye contact and speech or goal-oriented action, were present, but in response to nonsocial events, the TD toddlers showed relatively greater variability. Similarly to the TD group, the DD group showed higher-than-chance proportions of HCTFs in the Dyadic Bid condition and lower-than-chance proportions in Animated Toys. However, unlike the TD group, the proportion of HCTFs during the Sandwich condition in the DD group was at chance level. This finding is consistent with toddlers with developmental delays exhibiting gaze patterns more similar to younger TD toddlers, who spend more time looking at faces, as compared to older TD children, who spend more time looking at hands performing goal-oriented activities [38]. Alternatively, it is possible that variability in gaze patterns in the Sandwich condition in the DD group could be attributed to group heterogeneity in the understanding of daily living skills and activities [5]. By comparison, the ASD group had greater-than-chance proportions of HCTFs in the Animated Toys and Sandwich conditions and, in stark contrast to the TD and DD groups, lower-than-chance proportions of HCTFs in the Dyadic Bid condition. These findings may suggest that within the ASD group, attention was driven more toward perceptually salient nonsocial events.

In the normative cohesion model, one may notice that the TD group had no HCTFs in the Joint Attention condition. Joint attention induces a dynamic process of following the gaze direction of the person on the screen, which is not well-captured by the cohesion model. For example, two participants could both look back and forth between the actress and the target of attention while being locked completely out of phase (one looking at the target when the other is looking at the actress), and thus contribute to low spatial cohesion, despite a similar underlying strategy of attention [39] (see also Additional file 1: Material 1, Fig. S2). In addition, Joint Attention is a complex phenomenon that has high variability depending on age, developmental level, and temperamental factors, indexing a skill which is in rapid development during this period [40]. Future work will consider modifications to the cohesion model which can better account for cohesion effects during displays of complex social behavior.

There are several limitations in this study. First, we only applied this method to one video stimulus, and we acknowledge that this approach needs to be validated on additional stimuli and under different experimental contexts. Second, our correlation analysis between typicality score and autism-related symptoms in the ASD group is exploratory and uncorrected for multiple comparisons. Third, for consistency, we applied the same 10% cutoff criterion used for identifying HCTFs in the TD group for all groups but acknowledge that the mapping of 10% to distances/visual angles differs for the ASD (1.9°) or DD (1.6°) groups. Finally, this study involved very young children at the toddler age, and it is not clear whether these methods would be fully applicable across the lifespan. In the future, we hope to employ this technique for other research applications and to further explore the impact of variation in methodological parameters on different participant groups.

Conclusions

In summary, using our cohesion approach, we identified canonical gaze patterns in response to complex visual scenes and quantified the degree of consistency with which attention is drawn to specific features in the scene within different diagnostic groups. We also evaluated the clinical significance of individual differences from these canonical gaze patterns. Our results showed that this data-driven approach indexed atypical looking in the ASD group compared to the DD and TD control groups in socially charged experimental scenarios. Furthermore, atypical looking patterns during social conditions stratified children with ASD by level of autism symptoms. Finally, our results showed that ASD toddlers as a group exhibited more cohesive behaviors during non-social conditions and less during social conditions—a pattern reversed for DD and TD toddlers. These findings are consequential for understanding individual differences in attention to social targets in toddlers with ASD and for designing more sensitive biomarkers capable of measuring response to treatment.

Abbreviations
ADOS: Autism diagnostic observation schedule; ASD: Autism spectrum disorder; CBE: Clinical best estimate; DB: Dyadic Bid (video condition); DD: Developmental delay; DQ: Developmental quotient; HCTF: High-cohesion time frames; JA: Joint Attention (video condition); MSEL: Mullen Scales of Early Learning; NV: Non-verbal; ROI: Regions of interest; RRB: Restricted and repetitive behaviors; SA: Social affect; SD: Standard deviation; SW: Sandwich (video condition); TD: Typical development; Toy: Animated Toys (video condition); V: Verbal

Acknowledgements
We thank Kelly K. Powell, Scuddy Fontenelle IV, So Hyun Kim, Tina R. Goldsmith, Amanda Mossman Steiner, Ty W. Vernon, Anne Snow Gallagher, Grace Gengoux, Megan Lyons, Elizabeth Schoen Simmons, Karyn Bailey, Karen Bearss, Amy Giguere-Carney, Katherine Tsatsanis, and Rhea Paul for their contribution to sample characterization; Benjamin D. Oakes for his theoretical and computational contributions to this work; Carla A. Wall, Erin Barney, Claire E. Foster, Yeojin Amy Ahn, Minah Kim, and Lauren DiNicola for helpful edits; and Finola Kane-Grade, Perrine Heymann, Anna Milgramm, Emily Hilton, Lauren DiNicola, Gabriella Greco, Lilli Flink, Emily B. Prince, Eugenia Gisin, Alexandra C. Dowd, Grace Chen Wu, Marika C. Coffman, Mairin Batten, Brittany Butler, Jessa Reed, Jessica Bradshaw, Rebecca Doggett, Sarah Laughlin, Paula L. Ogston-Nobile, and Joslin Latz Davis for their help in data collection and experimental development.

Funding
This article were made possible through funding, resources, and experiences provided by NIH awards R21 MH102572, K01 MH104739, CTSA UL1 RR024139, R03 MH092618, NIH R01 MH100182, R01 MH087554, P50 MH081756, P01 HD003008; NSF CDI #0835767, DOD W81XWH-12-ARP-IDA, Autism Speaks Meixner Postdoctoral Fellowship (to both Q. Wang and D. Campbell) and the Associates of the Yale Child Study Center. Views in this article are those of the authors and do not reflect the opinions of any funding agency.

Authors' contributions
Drs. KC, SM, and FS contributed to the creation of stimuli used in this study and were involved in data acquisition. Drs. QW, DJC, and FS developed the mathematical/computational framework for analyses. Drs. QW, KC, and FS were involved in the data analysis, interpretation, and drafting of the manuscript. All authors contributed to the overarching design of the work, revising the manuscript, and read and approved the final manuscript.

Competing interests

Drs. Quan Wang, Suzanne Macari, and Katarzyna Chawarska report no biomedical financial interests or potential conflicts of interest. Dr. Campbell is employed by Vertex Pharmaceuticals Inc. Dr. Shic has previously received research funding from and/or acts as a consultant to F. Hoffmann-La Roche Ltd. and Janssen Research & Development, LLC.

Author details

[1]Child Study Center, Yale School of Medicine, 40 Temple St Suite 7D, New Haven, CT 06510, USA. [2]Vertex Pharmaceuticals Incorporated, 50 Northern Ave, Boston, MA 02210, USA. [3]Center for Child Health, Behavior and Development, Seattle Children's Research Institute, 2001 8th Ave Suite 400, Seattle, WA 98121, USA. [4]Department of Pediatrics, University of Washington, Seattle, WA, USA.

References

1. Chita-Tegmark M. Social attention in ASD: a review and meta-analysis of eye-tracking studies. Res Dev Disabil. 2016;48:79–93.
2. Aslin RN, McMurray B. Automated corneal-reflection eye tracking in infancy: methodological developments and applications to cognition. Infancy. 2004;6:155–63.
3. Chawarska K, Macari S, Shic F. Context modulates attention to social scenes in toddlers with autism. J Child Psychol Psychiatry. 2012;53:903–13.
4. Jones W, Carr K, Klin A. Absence of preferential looking to the eyes of approaching adults predicts level of social disability in 2-year-old toddlers with autism spectrum disorder. Arch Gen Psychiatry. 2008;65:946–54.
5. Shic F, Bradshaw J, Klin A, Scassellati B, Chawarska K. Limited activity monitoring in toddlers with autism spectrum disorder. Brain Res. 2011;1380:246–54.
6. Bedford R, Elsabbagh M, Gliga T, Pickles A, Senju A, Charman T, et al. Precursors to social and communication difficulties in infants at-risk for autism: gaze following and attentional engagement. J Autism Dev Disord. 2012;42:2208–18.
7. Falck-Ytter T, Fernell E, Gillberg C, Von Hofsten C von. Face scanning distinguishes social from communication impairments in autism. Dev Sci 2010;13(6):864–75.
8. Frazier TW, Strauss M, Klingemier EW, Zetzer EE, Hardan AY, Eng C, et al. A meta-analysis of gaze differences to social and nonsocial information between individuals with and without autism. J Am Acad Child Adolesc Psychiatry. 2017;56:546–55.
9. Campbell DJ, Shic F, Macari S, Chawarska K. Gaze response to dyadic bids at 2 years related to outcomes at 3 years in autism spectrum disorders: a subtyping analysis. J Autism Dev Disord. 2014:44:431–42.
10. Frank MC, Vul E, Johnson SP. Development of infants' attention to faces during the first year. Cognition. 2009;110:160–70.
11. Gluckman M, Johnson SP. Attentional capture by social stimuli in young infants. Front Psychol. 2013;4:527.
12. Di Giorgio E, Turati C, Altoè G, Simion F. Face detection in complex visual displays: an eye-tracking study with 3- and 6-month-old infants and adults. J Exp Child Psychol. 2012;113:66–77.
13. Farroni T, Johnson MH, Menon E, Zulian L, Faraguna D, Csibra G. Newborns' preference for face-relevant stimuli: effects of contrast polarity. Proc Natl Acad Sci U S A. 2005;102:17245–50.
14. Lewkowicz DJ, Hansen-Tift AM. Infants deploy selective attention to the mouth of a talking face when learning speech. Proc Natl Acad Sci. 2012;109:1431–6.
15. Tenenbaum EJ, Shah RJ, Sobel DM, Malle BF, Morgan JL. Increased focus on the mouth among infants in the first year of life: a longitudinal eye-tracking study. Infancy. 2012;18:534–53.
16. Young GS, Merin N, Rogers SJ, Ozonoff S. Gaze behavior and affect at 6 months: predicting clinical outcomes and language development in typically developing infants and infants at risk for autism. Dev Sci. 2009;12:798–814.
17. Hessels RS, Kemner C, van den Boomen C, Hooge ITC. The area-of-interest problem in eyetracking research: a noise-robust solution for face and sparse stimuli. Behav Res Methods. 2016;48:1694–712.
18. Holmqvist K, Nyström M, Andersson R, Dewhurst R, Jarodzka H, Van de Weijer J. Eye tracking: a comprehensive guide to methods and measures. New York: Oxford University Press Inc.; 2011.
19. Mullen EM. Mullen scales of early learning. Circ Pines MN Am Guid Serv. 1995;
20. Lord C, Risi S, Lambrecht L, Cook EH, Leventhal BL, DiLavore PC, et al. The autism diagnostic observation schedule—generic: a standard measure of social and communication deficits associated with the spectrum of autism. J Autism Dev Disord. 2000;30:205–23.
21. Lord C, Rutter M, DiLavore PC, Risi S, Gotham K, Bishop S. Autism diagnostic observation schedule: ADOS-2. CA: Western Psychological Services Los Angeles; 2012.
22. Zimmerman IL, Steiner VG, Pond RE. Preschool language scales, –Australian and New Zealand language adapted edition (PLS-5). Camberwell Aust Pearson Aust Group 2012.
23. Sparrow SS, Cicchetti DV, Balla DA. Vineland adaptive behavior scales, (Vineland-II). AGS Circ Pines MN. 2005;
24. Rutter M, LeCouteur A, Lord C. Autism diagnostic interview-revised (ADI-R). West Psychol Serv Los Angel CA. 2003;
25. Chawarska K, Shic F. Looking but not seeing: atypical visual scanning and recognition of faces in 2 and 4-year-old children with autism spectrum disorder. J Autism Dev Disord. 2009;39:1663–72.
26. Guthrie W, Swineford LB, Nottke C, Wetherby AM. Early diagnosis of autism spectrum disorder: stability and change in clinical diagnosis and symptom presentation. J Child Psychol Psychiatry. 2013;54:582–90.
27. Kim SH, Macari S, Koller J, Chawarska K. Examining the phenotypic heterogeneity of early autism spectrum disorder: subtypes and short-term outcomes. J Child Psychol Psychiatry. 2016;57:93–102.
28. Chawarska K, Ye S, Shic F, Chen L. Multilevel differences in spontaneous social attention in toddlers with autism spectrum disorder. Child Dev. 2015;
29. Duchowski AT. Eye tracking methodology: theory and practice. 1st edition: Springer; 2003.
30. Shic F. Computational methods for eye-tracking analysis: applications to autism: Ph.D. thesis. Yale University; 2008.
31. Holm S. A simple sequentially rejective multiple test procedure. Scand J Stat. 1979:65–70.
32. Bird AC, Weale RA. On the retinal vasculature of the human fovea. Exp Eye Res. 1974;19:409–17.
33. Hildebrand GD, Fielder AR. Anatomy and Physiology of the Retina. In: Pediatric Retina. Springer, Berlin, Heidelberg; 2011. p. 39–65.
34. Althoff R, Cohen N. Eye-movement-based memory effect: a reprocessing effect in face perception. J Exp Psychol Learn Mem Cogn. 1999;25:997–1010.
35. Nothdurft H-C. Salience from feature contrast: additivity across dimensions. Vis Res. 2000;40:1183–201.
36. Itti L, Koch C. Computational modelling of visual attention. Nat Rev Neurosci. 2001;2:194–203.
37. Hillstrom AP, Yantis S. Visual motion and attentional capture. Atten Percept Psychophys. 1994;55:399–411.
38. Frank MC, Vul E, Saxe R. Measuring the development of social attention using free-viewing. Infancy. 2012;17:355–75.
39. Shic F, Scassellati B. A behavioral analysis of computational models of visual attention. Int J Comput Vis. 2007;73:159–77.
40. Mundy P, Gomes A. Individual differences in joint attention skill development in the second year. Infant Behav Dev. 1998;21:469–82.

Prenatal mercury exposure and features of autism

Jean Golding[1]* , Dheeraj Rai[2], Steven Gregory[1], Genette Ellis[1], Alan Emond[1], Yasmin Iles-Caven[1], Joseph Hibbeln[3] and Caroline Taylor[1]

Abstract

Background: Mercury (Hg) has been suspected of causing autism in the past, especially a suspected link with vaccinations containing thiomersal, but a review of the literature shows that has been largely repudiated. Of more significant burden is the total quantity of Hg in the environment. Here, we have used the Avon Longitudinal Study of Parents and Children (ALSPAC) to test whether prenatal exposure from total maternal blood Hg in the first half of pregnancy is associated with the risk of autism or of extreme levels of autistic traits. This is the largest longitudinal study to date to have tested this hypothesis and the only one to have considered early pregnancy.

Methods: We have used three strategies: (1) direct comparison of 45 pregnancies resulting in children with diagnosed autism from a population of 3840, (2) comparison of high scores on each of the four autistic traits within the population at risk (n~2800), and (3) indirect measures of association of these outcomes with proxies for increased Hg levels such as frequency of fish consumption and exposure to dental amalgam ($n > 8000$). Logistic regression adjusted for social conditions including maternal age, housing circumstances, maternal education, and parity. Interactions were tested between risks to offspring of fish and non-fish eaters.

Results: There was no suggestion of an adverse effect of total prenatal blood Hg levels on diagnosed autism (AOR 0.89; 95% CI 0.65, 1.22) per SD of Hg ($P = 0.485$). The only indication of adverse effects concerned a measure of poor social cognition when the mother ate no fish, where the AOR was 1.63 [95% CI 1.02, 2.62] per SD of Hg ($P = 0.041$), significantly different from the association among the offspring of fish-eaters (AOR = 0.74 [95% CI 0.41, 1.35]).

Conclusion: In conclusion, our study identifies no adverse effect of prenatal total blood Hg on autism or autistic traits provided the mother ate fish. Although these results should be confirmed in other populations, accumulating evidence substantiates the recommendation to eat fish during pregnancy.

Keywords: ALSPAC, Prenatal mercury, Fish consumption, Autism, Autistic traits, Social cognition, Dental amalgam

Background

The possible link between Hg exposure and autism has attracted much controversy and debate over many years, largely related to suggestions that the Hg containing the additive thiomersal (thimerosal) in immunizations was causing harm (e.g., [1]). Reviews of the literature of accumulated evidence have since indicated a lack of association [2–4], and these have gradually reduced the general fear of having the baby immunized. In actual fact, the amount of Hg in thiomersal was relatively low compared with the amount absorbed from the atmosphere, the diet, and dental amalgam [5]. Nevertheless, there is still a fear concerning exposure to mercury among pregnant women, particularly focused around the consumption of seafood [6].

Although there are undoubtedly severe adverse effects with exposure to very high levels of mercury, prospective studies (summarized in the "Discussion" section of this paper) have mostly shown no adverse effects at a population level. Nevertheless, there is still confusion worldwide between the possible adverse effects on the offspring of low levels of mercury in pregnancy, especially when the exposure is from seafood. We have carried out a series of studies that have compared the levels

* Correspondence: jean.golding@bristol.ac.uk
[1]Centre for Child and Adolescent Health, Bristol Medical School, University of Bristol, Oakfield House, Oakfield Grove, Bristol BS8 2BN, UK
Full list of author information is available at the end of the article

of total mercury in maternal prenatal blood and shown that among children born to mothers who ate fish, there were no adverse associations with outcomes such as child development, child behavior, high blood pressure, or suboptimal IQ level [7–10].

Methods

The aim

Since there have been relatively few studies determining whether there is any association between total prenatal Hg exposure during pregnancy and autism, we have used a large population-based study in England, to determine whether (1) maternal prenatal whole blood Hg levels or (2) indirect measures of fetal exposure to Hg were associated with either a diagnosis of autism or the component traits of autism.

The population

Avon Longitudinal Study of Parents and Children (ALSPAC) is a pre-birth cohort study that enrolled ~ 80% of pregnant women resident in the Avon area of the UK in 1991–1992. The aim of the study was to assess ways in which the environment (defined in its broadest sense) interacted with genetics to influence the health, development, and well-being of the offspring. To this end, data collection used a variety of methodologies including direct examination of the offspring; self-completion questionnaires administered to the parents, the children, and their teachers; collection and assays of biological samples (including DNA); and linkage to health and education records [11, 12]. The study website contains details of all the data that are available through a fully searchable data dictionary: [http://www.bris.ac.uk/alspac/researchers/data-access/data-dictionary/].

The exposures

Prenatal measures of total mercury

Blood samples deliberately collected in acid-washed containers for determination of trace metals were obtained from 4484 women residing in two of the three Health Authority areas of the recruitment region. Samples were collected by midwives as early as possible in pregnancy. The sociodemographic characteristics of the women who donated samples were comparable to those of the rest of the ALSPAC study population apart from including a slight excess of older and more educated mothers [13]. Gestational age at sample collection [known for 4472 mothers (99.7%)] had a median value of 11 weeks and mode of 10 weeks. The interquartile range (IQR) was 9–13 weeks, and 93% of the samples were collected at < 18 weeks gestation. Samples were stored for 0–4 days at 4 °C at the collection site before being sent to the central Bristol laboratory. Samples were transported at room temperature for up to 3 h and stored at 4 °C

as whole blood in the original collection tubes for 18–19.5 years before analysis [14].

Analysis of the blood samples for whole blood Hg were carried out by the laboratory of Dr. Robert Jones at the Centers for Disease Control and Prevention (CDC) [CDC method 3009.1; unpublished information]. Clotted whole blood was digested to remove all clots, before being analyzed using the inductively coupled plasma dynamic reaction cell mass spectrometry (ICP-DRC-MS) [15, 16]. The entire amount of clotted whole blood was transferred to a digestion tube using concentrated nitric acid with the volume estimated from the weight. The blood sample was heated in a microwave oven at a controlled temperature and time, during which the organic matrix of the blood was digested removing the clots. ICP-DRC-MS internal standards (iridium and tellurium) were added at a constant concentration to all blanks, calibrators, and samples (at the time of 1:9 dilution of digestate) to facilitate correction for instrument noise and drift. The standard additions method of calibration was used to optimize the analytical sensitivity of the method for the whole blood samples. A recovery spike was included in each analytical run for calibration verification and as a blind quality control (QC) sample. The ICP-DRC-MS was operated in the DRC mode using oxygen when analyzing for Hg. QC materials as well as in-house QC samples with control limits unknown to the analysts were used for daily quality control. The level of detection (LOD) for Hg was 0.24 µg/L; three samples were below this level and were ascribed a value of 0.7 times the LOD (since the frequency distribution of Hg had evidence of a lower tail, a factor greater than 0.5 was deemed appropriate to reflect the likelihood that more of these three results would be closer to the LOD than zero). The maternal blood Hg levels ranged from 0.17 to 12.76 µg/L, with 5th, 10th, 50th, 90th, and 95th centiles of 0.81, 0.99, 1.86, 3.33, and 4.02 µg/L, respectively.

Proxy exposure measures

We have shown elsewhere that the blood Hg level increased if the woman ate fish during pregnancy [14] and with the number of amalgam fillings in the mouth and whether she had dental treatment involving amalgam during pregnancy [17] (see Additional file 1). We have therefore analyzed these variables as proxies for maternal Hg level.

The measures of fish consumption were obtained during pregnancy and comprised three questions concerning the frequency with which the mother ate (a) white fish, (b) oily fish, and (c) shellfish. Options given were as follows: not at all, about once in 2 weeks, 1–3 times a week, 4–7 times a week, and more than once a day. Dental exposures were also obtained from questionnaires completed by the woman in her own home and posted back to the study. They comprised questions concerning (i) whether she had an amalgam filling inserted during pregnancy, (ii) whether she had an amalgam filling extracted during pregnancy, and (iii) approximately how many amalgam fillings were in the woman's mouth at the time she was pregnant.

Outcome measures

Autistic traits

We have used the four independent trait predictors of autism identified previously as most predictive of autism in this cohort and described in the Appendix. They include measures of social communication at age 7 (using the Social and Communication Disorders Checklist (SCDC)), coherent speech (using the Child Communication Checklist) at age 9, sociability (using the Emotionality, Activity, Sociability temperament traits (EAS) temperament scale) at 3 years, and a derived repetitive behavior measure at 5. Each has been shown to be an independent predictor of clinically identified autism in ALSPAC using health records [18, 19]. Since these continuous scales were highly skewed and not easily amenable to transformation, we dichotomized them in order to identify children with approximately the worst 10% scores as described elsewhere [20] (details also provided in the Appendix). These extreme 10% subgroups of the traits are referred to as having poor social cognition, poor coherence, poor sociability, and repetitive behavior.

Identification of autism

In order to identify the children with autism, we used the following sources: (a) a review of all children given a statement for special educational provision in the Avon area to identify children diagnosed as on the autism spectrum using the ICD-10 criteria [18]; (b) the mother's answer to the question at age 9 "Have you ever been told that your child has autism, Asperger's syndrome or autistic spectrum disorder"; (c) classification as Pervasive Development Disorder using questions from the DAWBA questionnaire at 91 months [21], with the answers to the questionnaire classified by a child psychiatrist; (d) text responses to any question on diagnoses given to the child in questionnaires from 6 months to 11 years; and (e) letters from parents to the Study Director with details of the child's diagnosis. We used all sources. We have previously cross-validated ASD cases confirmed only by maternal report by showing that they have strong associations with various autistic trait measures [20]. This method identified 177 offspring (139 boys, 38 girls) with a presumed diagnosis of autism by age 11, giving a prevalence of 1.3%.

Confounders used in the adjusted analyses

The following factors collected using self-completion questionnaires during pregnancy were used as potential confounders in the analyses of autistic traits: maternal age, parity (number of previous pregnancies resulting in a live or stillbirth), family adversity index, housing tenure, household crowding, life events, smoking in pregnancy, and prenatal alcohol consumption. In addition, we took account of whether the child was breastfed, as in our previous studies [7, 10]. Although there were too few children with diagnosed autism to allow for a large number of confounders, we have allowed for the key variables collected prenatally that have influenced whether a diagnosis has been given; these comprise mother's age, education level, housing tenure, time lived in Avon, and maternal locus of control.

Statistical analyses

There were two sets of analyses:

Analyses A comprised the assessment of maternal prenatal total blood mercury in regard to autistic outcomes.

Analyses B examined the associations between proxies for mercury exposure (seafood consumption and dental amalgam) and the autistic outcomes.

The five outcomes in both sets of analyses comprised the binary measures involving the most extreme 10% of the autistic traits as well as the children with diagnosed autism. Logistic regression was used to assess the association between each of the five outcomes and (A) direct maternal total blood mercury levels in pregnancy and (B) the proxy measures indicating increased levels of blood mercury.

For adjustment using analyses A for the autistic traits, the models first included the confounders outlined above and then added the measure of mercury. In addition, since we have shown interactions between prenatal fish consumption and total blood Hg in predicting the offspring IQ [7], we stratified by maternal fish consumption and examined the results for interactions between Hg levels and whether the mother consumed fish, for each autistic trait. Further analyses using proxies for Hg exposure in pregnancy (seafood intake and dental amalgam experience) adjusted for the same set of possible confounders but did not look for interactions (see Table 4).

Results

Biases between the population for whom blood mercury was available and the rest of the cohort

We have shown elsewhere that there were no differences between the women for whom a trace metal result was obtained and the rest of the population in relation to their seafood intake [14], dental treatment [17], social conditions, and lifestyle [9], with two exceptions: more educated and older women were more likely to have had blood taken for trace metal analyses.

Variation of diagnosed autism with prenatal whole blood mercury

Of the 177 pregnancies that resulted in a child diagnosed with autism, 45 had a measure of total blood Hg. The mean blood level of Hg in this group [2.15 (SD 0.95) μg/L] was similar to the level in the remaining 3840 pregnancies [2.08 (SD 1.09) μg/L, $P = 0.655$].

Table 1 demonstrates the distribution of the pregnancies within quintiles of maternal prenatal total blood Hg (with the upper quintile divided into the two upper deciles) by autism outcome. There was no evidence for a trend of increasing prevalence with increasing level of blood Hg, and the highest decile of the distribution (> 3.39 μg/L) had one of the lowest prevalences of autism (1.09% of children of women with the highest levels compared with 1.34% of the children of women with the lowest blood mercury levels were diagnosed with autism). The adjusted regression analysis for autism using the five possible confounders (mother's age, education level, housing tenure, time lived in Avon, and maternal locus of control) found no evidence of an association between increased Hg levels and an autism diagnosis [adjusted OR 0.89; 95% CI 0.65, 1.22 per SD increase in Hg ($P = 0.485$)].

Associations of autism traits with prenatal blood mercury

The correlation coefficients [95% confidence interval] between increasing maternal mercury level and increasing level of autistic trait were as follows: social cognition $r = -0.02$ [-0.06, $+0.02$]; sociability $r = -0.04$ [-0.08, -0.01]; coherence $r = -0.03$ [-0.07, $+0.01$]; and repetitive behavior $r = -0.04$ [-0.08, $+0.001$]. Thus, all correlations indicated that with increasing levels of mercury, the signs of autism were slightly less, but none were statistically significant. It was also apparent from Table 1 that there was no evidence of an increasing prevalence of any of the extreme levels of autistic traits with increasing prenatal blood Hg. Table 2 shows the unadjusted and adjusted odds of total Hg levels with the dichotomized autism trait measures; the associations significant at the 10% level are italicized. For poor sociability, there were many

significant unadjusted associations with Hg level, but only one survived adjustment—and that was only of borderline significance ($P = 0.073$); all the results indicated that high levels of prenatal Hg were associated with reduced risk of poor sociability. Neither poor coherence nor repetitive behavior was associated with prenatal Hg at the 0.10 level of significance. The only adjusted association of statistical significance at the 0.05 level concerned the relationship between Hg and poor social cognition among the offspring of women who did not eat fish; this relationship was significantly different from the women who did eat fish.

Associations with proxies of mercury level

Table 3 shows the prevalence of diagnosed autism and the extreme levels of autism traits according to the frequency with which the pregnant women ate white fish, oily fish, and shellfish. No differences were apparent for diagnosed autism or the repetitive behavior trait, but children with mothers reporting eating no white fish appeared to have the highest prevalence of impairments in social cognition (16.1% vs 12.5 and 11.9%; $P < 0.001$) and coherence (12.1% vs 9.4 and 9.7%; $P = 0.026$). There were mixed findings for poor sociability.

In regard to dental features, poor sociability appeared to show significant relationships, but all were such that increased maternal exposure to dental amalgam was associated with lower rates of extreme levels of autistic traits. Upon adjustment (Table 4), there were four significant associations at the 10% level; all indicated a protective effect associated with the exposures that would have increased the mothers' Hg level (see Additional file 1).

Discussion

In this large birth cohort study with prospectively collected information, we found no evidence to suggest that prenatal exposure to total maternal blood Hg, measured

Table 1 Proportion of children to have diagnosed autism or extreme levels on autistic trait measures within each group of increasing prenatal total mercury levels

Prenatal blood mercury (μg/L)[a]	Diagnosed autism, % (n)	Autistic traits, % (n)			
		Poor social cognition	Poor sociability	Poor coherence	Repetitive behavior
≤ 1.28	1.34 (11)	12.7 (51)	12.7 (68)	12.4 (48)	6.6 (30)
1.29–1.68	0.51 (4)	12.2 (53)	12.6 (70)	10.7 (45)	6.9 (32)
1.69–2.10	0.67 (5)	11.8 (56)	11.3 (66)	7.8 (35)	4.7 (24)
2.11–2.74	1.81 (14)	11.3 (58)	11.1 (68)	9.4 (46)	5.9 (33)
2.75–3.39	1.79 (7)	9.6 (24)	10.4 (32)	12.3 (31)	7.4 (20)
> 3.39	1.09 (4)	13.0 (34)	10.5 (32)	8.4 (21)	2.6 (7)
All affected[b]	1.16 (45)	11.8 (276)	11.6 (336)	10.0 (226)	5.8 (146)
Total N	3885	2333	2902	2249	2529
P (5df)	0.112	0.840	0.827	0.181	0.102

df degrees of freedom

[a]First four quintiles and the last two deciles

[b]Note that overall the percentage of extreme autistic traits varies—it is as near to 10% as possible

Table 2 Unadjusted and adjusted odds ratios (OR [95%CI] per SD of mercury) between prenatal total blood mercury and the extreme levels of autistic traits are shown together with the results of separate analyses for children of mothers who did and those who did not eat fish during pregnancy

Population	Autistic trait			
	Poor social cognition	Poor sociability	Poor coherence	Repetitive behavior
All offspring				
Unadjusted	0.96 [0.87, 1.06]	*0.83 [0.74, 0.93]*	0.96 [0.86, 1.07]	0.94 [0.87, 1.02]
N (P)	2331 (0.432)	*2898 (0.002)*	2249 (0.411)	2528 (0.167)
Adjusted	0.96 [0.85, 1.08]	*0.88 [0.77, 1.01]*	1.01 [0.89, 1.14]	0.94 [0.86, 1.04]
N (P)	1991 (0.459)	*2422 (0.073)*	1938 (0.912)	2162 (0.234)
Mother ate fish				
Unadjusted	0.95[0.84, 1.06]	*0.85 [0.75, 0.97]*	1.00 [0.89, 1.13]	0.95 [0.86, 1.04]
N (P)	1945 (0.355)	*2389 (0.015)*	1873 (0.985)	2095 (0.228)
Adjusted	0.92[0.80, 1.05][a]	0.89 [0.76, 1.03]	1.04 [0.91, 1.19]	0.93 [0.84, 1.03]
N (P)	1744 (0.220)	2104 (0.106)	1698 (0.560)	1884 (0.150)
Mother ate no fish				
Unadjusted	1.26 [0.84, 1.87]	*0.64 [0.39, 1.05]*	0.96 [0.64, 1.45]	1.22[0.90, 1.64]
N (P)	285 (0.261)	*373 (0.079)*	273 (0.850)	317 (0.197)
Adjusted	*1.63 [1.02, 2.62][b]*	0.74 [0.41, 1.35]	0.87 [0.51, 1.48]	1.16 [0.81, 1.66]
N (P)	*240 (0.041)*	280 (0.327)	231 (0.598)	272 (0.425)

All associations with $P < 0.10$ are italicized
[a]Adjusted for maternal age, parity, family adversity index, housing tenure, household crowding, life events, smoking in pregnancy, prenatal alcohol consumption, and whether child was breastfed
[b]Significant interaction between adjusted results for offspring of fish and non-fish eaters

directly in whole blood, and indirectly through fish consumption and dental amalgam fillings, was associated with autism or increased autism symptoms in the offspring.

There is increasing recognition that trying to find a biological basis for syndromes such as autism is probably best served by studying the component traits [22, 23], on the assumption that particular component traits may be influenced by different environmental and/or genetic factors. Here, we have shown a differential relationship between the social cognition trait and prenatal Hg exposure, such that there was a significant difference in apparently protective effects contingent upon whether the mother ate fish. This was not found for the other traits and may imply that this trait is particularly influenced by the beneficial components of fish such as the omega-3 fatty acids, iodine, and vitamins D and B2.

Comparison with the literature
There have been several reviews showing no adverse associations between autism and ethyl Hg in thiomersal, but they have pointed out that the studies looking at other Hg exposures tend to have concentrated on either air pollutants or dental or dietary exposures but rarely looked at Hg biomarkers [24, 25] apart from one study of 84 cases of autism and 158 controls which showed no difference in mid-pregnancy serum or cord blood Hg

levels [26]. Our study is consistent with these prior null findings, with the additional advantage of being able to assess the effect of direct as well as indirect measures of Hg exposure on the diagnosis as well as on four different autistic traits.

Although it did not consider diagnosed autism, a study that bears the closest resemblance to our own analyzed data comprising a longitudinal birth cohort in the Seychelles where the consumption of ocean fish is almost universal and the prenatal Hg levels are about 10 times those of the USA. Hair collected from 537 mothers shortly after birth was assayed for Hg, and levels were assumed to be a proxy for prenatal Hg exposure of the fetus. The study found no evidence of a deleterious effect of these Hg levels or of fish consumption with measures of social interaction or communication in the offspring [27].

Our findings of an interaction with prenatal fish consumption are mirrored by a study of 2062 children tested for IQ using the WISC at 8 years of age [9]; after detailed adjustment, there was a difference of 3 IQ points per SD of Hg between children of fish eaters (+ 0.83) and non-fish eaters (− 2.22) ($P = 0.043$). This difference, and that with social cognition found here, suggests that the benefits of nutrients in fish counteract any possible adverse cognitive and behavioral differences that may be caused by prenatal exposure to Hg.

Table 3 Proportion of children with diagnosed autism or extreme levels of autistic traits by proxies for increased mercury exposure

Proxy for mercury exposure	Diagnosed autism, % (n)	Autistic traits, % (n)			
		Poor social cognition	Poor sociability	Poor coherence	Repetitive behavior
White fish frequency[a]					
Not at all	1.21 (27)	*16.1 (204)*	*11.6 (191)*	*12.1 (147)*	6.5 (90)
Once in 2 weeks	1.33 (65)	*12.5 (386)*	*10.4 (397)*	*9.4 (277)*	6.0 (199)
> once a week	1.37 (69)	*11.9 (397)*	*12.3 (494)*	*9.7 (314)*	5.6 (197)
P (2df)	0.640	*< 0.001*	*0.029*	*0.026*	0.481
Oily fish frequency[a]					
Not at all	1.23 (63)	*13.8 (407)*	*12.6 (480)*	*10.9 (308)*	6.0 (195)
Once in 2 weeks	1.49 (60)	*13.2 (354)*	*10.3 (334)*	*10.0 (256)*	5.8 (165)
> once a week	1.27 (38)	*11.1 (226)*	*11.0 (268)*	*8.7 (174)*	5.9 (126)
P (2df)	0.672	*0.017*	*0.010*	*0.044*	0.971
Shellfish frequency[a]					
Not at all	1.35 (132)	13.0 (801)	*11.0 (834)*	10.2 (598)	5.8 (384)
Any	1.23 (29)	12.1 (186)	*13.1 (248)*	9.4 (140)	6.3 (102)
P (2df)	0.527	0.352	*0.008*	0.414	0.438
Had amalgam fillings inserted in pregnancy					
Yes	1.09 (12)	12.8 (222)	*10.0 (213)*	10.0 (169)	*6.7 (127)*
No	1.52 (67)	12.8 (700)	*11.7 (786)*	9.9 (516)	*5.7 (332)*
P (1df)	0.283	0.995	*0.029*	0.920	*0.092*
Had amalgam fillings removed in pregnancy					
Yes	1.03 (15)	13.8 (155)	*9.1 (126)*	10.6 (118)	6.0 (73)
No	1.58 (126)	12.6 (767)	*11.7 (873)*	9.8 (567)	5.9 (386)
P (1df)	0.110	0.284	*0.006*	0.405	0.865
Number of amalgams in mouth in pregnancy					
0	1.62 (11)	13.5 (60)	*12.4 (77)*	11.4 (47)	6.7 (34)
1–3	1.29 (25)	13.5 (188)	*14.0 (250)*	8.6 (112)	6.8 (101)
4+	1.57 (96)	12.6 (612)	*10.4 (600)*	9.9 (463)	5.9 (305)
P (2df)	0.677	0.653	*< 0.001*	0.196	0.355

All associations with P < 0.10 are italicized
df degrees of freedom
[a]Amount consumed by mother as reported at 32 weeks gestation

Strengths and limitations

There are a number of limitations of this study: (i) Despite the large sample, the numbers of autism cases with prenatal total blood Hg measured were relatively low, limiting statistical power. (ii) Although we accounted for several important confounders which are relevant to Hg levels and autism, the possibility of unmeasured confounding cannot be ruled out. (iii) The measures of Hg were obtained from whole blood in the first half of pregnancy—while having measures of Hg in early pregnancy may be a strength considering many teratogens are known to affect development at this stage, it may also be possible that exposure at later time points is more deleterious in regard to the autism spectrum. (iv) The data collected on fish consumption distinguished between oily and white fish but did not further characterize the types of fish consumed. Thus, we cannot identify the mothers who consumed fish at the extreme end of the food chain such as shark. However, although the levels of mercury in these fish are considerably greater than that in less predatory fish, there is no evidence of harmful effects to the fetus from eating such fish, as evidenced by the findings in this study of a lack of increasing risk to autism or autistic traits with increasing levels of maternal mercury. (v) The levels of total blood Hg in this population may be different from other populations, and therefore, caution is required before generalizing the results. For example, the median total blood Hg level in ALSPAC was 1.86 μg/L compared with 0.89 μg/L in the National Health and Nutrition Examination Survey (NHANES) in 1999–2000, but the proportion of women with higher than the

Table 4 Adjusted associations between prenatal mercury and offspring diagnosed autism and extreme levels of autistic traits. Odds ratios [95%CI] adjusted for maternal age, family adversity index, prenatal life events, smoking and alcohol in pregnancy, maternal locus of control, and maternal education

Proxy for Hg exposure[a]	Diagnosed autism, OR [95% CI]	Autistic trait, OR [95% CI]			
		Poor social cognition	Poor sociability	Poor coherence	Repetitive behavior
White fish	1.39 [0.80, 2.40]	*0.85 [0.71 ,1.03]*	0.93 [0.77, 1.11]	0.90 [0.78, 1.04]	1.01 [0.88, 1.16]
	(P = 0.238)	*(P = 0.092)*	(P = 0.399)	(P = 0.163)	(P = 0.886)
Oily fish	1.00 [0.68, 1.47]	0.98 [0.84, 1.14]	0.90 [0.78, 1.04]	1.01 [0.90, 1.14]	1.03 [0.92, 1.15]
	(P = 0.994)	(P = 0.774)	(P = 0.150)	(P = 0.853)	(P = 0.613)
Shellfish	0.86 [0.54, 1.38]	0.92 [0.77, 1.11]	0.91 [0.76, 1.08]	0.94 [0.81, 1.08]	1.03 [0.90, 1.17]
	(P = 0.542)	(P = 0.401)	(P = 0.284)	(P = 0.351)	(P = 0.707)
Amalgam inserted	*0.62 [0.37, 1.03]*	0.99 [0.83, 1.18]	1.14 [0.97, 1.34]	1.07 [0.94, 1.22]	1.02 [0.90, 1.16]
	(P = 0.067)	(P = 0.905)	(P = 0.119)	(P = 0.320)	(P = 0.761)
Amalgam extracted	*0.47 [0.24, 0.93]*	1.09 [0.89, 1.33]	1.14 [0.94, 1.38]	1.10 [0.94, 1.28]	1.04 [0.89, 1.20]
	(P = 0.031)	(P = 0.424)	(P = 0.178)	(P = 0.237)	(P = 0.647)
No. of amalgam fillings	0.96 [0.76, 1.21]	1.00 [0.91, 1.09]	*0.91 [0.84, 0.99]*	1.01 [0.94, 1.09]	0.95 [0.89, 1.01]
	(P = 0.730)	(P = 0.965)	*(P = 0.033)*	(P = 0.790)	(P = 0.122)
No. in analyses	7498–10,452	5888–6972	7119–8512	5646–6690	6302–7477

All associations with P < 0.10 are italicized
[a]Categorization of variables as shown in Table 3. Significance levels calculated testing for a linear trend

recommended USA action level (5.8 μg/L) [28] was 8% in NHANES compared with only 1% in ALSPAC [14]. (vi) The blood used for analysis had been kept in the vacutainers in which they were collected for 19 years before assay. It is conceivable that some of the mercury might have leaked through the rubber stoppers. However, this is unlikely to have been differential in relation to the outcomes being studied and therefore could theoretically bias the relationship between maternal mercury and offspring outcome towards the null. (vii) The identification of cases of autism was not carried out using a specific examination but rather used a multisource ascertainment approach; consequently, the possibility of outcome misclassification cannot be ruled out. Nevertheless, we have previously validated additional cases identified against autistic symptoms [20] and have also found that polygenic risk scores for ASD from the most recent genome-wide association study with publicly available summary data [29] are associated with the ASD diagnosis identified in ALSPAC (paper under review).

On the other hand, this study provides a number of advantages: (a) it is based on a geographic population with a high enrolment rate (∼ 80%) and consequently may be more generalizable to areas with similar distributions of blood Hg among pregnant women; (b) a relatively large number of confounders were available to be taken into account, thus diminishing the likelihood of bias in the results; (c) the prenatal data were collected prospectively with no knowledge as to how the child would develop, again reducing the likelihood of possible bias; and

(d) sufficient numbers were available to allow comparison between offspring of fish and non-fish consumers for autistic traits (although not for diagnosed autism).

Conclusions

In conclusion, this study did not find evidence to suggest that total prenatal blood Hg levels, or proxies for Hg levels, were important in relation to offspring diagnosis of autism. Although the results for the social communication trait mirrored results we have found for suboptimal IQ in showing an adverse effect of blood mercury if the mother ate no fish, but a beneficial association when fish was eaten, it is important that this be tested in other populations. There is no consistent evidence from this study to implicate prenatal exposure to mercury in the etiology of autism.

This is the largest prospective population study to date to address this question. It is the only study to compare total blood mercury levels in the first half of pregnancy among offspring with autism or high scores on autistic traits. It is also the only study to determine whether the exposures known to result in increased mercury levels were associated with autistic outcomes in the offspring.

Appendix

Independent trait descriptors of autism used in ALSPAC
The social communication trait
We used the 12-item Social and Communication Disorders Checklist (SCDC), developed by [30]. They showed that the internal consistency was excellent (0.93) and the test-retest reliability was high (0.81). The method was

developed on clinical samples, and when later used on the ALSPAC population at age 7.7 years, the high end of the scale was shown to predict a variety of adverse outcomes but was most specific for autism spectrum disorder [31]. Further research with ALSPAC data showed that the measure was reasonably stable over time [32].

For the present analysis, we have used the prorated score, which was calculated when any items were missing a response by using the average of the items that had been answered by the individual (2.7% of the population, almost all of whom had just one item missing). If all items were missing, the score was put to missing. The measure ranged from 0 to 24; the higher the score the more impaired was the child's social cognition. The distribution was skewed with a long upper tail. (12.8% had a score of over 6 and comprise the abnormal group for these analyses.)

The coherence measure

At age 9, the study mother completed a questionnaire which included seven of the nine scales of the first version of the Children's Communication Checklist (CCC) [33]. This checklist was designed to assess aspects of communication that are not readily assessed by conventional standardized tests including aspects of speech and syntax, as well as pragmatic aspects such as over-literal interpretation of stereotyped language. Although the CCC was initially designed to identify pragmatic difficulties, it has been shown to be good at discriminating a wide range of language and communication problems from typical development [34]. Analyses of traits predictive of autism in ALSPAC showed that the Coherence scale performed better than the other scales [19] and consequently it is used here. The scale comprises eight items (e.g., "It is sometimes hard to make sense of what she is saying because it seems illogical or disconnected" and "She has difficulty in telling a story, or describing what she has done in a sequence of events"). The score ranged from 20 to 36, with higher scores indicating more typical behavior. The score had a skewed distribution. The lower tail used in this analysis comprised those children scoring ≤ 33 points (10.0% of the population).

Abnormal and repetitive behavior

This scale was developed from the answer to four questions in the questionnaire sent to the mother at 69 months; these were as follows: "How often does he/she (a) repeatedly rock his head or body for no reason; (b) have a tic or twitch; (c) have other unusual behavior"; or (d) "Does he/she stumble or get stuck on words, or repeat them many times? (e.g., I I I I want a sweet)"? The responses to each question were coded as often/always = 3; sometimes = 2; never = 1 and summed. The resultant scale had a range from 4 to 12, with 22% scoring 5 and only 5.9% scoring

more than 5. Thus, it was impossible to approximate to a 10% cut-off; we therefore used > 5 as our abnormal group.

Sociability temperament

The questionnaire concerning the child sent to the study mothers when the child was 38 months of age included the 20 questions of the EAS temperament scale [35] and measured four traits—emotionality, activity, shyness and sociability—each based on the answers to 5 questions. The range of the Sociability sub-score was from 5 to 25 and the frequency distribution was approximately normal, a high score indicating a high level of sociability. The prorated scale was calculated for missing values as in the scales mentioned above. We then selected the lowest 11.4% of the children for our analyses (score < 8) as being the nearest to 10%.

Abbreviations

ALSPAC: Avon Longitudinal Study of Parents and Children; AOC: Adjusted odds ratio; CDC: Centers for Disease Control and Prevention; CI: Confidence interval; DAWBA: Development and well-being assessment; DNA: Deoxyribonucleic acid; EAS: Emotionality, Activity, Sociability temperament traits; ICD-10: International Classification of Diseases, 10th Edition; ICP-DRC-MS: Inductively coupled plasma dynamic reaction cell mass spectrometry; IQ: Intelligence quotient; IQR: Interquartile range; LOD: Level of detection; NHANES: National Health and Nutrition Examination Survey; OR: Odds ratio; QC: Quality control; SD: Standard deviation

Acknowledgements

We are extremely grateful to all the families who took part in this study, the midwives for their help in recruiting them, and the whole ALSPAC team, which includes interviewers, computer and laboratory technicians, clerical workers, research scientists, volunteers, managers, receptionists, and nurses.

Funding

The UK Medical Research Council and the Wellcome Trust (grant ref.: 102215/2/13/2) and the University of Bristol currently provide core support for ALSPAC. CMT was supported by a Wellcome Trust Career Re-Entry Fellowship (grant ref.: 104077/Z/14/Z). The assays of the maternal blood samples were carried out at the Centers for Disease Control and Prevention with funding from NOAA, and the statistical analyses were carried out in Bristol with funding from NOAA and support from the Intramural Research Program of NIAAA, NIH. This study was also supported by the NIHR Biomedical Research Centre at the University Hospitals Bristol NHS Foundation Trust and the University of Bristol.
The funders had no role in the data collection, research, nor subsequent decision to publish. The findings and conclusions in this report are those of the authors and do not necessarily represent the views of the funders. The authors had full access to all the data from the study and had final responsibility for the content of this paper and decision to submit for publication. Jean Golding and Steven Gregory will serve as guarantors for the contents of this paper.

Authors' contributions

JG conceived the idea and wrote the first draft. DR reviewed drafts of the paper. SG was responsible for data curation and formal analyses. GE was responsible for formal analyses. AE reviewed drafts of the paper. YIC assisted with writing, reviewing, and editing. JH and CT reviewed drafts of the paper. All authors read and approved the final manuscript.

Competing interests
The authors declare that they have no competing interests.

Author details
[1]Centre for Child and Adolescent Health, Bristol Medical School, University of Bristol, Oakfield House, Oakfield Grove, Bristol BS8 2BN, UK. [2]Centre for Academic Mental Health, Bristol Medical School, University of Bristol, Oakfield House, Oakfield Grove, Bristol BS8 2BN, UK. [3]Section on Nutritional Neurosciences, LMBB, National Institute on Alcohol Abuse and Alcoholism, National Institutes of Health, 31 Center Drive 1B/58, Bethesda, MD 20892, USA.

References
1. Geier DA, Geier MR. An evaluation of the effects of thimerosal on neurodevelopmental disorders reported following DTP and Hib vaccines in comparison to DTPH vaccine in the United States. J Toxicol Environ Health A. 2006;69:1481-95.
2. Schultz ST. Does thimerosal or other mercury exposure increase the risk for autism. Acta Neurobiol Exp. 2010;70:187-95.
3. DeStefano F. Vaccines and autism: evidence does not support a causal association. Clin Pharmacol Ther. 2007;82:756-9.
4. Taylor LE, Swerdfeger AL, Eslick GD. Vaccines are not associated with autism: an evidence-based meta-analysis of case-control and cohort studies. Vaccine. 2014;32:3623-9.
5. Clements CJ. The evidence for the safety of thiomersal in newborn and infant vaccines. Vaccine. 2004;22(15):1854-61.
6. Oken E, Kleinman KP, Berland WE, Simon SR, Rich-Edwards JW, Gillman MW. Decline in fish consumption among pregnant women after a national mercury advisory. Obstet Gynecol. 2003;102(2):346-51.
7. Golding J, Gregory S, Emond A, Iles-Caven Y, Hibbeln J, Taylor C. Prenatal mercury exposure and offspring behaviour in childhood and adolescence. Neurotoxicol. 2016c;57:87-94.
8. Gregory S, Iles-Caven Y, Hibbeln JR, Taylor CM, Golding J. Are prenatal mercury levels associated with subsequent blood pressure in childhood and adolescence? The Avon prebirth cohort study. BMJ Open. 2016;6(10):e012425.
9. Golding J, Gregory S, Iles-Caven Y, Emond A, Hibbeln J, Taylor CM. Maternal prenatal blood mercury is not adversely associated with offspring IQ at 8 years provided the mother eats fish: a British prebirth cohort study. Int J Hyg Environ Health. 2017; https://doi.org/10.1016/j.ijheh.2017.07.004
10. Golding J, Gregory S, Iles-Caven Y, Hibbeln J, Emond A, Taylor CM. Associations between prenatal mercury exposure and early child development in the ALSPAC study. NeuroToxicol. 2016;53:215-22.
11. Golding J, Pembrey M, Jones R, ALSPAC Study Team. ALSPAC—the Avon Longitudinal Study of Parents and Children. I. Study methodology. Paediatr Perinatal Epidemiol. 2001;15:74-87.
12. Boyd A, Golding J, Macleod J, Lawlor DA, Fraser A, Henderson J, Molloy L, et al. Cohort profile: the 'children of the 90s'—the index offspring of the Avon Longitudinal Study of Parents and Children. Int J Epidemiol. 2013;42:111-27. https://doi.org/10.1093/ije/dys066.
13. Taylor CM, Golding J, Hibbeln J, Emond A. Environmental factors predicting blood lead levels in pregnant women in the UK: the ALSPAC study. PLoS One. 2013;8:e72371.
14. Golding J, Steer CD, Hibbeln JR, Emmett PM, Lowery T, Jones R. Dietary predictors of maternal prenatal blood mercury levels in the ALSPAC birth cohort. Environ Health Pers. 2013;121:1214-8.
15. Tanner SD, Baranov VI. Theory, design and operation of a dynamic reaction cell for ICP-MS. Atomic Spectrosc. 1999;20:45-52.
16. Tanner SD, Baranov VI, Bandura DR. Reaction cells and collision cells for ICP-MS: a tutorial review. Spectrochim Acta A Mol Biomol Spectrosc. 2002;57:1361-452.
17. Golding J, Steer CD, Gregory S, Lowery T, Hibbeln JR, Taylor CM. Dental associations with blood mercury in pregnant women. Community Dent Oral Epidemiol. 2016a;44:216-22.
18. Williams E, Thomas K, Sidebotham H, Emond A. Prevalence and characteristics of autistic spectrum disorders in the ALSPAC cohort. Dev Med Child Neurol. 2008;50:672-7.
19. Steer CD, Golding J, Bolton PF. Traits contributing to the autistic spectrum. PLoS One. 2010;5:e12633. https://doi.org/10.1371/journal.pone.0012633.
20. Guyatt AL, Heron J, Le Cornu KB, Golding J, Rai D. Digit ratio and autism spectrum disorders in the Avon Longitudinal Study of Parents & Children: a birth cohort study. BMJ Open. 2015;5:e007433. https://doi.org/10.1136/bmjopen-2014-007433.
21. Goodman R, Ford T, Richards H, Gatward R, Meltzer H. The Development and Well-Being Assessment: description and initial validation of an integrated assessment of child and adolescent psychopathology. J Child Psychol Psychiatr. 2000;41:645-55.
22. Happé F, Ronald A, Plomin R. Time to give up on a single explanation for autism. Nature Neurosci. 2006;9:1218-20.
23. Levy Y, Ebstein RP. Research review: crossing syndrome boundaries in the search for brain endophenotypes. J Child Psychol Psychiatr. 2009;50:657-68.
24. Yoshimasu K, Kiyohara C, Takemura S, Nakai K. A meta-analysis of the evidence on the impact of prenatal and early infancy exposures to mercury on autism and attention deficit/hyperactivity disorder in the childhood. Neurotoxicol. 2014;44:121-31.
25. Ornoy A, Weinstein-Fudim L, Ergaz Z. Prenatal factors associated with autism spectrum disorder (ASD). Reprod Toxicol. 2015;56:155-69.
26. Yau VM, Green PG, Alaimo CP, Yoshida CK, Lutsky M, Windham GC, et al. Prenatal and neonatal peripheral blood mercury levels and autism spectrum disorders. Env Res. 2014;133:294-303.
27. van Wijngaarden E, Davidson PW, Smith TH, Evans K, Yost K, Love T, et al. Autism spectrum disorder phenotypes and prenatal exposure to methylmercury. Epidemiology. 2013;24:651-9.
28. Committee on the Toxological Effects of Methylmercury, Board on Environmental Studies and Toxicology, National Research Council. Toxicological effects of methylmercury. 2000; http://www.nap.edu/catalog/9899.html Accessed 30 Mar 2017.
29. Cross-Disorder Group of the Psychiatric Genomics Consortium. Genetic relationship between five psychiatric disorders estimated from genome-wide SNPs. Nat Genet. 2013;45(9):984-94. https://doi.org/10.1038/ng.2711.
30. Skuse DH, Mandy WP, Scourfield J. Measuring autistic traits: heritability, reliability and validity of the Social and Communication Disorders Checklist. Br J Psychiatry. 2005;187:568-72. https://doi.org/10.1192/bjp.187.6.568.
31. Skuse DH, Mandy W, Steer C, Miller LL, Goodman R, Lawrence K, Emond A, Golding J. Social communication competence and functional adaptation in a general population of children: preliminary evidence for sex-by-verbal IQ differential risk. J Am Acad Child Adolesc Psychiatr. 2009;48:128-37. https://doi.org/10.1097/CHI.0b013e31819176b8.
32. Pourcain BS, Mandy WP, Heron J, Golding J, Davey Smith G, Skuse DH. Links between co-occurring social-communication and hyperactive-inattentive trait trajectories. J Am Acad Child Adolesc Psychiatr. 2011;50:892-902.
33. Bishop DVM. Development of the Children's Communication Checklist (CCC): a method for assessing qualitative aspects of communicative impairment in children. J Child Psychol Psychiatr. 1998;39:879-91.
34. Bishop DVM, Baird G. Parent and teacher report of pragmatic aspects of communication: use of the Children's Communication Checklist in a clinical setting. Dev Med Child Neurol. 2001;43:809-18.
35. Buss AH, Plomin R. Temperament: early developing personality traits. Hillsdale: Lawrence Erlbaum; 1984.

Impairment of social behaviors in *Arhgef10* knockout mice

Dai-Hua Lu[1], Hsiao-Mei Liao[2], Chia-Hsiang Chen[3,4], Huang-Ju Tu[1], Houng-Chi Liou[1], Susan Shur-Fen Gau[2*] and Wen-Mei Fu[1*]

Abstract

Background: Impaired social interaction is one of the essential features of autism spectrum disorder (ASD). Our previous copy number variation (CNV) study discovered a novel deleted region associated with ASD. One of the genes included in the deleted region is *ARHGEF10*. A missense mutation of *ARHGEF10* has been reported to be one of the contributing factors in several diseases of the central nervous system. However, the relationship between the loss of ARHGEF10 and the clinical symptoms of ASD is unclear.

Methods: We generated *Arhgef10* knockout mice as a model of ASD and characterized the social behavior and the biochemical changes in the brains of the knockout mice.

Results: Compared with their wild-type littermates, the *Arhgef10*-depleted mice showed social interaction impairment, hyperactivity, and decreased depression-like and anxiety-like behavior. Behavioral measures of learning in the Morris water maze were not affected by *Arhgef10* deficiency. Moreover, neurotransmitters including serotonin, norepinephrine, and dopamine were significantly increased in different brain regions of the *Arhgef10* knockout mice. In addition, monoamine oxidase A (MAO-A) decreased in several brain regions.

Conclusions: These results suggest that *ARHGEF10* is a candidate risk gene for ASD and that the *Arhgef10* knockout model could be a tool for studying the mechanisms of neurotransmission in ASD.

Keywords: ARHGEF10, Autism spectrum disorder, Social deficits, Serotonin, Norepinephrine

Background

Autism spectrum disorder (ASD) is a common neurodevelopmental disorder marked by lifetime social functional impairment [1, 2]. The essential features of ASD include impairment in reciprocal social communication; a deficit in communication ability; and restricted, repetitive behavior and interests [1]. ASD occurs at a higher incidence in males than females, with a common consensus ratio of 4:1 [3]. The prevalence of ASD has been estimated at approximately 1.5% and has increased dramatically over the past few decades [4, 5]. Various genetic studies have provided convincing evidence that ASD is a complex and highly polygenic disease [6]. However, the genetic underpinnings of ASD remain unclear, which impedes understanding of the disease pathology and the search for treatments.

Our previous study identified two novel chromosomal deletions in two unrelated ASD patients [7]. One of the deletions, which spans 8p23.3-pter, contains three genes––*DLGAP2*, *CLN8*, and *ARHGEF10*––that may be relevant to neurological functions. The functional loss of these genes might contribute to the clinical symptoms of ASD [8, 9]. In this study, we target the gene *ARHGEF10* to further investigate the impacts of its functional loss. ARHGEF10, as a rho guanine nucleotide exchange factor (GEF), regulates rho GTPases by catalyzing the exchange of G-protein-bound GDP for GTP. There are over 60 rho GEFs identified in the human genome. However, few have been functionally evaluated in animal models. The Thr109Ile mutation of the rho GEF 10 (*ARHGEF10*)

* Correspondence: gaushufe@ntu.edu.tw; wenmei@ntu.edu.tw
[2]Department of Psychiatry, National Taiwan University Hospital and College of Medicine, Taipei, Taiwan
[1]Pharmacological Institute, College of Medicine, National Taiwan University, Taipei, Taiwan
Full list of author information is available at the end of the article

gene was found in a family of patients with slow nerve conduction and thinly myelinated peripheral nerves [10]. In addition to its possible role in the myelination process, the single nucleotide polymorphism of ARHGEF10 has also been reported to be associated with schizophrenia [11]. GEFs are the main regulators that facilitate the activation of rho GTPases by converting them from the GDP-bound state to an active GTP-bound state. Rho GTPases have been widely studied in neuronal development and neuronal diseases [12]. Given the importance of rho GTPases in the nervous system, dysregulation of rho GEFs is believed to be involved in neurodevelopmental diseases. For example, a mutation of *ARHGEF6* has been associated with intellectual disability [13]. These findings encouraged us to further study the possible role of *ARHGEF10* in ASD.

To explore the role of *ARHGEF10* in ASD and to further understand the impacts of *ARHGEF10* deletion on the molecular mechanisms of neurological function, we generated an *Arhgef10* knockout mouse model by deleting exons 4 and 5 of the mouse *Arhgef10* gene. The mice without the *Arhgef10* gene have normal fertility and body weight gain. The *Arhgef10* knockout mice were then subjected to tests measuring their startle responses, motor behavior, spatial learning, and social behavior. Behavioral changes may reflect a disturbance of neurotransmission. Previous studies have shown that the dysregulation of biosynthesis, transportation, and degradation of neurotransmitters could be associated with ASD [14]. In addition, genetic association studies have identified some genes that encode the transporters or degradation enzymes of neurotransmitters as contributing to the risk of ASD [15]. For instance, monoamine oxidase A (MAO-A), an enzyme that is important for the metabolism of serotonin and norepinephrine, is associated with ASD in a population-based study [15]. Another population-based association study also indicates that changes in monoamine oxidase B (MAO-B) activity increase ASD risk in males [16]. Based on those findings, we evaluated the levels of monoamines in *Arhgef10* knockout mice to understand the possible roles of *Arhgef10* in the serotonergic system.

In this study, we found that *Arhgef10* knockout mice exhibited impaired social interaction and social recognition, representing the key characteristics of ASD. In addition, *Arhgef10* knockout mice also displayed reduced anxiety-like and depression-like behaviors and increased locomotor activity. Additionally, serotonin, norepinephrine, and dopamine were elevated in the frontal cortex, hippocampus, and amygdala in *Arhgef10* knockout mice. Moreover, MAO-A, a molecule that regulates the levels of certain neurotransmitters, was also reduced in *Arhgef10* knockout mice. Behavioral studies and biochemical examination showed that ARHGEF10 not only plays a critical role in social behavior but also participates in the regulation of neurotransmitters.

Methods

Animals and experimental design

Arhgef10 knockout mice were generated by the deletion of exon 4 and exon 5 using the Cre-loxP site-specific knockout according to a method described previously [8]. The strategy for generating *Arhgef10* knockout mice is shown in Additional file 1: Figure S1. In brief, exons 4 and 5 of ARHGEF10 in embryonic stem cells from the 129S1/Sv mouse strain were replaced with a construct containing ARHGEF10 exons 4 and 5 interposed between two loxP sites and a NEO cassette to produce Cre-induced homologous recombination. *Arhgef10* knockout mice were then backcrossed for at least ten generations with C57BL/6J mice. The *Arhgef10* knockout mice used in this study were produced by heterozygous breeding pairs in a trio breeding format. All mice were kept under standard temperature, humidity, and timed lighting conditions and provided with mouse chow and water ad libitum. *Arhgef10* knockout mice and their control littermates were housed in groups (3–5 mice per cage).

Behavioral tests were conducted during the light cycle (07:00–19:00) in a testing room next to the mouse housing room. Eight- to twelve-week-old male *Arhgef10* KO mice and their WT littermates were used in this study. All behavioral tests were carried out with male mice. Animals in the same littermates were used in the same behavioral test, except for the plus maze, open field, and water maze tests. In these three tests, the intervals between tests were approximately 7 days each. The open field test was conducted first, followed by the plus maze and then the water maze. Mice were transported to the testing room and habituated for 30 min before behavioral testing. All animal experiments were approved by the Ethical Committee for the Animal Research of National Taiwan University.

Sample preparation

Mice were anesthetized with isoflurane and then decapitated. For Nissl staining, the brains of 10-week-old mice were removed after saline perfusion and post-fixed with 4% paraformaldehyde (PFA) overnight. Tissue samples for Western blots and high-performance liquid chromatography (HPLC) were prepared by dissecting four parts from the fresh brains of 10- to 12-week-old mice: frontal cortex, striatum, hippocampus, and amygdala. These tissues were then weighed and homogenized.

Nissl staining

Nissl staining was performed as previously described [17]. In brief, 40-μm-thick frozen brain sections from

WT and *Arhgef10* knockout mice were mounted on gelatin-coated slides and air-dried overnight. The slices were then placed directly into xylene for 3 min and then rehydrated with 100, 95, and 85% alcohol, followed by distilled water. The slices were stained with 0.02% crystal violet (Sigma-Aldrich, St. Louis, MO, USA) solution for 25–35 min and then rinsed quickly in distilled water. Finally, the slices were soaked in xylene and mounted with permanent mounting medium.

Open field test
Mice were placed in an open plastic chamber (40 × 40 × 38 cm), and locomotor activity was monitored for 1 h. The central region of the open field was defined as a region of 20×20 cm^2, and all activity was measured by a 16×16 photobeam sensor connected to an automated tracking program (PAS-Open Field, San Diego Instruments). The number of beam breaks were used as an indicator of locomotor activity.

Elevated plus maze test
The elevated plus maze (EPM) apparatus (made of white Plexiglas) was elevated 40 cm above the floor and consisted of two open arms alternating with two closed arms. The open arms and closed arms were made of plastic and measured 25 cm long × 5 cm wide. The two closed arms were protected by 15-cm-high walls. Mice were placed in the EPM for 5 min, and the time spent in each arm and frequency of entry into each arm were recorded by Noldus EthoVision 3.0 (EthoVision˚, Noldus Information Technology).

Tests for sociability and social novelty preference in a three-chamber apparatus
The tests for sociability and social novelty preference were performed in a three-chamber apparatus as previously described with minor modification [18, 19]. The animals used here were all age- and sex-matched littermates; C57BL/6J mice were used as the stranger mice. All animals were habituated to the test chamber for 30 min 1 day before the behavioral test. The three-chamber apparatus was a 21 cm (height) × 25 cm (width) × 48 cm (length) black plastic box. Before the sociability test, the animal was free to explore the apparatus for 5 min. In the sociability test session, an unfamiliar same-sex mouse, designated as stranger 1, was placed in the plastic cylinder; an empty cylinder was placed in the opposite chamber. The cylinders (13 cm in height, 10 cm in diameter) were transparent, and their walls contained holes that allowed the mice to sniff each other. The test mouse was placed in the central chamber and allowed to freely explore these three chambers for 10 min. In the social novelty preference test, a second novel mouse, stranger 2, was placed in the opposite chamber, which was empty in the previous session. The test mouse was allowed to freely explore the chambers for 10 min in this session. The time spent in each chamber and the time spent sniffing or interacting with the stranger mouse were recorded. In addition, the number of entries into all chambers were analyzed using EthoVision.

Tail suspension test and forced swim test
The tail suspension test (TST) [20] and the forced swim test (FST) are the most commonly used tests to evaluate depression-like behavior in rodents. In the TST, the animals were suspended by the tail with adhesive tape for 6 min. In the FST, the animals were placed in a plastic cylinder tank (30 cm in height × 15 cm in diameter) filled with 25 ± 2 °C water for 6 min. The complete TST and FST sessions were all videotaped for analysis. Immobility was defined as a lack of motion of the whole body at 2–6 min, when the mice ceased struggling and began passively floating, making only the movements necessary to keep the head above water.

Pre-pulse inhibition test
Pre-pulse inhibition (PPI) was tested in an acoustic startle chamber (SR Lab, San Diego Instruments, San Diego, CA). The chamber contained a Plexiglas cylinder (12.6 cm in length × 4.0 cm in internal diameter) fixed on a platform under which a piezoelectric accelerometer recorded and transduced the motion of the tube. The sensor transmitted the digitized signals to a computer interfaced with the startle apparatus. To provide a consistent acoustic environment and mask external noise, we maintained a continuous background of 65-dB white noise within each chamber throughout the PPI tests. The inter-trial interval was between 10 and 20 s. Each startle trial consisted of a single 120-dB white noise burst lasting 40 ms. Each PPI trial consisted of a pre-pulse (20 ms burst of white noise with an intensity of 70, 74, or 82 dB) followed by the startle stimulus 100 ms later (120 dB, 40 ms of white noise). Each of the three types of pre-pulse trials (70, 74, and 82 dB) was presented 10 times. The percentage of PPI was calculated according to the following formula: %PPI = (S − (P + S))/ S × 100%, where P + S is the recorded response amplitude for pre-pulse plus startle pulse trials, and S is the recorded response amplitude for startle pulse-only trials.

Morris water maze test
Spatial learning was evaluated behaviorally using the Morris water maze. The maze consisted of a circular pool of water, 105 cm in diameter and 21 cm in height. The pool was divided into four equal quadrants: the target zone, two adjacent zones, and the opposite zone. The pool was filled with water at 22 ± 0.5 °C. A circular

platform of 10 cm diameter was placed at the center of the target quadrant, and approximately 1.5 cm below the surface of the water. The maze was surrounded by four simple visual cues external to the maze. The movements of the mice were recorded with a video camera placed on the ceiling over the center of the maze, and the paths of the mice were analyzed using EthoVision. The training was started by acclimating the mice to the task environment with 1 day of free swimming in the pool without the platform. Each mouse underwent four consecutive training trials per day for 4 days. In each trial, the mice were placed along the edge of one quadrant of the maze; all quadrants except the target quadrant were used as starting locations. The duration from the time when the mouse entered the water until it climbed onto the platform was recorded as escape latency, and the mean latency to find the hidden platform was calculated for each individual mouse on each day. The maximum duration of each trial was 1 min, and the mice were removed from the pool by the experimenter after each trial. If the mice failed to find the platform within 1 min, they would be placed on the platform, where they were allowed to remain for 15 s. For the probe trial, 24 h after the final trial, the platform was removed. Each mouse was placed in the water maze at the edge of the former platform location and allowed to swim freely for 60 s. The total time that each mouse spent in each quadrant of the tank was recorded.

High-performance liquid chromatography

The levels of serotonin, norepinephrine, and dopamine in the frontal cortex, striatum, hippocampus, and amygdala were measured by HPLC analysis. Four different mouse brain areas were dissected from the cerebral hemisphere, weighed, and homogenized in 0.1 N perchloric acid by sonication. The homogenates were then centrifuged at $14,500 \times g$ for 30 min at 4 °C, and the supernatants were collected for HPLC analysis. HPLC–ECD (Sykam, Gilching, Germany) was used to evaluate levels of monoamines, including dopamine, 5-HT, and NE and their metabolites, in the samples (20 μl). The chromatogram peaks corresponding to the monoamines were identified by their retention times compared with the elution times of monoamine standards (Sigma, St. Louis, MO). The levels of dopamine, 5-HT and NE, were then estimated by the ratios of the peak heights to those of the internal standards and expressed as nanograms of neurotransmitter per gram of tissue.

Western blotting

Western blot analysis was performed to characterize ARHGEF10 (Proteintech Group, IL, USA; 11112-1-AP), GAPDH (Santa Cruz, Dallas, TX, USA; sc25778), β-actin (Sigma-Aldrich, St. Louis, MO, USA; A5316), MAO-A (Abcam, Cambridge, UK; ab126751), monoamine oxidase B (MAO-B) (Abcam, Cambridgeshire, UK; ab137778), dopamine ß-hydroxylase (DβH) (Abcam, Cambridge, UK; ab108384), and tryptophan hydroxylase (TPH) (Abcam, Cambridge, UK; ab52954) expression in the brains of WT and ARHGEF10 knockout mice. Mouse brain tissues were lysed in RIPA buffer (150 mM NaCl, 50 mM Tris–HCl, 1 mM EGTA, 1% Nonidet P-40, 0.25% deoxycholate, 1 mM sodium fluoride, 50 mM sodium orthovanadate) supplemented with Halt protease inhibitor cocktail (Thermo, IL, USA). Proteins were separated by SDS-PAGE, transferred to PVDF membranes, and blocked with 5% non-fat milk for 1 h. The membranes were then incubated with primary antibodies at 4 °C overnight followed by the appropriate secondary antibodies at room temperature for 1 h. The protein bands were visualized using enhanced chemiluminescence (ECL) (Millipore, MA, USA) reagent, and blot images were captured using a UVP imaging system with LabWorks Software (Upland, CA, USA).

Data analysis

Throughout the study, parametric analysis was performed by one- or two-way ANOVA, using a between-group factor of genotype and a within-group factor of each behavioral parameter. If the overall ANOVA showed a significant difference, Tukey's test was used for post hoc comparisons. Statistical analysis was conducted using SPSS (IBM Inc., Somers, NY, USA) and GraphPad Prism (San Diego, CA, USA) software. Graphs of the data were also created using GraphPad Prism. The data were represented as the mean ± standard error.

Results

ARHGEF10 expression in different brain regions

To examine ARHGEF10 expression in the central nervous system, we measured the protein level by Western blot analysis. As shown in Fig. 1a, ARHGEF10 protein was widely expressed in the wild-type (WT) mouse brain, especially in the frontal cortex and amygdala. Notably, the absence of ARHGEF10 protein in the knockout mouse brain was confirmed by Western blotting (Fig. 1b). Nissl staining of serial coronal brain sections revealed a similar brain structure between WT and *Arhgef10* knockout mice (Fig. 1c).

Arhgef10 knockout mice display social deficits in the three-chamber test

To explore whether *Arhgef10* knockout affects social interaction, we employed the three-chamber paradigm to test sociability and social recognition. After habituation, a novel same-sex mouse was placed within the plastic cylinder (stranger mouse 1) in one chamber, and one empty cylinder was placed in another chamber. We found that WT mice

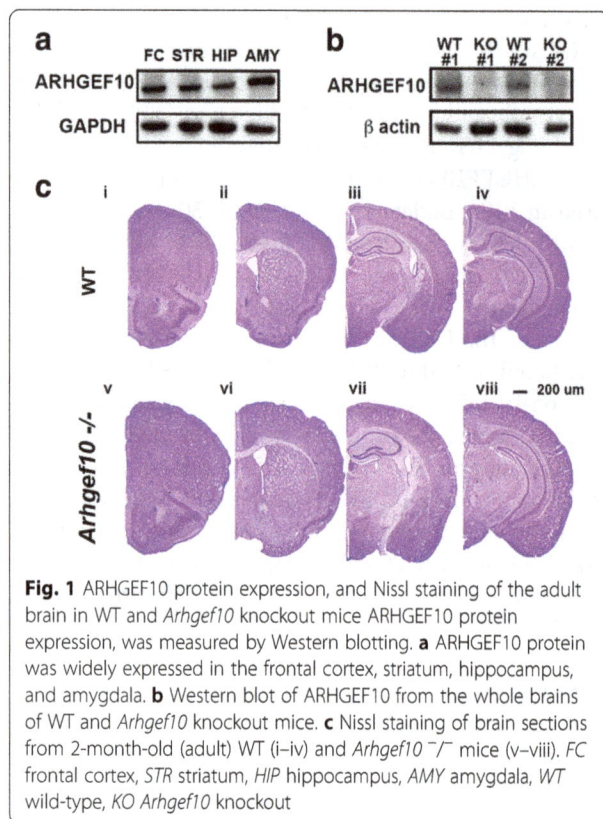

Fig. 1 ARHGEF10 protein expression, and Nissl staining of the adult brain in WT and *Arhgef10* knockout mice ARHGEF10 protein expression, was measured by Western blotting. **a** ARHGEF10 protein was widely expressed in the frontal cortex, striatum, hippocampus, and amygdala. **b** Western blot of ARHGEF10 from the whole brains of WT and *Arhgef10* knockout mice. **c** Nissl staining of brain sections from 2-month-old (adult) WT (i–iv) and *Arhgef10* $^{-/-}$ mice (v–viii). *FC* frontal cortex, *STR* striatum, *HIP* hippocampus, *AMY* amygdala, *WT* wild-type, *KO Arhgef10* knockout

spent a significantly longer time in the chamber with a stranger mouse than in the empty chamber (Fig. 2a; $F_{1,22} = 36.517$, $p < 0.001$ for genotype × chamber by two-way ANOVA; $F_{1,22} = 24.831$, $p < 0.001$ for chamber; Tukey's post hoc comparisons were used to examine the differences between the empty cylinder and stranger mouse 1, WT: $p < 0.05$; KO: $p > 0.05$; $n = 12$ for each). However, *Arhgef10* knockout mice did not spend a longer time in the chamber with the stranger mouse (Fig. 2a). Upon further evaluation of the social interactions, we found that WT mice spent significantly and markedly more time in close interaction with the stranger mouse by sniffing the holes of the cylinder, indicating normal social ability (Fig. 2b; $F_{1,22} = 52.971$, $p < 0.001$ for genotype × chamber by two-way ANOVA; $p < 0.05$ for post hoc comparisons between the empty cylinder and the stranger mouse, $n = 12$). *Arhgef10* knockout mice showed no significant preference between these two cylinders, indicating that they did not exhibit interest in the stranger mouse (Fig. 2b; $p > 0.05$ for post hoc comparisons between the empty cylinder and the stranger mouse, $n = 12$). Since enhanced locomotor activity may increase the possibility of contacts between mice, we further examined the number of entries into each chamber. We found that the number of entries into these two chambers were similar in WT mice and *Arhgef10* knockout mice (Fig. 2c; $F_{1,22} = 1.607$, $p = 0.218$ for genotype × chamber, by two-way ANOVA).

In the test for social novelty preference, we further examined social recognition in WT and *Arhgef10* knockout mice. Mice naturally exhibit a preference for social novelty, spending more time with a new mouse than with a familiar mouse as a social stimulus. In addition to stranger 1 in the original cylinder, another stranger mouse (stranger 2) was placed in the second cylinder. WT mice showed a preference for exploring the compartment with the novel mouse, stranger 2, compared with the chamber containing stranger 1 (Fig. 2d and e; $F_{1,22} = 5.843$, $p = 0.024$ for genotype × chamber, by two-way ANOVA; post hoc for comparisons between stranger 1 and stranger 2 revealed $p < 0.05$, $n = 12$ for WT, and $p < 0.05$, $n = 12$ for KO). Although *Arhgef10* knockout mice spent more time in the chamber with the first stranger mouse than in the chamber with the second stranger mouse (Fig. 2d), the time spent in social interactions, such as sniffing or tail rattling or time spent near the cylinder containing the stranger mice was similar between the first and the second stranger mouse (Fig. 2e). Keeping up with the decreased social interaction in sociability test, it was found that the social novelty preference was affected in *Arhgef10* knockout mice. However, the longer time spent in the chamber with the first stranger mouse without more social interaction may imply that *Arhgef10* knockout mice need more time to become familiar with the stranger mouse during the experiment. Both WT and *Arhgef10* knockout mice showed a comparable number of entries into the compartment with stranger 1 and the one with the novel mouse, stranger 2 (Fig. 2f; $F_{1,22} = 0.983$, $p = 0.602$ for genotype × chamber, by two-way ANOVA).

Increased locomotor activity in *Arhgef10* knockout mice

The open field test was used to evaluate the general locomotor and exploratory activity of the mice. *Arhgef10* knockout mice showed a higher level of locomotor activity in open field ($F_{1,30} = 12.296$, $p = 0.001$, $n = 16$) (Fig. 3a). In a 60-min open field test, *Arhgef10* knockout mice exhibited significantly enhanced locomotor activity compared with WT mice at 0–5, 30–35, and 45–50 min (Fig. 3b, Tukey's test for multiple comparisons, $p < 0.05$). There was no significant difference in rearing activity between WT and knockout mice (Fig. 3c). In addition, there was no significant difference between WT and *Arhgef10* knockout mice in the amount of activity occurring in the center of the field (Fig. 3d).

Reduction of anxiety-like behavior in *Arhgef10* knockout mice

The EPM was used to measure the level of anxiety-like behavior in the mice. The time spent in the open

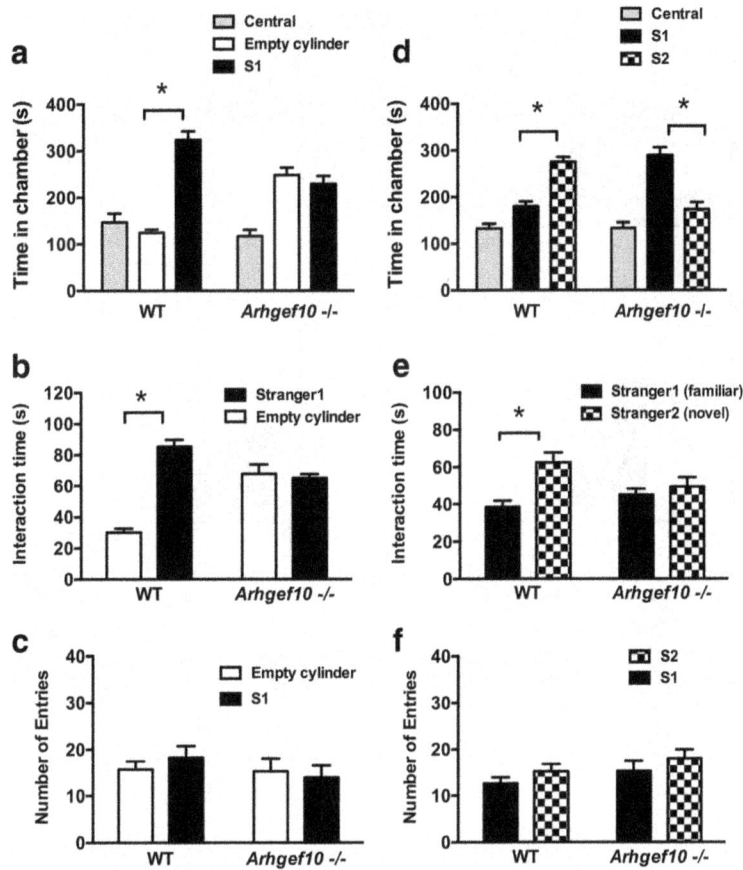

Fig. 2 *Arhgef10* knockout mice exhibit social impairment in the three-chamber test. **a** The time spent in each of the three compartments was analyzed using EthoVision. **b** The active interaction times with the empty cylinder and an unfamiliar mouse (stranger 1) in the session were also evaluated. WT mice (*n* = 12) spent much more time in the chamber with stranger 1 than in the empty cylinder, and displayed more interaction with the mouse than with the empty cylinder, indicating normal sociability (*p* < 0.001). However, Arhgef10 $^{-/-}$ mice (*n* = 12) spent equal durations of both total time and active interaction time in the chamber with empty cylinder and stranger 1. **d** In the preference for social novelty test, the time spent in each chamber was analyzed as in the previous test. WT mice spent more time in the chamber with a novel mouse (stranger 2) than in the compartment with stranger 1. However, Arhgef10 –/– mice spent less time in the chamber with stranger 2 than in the chamber with stranger 1. **e** The duration of contact time was measured with stranger 1 and the novel mouse stranger 2. WT mice displayed a significant increase in the duration of close interaction with stranger 2 compared with stranger 1 (*p* < 0.001). However, Arhgef10 –/– mice did not show a preference for novel stranger 2

arms or closed arms is used as an index to define the level of anxiety-like behavior. It was found that *Arhgef10* knockout mice displayed less anxiety-like behavior. The time spent in the open arms was significantly increased in *Arhgef10* knockout mice (open arms: $F_{1,23}$ = 11.04, *p* = 0.003; closed arms: $F_{1,23}$ = 14.481, *p* = 0.001, *n* = 13 for WT vs *Arhgef10* KO) (Fig. 4a), indicating that anxiety-like behavior was reduced in knockout mice. Upon analyzing the number of entries into each arm, we found that the number of entries into the open arms was significantly increased in *Arhgef10* knockout mice (open arms: $F_{1,23}$ = 6.301, *p* = 0.02; closed arms: $F_{1,23}$ = 2.431, *p* = 0.134 for WT vs *Arhgef10* KO) (Fig. 4b). The results demonstrated that there was a reduction of anxiety-like behavior in *Arhgef10* KO mice.

Reduction of depression-like behavior in *Arhgef10* knockout mice

To further examine whether other mood-related behaviors were also affected in *Arhgef10* knockout mice, animals were subjected to the tail suspension test (TST) and the forced swim test (FST). Increased immobility and floating time are indicative of depression-related behavior. Interestingly, *Arhgef10* knockout mice showed a significant reduction of immobility in both the FST (151.1 ± 9.47 s, and 62.43 ± 1.5 s for WT and KO mice, respectively) and TST (207.0 ± 6.013 s and 131.2 ± 13.47 for WT and KO, respectively) (Fig. 4c, d). The duration of immobility time in both the FST and the TST was significantly shorter in *Arhgef10* knockout mice than in WT mice ($F_{1,17}$ = 39.175, *p* < 0.0001 in FST; $F_{1,17}$ = 24.109, *p* = 0.0013 in

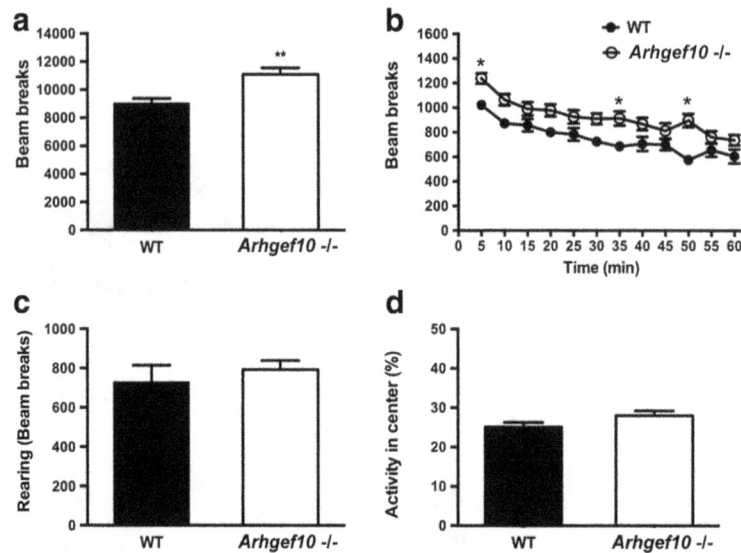

Fig. 3 *Arhgef10* knockout mice display spontaneous locomotor hyperactivity in the open field test. Spontaneous locomotor activity was tested in an open field for 60 min. **a** Total ambulatory locomotion ($p = 0.001$). **b** Time course of locomotor activity. Note that locomotor activity was greater in *Arhgef10* knockout mice. **c** No difference between WT mice and *Arhgef10* $^{-/-}$ mice in total rearing was observed. **d** No difference in percent of activity in the central part of the open field was observed between WT mice and *Arhgef10* $^{-/-}$ mice. The bar graph shows mean ± SEM ($n = 16$ per genotype for WT mice and KO mice); * $p < 0.05$ compared with WT mice by one-way ANOVA

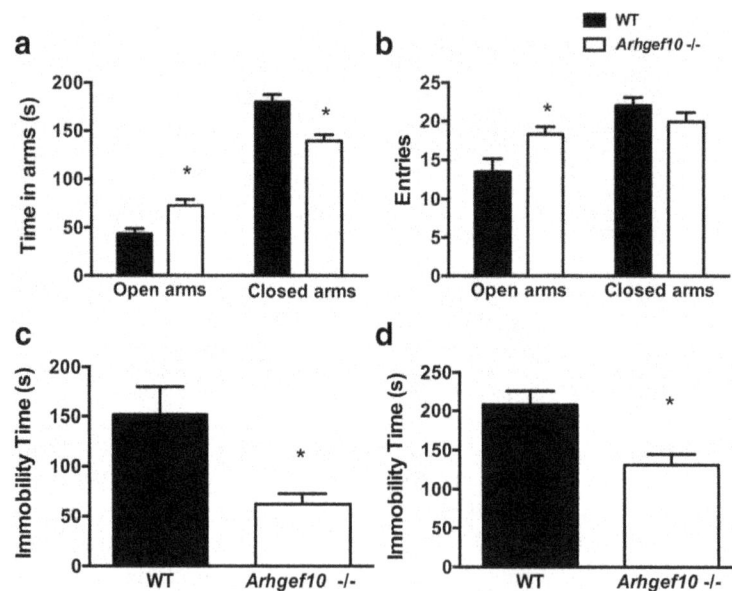

Fig. 4 Reduced anxiety-like and depression-related behavior in *Arhgef10* $^{-/-}$ mice. Anxiety-like behavior was tested in an elevated plus maze (EPM) for 5 min. For depression-related behavior, immobility was measured between 2 and 6 min in the forced swim test (FST) and the tail suspension test (TST). **a** *Arhgef10* $^{-/-}$ mice spent more time in open arms than WT mice ($n = 13$ for each) in the EPM. **b** Total entries into open arms and closed arms of the EPM in WT and *Arhgef10* $^{-/-}$ mice. **c** Reduced immobility time was observed in *Arhgef10* $^{-/-}$ mice ($n = 9$ and 10 for WT and KO, respectively) during the FST. **d** *Arhgef10* $^{-/-}$ mice also displayed reduced immobility time compared with WT mice during the TST ($n = 9$ and 10 for WT and KO, respectively). The bar graph shows the mean ± SEM. *$p < 0.05$ compared with WT

TST; $n = 9$ and 10 for WT and KO, respectively). These results indicated that there was reduction of depression-like behavior in *Arhgef10* KO mice.

Pre-pulse inhibition is unaffected in *Arhgef10* knockout mice

The pre-pulse inhibition (PPI) test is used to evaluate sensory gating in mice. Acoustic startle responses provide information on the sensorimotor processes of the animal in response to acoustic stimuli. *Arhgef10* knockout mice had a normal startle amplitude in response to 120 dB acoustic stimuli, indicating that the reflexive contraction of the muscles in response to acoustic stimuli was normal ($F_{1.9} = 1. 171$, $p = 0.337$, $n = 5–6$) (Fig. 5a). Moreover, *Arhgef10* knockout mice also exhibited a reduced acoustic startle response when the acoustic startle stimulus was preceded by a weaker acoustic stimulus, indicating a normal PPI response in comparison with WT mice (two-way ANOVA for genotype × pre-pulse dB, main effect of genotype: $F_{1.9} = 1. 0366$, $p = 0.8524$; main effect of pre-pulse dB: $F_{2,18} = 25.27$, $p < 0.001$.) (Fig. 5b).

Arhgef10 knockout mice exhibit normal spatial learning in the Morris water maze test

Spatial learning behavior was measured using the Morris water maze test. For four training days, *Arhgef10* knockout mice displayed normal learning ability with typical decreases in escape latency ($F = 0.260$, $p = 0.618$, $n = 6–$

7) (Fig. 5c). In the probe test, both WT and *Arhgef10* knockout mice spent much more time in the target quadrant than in opposite or adjacent quadrants (Fig. 5d), indicating that *Arhgef10* knockout mice exhibited normal spatial learning.

Increased norepinephrine (NE) and serotonin (5-HT) levels in the frontal cortex and amygdala of *Arhgef10* knockout mice

To further explore the possible underlying mechanisms leading to the behavioral changes caused by functional loss of ARHGEF10, we investigated the neurochemical composition of different brain regions of *Arhgef10* knockout mice. The frontal cortex, striatum, hippocampus, and amygdala from WT and KO mice were analyzed by HPLC with electrochemical detection (ECD) to determine the content of dopamine, 5-HT, NE, and their metabolites. The content of NE in the frontal cortex and amygdala was significantly elevated in *Arhgef10* knockout mice (two-way ANOVA for genotype × brain regions, main effect of genotype: $F_{1, 10} = 6.776$, $p = 0.0264$ and brain regions $F_{3, 30} = 3.250$, $p = 0.0354$; interaction: $F_{3, 30} = 2.764$, $p = 0.0591$). Post hoc comparisons between WT and KO revealed significant differences in the frontal cortex and amygdala (Fig. 6a). Serotonin content in the amygdala and hippocampus was also increased in *Arhgef10* knockout mice compared with WT mice (two-way ANOVA for genotype × brain regions, main effect of genotype: $F_{1, 10} =$

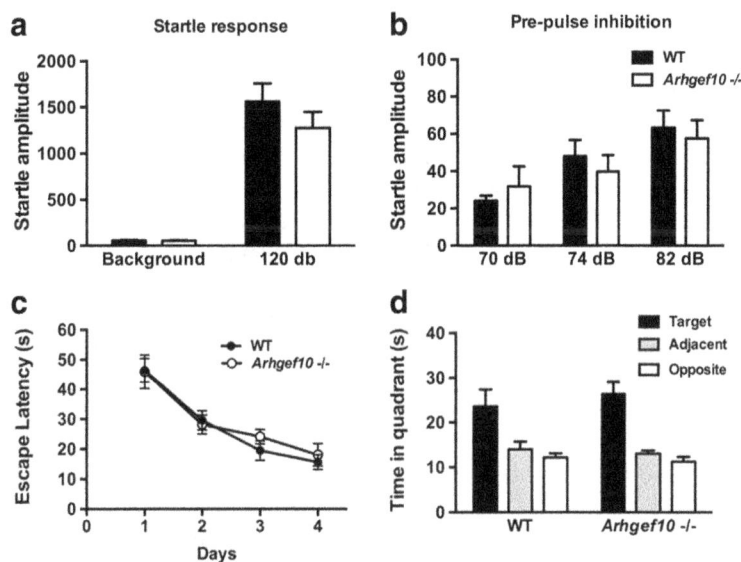

Fig. 5 *Arhgef10* knockout does not affect the startle response, pre-pulse inhibition (PPI) or learning. The startle reflex response was measured as startle amplitude, and PPI is the reduction of this response when an acoustic startle (120 dB) is preceded by a stimulus of 70, 74, or 82 dB. **a** There was no difference between WT and *Arhgef10 −/−* mice in startle responses to a 120-dB acoustic stimulus. **b** *Arhgef10 −/−* mice did not show a PPI deficit for a pre-pulse of 70, 74, or 82 dB ($n = 5–6$). **c** In the Morris water maze test, all mice were trained for 4 days to reach the platform. **d** On day 5, the platform was removed for the probe test to examine the memory of the animals. Note that *Arhgef10 −/−* mice exhibit the same normal acquisition curve as WT mice. Both WT and *Arhgef10 −/−* mice spent much more time in the target zone than in any other zone in the probe test. The bar graph shows the mean ± SEM ($n = 6–7$). *$p < 0.05$ compared with adjacent or opposite quadrants

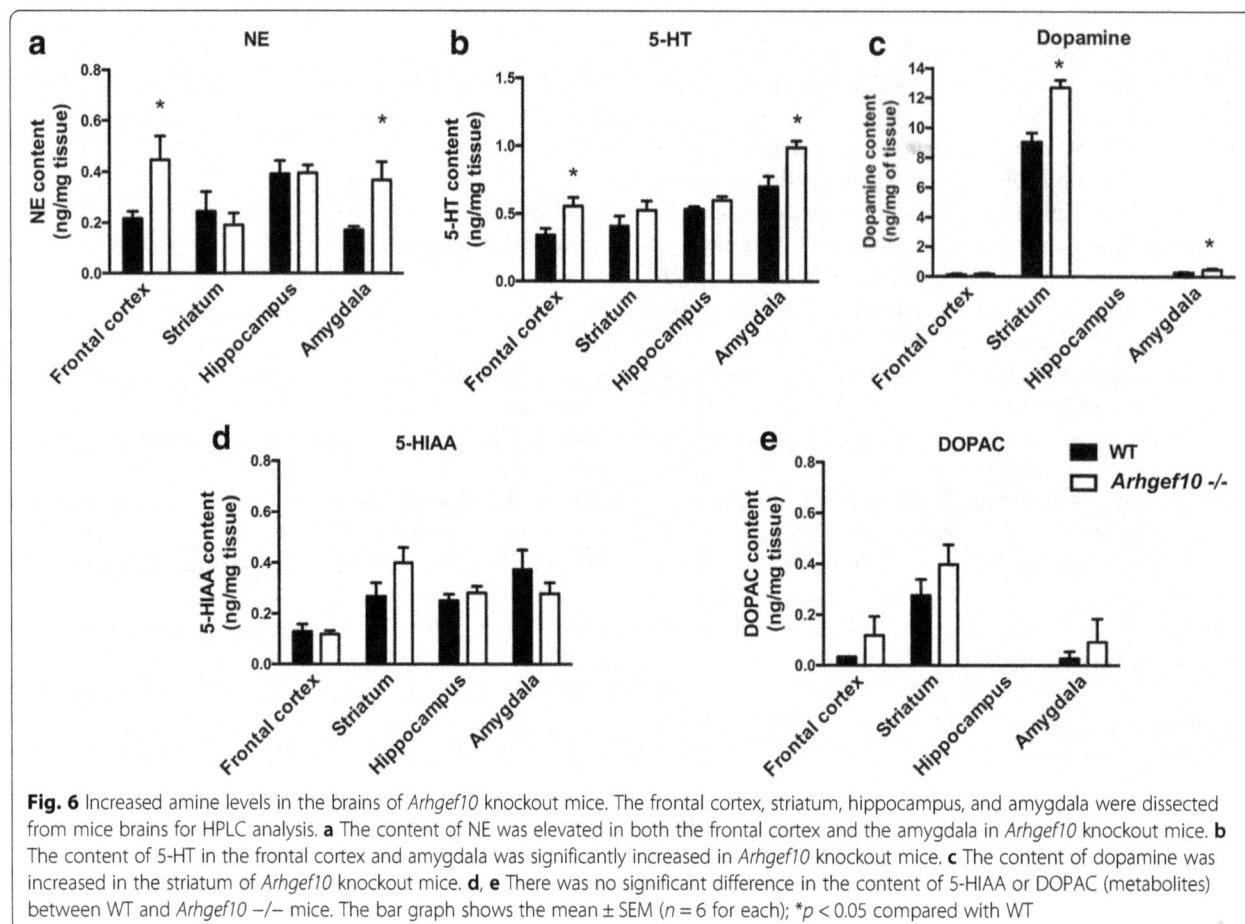

Fig. 6 Increased amine levels in the brains of *Arhgef10* knockout mice. The frontal cortex, striatum, hippocampus, and amygdala were dissected from mice brains for HPLC analysis. **a** The content of NE was elevated in both the frontal cortex and the amygdala in *Arhgef10* knockout mice. **b** The content of 5-HT in the frontal cortex and amygdala was significantly increased in *Arhgef10* knockout mice. **c** The content of dopamine was increased in the striatum of *Arhgef10* knockout mice. **d, e** There was no significant difference in the content of 5-HIAA or DOPAC (metabolites) between WT and *Arhgef10* −/− mice. The bar graph shows the mean ± SEM ($n = 6$ for each); $*p < 0.05$ compared with WT

11.57, $p = 0.0068$ and brain regions ($F_{3,\ 30} = 24.650$, $p < 0.0001$; interaction: $F_{3,\ 30} = 1.814$, $p = 0.1659$). Post hoc comparisons between WT and KO revealed significant differences in the frontal cortex and amygdala. Dopamine in the striatum was also increased in *Arhgef10* knockout mice compared with WT mice (two-way ANOVA for genotype × brain regions, main effect of genotype: $F_{1,\ 10} = 23.47$, $p = 0.0007$ and brain regions $F\ (3,\ 30) = 731.5$, $p < 0.0001$; interaction: $F_{3,\ 30} = 20.36$, $p < 0.0001$). Post hoc comparisons between WT and KO revealed a significant difference in the striatum (Fig. 6c). However, there were no differences in the metabolites of these monoamines between WT and *Arhgef10* knockout mice (Fig. 6d, e).

Reduction of MAO-A expression in *Arhgef10* knockout mice

Since NE and 5-HT levels were significantly elevated in *Arhgef10* knockout mice, we measured the expression of MAO-A and MAO-B, the key enzymes that degrade NE and 5-HT, in the corresponding brain areas using Western blotting. MAO-A levels between WT and *Arhgef10* knockout mice were evaluated by two-way ANOVA (two-way ANOVA for genotype × brain regions, main effect of genotype: $F_{1,\ 12} = 4.305$, $p = 0.0602$ and brain

regions $F_{3,\ 36} = 2.286$, $p = 0.0953$; interaction: $F_{3,\ 36} = 2.324$, $p = 0.0913$). Post hoc comparisons between WT and KO revealed significant differences in frontal cortex and amygdala. Further comparison of these differences found significantly reduced MAO-A levels in the frontal cortex and amygdala (Fig. 7a). In contrast with MAO-A levels, no statistically significant difference was found in MAO-B levels between WT and *Arhgef10* knockout mice (two-way ANOVA for genotype × brain regions, main effect of genotype: $F_{1,\ 4} = 3.163$, $P = 0.1499$ and brain regions $F_{3,\ 12} = 2.688$, $p = 0.0934$; interaction: $F_{3,\ 12} = 0.3990$, $p = 0.7563$) (Fig. 7b). Furthermore, we also examined the enzymes dopamine β-hydroxylase (DBH) and tryptophan hydroxylase (TPH), which are involved in the synthesis of NE and 5-HT, respectively. WT and *Arhgef10* knockout mice had similar protein levels of both DBH (two-way ANOVA for genotype × brain regions, main effect of genotype: $F_{1,\ 4} = 0.03559$, $p = 0.8595$ and brain regions $F_{3,\ 12} = 7.614$, $p = 0.0041$; interaction: $F_{3,\ 12} = 0.2854$, $p = 0.8350$) and TPH (two-way ANOVA for genotype × brain regions, main effect of genotype: $F_{1,\ 4} = 0.5692$, $p = 0.4926$ and brain regions $F_{3,\ 12} = 6.591$, $p = 0.0070$; interaction: $F_{3,\ 12} = 1.190$, $P = 0.3549$) in the tested brain regions (Fig. 7c, d).

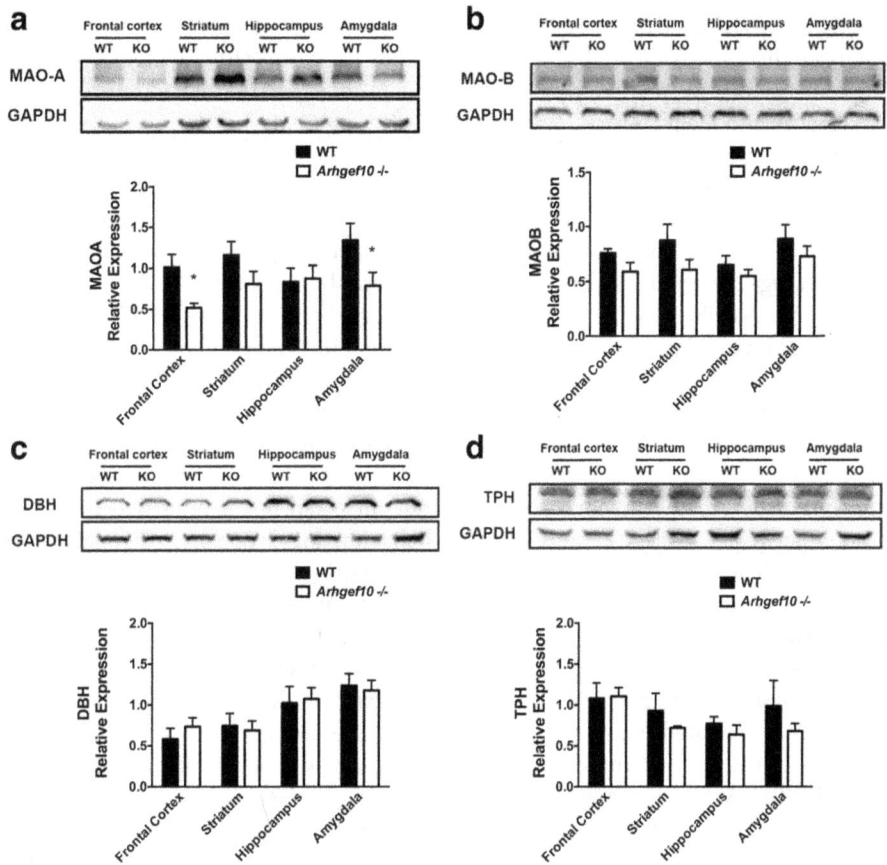

Fig. 7 MAO-A is decreased in *Arhgef10* $^{-/-}$ mice. The main degradation enzymes 5-HT and NE were analyzed by Western blotting. **a** MAO-A expression was decreased in the frontal cortex and amygdala of *Arhgef10* $^{-/-}$ mice. Another metabolizing enzyme, MOA-B, did not show a significant difference between WT and KO mice **b**. The main enzymes for the synthesis of the amine neurotransmitters were also analyzed by Western blotting. The protein levels of both DBH **c** and TPH **d** were similar between WT and KO mice in the examined brain areas. *$p < 0.05$ compared with WT. *MAO-A* monoamine oxidase A, *MAO-B* monoamine oxidase B, *DBH* dopamine β-hydroxylase, *TPH* tryptophan hydroxylase

Discussion

In a previous clinical study, we found a terminal deletion containing the gene *ARHGEF10* on chromosome 8 in autistic patients. The current study demonstrates that loss of function of *Arhgef10* leads to impairment of social behavior and altered mood-related behavior in mice. Importantly, *Arhgef10* knockout mice showed indifference toward the novel objects and stranger mice in the free social interaction assay, as well as a lack of preference between the novel mouse and the familiar mouse during the social recognition test. Overall, *Arhgef10* knockout mice displayed no preference between the empty chamber and stranger mouse 1 and showed no preference for social interaction with the novel mouse, stranger 2. These results indicate that ARHGEF10 deficiency might cause a deficit in social interaction and social recognition. Interestingly, although *Arhgef10* knockout mice stayed longer in the chamber with the first stranger mouse than the chamber with the second

stranger mouse (Fig. 2d), there was no difference in the time of social interaction between the two chambers containing stranger mice (Fig. 2e). These results suggest that *Arhgef10* knockout mice lacked interest in interaction with stranger mice. Moreover, *Arhgef10* knockout mice exhibited a decreased tendency to explore the area with the second mouse. This decreased tendency to investigate the area with a novel stranger mouse may correlate with an aloof character typical of autism. The reduced social interaction and lack of preference for social novelty observed in the three-chamber social behavior tests support our speculation that the deletion of ARHGEF10 might partly be correlated with clinical manifestations in individuals with ASD.

Several published observations have shown that children with ASD are at a high risk of anxiety disorders [21]. In this study, a reduced anxiety level was found in knockout mice, compared with WT mice, in the EPM test. *Arhgef10* knockout mice spent a longer duration in the open arms than WT mice, implying reduced anxiety-like behavior in *Arhgef10* knockout mice. Moreover, the reduced anxiety-like behavior in EPM could result from the decreased innate fear responses to elevated and open areas. Additionally, *Arhgef10* knockout mice entered the open arm more frequently than WT, which suggests *Arhgef10* deficiency did not affect the natural tendency to explore novel places. However, in the three-chamber test, the tendency to investigate the place with a novel stranger was reduced in *Arhgef10* knockout mice, indicating possible social withdrawal behavior. Although the finding of a lower level of anxiety in *Arhgef10* knockout mice is inconsistent with another reported autism-like mouse strains [22, 23], the reduced anxiety in *Arhgef10* knockout mice indicates that social interaction defects were not caused by anxiety-like behavior. The reduction of anxiety-like behavior strengthened the correlation between *Arhgef10* and social behavior and suggests the involvement of *Arhgef10* in anxiety-related behavior.

We further evaluated specific depression-like behavior using the FST and the TST, to verify that social deficits in *Arhgef10* knockout mice are not caused by depression-related effects. Compared with WT mice, *Arhgef10* knockout mice exhibited lower immobility time in the FST and the TST than WT mice, suggesting that *Arhgef10* KO reduces depression-like behavior. These results revealed that ARHGEF10 is also involved in the regulation of depression-like behavior. The lower levels of anxiety-like and depression-like behavior further demonstrated that the social traits in *Arhgef10* knockout mice were not the results of mood-related behavioral abnormalities. In addition, *Arhgef10* knockout mice exhibited enhanced locomotor activity in a novel open field, which might be a reflection of the hyperactivity that is often observed clinically in autistic patients. The features of hyperactivity have also been reported in other animal models of autism [24–26]. Although *Arhgef10* knockout mice displayed characteristic hyperactivity, the number of entries into each compartment was not increased in the three-chamber tests, indicating that the reduced social behavior was not a result of hyperactivity. When the results of social impairment and hyperactivity are taken together, the ASD-associated social inability observed in the *Arhgef10* deficiency mice appears not to result from low levels of spontaneous activity. The reduced anxiety-like behavior and hyperactivity phenotype observed in *Arhgef10* knockout mice may be a sign of increased impulsive behavior. We thus further evaluated impulsive behavior using the electro-foot shock aversive water drinking test (EFSDT) [27]. *Arhgef10* knockout mice displayed no obvious impulsive behaviors in comparison with WT mice (Additional file 2: Figure S2-2).

Although some studies suggest that autism features sensorimotor deficits [28], we did not find any PPI deficit in *Arhgef10* knockout mice. No abnormalities were found in the startle response or sensory gating, indicating that the *Arhgef10* knockout does not affect the sensory gating system in mice. Moreover, escape latencies were comparable between WT and *Arhgef10* knockout mice in the Morris water maze, suggesting that the deletion of ARHGEF10 does not impair spatial-learning-based behavior.

Social behavior can be affected by many behavioral factors, including anxiety levels, spontaneous activity, depression, sensory perception, memory, and cognition. *Arhgef10* knockout mice displayed normal sensorimotor responses in the PPI test and normal spatial learning behavior in the water maze. Moreover, *Arhgef10* knockout mice did not exhibit depression-like or anxiety-like behavior, suggesting that the social deficit was not confounded by these factors. Our study demonstrated that the loss of function of ARHGEF10 mainly caused social impairment in mice.

In this study, changes in neurotransmitter levels were observed as well. Serotonin and norepinephrine levels were significantly increased in the frontal cortex and amygdala of *Arhgef10* knockout mice. The amygdala has been implicated in various functions concerning emotion and social behavior. Several studies in primates and other mammalian species have implicated the amygdala as an important contributor to social behavior [29, 30]. Neonatal lesions of the amygdala in rats results in a social behavior deficit, and these rats exhibit autistic-like symptoms [31]. Furthermore, an early bilateral lesion of the amygdala in rhesus monkeys leads to reduced social interactions with other monkeys [32]. On the basis of the biological function of the amygdala, it is proposed to be one of the main regulatory brain regions driving the pathology of ASD [33]. Furthermore, the frontal cortex is the region responsible for emotion control and decision making and has been reported to be associated with the cognitive and anatomical abnormalities in patients with autism [34]. Based on the distinctive roles of the frontal cortex and amygdala in autism, the neurochemical changes in these brain regions may be linked to the observed phenomena in *Arhgef10* knockout mice. The neurochemical study of autism began with a report of changes in serotonin [35]. An elevated serotonin level in whole blood is a well-characterized biomarker in autism research [6]. Additionally, increased serotonin synthesis capacity has been reported in autistic children, suggesting that serotonin may play an important role in the development of autism [36]. The elevated serotonin levels found in the brains of *Arhgef10* knockout mice correlate with attenuated depression-like behaviors observed in the FST and the TST. These findings also support the role of the serotonin system in some autism patient symptoms. Apart from serotonin, norepinephrine is also an important monoamine associated with neuronal functions and levels of anxiety, arousal, and stress sensitivity, and many of these functions are also impaired in ASD. Evidence for involvement of norepinephrine in ASD comes from a report indicating that patients with autism and their families showed elevated plasma levels of NE and low enzyme activity [37]. The Angelman syndrome mouse model, which exhibits autistic-like behavior, shows increased norepinephrine and serotonin levels in different brain regions [23]. In addition, the elevated serotonin level in brain found in *Arhgef10* knockout mice can also explain their attenuated depression-like behaviors in the FST and the TST. The changes of serotonin and norepinephrine in the frontal cortex and amygdala indicate that ARHGEF10 might play a role in linking the phenotype of social impairment to the balance of monoamines. Therefore, the loss of homeostasis of serotonin and norepinephrine in the frontal cortex and amygdala of the *Arhgef10* knockout mice might be the basis of their autistic-like behaviors.

We sought to further understand the underlying mechanisms that contribute to the increased level of amine neurotransmitters. Therefore, we examined MAO-A and MOA-B, which are the key enzymes responsible for catalyzing the metabolism of monoamines, including serotonin and norepinephrine. In addition, the enzymes dopamine β-hydroxylase (DBH), and tryptophan hydroxylase (TPH), which are responsible for the synthesis of norepinephrine and serotonin, respectively, were also examined using Western blot. MAO-A was decreased in the frontal cortex and amygdala in *Arhgef10* knockout mice. However, the levels of DBH and TPH were comparable to those of WT littermates, indicating that the synthesis of the corresponding neurotransmitters was not affected by the *Arhgef10* knockout. The lower level of MAO-A may reduce the capacity for serotonin and NE degradation. The decreased MAO-A in *Arhgef10* knockout mice provides a possible explanation for the higher levels of serotonin and norepinephrine in the frontal cortex and amygdala. Recently, a study demonstrated that patients with autism had decreased MAO-A activity in the frontal cortex and cerebellum [38]. Moreover, mice lacking MAO-A displayed increased serotonin and norepinephrine levels and aggressive behavior [39]. Another knockout mouse lacking MAO-A/B also exhibited elevated serotonin levels and autistic-like features [40]. These previous reports support our findings in *Arhgef10* knockout mice, which implied that the reduced MAO-A levels and elevated amine levels might be the causes of social impairment. Although the phenotypes might result from changes in amine levels in the frontal cortex and amygdala, further study of the neurotransmitters and related molecules

that are regulated by ARHGEF10 is required to clarify the underlying mechanism.

Conclusion

In conclusion, this study demonstrated the behavioral and neurochemical changes of *Arhgef10* knockout mice. These mice exhibited social inability in the three-chamber test, reflecting the social impairment observed in humans with ASD. On the other hand, *ARHGEF10* knockout mice displayed hyperactivity in the locomotor test, reduced anxiety-like behavior in the EPM, and reduced depression-like behavior in the FST and TST. These behavioral changes further confirmed that the social deficits in *Arhgef10* knockout mice were not confounded by mood disorders. Moreover, neurochemical changes such as elevated serotonin and norepinephrine levels were also found in the frontal cortex and amygdala in *Arhgef10* knockout mice. Further analysis of MAO-A and MAO-B, the key enzymes that degrade norepinephrine and serotonin, revealed that the loss of function of ARHGEF10 decreased the expression of MAO-A in the frontal cortex and amygdala. These results suggest that *ARHGEF10* is a risk gene for ASD, especially correlated with the symptom of social activity impairment.

Abbreviations

5-HT: Serotonin; ARHGEF10: A rho guanine nucleotide exchange factor 10; ASD: Autism spectrum disorder; CNV: Copy number variation; DBH: Dopamine ß-hydroxylase; EFSDT: Electro-foot shock aversive water drinking test; EPM: Elevated plus maze; FST: Forced swimming test; GAPDH: Glyceraldehyde-3-phosphate dehydrogenase; GEF: Guanine nucleotide exchange factor; KO: Knockout; MAO-A: Monoamine oxidase A; MAO-B: Monoamine oxidase B; NE: Norepinephrine; PPI: Pre-pulse inhibition; TPH: Tryptophan hydroxylase; TST: Tail suspension test; WT: Wild-type

Acknowledgements
Not applicable

Funding
This work was supported by the National Science Council (NSC 99-3112-B-002-036 and NSC 101-2314-B-002-136-MY3), Taiwan, National Taiwan University (AIM for Top University Excellent Research Project, 10R81918-03,101R892103, 102R892103, 103R892103), and Ministry of Science and Technology (MOST 105-2321-B-002-020), Taiwan. We thank the technical services provided by the Transgenic Mouse Model Core Facility of the National Core Facility Program for Biotechnology, the National Science Council, and the Gene Knockout Mouse Core Laboratory of National Taiwan University Center for Genomic Medicine.

Authors' contributions

SS-FG initiated this research. SS-FG, H-ML, and C-HC generated and verified the mutant mice. D-HL and W-MF designed the experiments in this paper. D-HL, H-JT, and H-CL performed the experiments. D-HL analyzed the data. D-HL, H-ML, W-MF, and SS-FG interpreted the results. D-HL drafted the manuscript. H-ML, W-MF, and SS-FG revised the manuscript. SS-FG and W-MF supervised the studies and edited the manuscript for resubmission. All the authors approved the final version of the manuscript.

Competing interests

The authors declare no competing finance interests.

Author details

[1]Pharmacological Institute, College of Medicine, National Taiwan University, Taipei, Taiwan. [2]Department of Psychiatry, National Taiwan University Hospital and College of Medicine, Taipei, Taiwan. [3]Department of Psychiatry, Chang Gung Memorial Hospital Linkou, Taoyuan, Taiwan. [4]Department and Graduate Institute of Biomedical Sciences, Chang Gung University, Taoyuan, Taiwan.

References

1. American Psychiatric Association. Diagnostic and statistical manual of mental disorders. Fifth ed. Arlington: American Psychiatric Association; 2013.
2. Yin CL, Chen HI, Li LH, Chien YL, Liao HM, Chou MC, et al. Genome-wide analysis of copy number variations identifies PARK2 as a candidate gene for autism spectrum disorder. Mol Autism. 2016;7:23. https://doi.org/10.1186/s13229-13016-10087-13227. eCollection 12016
3. Werling DM, Geschwind DH. Sex differences in autism spectrum disorders. Curr Opin Neurol. 2013;26:146–53.
4. Baxter AJ, Brugha TS, Erskine HE, Scheurer RW, Vos T, Scott JG. The epidemiology and global burden of autism spectrum disorders. Psychol Med. 2015;45:601–13.
5. Lyall K, Croen L, Daniels J, Fallin MD, Ladd-Acosta C, Lee BK, et al. The Changing Epidemiology of Autism Spectrum Disorders. Annu Rev Public Health. 2017;38:81-102.
6. Ruggeri B, Sarkans U, Schumann G, Persico AM. Biomarkers in autism spectrum disorder: the old and the new. Psychopharmacology. 2014;231:1201–16.
7. Chien WH, Gau SS, Wu YY, Huang YS, Fang JS, Chen YJ, et al. Identification and molecular characterization of two novel chromosomal deletions associated with autism. Clin Genet. 2010;78:449–56.
8. Jiang-Xie LF, Liao HM, Chen CH, Chen YT, Ho SY, Lu DH, et al. Autism-associated gene Dlgap2 mutant mice demonstrate exacerbated aggressive behaviors and orbitofrontal cortex deficits. Mol Autism. 2014;5:32. https://doi.org/10.1186/2040-2392-1185-1132. eCollection 2014
9. Chien WH, Gau SS, Liao HM, Chiu YN, Wu YY, Huang YS, et al. Deep exon resequencing of DLGAP2 as a candidate gene of autism spectrum disorders. Mol Autism. 2013;4:26. https://doi.org/10.1186/2040-2392-1184-1126.
10. Verhoeven K, De Jonghe P, Van de Putte T, Nelis E, Zwijsen A, Verpoorten N, et al. Slowed conduction and thin myelination of peripheral nerves associated with mutant rho Guanine-nucleotide exchange factor 10. Am J Hum Genet. 2003;73:926–32.
11. Jungerius BJ, Hoogendoorn ML, Bakker SC, Van't Slot R, Bardoel AF, Ophoff RA, et al. An association screen of myelin-related genes implicates the chromosome 22q11 PIK4CA gene in schizophrenia. Mol Psychiatry. 2008;13:1060–8.
12. Stankiewicz TR, Linseman DA. Rho family GTPases: key players in neuronal development, neuronal survival, and neurodegeneration. Front Cell Neurosci. 2014;8:314.
13. Kutsche K, Yntema H, Brandt A, Jantke I, Nothwang HG, Orth U, et al. Mutations in ARHGEF6, encoding a guanine nucleotide exchange factor for Rho GTPases, in patients with X-linked mental retardation. Nat Genet. 2000;26:247–50.
14. Lam KS, Aman MG, Arnold LE. Neurochemical correlates of autistic disorder: a review of the literature. Res Dev Disabil. 2006;27:254–89.
15. Tassone F, Qi L, Zhang W, Hansen RL, Pessah IN, Hertz-Picciotto I. MAOA, DBH, and SLC6A4 variants in CHARGE: a case-control study of autism spectrum disorders. Autism Res. 2011;4:250–61.
16. Chakraborti B, Verma D, Karmakar A, Jaiswal P, Sanyal A, Paul D, et al. Genetic variants of MAOB affect serotonin level and specific behavioral attributes to increase autism spectrum disorder (ASD) susceptibility in males. Prog Neuro-Psychopharmacol Biol Psychiatry. 2016;71:123–36.
17. Kadar A, Wittmann G, Liposits Z, Fekete C. Improved method for combination of immunocytochemistry and Nissl staining. J Neurosci Methods. 2009;184:115–8.
18. Moy SS, Nadler JJ, Perez A, Barbaro RP, Johns JM, Magnuson TR, et al. Sociability and preference for social novelty in five inbred strains: an approach to assess autistic-like behavior in mice. Genes Brain Behav. 2004;3:287–302.
19. Li J, Chai A, Wang L, Ma Y, Wu Z, Yu H, et al. Synaptic P-Rex1 signaling regulates hippocampal long-term depression and autism-like social behavior. Proc Natl Acad Sci U S A. 2015;112:E6964–72.
20. Cryan JF, Markou A, Lucki I. Assessing antidepressant activity in rodents: recent developments and future needs. Trends Pharmacol Sci. 2002;23:238–45.
21. van Steensel FJ, Bogels SM, Perrin S. Anxiety disorders in children and adolescents with autistic spectrum disorders: a meta-analysis. Clin Child Fam Psychol Rev. 2011;14:302–17.
22. McFarlane HG, Kusek GK, Yang M, Phoenix JL, Bolivar VJ, Crawley JN. Autism-like behavioral phenotypes in BTBR T+tf/J mice. Genes Brain Behav. 2008;7:152–63.
23. Farook MF, DeCuypere M, Hyland K, Takumi T, LeDoux MS, Reiter LT. Altered serotonin, dopamine and norepineperine levels in 15q duplication and Angelman syndrome mouse models. PLoS One. 2012;7:e43030.
24. Penagarikano O, Abrahams BS, Herman EI, Winden KD, Gdalyahu A, Dong H, et al. Absence of CNTNAP2 leads to epilepsy, neuronal migration abnormalities, and core autism-related deficits. Cell. 2011;147:235–46.
25. Radyushkin K, Hammerschmidt K, Boretius S, Varoqueaux F, El-Kordi A, Ronnenberg A, et al. Neuroligin-3-deficient mice: model of a monogenic heritable form of autism with an olfactory deficit. Genes Brain Behav. 2009;8:416–25.
26. Schmeisser MJ, Ey E, Wegener S, Bockmann J, Stempel AV, Kuebler A, et al. Autistic-like behaviours and hyperactivity in mice lacking ProSAP1/Shank2. Nature. 2012;486:256–60.
27. Yang MT, Lu DH, Chen JC, Fu WM. Inhibition of hyperactivity and impulsivity by carbonic anhydrase inhibitors in spontaneously hypertensive rats, an animal model of ADHD. Psychopharmacology. 2015;232:3763–72.
28. Perry W, Minassian A, Lopez B, Maron L, Lincoln A. Sensorimotor gating deficits in adults with autism. Biol Psychiatry. 2007;61:482–6.
29. Amaral DG. The amygdala, social behavior, and danger detection. Ann N Y Acad Sci. 2003;1000:337–47.
30. Adolphs R, Tranel D, Damasio AR. The human amygdala in social judgment. Nature. 1998;393:470–4.
31. Diergaarde L, Gerrits MA, Stuy A, Spruijt BM, van Ree JM. Neonatal amygdala lesions and juvenile isolation in the rat: differential effects on locomotor and social behaviour later in life. Behav Neurosci. 2004;118:298–305.
32. Moadab G, Bliss-Moreau E, Bauman MD, Amaral DG. Early amygdala or hippocampus damage influences adolescent female social behavior during group formation. Behav Neurosci. 2017;131:68–82.
33. Baron-Cohen S, Ring HA, Bullmore ET, Wheelwright S, Ashwin C, Williams SC. The amygdala theory of autism. Neurosci Biobehav Rev. 2000;24:355–64.
34. Carper RA, Courchesne E. Inverse correlation between frontal lobe and cerebellum sizes in children with autism. Brain. 2000;123(Pt 4):836–44.
35. Schain RJ, Freedman DX. Studies on 5-hydroxyindole metabolism in autistic and other mentally retarded children. J Pediatr. 1961;58:315–20.
36. Chugani DC. Role of altered brain serotonin mechanisms in autism. Mol Psychiatry. 2002;7(Suppl 2):S16–7.
37. Lake CR, Ziegler MG, Murphy DL. Increased norepinephrine levels and decreased dopamine-beta-hydroxylase activity in primary autism. Arch Gen Psychiatry. 1977;34:553–6.
38. Gu F, Chauhan V, Chauhan A. Monoamine oxidase-A and B activities in the cerebellum and frontal cortex of children and young adults with autism. J Neurosci Res. 2017;95:1965-1972.

Risk markers for suicidality in autistic adults

Sarah Cassidy[1,2,3*] ⓘ, Louise Bradley[2], Rebecca Shaw[2,4] and Simon Baron-Cohen[3,5]

Abstract

Background: Research has shown high rates of suicidality in autism spectrum conditions (ASC), but there is lack of research into *why* this is the case. Many common experiences of autistic adults, such as depression or unemployment, overlap with known risk markers for suicide in the general population. However, it is unknown whether there are risk markers unique to ASC that require new tailored suicide prevention strategies.

Methods: Through consultation with a steering group of autistic adults, a survey was developed aiming to identify unique risk markers for suicidality in this group. The survey measured suicidality (SBQ-R), non-suicidal self-injury (NSSI-AT), mental health problems, unmet support needs, employment, satisfaction with living arrangements, self-reported autistic traits (AQ), delay in ASC diagnosis, and 'camouflaging' ASC. One hundred sixty-four autistic adults (65 male, 99 female) and 169 general population adults (54 males, 115 females) completed the survey online.

Results: A majority of autistic adults (72%) scored above the recommended psychiatric cut-off for suicide risk on the SBQ-R; significantly higher than general population (GP) adults (33%). After statistically controlling for a range of demographics and diagnoses, ASC diagnosis and self-reported autistic traits in the general population significantly predicted suicidality. In autistic adults, non-suicidal self-injury, camouflaging, and number of unmet support needs significantly predicted suicidality.

Conclusions: Results confirm previously reported high rates of suicidality in ASC, and demonstrate that ASC diagnosis, and self-reported autistic traits in the general population are independent risk markers for suicidality. This suggests there are unique factors associated with autism and autistic traits that increase risk of suicidality. Camouflaging and unmet support needs appear to be risk markers for suicidality unique to ASC. Non-suicidal self-injury, employment, and mental health problems appear to be risk markers shared with the general population that are significantly more prevalent in the autistic community. Implications for understanding and prevention of suicide in ASC are discussed.

Keywords: Autism spectrum condition, Autistic traits, Suicidality, Non-suicidal self-injury, NSSI, SBQ-R, NSSI-AT, Risk markers, Mental health, Depression, Anxiety

Background

There are elevated rates of suicidality in adults diagnosed with autism spectrum conditions (ASC) [1–5]. However, suicidality in ASC is poorly understood, and there is a paucity of research exploring *why* adults with ASC (henceforth, autistic adults) may be at increased risk [6]. Although a number of studies have explored suicidality in autistic adults, no study has yet utilised a suicidality assessment tool with evidence of validity [4, 7, 8]. Non-suicidal self-injury (NSSI) is a risk factor for

suicide attempts in the general population [9]. However, to our knowledge, only one study has ever explored NSSI in a small sample of autistic adults using a validated instrument but did not explore associations with suicidality [10]. Clearly, it is crucial to better understand suicidality in autistic adults, and associated risk markers, using instruments with evidence of validity (albeit not yet in autistic adults). Given the paucity of literature in the area of suicide in ASC research, it is important to engage with the autistic community in the refinement of research priorities to speed up progress and benefit the end users of research [11]. This is the aim of the current study.

Suicidal thoughts and behaviours are significantly increased in autistic adults compared to the general population and other clinical groups. In a large sample of 374 adults newly diagnosed with Asperger syndrome

* Correspondence: Sarah.Cassidy@Nottingham.ac.uk
[1]School of Psychology, University of Nottingham, University Park, Nottingham NG7 2RD, UK
[2]Centre for Innovative Research across the Life Course, Coventry University, Coventry, UK
Full list of author information is available at the end of the article

(AS; autism without language delay or intellectual disability), 66% had contemplated suicide, significantly higher than the general population (17%) and patients with psychosis (59%); 35% had planned or attempted suicide [2], higher than previous estimates of attempted suicide in general and university populations (2.5–10%) [12–14]. Only one study has ever explored whether autistic people are more at risk of dying by suicide than the general population; this population study in Sweden showed that autistic people were significantly more likely to die by suicide (0.31%) compared to the general population (0.04%) [15].

Traits characteristic of autism are also significantly associated with suicidality in those with [2], and without ASC diagnosis [16–18]. ASC diagnosis has also recently been found to be an independent risk marker for suicide attempts independent of demographic characteristics and co-occurring diagnoses [19]. These findings suggest that ASC explains additional variance in suicidality, not accounted for by other well-known risk markers in the general population which are more prevalent in ASC, such as depression [20–22] or social isolation [23, 24], which have been associated with increased risk of suicidality in ASC [2, 15, 17, 25, 26]. Hence, there may be as yet unknown unique risk markers for suicidality in ASC that are not shared with the general population or other clinical groups, requiring adapted suicide prevention strategies [6].

Studies exploring the characteristics of suicidality in ASC could provide important clues for possible unique risk markers in this group. For example, the highest rates of suicidal ideation (66%) were reported in adults newly diagnosed with AS, who had struggled without support [2]. Age of diagnosis and adequate access to post-diagnostic support could therefore be particularly important in preventing suicidality in ASC [2]. However, many children and adults diagnosed with ASC not only struggle to obtain their diagnosis, but also struggle to obtain post-diagnostic support [27–29]. Lack of tangible social support has been associated with increased risk of suicidality, indirectly through depression [25].

In the general population, the global male to female ratio of deaths by suicide is estimated to be 1.7 [30], indicating that males are more likely to die by suicide than females. However, in the one available study exploring death by suicide in the autistic community, autistic females without intellectual disability (ID) were more at risk of dying by suicide (0.32%) compared to autistic males (0.3%); opposite to the general population where males (0.05%) were more likely to die by suicide than females (0.03%) [15]. Autistic females have been under-researched, and it has been recognised that this group may also be under-diagnosed [29, 31, 32]. Autistic people report attempting to camouflage their ASC in order to try and fit in in social situations, which may delay obtaining a timely ASC diagnosis and negatively affect their mental

health [31–33]. However, no study has quantitatively measured associations between 'camouflaging' and risk of mental health difficulties or suicidality in both autistic males and females.

In addition to lack of research into possible autism specific risk markers for suicidality, some potentially common risk factors for suicidality in those with and without ASC diagnosis have very different conceptualisations that have resulted in them being overlooked by researchers and clinicians. For example, self-injurious behaviour in ASC [34] is conceptualised rather differently than NSSI in the general population, as primarily a restricted and repetitive behaviour characteristic of ASC [35]. By contrast NSSI in the general population is considered a possible risk marker for later suicide attempts [9]. Only one study has explored NSSI in autistic adults without co-occurring ID using a tool validated for online research in non-clinical populations [10] (non-suicidal self-injury assessment tool (NSSI-AT)) [36]. The rate of NSSI in ASC was elevated (50%) compared to college students (17%) and adult community samples (23%), but the phenomenology of NSSI was broadly similar between those with and without ASC [10]. Importantly, this suggests that NSSI could be more prevalent in ASC than that in the general population, and could potentially be a previously unexplored common risk factor for suicidality in ASC and the general population.

Previous research has taken a piecemeal approach to furthering our understanding of suicidality in ASC. Important limitations include the fact that no suicidality studies in ASC have used a suicidality assessment tool with evidence of validity in this group [7, 8], and very few studies have included a comparison group [3]. Studies have also failed to disentangle common shared and unique risk markers for suicidality in autistic and general populations, which is key to understanding and preventing suicide in ASC [6].

The current study thus aimed to address these pitfalls in previous suicidality in ASC research. First, we used both a review of the available literature, and consultation with a steering group of autistic adults who have experienced suicidality, to ensure that we identified a range of high priority risk markers for suicidality in autism, some of which may be unique to this group. Second, we are the first to utilise a well-validated suicidality assessment tool (the Suicide Behaviours Questionnaire-Revised (SBQ-R)) [37] in autistic adults (confirmed in a systematic review) [7], and NSSI assessment tool previously utilised in autistic adults (NSSI-AT) [10]. We also include a general population comparison group. Hence, we are able to explore whether autistic adults are at increased risk of suicidality compared to the general population, while controlling for known common risk factors for suicidality (e.g. age, sex, mental health problems, employment, living situation). We also explore for the first time a potentially unique risk marker for suicidality and NSSI in ASC males and ASC females—camouflaging ASC in order to cope in social situations—as well as age of ASC diagnosis, and unmet support needs. We also explore whether NSSI is an independent risk marker for suicidality in those with and without ASC, and whether autistic traits are an independent risk marker for suicidality in the general population without ASC diagnosis.

Method
Participants
The ASC group comprised 164 adults (65 males; 99 females) who self-reported a diagnosis of ASC from a trained clinician, and a majority (81.1%) confirmed the clinic where this diagnosis was obtained. The general population group comprised 169 adults (54 males; 115 females). Participants were aged between 20 and 60 years old (Table 1). There were no significant differences in age ($t(331) = .657$, $p = .511$) or sex ratio ($\chi^2 (1) = 2.14$, $p = .14$) between the ASC and general population group. The ASC group scored significantly higher on the Autism-Spectrum Quotient (AQ) (36.42) than the general population group (19.87) ($t(331) = .657$, $p < .001$). See Table 1 for group demographics.

Participants were recruited from research volunteers databases located in the Autism Research Centre at the University of Cambridge. Autistic adults and their family members across the UK and internationally register in the Cambridge Autism Research Database (CARD) (https://www.autismresearchcentre.net/). General population adults without an autism diagnosis or autistic family members register at a separate website (https://www.cambridgepsychology.com/login). Volunteers register in these databases to receive information about a variety of psychology research projects and not mental health specifically. Additionally, participants were recruited from online adverts.

Measures
Survey development
An online questionnaire exploring mental health, self-injury, and thoughts of ending life was developed for the current study in partnership with a steering group of eight adults diagnosed with ASC (6 females, 2 males) through a series of 6 focus groups. Given the topic of the survey, all steering group members were recruited by advertising for autistic adults who would like to share their experience to influence research and improve support for mental health problems, self-injury, and suicidality. The first three focus groups developed the topics to be captured in the questionnaire. First, the researchers proposed a number of topics thought to be important contributors to mental health and suicidality in autism, and the focus group fed back on the relevance and importance of these proposed topics, and whether any important topics were missing. This ensured that a large array of possible risk markers was prioritised for the study. Subsequent focus groups discussed participants' experiences of the topics. The researchers then developed a survey to capture these topics and experiences. The steering group provided feedback on three drafts of the survey to ensure that the questions were comprehensive, relevant, and clear.

Demographics
Participants who completed the online survey provided information on age, biological birth sex, education, employment, living situation, diagnosed developmental and mental health conditions, current medication, whether they were currently receiving any treatment for mental health problems, suicidal thoughts, self-injury or other reason. Participants also reported whether they need or currently receive support, and if yes, were asked (a) in which areas they would ideally like support in (in the home, with employment, health care, mental health care, finance, social activities, in the community, organisation, mentoring, education, other); and (b) in which of these areas they actually receive support. Unmet support needs were thus calculated as the mismatch between the number of areas participants actually received support, compared to the number of areas participants would ideally like support (unmet support needs = n areas support ideally liked—n areas support actually received) (Table 1).

Camouflaging
A brief set of four questions were designed to quantify tendency to camouflage in the current study. Autistic adults were asked "Have you ever tried to camouflage or mask your characteristics of ASC to cope with social situations? For example, have you ever tried to copy or mimic other people's behaviour to try and fit in (e.g. copying another person's accent or mannerisms), or tried to mask or hide your symptoms of ASC from other people?" If participants responded yes, they subsequently (a) specified the areas in which they camouflage (work, educational settings, social gatherings, when visiting the doctors, when visiting a health professional, at home, with friends, other); (b) the overall frequency they camouflage on a scale from 1 (never) to 6 (always (over 90% of social situations)); and (c) overall amount of the day they spend camouflaging on a scale from 1 (none of my waking time) to 6 (all of my waking time (over 90% of social situations)). Scores were calculated as the sum of number of areas (maximum 8), overall frequency (maximum 6), and overall amount (maximum 6), with a maximum score of 20 overall. Internal consistency for the whole scale was acceptable in the ASC group ($\alpha = .75$).

Table 1 Participant characteristics

Variables	Group			
	GP male (*n* = 54) Mean (SD)/*n* (%)	GP female (*n* = 115)	ASC male (*n* = 65)	ASC female (*n* = 99)
Age	39.11 (10.09)	41.48 (11.18)	41.52 (11.73)	38.89 (10.47)
AQ total score	22.96 (8.56)	18.43 (7.12)	35.38 (7.5)	37.1 (8.33)
Age diagnosed with ASC	–	–	34.55 (14.75)	35.06 (11.83)
% Lifetime 'camouflage'	–	–	58 (89.2)	90 (90.9)
Camouflage total score	–	–	12.9 (4.06)	14.7 (3.61)
% Non-suicidal self-injury	18 (33.3)	32 (28.1)	35 (53.8)	71 (74)
Suicidality				
SBQ-R total score	7.48 (3.7)	6.36 (3.08)	10.14 (3.99)	10.56 (3.98)
% ≥ general population cut off	27 (50)	49 (42.6)	52 (80)	79 (79.8)
% ≥ psychiatric population cut-off	22 (40.7)	35 (30.4)	45 (69.2)	73 (73.7)
% Lifetime suicide attempt	7 (13)	7 (6.1)	21 (32.3)	42 (42.4)
ASC subtype				
HFA/AS	–	–	51 (78.5)	85 (85.9)
Autism/classic autism	–	–	0 (0)	2 (2)
ASC	–	–	7 (10.8)	7 (6.9)
PDD/PDD-NOS	–	–	1 (1.5)	1 (1)
Other	–	–	6 (9.2)	4 (4)
Education type				
Mainstream	53 (98.1)	113 (98.3)	59 (98.1)	88 (88.9)
Home	1 (1.9)	2 (1.7)	1 (1.5)	2 (2)
Special	0 (0)	0 (0)	3 (4.6)	4 (4)
Private/boarding	0 (0)	0 (0)	2 (3.1)	5 (5.1)
Support				
Need/receive support	16 (29.6)	36 (31.3)	51 (78.5)	75 (76.5)
Unmet support needs*	2.12 (1.78)	1.3 (1.47)	3.1 (2.44)	3.43 (2.25)
Treatment				
Current treatment (total)	28 (51.9)	60 (53.1)	51 (78.5)	77 (77.8)
For mental health	27 (93.1)	51 (76.1)	44 (77.2)	71 (76.3)
For suicidal thoughts	9 (31)	8 (11.9)	14 (24.6)	25 (26.9)
For self-injury	3 (10.3)	2 (3)	4 (7)	9 (9.7)
Other	2 (6.9)	6 (9)	8 (14)	14 (14)
Living arrangements				
Living independently	15 (27.8)	26 (22.6)	18 (27.7)	30 (30.3)
Living with parents	5 (9.3)	5 (4.3)	15 (23.1)	15 (15.2)
Living with flatmate(s)	4 (7.4)	8 (7)	2 (3.1)	3 (3)
Live with friend(s)	0 (0)	3 (2.6)	1 (1.5)	0 (0)
Living with a partner and/or dependent(s)	29 (53.7)	71 (61.7)	21 (32.3)	44 (44.4)
Living in supported accommodation	0 (0)	0 (0)	2 (3.1)	1 (1)
Living with a carer	0 (0)	0 (0)	1 (1.5)	1 (1)
Other	1 (1.9)	2 (1.7)	5 (7.7)	5 (5.1)
Occupational status				
Employed	41 (75.9)	94 (81.7)	30 (46.2)	51 (51.5)

Table 1 Participant characteristics *(Continued)*

Variables	Group			
	GP male (*n* = 54)	GP female (*n* = 115)	ASC male (*n* = 65)	ASC female (*n* = 99)
	Mean (SD)/*n* (%)			
Volunteering	2 (3.7)	6 (5.2)	3 (4.6)	9 (9.1)
Student	5 (9.3)	6 (5.2)	6 (9.2)	15 (15.2)
Unemployed/unable to work	4 (7.4)	9 (7.8)	25 (38.5)	22 (22.2)
Retired	2 (33.3)	0 (0)	1 (1.5)	2 (2)
Mental health or other condition				
≥1 mental health or other condition	29 (53.7)	66 (57.4)	51 (78.5)	92 (92.9)
Current medication for mental health condition	10 (34.5)	26 (39.4)	26 (51)	56 (60.9)
Depression	25 (46.3)	51 (44.3)	47 (72.3)	84 (84.8)
Anxiety	19 (35.2)	42 (36.5)	40 (61.5)	77 (77.8)
Obsessive compulsive disorder	0 (0)	3 (2.6)	7 (10.8)	17 (17.2)
Bipolar disorder	1 (1.9)	2 (1.7)	2 (1.7)	6 (3.7)
Personality disorder	1 (1.9)	4 (3.5)	5 (7.7)	18 (18.2)
Schizophrenia	0 (0)	0 (0)	2 (3.1)	4 (4)
Anorexia nervosa	0 (0)	4 (3.5)	1 (1.5)	8 (8.1)
Bulimia	0 (0)	1 (0.9)	0 (0)	2 (2)
Myalgic encephalopathy	0 (0)	3 (2.6)	3 (4.6)	10 (10.1)
Tourettes	0 (0)	0 (0)	2 (3.1)	2 (2)
Epilepsy	1 (1.9)	4 (3.5)	1 (1.5)	4 (4)
Other	4 (7.4)	4 (3.5)	10 (15.4)	21 (21.2)
Developmental condition				
≥1 developmental condition	2 (3.7)	1 (0.9)	15 (23.1)	22 (22.2)
Dyspraxia	1 (1.9)	1 (0.9)	7 (3.9)	11 (11.1)
Learning disability	1 (0)	0 (0)	1 (1.5)	0 (0)
Learning difficulty	0 (0)	0 (0)	0 (0)	2 (2)
Dyscalculia	0 (0)	0 (0)	2 (31)	1 (1)
Dyslexia	2 (3.7)	0 (0)	5 (7.7)	8 (8.1)
Attention deficit hyperactivity disorder	0 (0)	0 (0)	2 (3.1)	9 (9.1)
Developmental delay	0 (0)	0 (0)	0 (0)	1 (1)
Other	0 (0)	1 (0.9)	2 (3.1)	4 (4)

NB, unmet support needs calculated by (total *n* areas support ideally liked—total *n* areas support actually received)

Autism-Spectrum Quotient (AQ)

The Autism-Spectrum Quotient (AQ) is a 50-item questionnaire assessing the number of self-reported autistic traits [38]. The AQ has been shown to reliably distinguishing those with and without a diagnosis of ASC [38, 39], with scores ≥ 26 indicating potential diagnosis of ASC [40].

Non-suicidal self-injury (NSSI)

The non-suicidal self-injury assessment tool (NSSI-AT) [36] was used to screen for presence of any form of lifetime NSSI in the current sample. Participants were first asked the screening question "Have you ever hurt your body (e.g. cut, carve, burn, scratch really hard, punch) on purpose but without wanting to end your life?" If yes, participants then completed sections A–B of the NSSI-AT to confirm that suicidality was not the primary reason for their self-harm. Subsequently, responses were classified as endorsing lifetime NSSI, or no lifetime NSSI.

The NSSI-AT was developed as a research tool to assess NSSI online in non-clinical populations and has previously been shown to have adequate measurement properties in college students; test-retest reliability for any form of NSSI was 0.74, with moderate correlations with related behavioural problems [36]. One study has previously used the NSSI-AT in an ASC adult sample and found evidence in support of similar phenomenology of NSSI in those with and without ASC [10].

Suicidality

Participants completed the Suicide Behaviours Questionnaire-Revised (SBQ-R) [37], a 4-item self-report questionnaire that assesses lifetime suicidal behaviour, suicide ideation over the past 12 months, threat of suicide attempt, and likelihood of suicidal behaviour in the future. The SBQ-R has been validated for use in general population and clinical samples to reliably distinguish suicide attempters from non-attempters [37], and is widely used in research, with moderate-strong evidence in support of internal consistency, structural validity, hypothesis testing, and criterion validity in clinical and non-clinical samples [7]. Internal consistency for the whole scale was acceptable in both autistic adults ($\alpha = .76$) and general population adults ($\alpha = .768$).

Ethical approval

The current study received ethical approval from Coventry University Psychology Ethics Committee and was approved by the autism steering group who fed back on the questionnaire, and the scientific advisory group at the Autism Research Centre, University of Cambridge, prior to recruiting participants registered in the Cambridge Autism Research Database (CARD).

Procedure

Participants with and without ASC diagnosis were invited to complete an online survey about understanding and preventing mental health problems, self-injury, and suicidality. Participants could take part regardless of prior experience of mental health difficulties, self-injury or suicidality. Participants read the participant information and indicated informed consent to participate via an online form. Participants were fully briefed about the nature of the research, that they could skip sections and/or questions that made them feel uncomfortable, and were provided information about relevant support services before and after taking part in the study. Participants subsequently completed questions on demographics, diagnoses (mental health, developmental conditions, and ASC), NSSI-AT, camouflaging, AQ, SBQ-R, current treatment (for mental health, self-injury, or suicidality), and support (areas in which support was actually received and ideally liked but not yet received).

Analysis approach

Data were analysed using SPSS 24. Chi-square analysis was used to explore group differences in frequency of lifetime NSSI, lifetime experience of camouflaging, and demographics, with odds ratios (with 95% confidence intervals) calculated as a measure of effect size. Independent samples t tests were used to compare total scores on the SBQ-R, AQ, and camouflaging questionnaires between groups, with Cohen's d as a measure of effect size (where

0.2 = small, 0.5 = medium, and 0.8 = large effect) [41]. One sample t tests compared SBQ-R total scores to established cut-offs in general and psychiatric populations. Spearman's correlations were used to explore inter-correlations between all variables in each group (where 0.1 = small, 0.3 = medium, and 0.5 = large effect). Multiple hierarchical regressions subsequently explored whether significant associations between demographics and diagnoses with suicidality remained when controlling for significant covariates.

The SBQ-R was non-normally distributed. Analyses were therefore undertaken using bootstrapping techniques, a robust analysis technique which is reliable even when assumptions of a symmetric distribution are not met [42]. Utilising this robust analysis technique did not alter the pattern of results, with similar direction and magnitude of effects and statistical significance found using bootstrapping or normal analytic approach; therefore, untransformed results are reported for ease of interpretation.

Results

Group comparisons

Suicidality

There was no significant difference in total SBQ-R scores between autistic males and autistic females ($t(162) = .671$, $p = .503$), so results were pooled. A one sample t test showed that autistic adults SBQ-R total scores were significantly higher than the recommended cut-off for the general population (7) ($t(163) = 10.92$, $p < .001$), and psychiatric populations (8) ($t(163) = 7.71$, $p < .001$) [33]. A majority (72%) of autistic adults scored at or above the cut-off for psychiatric populations (8) (Table 1).

There was a significant difference in total SBQ-R scores between general population (GP) males and females ($t(167) = 2.06$, $p = .041$), so data from males and females were analysed separately. One sample t tests showed that GP males SBQ-R scores were not significantly different from the recommended cut-off for the general ($t(53) = .956$, $p = .343$) or psychiatric population ($t(162) = .671$, $p = .503$). GP females scored significantly lower than the recommended cut off for the general ($t(114) = 2.211$, $p = .029$) and psychiatric population ($t(114) = 5.694$, $p < .001$) (Table 1).

Autistic adults scored significantly higher on the SBQ-R than GP adults ($t(331) = 9.131$, $p < .001$, $d = 1$) and were significantly more likely to score above the psychiatric cut-off for suicide risk (72%) than GP adults (33.7%) ($\chi^2(1) = 48.77$, $p < .001$, OR 5.04, 95% CI 3.16–8.04) (Table 1).

NSSI

Significantly more autistic females (74%) reported NSSI than autistic males (53.8%) ($\chi^2(1) = 6.97$, $p < .01$, OR 2.43, 95% CI 1.25–4.74). There was no significant sex difference in NSSI in the GP group ($\chi^2(1) = .486$, $p = .486$). Autistic adults were significantly more likely to report lifetime NSSI (65%) than GP adults (29.8%) ($\chi^2(1) = 42.91, p < .001$, OR 4.55, 95% CI 2.86–7.23) (Table 1).

Demographics

Compared to the general population, autistic adults reported significantly lower satisfaction with their living arrangements ($t(146) = 2.82, p = .005; d = .4$) were significantly more likely to be unemployed ($\chi^2(1) = 33.95, p < .001$, OR 4.07, 95% CI 2.5–6.61), be diagnosed with at least one co-occurring developmental condition ($\chi^2(1) = 34.02, p < .001$, OR 16.12, 95% CI 4.86–53.47), at least one mental health or other condition ($\chi^2(1) = 39.18, p < .001$, OR 5.3, 95% CI 3.06–9.19), depression ($\chi^2(1) = 43.1, p < .001$, OR 4.86, 95% CI 2.98–7.91), anxiety ($\chi^2(1) = 41.56, p < .001$, OR 4.41, 95% CI 2.78–6.99), and report higher unmet support needs ($t(176) = 4.91, p < .001; d = .87$) (Table 1).

Camouflaging

There was no significant difference between autistic males (89.2%) and autistic females (90.9%) in terms of whether they attempted to camouflage their ASC in order to fit in in social situations ($\chi^2(1) = .126, p = .723$). However, autistic females scored significantly higher on the camouflaging questionnaire overall (14.7, SD 3.61) than autistic males (12.9, SD 4.06) ($t(146) = 2.82, p = .005; d = .47$) (Table 1).

Predictors of suicidality in ASC

Table 2 shows the results of all inter correlations between variables in the ASC group. Lifetime NSSI, camouflaging, ADHD, depression, anxiety, unmet support needs, and satisfaction with living arrangements all significantly correlated with suicidality (total SBQ-R scores). However, age of diagnosis was not significantly correlated with any other variables.

Hierarchical regression models were performed with total SBQ-R scores as the outcome variable. To statistically control for these variables, age at testing and gender were entered into the first step, and employment, satisfaction with living arrangements, developmental conditions, depression, and anxiety entered into the second step. The third step explored additional variance accounted for by the predictor variable. Separate models explored the additional predictive contribution of ASC diagnosis (in the combined ASC and GP groups), lifetime experience of NSSI, camouflaging questionnaire total scores, and unmet support needs (in the ASC sub-group), to the model. Age of ASC diagnosis was not explored further as a unique predictor given that this did not significantly correlate with any other variables (Table 2).

ASC diagnosis

In step one, the regression model containing sex and age significantly predicted SBQ-R scores ($F(2,330) = 6.99, p < .001$), accounting for 4.1% of the variance. In step two, employment, satisfaction with living arrangements, presence of at least one developmental condition, depression, and anxiety accounted for significantly more of the variance (33.4%) in SBQ-R scores ($F(5,325) = 34.79, p < .001$). In step three, autism diagnosis accounted for significantly more of the variance (4.5%) in SBQ-R scores ($F(1,324) = 24.9, p < .001$) (Table 3).

NSSI

In step one, the regression model containing sex and age did not significantly predict SBQ-R scores ($F(2,158) = 1.99, p = .141$), accounting for only 2.5% of the variance. In step two, employment, satisfaction with living arrangements, presence of at least one developmental condition, depression, and anxiety accounted for significantly more of the variance (19.9%) in SBQ-R scores ($F(5,153) = 7.84, p < .001$). In step three, NSSI accounted for significantly more of the variance (4%) in SBQ-R scores ($F(1,152) = 6.78, p = .005$) (Table 4).

Camouflaging

In step one, the regression model containing sex and age did not significantly predict SBQ-R scores ($F(2,145) = .529, p = .59$), accounting for only 0.7% of the variance. In step two, employment, satisfaction with living arrangements, at least one developmental condition, depression, and anxiety accounted for significantly more of the variance (20.7%) in SBQ-R scores ($F(5,140) = 7.39, p < .001$). In step three, camouflaging total scores accounted for significantly more of the variance (3.5%) in SBQ-R scores ($F(1,139) = 6.56, p = .01$) (Table 5).

Unmet support needs

In step one, the regression model containing sex and age did not significantly predict SBQ-R scores ($F(2,123) = .233, p = .793$), accounting for only 0.4% of the variance. In step two, employment, satisfaction with living arrangements, at least one developmental condition, depression, and anxiety accounted for significantly more of the variance (13.5%) in SBQ-R scores ($F(5,118) = 3.7, p = .004$). In step three, unmet support needs accounted for significantly more of the variance (3.1%) in SBQ-R scores ($F(1,117) = 4.32, p = .04$) (Table 6).

Predictors of suicidality in the general population

Table 7 shows the results of all inter correlations between variables in the GP group. Self-reported autistic traits (AQ total scores), lifetime NSSI, depression, anxiety, satisfaction with living arrangements and employment all significantly correlated with suicidality (total SBQ-R scores).

Table 2 Means, standard deviations and inter-correlations for all variables in the ASC group

Variable	AQ	Age of ASC diagnosis	SBQ-R	NSSI	Lifetime camouflage	Camouflage score	Unmet support needs	≥1 developmental condition	ADHD	≥1 mental health/other condition	Depression	Anxiety	Satisfaction with living arrangements	Employed	Sex	Age at testing
AQ	–															
Age of ASC diagnosis	.147	–														
SBQ-R	.099	−.138	–													
NSSI	.126	−.125	.277*	–												
Lifetime camouflage	.053	−.048	.245*	.33*	–											
Camouflage score	.058	.107	.164*	.085	–	–										
Unmet support needs	.101	−.087	.247*	.109	.088	.085	–									
≥1 developmental condition	−.008	−.201*	.064	.009	.068	.073	−.023	–								
ADHD	−.02	−.113	.182*	.077	.088	.001	.058	.497*	–							
≥1 mental health/other condition	.259*	−.035	.365*	.188*	.182*	.112	.063	.032	.103	–						
Depression	.199*	.128	.322*	.088	.143	.076	−.035	−.093	−.048	.764*	–					
Anxiety	.161*	.012	.325*	.286*	.201*	.119	.079	.084	.062	.605	.59*	–				
Satisfaction with living arrangements	−.072	.081	−.257*	−.047	.003	.170*	−.386*	−.063	−.054	.034	.037	−.15	–			
Employed	−.174*	.023	−.114	.078	.037	.044	−.096	.021	.076	−.205*	−.143	−.102	.135	–		
Sex	.105	.105	.053	.208*	.028	.228*	.07	−.01	.118	.212*	.153	.176*	.212*	.052	–	
Age at testing	.104	.91*	−.137	−.152	−.073	.096	−.141	−.2*	−.134	−.017	.131	.028	.076	.03	−.117	–
Mean/%	36.42	34.85	10.4	64.63	90.2	13.99	3.29	22.5	6.7	87.19	79.88	71.34	68.47	28.66	39.63	39.93
SD	8.03	13.03	3.98	–	–	3.88	2.33	–	–	–	–	–	26.67	–	–	11.03

Note: AQ, Autism-Spectrum Quotient (total score); SBQ-R, Suicidal Behaviours Questionnaire-Revised (total score); *Lifetime camouflage*, attempting to camouflage autism in order to fit in in social situations; *Camouflage score*, total score on the camouflaging questionnaire; *Mismatch*, (*n* areas of support ideally liked – <u>n</u> areas actually received); *≥1 developmental condition*, at least one co-occurring developmental condition; *≥1 mental health/other condition*, at least one co-occurring mental health or other condition; *Sex*, % autistic male; *Age at testing*, age in years at testing. *Significant correlations *p* < .05

Table 3 Hierarchical regression with diagnostic group (ASC vs. general population) predicting SBQ-R

	B	SE B	β
Step 1			
Constant	12.408	1.135	
Sex	−.635	.460	− .074
Age	−.070	.020	− .188*
Step 2			
Constant	13.591	1.382	
Employed	−.768	.395	− .090
Satisfaction with living arrangements	−.045	.008	− .280*
≥1 developmental condition	.827	.567	.066
Depression	2.856	.482	.339*
Anxiety	.898	.474	.110
Step 3			
Constant	8.918	1.630	
Diagnostic group	2.038	.408	.249*

Note: R^2 = .041 for step 1, ΔR^2 = .334 for step 2, ΔR^2 = .045 for step 3 (p < .001).
*p < .001. N = 333

Table 5 Hierarchical regression with camouflaging total scores predicting SBQ-R in the ASC group

	B	SE B	β
Step 1			
Constant	11.139	1.730	
Sex	.335	.668	.042
Age at testing	− .024	.030	− .068
Step 2			
Constant	12.033	2.043	
Employed	− .291	.599	− .037
Satisfaction with living arrangements	− .045	.012	− .307*
≥ 1 developmental condition	.275	.736	.029
Depression	2.725	.971	.270*
Anxiety	.803	.850	.090
Step 3			
Constant	10.217	2.126	
Camouflage score	.200	.078	.198*

Note: R^2 = .006 for step 1, ΔR^2 = .207 for step 2, ΔR^2 = .035 for step 3 (p = .01).
*p < .01. N = 148

A hierarchical regression model was thus performed with total SBQ-R scores as the outcome variable. To statistically control for these variables, age at testing and gender were entered into the first step. To statistically control for additional co-variates, employment, satisfaction with living arrangements, developmental conditions, depression, and anxiety were entered into the second step. The third and final step explored much additional variance in suicidality was explained by self-reported autistic traits.

Autistic traits

In step one, the regression model containing sex and age significantly predicted SBQ-R scores ($F(2,166) = 7.57$, $p < .001$), accounting for 8.4% of the variance. In step two, employment, satisfaction with living arrangements, presence of at least one developmental condition, depression, and anxiety accounted for significantly more of the variance (31.5%) in SBQ-R scores ($F(5,161) = 16.85$, $p < .001$). In step three, self-reported autistic traits accounted for

Table 4 Hierarchical regressions with NSSI predicting SBQ-R in the ASC group

	B	SE B	β
Step 1			
Constant	12.283	1.661	
Sex	.153	.642	.019
Age at testing	− .055	.029	−.153
Step 2			
Constant	12.822	1.896	
Employed	− .261	.578	−.033
Satisfaction with living arrangements	− .037	.011	−.251*
≥ 1 developmental condition	− .194	.707	−.020
Depression	2.716	.903	.276*
Anxiety	.971	.809	.111
Step 3			
Constant	12.131	1.869	
NSSI	1.803	.631	.215*

Note: R^2 = .012 for step 1, ΔR^2 = .199 for step 2, ΔR^2 = .04 for step 3 (p = .005).
*p < .01. N = 161

Table 6 Hierarchical regression with unmet support needs predicting SBQ-R in the ASC group

	B	SE B	β
Step 1			
Constant	11.738	1.759	
Sex	.142	.718	.018
Age at testing	− .020	.032	− .058
Step 2			
Constant	11.296	2.148	
Employed	.060	.690	.008
Satisfaction with living arrangements	− .028	.012	− .204*
≥ 1 developmental condition	.032	.830	.003
Depression	2.771	1.089	.264*
Anxiety	.826	.963	.090
Step 3			
Constant	8.394	2.537	
Unmet support needs	.329	.158	.195*

Note: R^2 = .004 for step 1, ΔR^2 = .135 for step 2, ΔR^2 = .031 for step 3 (p = .04).
*p < .05. N = 126

Table 7 Means, standard deviations and inter-correlations for all variables in the general population group

Variable	AQ	SBQ-R	NSSI	Unmet support needs	≥ 1 developmental condition	≥ 1 mental health/other condition	Depression	Anxiety	Satisfaction with living arrangements	Employed	Sex	Age at testing
AQ	–											
SBQ-R	.329*	–										
NSSI	.009	.233*	–									
Unmet support needs	.277	.205	−.191	–								
≥ 1 developmental condition	.116	.097	.011	–	–							
≥ 1 mental health/ other condition	.168*	.373*	.132	.052	.028	–						
Depression	.232*	.432*	193*	.091	−.059	.798*	–					
Anxiety	.206*	.301*	194*	−.136	.008	.663	.559*	–				
Satisfaction with living arrangements	.136	−.487*	−.119	−.193	−.005	.212*	−.181	−.173*	–			
Employed	.149	.185*	.029	.392	.044	.175*	.169*	−.115	.118	–		
Sex	−.269*	−.157*	−.054	−.238	.1	−.035	−.018	.013	.238*	.068	–	
Age at testing	−.15	−.257*	−.23*	−.121	.087	.082	−.032	−.148	.312*	.121	.102	–
Mean/%	19.86	6.72	29.8	1.56	2.9	56.2	44.97	19.24	78.44	7.69	31.95	42.72
SD	7.87	3.32	–	1.6	–	–	–	–	23.16	–	–	10.87

Note: AQ, Autism-Spectrum Quotient (total score); SBQ-R, Suicidal Behaviours Questionnaire-Revised (total score); Mismatch, (n areas of support ideally liked −n areas actually received); ≥ 1 developmental condition; ≥ 1 mental health/other condition, at least one mental health or other condition; Sex, % male; Age at testing, age in years at testing. *Significant correlations p < .05

significantly more of the variance (3.2%) in SBQ-R scores ($F(1,160) = 9.08$, $p = .003$) (Table 8).

Discussion

Previous research exploring suicidality in ASC has failed to include adequately sized samples, matched comparison groups, explore risk or protective factors [2, 3, 6], or include validated suicidality assessment tools [7]. The current study aimed to address these weaknesses of previous research, to identify common and unique risk markers for suicidality in ASC. Specifically, whether there are unique aspects of ASC and autistic traits that increase risk of suicidality, after statistically controlling for common risk factors such as age, sex, employment, or mental health. We then explored possible unique risk factors which could explain increased risk of suicide in ASC, identified by our steering group of autistic adults: camouflaging one's ASC in an attempt to fit in in social situations, age of ASC diagnosis, whether people felt they received the support they required, and NSSI. Previous studies have not systematically studied unique and common risk markers for suicidality in ASC compared to the general population, which has prevented development of tailored suicide prevention strategies for this group [6].

Results are consistent with previous findings that autistic adults are at significantly increased risk of suicidality compared to the general population [2]. A majority (72%) of

autistic adults scored significantly above the recommended cut-off for suicide risk in psychiatric populations, significantly higher than general population adults (33%) with similar age and gender composition. This significant

Table 8 Hierarchical regressions with autistic traits predicting SBQ-R in the general population group

Autistic traits	B	SE B	β
Step 1			
Constant	11.335	1.244	
Sex	−.940	.530	−.132
Age	−.074	.023	−.244*
Step 2			
Constant	5.690	3.193	
Employed	−.561	.517	−.068
Satisfaction with living Arrangements	−.051	.010	−.357*
≥ 1 developmental condition	3.410	1.554	.136*
Depression	2.321	.501	.349*
Anxiety	.119	.517	.017
Step 3			
Constant	2.597	3.281	
Autistic traits	.083	.027	.196*

Note: $R^2 = .084$ for step 1, $\Delta R^2 = .315$ for step 2, $\Delta R^2 = .032$ for step 3 ($p = .003$). *p < .05. N = 169

association between ASC diagnosis and suicidality remained when controlling for a number of demographics and diagnoses, known to increase or decrease risk of suicidality in the general population (employment, depression, anxiety, and satisfaction with living arrangements). Additionally, the significant association between self-reported autistic traits in the general population and suicidality remained after statistically controlling for these demographics and diagnoses. These results suggest that autism diagnosis and autistic traits explain significant additional variance in suicidality beyond a range of known risk factors, and are therefore independent risk markers for suicidality. This is consistent with research showing that ASC diagnosis is an independent risk marker for suicide attempts when controlling for a range of demographics and co-occurring diagnoses [19]. These findings suggest additional unique contributors to suicidality in ASC, which must be addressed in addition to important well-known factors such as mental health, employment, and living arrangements.

The current study explored a potentially unique risk marker for suicidality in ASC, identified by our steering group of autistic adults: tendency to camouflage one's ASC in order to cope in social situations. Previous research [29, 32] and discussions with our steering group identified camouflaging as an important potential barrier to timely ASC diagnosis, and having a negative impact on mental health and risk of suicidality. Previous research has also suggested that camouflaging is primarily experienced by autistic females [31, 33], which may at least in part explain why this group has been under-diagnosed [43]. Results from the current study however showed subtle differences in camouflaging behaviour between autistic males and females: there was no sex difference in reporting whether one engages in camouflaging behaviour, but autistic females tended to report that they camouflaged across more situations, more frequently and more of the time than autistic males.

Camouflaging significantly predicted suicidality in the ASC group, after controlling for age, sex, presence of at least one developmental condition, depression, anxiety, employment, and satisfaction with living arrangements. Camouflaging and age of ASC diagnosis, and suicidality and age of ASC diagnosis were not significantly correlated. This suggests that camouflaging is directly associated with suicidality rather than in combination with delay in ASC diagnosis. Camouflaging also explained significant additional variance in suicidality above depression or anxiety, suggesting that the association with suicidality is, at least in part, independent of mental health. This is the first evidence of camouflaging being a unique independent risk factor for suicidality in ASC.

In order to engage in camouflaging, one must have insight into one's own difficulties, how these may be negatively perceived by others, and have a strong motivation to adapt one's social behaviour to be accepted. Understanding associations between these factors with camouflaging, and the consequent impact on mental health would be valuable. For example, autistic people who have greater insight into their own difficulties are more likely to be depressed than those with less insight [44], and autistic people are able to accurately predict how family members perceive them, despite being different to their own view [45]. It would be interesting to explore whether perspective taking ability and insight into one's own difficulties increase likelihood of engaging in camouflaging behaviour with consequent negative impact on mental health and suicidality.

Importantly, our findings challenge the assumption that autistic people are socially unmotivated, consistent with calls for more accurate and useful autism research, embracing the unique nature of social interest in autism [46]. It is perhaps more accurate to acknowledge a "double empathy problem", where autistic people are misinterpreted by non-autistic people and vice versa [45, 47, 48], which contribute to feelings of isolation among autistic people [49]. Increasing acceptance of autistic people in society could therefore lead to a reduced need for camouflaging and increased feelings of belonging—a protective factor for suicidality [17, 23].

Contrary to expectations, and discussions with our autistic steering group, age of ASC diagnosis was not significantly correlated with any other variables, such as mental health problems, suicidality, or NSSI. However, this may have been due to the fact that the mean age of ASC diagnosis was 34 years, and therefore, participants represent autistic people diagnosed in adulthood. Future research will need to explore whether those diagnosed in childhood are significantly less likely to experience mental health problems of suicidality compared to those diagnosed in adulthood. Another important theme identified from discussions with our steering group was lack of access to support, which could compound mental health difficulties and suicidality. Previous research has shown that the autistic community is disconnected from psychiatric services [18], as many practitioners are not trained in ASC [50]. The current study therefore quantitatively explored the mismatch between the number of areas an individual would ideally like support, compared to the number of areas they actually received support. These unmet support needs significantly predicted suicidality in the ASC group when controlling for the aforementioned variables. Hence, a clear recommendation for policy and practice to reduce suicide risk in autistic adults, a high-risk group for dying by suicide [15], is to urgently identify and address unmet support needs in this group. Meeting this shortfall in support could, at least in part, help reduce high rates of suicidality and death by suicide in the autistic community. Research from our group is exploring in more depth barriers and enablers in accessing treatment and support in autistic adults, to help assist in service planning.

The rate of NSSI in the ASC group (63.6%) was significantly higher than the general population group (29.8%), and similar to the rate reported in previous research [10] (50%), which also utilised the NSSI-AT in autistic adults. NSSI also significantly predicted suicidality in autistic adults, after controlling for a range of known risk factors. Hence, NSSI should not continue to be overlooked, or seen as part of ASC, and rather must be addressed in its own right. Our findings are therefore an important call to action for the research community and clinicians to increase understanding and support for those with ASC experiencing NSSI. However, future studies will need to explore whether this rate of NSSI in ASC adults remains stable, and explore the measurement properties of NSSI assessment tools in ASC.

The current study has a number of strengths as well as limitations. This study is the first to use measures of suicidality (SBQ-R) and NSSI (NSSI-AT) that have good evidence of validity, albeit not yet in autistic adults [7, 10]. There is a paucity of validated outcome measures for autistic adults, and using tools validated for the general population is an important stop gap until tools adapted for autistic people become available [7, 10, 51–53]. The current study was only cross-sectional, and it is unclear for example whether unmet support needs are a cause or consequence of suicidality. The current study focused on adults, without intellectual disability (ID), and it is unknown whether autism and autistic traits would similarly be a unique risk marker for those with co-occurring ID. Although autism, autistic traits, unmet support needs, and camouflaging explained significant additional variance in suicidality when statistically controlling for a number of other factors, the additional variance explained was small.

ASC diagnosis was assessed by self-report only; however, a majority of participants confirmed the clinic where this diagnosis was obtained. Lifetime suicide attempts in the general population (8%) and ASC group (38%) are similar to previous studies [2, 17], which suggests that the sample was not biased in this respect. However, lifetime experience of depression in the general population (44.9%) and ASC group (80%) were much higher than previous estimates [2, 22, 54], despite participants not being recruited because of experience with mental health problems. The rate of mental health difficulties in the current sample therefore may not be representative of the general or autistic populations. A majority of participants in the steering group and online survey were female. Therefore, it could be argued that the topics explored in the survey and study findings apply mostly to autistic females and may not be generalisable to autistic males. However, a majority of autistic males and autistic females reported camouflaging, and regression analyses statistically controlled for sex, suggesting this and other risk markers apply to both sexes.

A key strength and novel aspect of the current study was the participatory research element with a group of autistic adults, who refined the focus of the study, and the content of the survey. This ensured that the study included a range of possible unique and common risk factors for suicidality not explored or considered in previous research on this topic. It also ensured high content validity of the survey, which was refined through three iterations of feedback from the steering group. Previous research has shown that the views of the autistic community which the research affects are rarely included, which can hamper the potential benefits of ASC research for the wider community [11]. Our study demonstrates the importance of including the voices of autistic people in important and sensitive research that can impact their lives.

Conclusions

The current study is the first to use validated assessment tools, and survey co-designed with autistic people, to explore unique risk factors for suicidality in this group. Results reiterate that rates of suicidality in autistic adults are higher than the general population, and ASC diagnosis and autistic traits are independent risk markers for suicidality. Importantly, unique risk markers for suicidality in ASC include camouflaging one's ASC in order to fit in in social situations and number of unmet support needs. These explain small but significant additional variance in suicidality in ASC, above a range of known risk factors common with the general population. Future research must further explore these and identify other unique mechanisms driving suicidality in ASC to develop new effective suicide prevention strategies for this group.

Abbreviations
ADHD: Attention deficit hyperactivity disorder; AQ: Autism-Spectrum Quotient; AS: Asperger syndrome; ASC: Autism spectrum condition; GP: General population; HFA: High functioning autism; ID: Intellectual disability; NSSI: Non-suicidal self-injury; NSSI-AT: Non-suicidal self-injury assessment tool; PDD: Pervasive developmental disorder; PDD-NOS: Pervasive Developmental Disorder Not Otherwise Specified; SBQ-R: Suicidal Behaviours Questionnaire-Revised

Acknowledgements
We would like to sincerely thank the members of the Coventry Autism steering group, who assisted the researchers in designing and advertising the study. We would also like to thank Paula Smith, database manager at the Autism Research Centre, University of Cambridge for her assistance with contacting participants registered in the Cambridge Autism Research Database. We would also like to thank everyone for taking part in the study. We appreciate that this is a difficult topic to think and talk about, and greatly appreciate their support in increasing understanding and prevention of suicide.

Funding
This work was supported by the Economic and Social Research Council [grant number ES/N000501/2]. This work also received support from a research pump prime award from Coventry University. SBC was supported by the Autism Research Trust, the MRC, and the National Institute for Health Research (NIHR) Collaboration for Leadership in Applied Health Research and Care East of England at Cambridgeshire and Peterborough NHS Foundation Trust. The views expressed are those of the authors and not necessarily those of the NHS, the NIHR, or the Department of Health.

Authors' contributions
SC conceived and designed the study, collected and analysed the data, and wrote the manuscript; LB helped design the study, collected the data, and provided critical feedback on the manuscript. RS helped design the study, collected the data, and provided critical feedback on the manuscript. SB helped design the study and provided critical feedback on the manuscript. All authors read and approved the final manuscript.

Competing interests
The authors declare that they have no competing interests.

Author details
[1]School of Psychology, University of Nottingham, University Park, Nottingham NG7 2RD, UK. [2]Centre for Innovative Research across the Life Course, Coventry University, Coventry, UK. [3]Autism Research Centre, University of Cambridge, Cambridge, UK. [4]Coventry and Warwickshire Partnership Trust, Coventry, UK. [5]Cambridge Lifetime Asperger Syndrome Service (CLASS), Cambridgeshire and Peterborough NHS Foundation Trust, Cambridge, UK.

References
1. Zahid S, Upthegrove R. Suicidality in autistic spectrum disorders: a systematic review. Crisis. 2017;38(4):237.
2. Cassidy S, Bradley P, Robinson J, Allison C, McHugh M, Baron-Cohen S. Suicidal ideation and suicide plans or attempts in adults with Asperger's syndrome attending a specialist diagnostic clinic: a clinical cohort study. Lancet Psychiatry. 2014;1(2):142–7.
3. Segers M, Rawana J. What do we know about suicidality in autism spectrum disorders? A systematic review. Autism Res. 2014;7(4):507–21.
4. Hedley D, Uljarević M. Systematic review of suicide in autism spectrum disorder: current trends and implications. Curr Dev Disord Rep. 2018;5(1):65-76.
5. Croen LA, Zerbo O, Qian Y, Massolo ML, Rich S, Sidney S, Kripke C. The health status of adults on the autism spectrum. Autism. 2015;19(7):814–23.
6. Cassidy S, Rodgers J. Understanding and prevention of suicide in autism. Lancet Psychiatry. 2017;4(6):e11.
7. Cassidy S, Bradley L, Wigham S, Bowen E, Rodgers J. Measurement properties of tools used to assess suicidality in adults with and without autism spectrum conditions: a systematic review. Clin Psychol Rev. In Press
8. Hannon G, Taylor EP. Suicidal behaviour in adolescents and young adults with ASD: Findings from a systematic review. Clinical psychology review. 2013;33(8):1197-204.
9. Ribeiro JD, Franklin JC, Fox KR, Bentley KH, Kleiman EM, Chang BP, Nock MK. Self-injurious thoughts and behaviors as risk factors for future suicide ideation, attempts, and death: a meta-analysis of longitudinal studies. Psychol Med. 2016;46(2):225–36.
10. Maddox BB, Trubanova A, White SW. Untended wounds: non-suicidal self-injury in adults with autism spectrum disorder. Autism. 2017;21(4):412–22.
11. Pellicano L, Dinsmore A, Charman T. A Future Made Together: Shaping autism research in the UK. 2013. http://discovery.ucl.ac.uk/1495583/1/A_Future_Made_Together_1.2_LR.pdf. Accessed 21 Feb 2018.
12. Nock MK, Borges G, Bromet EJ, Alonso J, Angermeyer M, Beautrais A, et al. Cross-national prevalence and risk factors for suicidal ideation, plans and attempts. Br J Psychiatry. 2008;192(2):98–105.
13. Kessler RC, Borges G, Walters EE. Prevalence of and risk factors for lifetime suicide attempts in the National Comorbidity Survey. Arch Gen Psychiatry. 1999;56(7):617–26.
14. O'Carroll PW. Attempted suicide among young adults: progress toward a meaningful estimate of prevalence. Am J Psychiatr. 1992;149:41.
15. Hirvikoski T, Mittendorfer-Rutz E, Boman M, Larsson H, Lichtenstein P, Bölte S. Premature mortality in autism spectrum disorder. Br J Psychiatry. 2016;208(3):232–8.
16. Upthegrove R, Abu-Akel A, Chisholm K, Lin A, Zahid S, Pelton M, Apperly I, Hansen PC, Wood SJ. Autism and psychosis: clinical implications for depression and suicide. Schizophr Res. 2018;195:80–5.
17. Pelton MK, Cassidy SA. Are autistic traits associated with suicidality? A test of the interpersonal-psychological theory of suicide in a non-clinical young adult sample. Autism Res. 2017;10(11):1891–904.
18. Takara K, Kondo T. Comorbid atypical autistic traits as a potential risk factor for suicide attempts among adult depressed patients: a case–control study. Ann General Psychiatry. 2014;13(1):33.
19. Chen MH, Pan TL, Lan WH, Hsu JW, Huang KL, Su TP, Li CT, Lin WC, Wei HT, Chen TJ, Bai YM. Risk of suicide attempts among adolescents and young adults with autism spectrum disorder: a Nationwide longitudinal follow-up study. J Clin Psychiatry. 2017;78(9):e1174–9.
20. Barraclough BJ, Bunch J, Nelson B, Sainsbury P. A hundred cases of suicide: clinical aspects. Br J Psychiatry. 1974;125(587):355–73.
21. Wigham S, Barton S, Parr JR, Rodgers J. A systematic review of the rates of depression in children and adults with high-functioning autism spectrum disorder. J Ment Health Res Intellect Disabil. 2017;10(4):267–87.
22. Lever AG, Geurts HM. Psychiatric co-occurring symptoms and disorders in young, middle-aged, and older adults with autism spectrum disorder. J Autism Dev Disord. 2016;46(6):1916–30.
23. Van Orden KA, Witte TK, Cukrowicz KC, Braithwaite SR, Selby EA, Joiner TE Jr. The interpersonal theory of suicide. Psychol Rev. 2010;117(2):575.
24. Orsmond GI, Shattuck PT, Cooper BP, Sterzing PR, Anderson KA. Social participation among young adults with an autism spectrum disorder. J Autism Dev Disord. 2013;43(11):2710–9.
25. Hedley D, Uljarević M, Wilmot M, Richdale A, Dissanayake C. Brief report: social support, depression and suicidal ideation in adults with autism spectrum disorder. J Autism Dev Disord. 2017;47(11):3669–77.
26. Hedley D, Uljarević M, Wilmot M, Richdale A, Dissanayake C. Understanding depression and thoughts of self-harm in autism: a potential mechanism involving loneliness. Res Autism Spectr Disord. 2018;46:1–7.
27. Crane L, Chester JW, Goddard L, Henry LA, Hill E. Experiences of autism diagnosis: a survey of over 1000 parents in the United Kingdom. Autism. 2016;20(2):153–62.
28. Jones L, Goddard L, Hill EL, Henry LA, Crane L. Experiences of receiving a diagnosis of autism spectrum disorder: a survey of adults in the United Kingdom. J Autism Dev Disord. 2014;44(12):3033–44.
29. Lai MC, Baron-Cohen S. Identifying the lost generation of adults with autism spectrum conditions. Lancet Psychiatry. 2015;2(11):1013–27.
30. World Health Organisation. (2018). World Health Statistics. Global Health Observatory data. Available from: http://apps.who.int/iris/bitstream/handle/10665/272596/9789241565585-eng.pdf?ua=1. Accessed 21 Feb 2018.
31. Lai MC, Lombardo MV, Ruigrok AN, Chakrabarti B, Auyeung B, Szatmari P, Happé F, Baron-Cohen S, MRC AIMS Consortium. Quantifying and exploring camouflaging in men and women with autism. Autism. 2017;21(6):690–702.
32. Hull L, Petrides KV, Allison C, Smith P, Baron-Cohen S, Lai MC, Mandy W. "Putting on my best normal": social camouflaging in adults with autism spectrum conditions. J Autism Dev Disord. 2017;47(8):2519–34.
33. Rynkiewicz A, Schuller B, Marchi E, Piana S, Camurri A, Lassalle A, Baron-Cohen S. An investigation of the 'female camouflage effect' in autism using a computerized ADOS-2 and a test of sex/gender differences. Mol Autism. 2016;7(1):10.
34. Duerden EG, Oatley HK, Mak-Fan KM, McGrath PA, Taylor MJ, Szatmari P, Roberts SW. Risk factors associated with self-injurious behaviors in children and adolescents with autism spectrum disorders. J Autism Dev Disord. 2012;42(11):2460–70.
35. South M, Ozonoff S, McMahon WM. Repetitive behavior profiles in Asperger syndrome and high-functioning autism. J Autism Dev Disord. 2005;35(2):145–58.

36. Whitlock J, Exner-Cortens D, Purington A. Assessment of nonsuicidal self-injury: development and initial validation of the non-suicidal self-injury–assessment tool (NSSI-AT). Psychol Assess. 2014;26(3):935.

37. Osman A, Bagge CL, Gutierrez PM, Konick LC, Kopper BA, Barrios FX. The Suicidal Behaviors Questionnaire-Revised (SBQ-R): validation with clinical and nonclinical samples. Assessment. 2001;8(4):443–54.

38. Baron-Cohen S, Wheelwright S, Skinner R, Martin J, Clubley E. The autism-spectrum quotient (AQ): evidence from Asperger syndrome/high-functioning autism, males and females, scientists and mathematicians. J Autism Dev Disord. 2001;31(1):5–17.

39. Ruzich E, Allison C, Smith P, Watson P, Auyeung B, Ring H, Baron-Cohen S. Measuring autistic traits in the general population: a systematic review of the Autism-Spectrum Quotient (AQ) in a nonclinical population sample of 6,900 typical adult males and females. Mol Autism. 2015;6(1):2.

40. Woodbury-Smith MR, Robinson J, Wheelwright S, Baron-Cohen S. Screening adults for Asperger syndrome using the AQ: a preliminary study of its diagnostic validity in clinical practice. J Autism Dev Disord. 2005;35(3):331–5.

41. Cohen J. Statistical power analysis for the behavioral sciences. 2nd ed. Hillsdale: Erlbaum Associates; 1988.

42. Field A. Discovering statistics using SPSS. London: Sage publications; 2009.

43. Ratto AB, Kenworthy L, Yerys BE, Bascom J, Wieckowski AT, White SW, Wallace GL, Pugliese C, Schultz RT, Ollendick TH, Scarpa A. What about the girls? Sex-based differences in autistic traits and adaptive skills. J Autism Dev Disord. 2018;48(5):1698-711.

44. Gotham K, Bishop SL, Brunwasser S, Lord C. Rumination and perceived impairment associated with depressive symptoms in a verbal adolescent–adult ASD sample. Autism Res. 2014;7(3):381–91.

45. Heasman B, Gillespie A. Perspective-taking is two-sided: misunderstandings between people with Asperger's syndrome and their family members. Autism. 2018;22(6):740–50. https://doi.org/10.1177/1362361317708287.

46. Jaswal VK, Akhtar N. Being vs. appearing socially uninterested: challenging assumptions about social motivation in autism. Behav Brain Sci. 2018;19:1–84.

47. Sasson NJ, Faso DJ, Nugent J, Lovell S, Kennedy DP, Grossman RB. Neurotypical peers are less willing to interact with those with autism based on thin slice judgments. Sci Rep. 2017;7:40700.

48. Milton DE. On the ontological status of autism: the 'double empathy problem'. Disabil Soc. 2012;27(6):883–7.

49. Milton D, Sims T. How is a sense of well-being and belonging constructed in the accounts of autistic adults? Disabil Soc. 2016;31(4):520–34.

50. Raja M. Suicide risk in adults with Asperger's syndrome. Lancet Psychiatry. 2014;1(2):99–101.

51. Cassidy SA, Bradley L, Bowen E, Wigham S, Rodgers J. Measurement properties of tools used to assess depression in adults with and without autism spectrum conditions: a systematic review. Autism Res. 2018;11(5):738–54.

52. McConachie H, Parr JR, Glod M, Hanratty J, Livingstone N, Oono IP, Robalino S, Baird G, Beresford B, Charman T, Garland D. Systematic review of tools to measure outcomes for young children with autism spectrum disorder. https://ore.exeter.ac.uk/repository/handle/10871/17760. Accessed 21 Feb 2018.

53. Wigham S, McConachie H. Systematic review of the properties of tools used to measure outcomes in anxiety intervention studies for children with autism spectrum disorders. PLoS One. 2014;9(1):e85268.

54. Kessler C, Berglund P, Demler O, Jin R, Merikangas R, Walters E. Lifetime prevalence and age-of-onset distributions of DSM-IV disorders in the national comorbidity survey replication. Arch Gen Psychiatry. 2005;62(6):593–602.

Abnormal coherence and sleep composition in children with Angelman syndrome: a retrospective EEG study

Hanna den Bakker[1,2,3†], Michael S. Sidorov[1,2,3†], Zheng Fan[4], David J. Lee[5], Lynne M. Bird[6,7], Catherine J. Chu[8,9] and Benjamin D. Philpot[1,2,3*] (iD)

Abstract

Background: Angelman syndrome (AS) is a neurodevelopmental disorder characterized by intellectual disability, speech and motor impairments, epilepsy, abnormal sleep, and phenotypic overlap with autism. Individuals with AS display characteristic EEG patterns including high-amplitude rhythmic delta waves. Here, we sought to quantitatively explore EEG architecture in AS beyond known spectral power phenotypes. We were motivated by studies of functional connectivity and sleep spindles in autism to study these EEG readouts in children with AS.

Methods: We analyzed retrospective wake and sleep EEGs from children with AS (age 4–11) and age-matched neurotypical controls. We assessed long-range and short-range functional connectivity by measuring coherence across multiple frequencies during wake and sleep. We quantified sleep spindles using automated and manual approaches.

Results: During wakefulness, children with AS showed enhanced long-range EEG coherence across a wide range of frequencies. During sleep, children with AS showed increased long-range EEG coherence specifically in the gamma band. EEGs from children with AS contained fewer sleep spindles, and these spindles were shorter in duration than their neurotypical counterparts.

Conclusions: We demonstrate two quantitative readouts of dysregulated sleep composition in children with AS—gamma coherence and spindles—and describe how functional connectivity patterns may be disrupted during wakefulness. Quantitative EEG phenotypes have potential as biomarkers and readouts of target engagement for future clinical trials and provide clues into how neural circuits are dysregulated in children with AS.

Keywords: Angelman syndrome, UBE3A, EEG, Coherence, Spindles, Biomarker

Background

Angelman syndrome (AS) is a neurodevelopmental disorder caused by loss of neuronal expression of the maternally inherited *UBE3A* gene. Symptoms of AS include severe intellectual disability, impaired speech and motor function, epilepsy, sleep abnormalities, and some phenotypic overlap with autism [1–3]. Consistent and widespread electroencephalographic (EEG) irregularities in AS include epileptiform discharges, intermittent theta waves, and enhanced rhythmic delta waves [4–7]. In a prior study, we established that quantitative methods can be successfully applied to retrospective EEG data to confirm prior clinical descriptions of rhythmic delta in AS [6]. Here, we sought to use quantitative approaches to identify novel EEG signatures in the same groups of retrospective EEG data. We assessed EEG coherence during wakefulness and non-rapid eye movement (NREM) sleep and quantified sleep spindles during NREM sleep.

* Correspondence: bphilpot@med.unc.edu
†Equal contributors
[1]Department of Cell Biology and Physiology, University of North Carolina, Chapel Hill, NC 27599, USA
[2]Carolina Institute for Developmental Disabilities, University of North Carolina, Chapel Hill, NC 27599, USA
Full list of author information is available at the end of the article

Coherence is a measure of how two simultaneously recorded EEG signals are correlated and represents a non-invasive approach to assess functional connectivity between brain areas [8]. We were motivated to study coherence in AS by the observation that individuals with autism show altered coherence patterns [9–17]. Autism has been recognized as a component feature of AS [18–22], and copy number increases in the 15q11-13 chromosomal region including *UBE3A* are also associated with syndromic autism [23, 24]. Some estimates suggest that up to ~ 50–80% of individuals with AS meet diagnostic criteria for autism [18]; however, these estimates vary greatly due to the difficulties assessing autism with standardized clinical tests in AS individuals. Traditionally, individuals with autism were thought to have comparatively high coherence between nearby electrode pairs (local hyperconnectivity) and low coherence between long-distance signals (global hypoconnectivity) [9–13], but this view has been challenged and become more nuanced in recent years [14–17, 25]. Thus, although specific connectivity patterns remain unclear, there is widespread consensus that EEG coherence is altered in autism. The phenotypic and genetic links between AS and autism led us to hypothesize that children with AS might also display irregularities in the relationship between long-range and short-range coherence.

Sleep abnormalities are common in individuals with AS [1–3, 26–34] and have also been reported in mouse models of the disorder [35, 36]. Sleep dysfunction includes arousal during sleep and short sleep duration, and has a major impact on the quality of life of individuals with AS and their caretakers [28–31]. We sought to identify quantitative EEG signatures underlying disrupted sleep patterns in children with AS. In addition to measuring coherence during sleep, we also quantified sleep spindles. Spindles are thalamocortical oscillations in the sigma band (~ 11–16 Hz) that occur during NREM sleep and are important for memory consolidation [37, 38]. Sleep spindle activity is decreased in a number of neurodevelopmental and neurodegenerative disorders, such as autism, intellectual disability, epilepsy, Alzheimer's disease, and schizophrenia [39–46]. Although there have not yet been reports of substantial impairments in sleep architecture in AS, we hypothesized that quantitative measures might reveal subtle impairments in spindles and in patterns of sleep coherence that might be otherwise difficult to detect manually in a clinical EEG review setting.

During wakefulness, we report increased long-range EEG coherence in children with AS. During sleep, we also find increased long-range coherence, but specifically in the gamma band. We also report that sleep spindles are less frequent and shorter in children with AS. Overall, these measures provide insights into circuit-level neurobiology in AS and may have value as biomarkers or measures of target engagement for future therapeutic interventions. As this study was exploratory in nature, future work is needed to confirm coherence and spindle dysregulation in additional cohorts and to link these EEG phenotypes with behavioral outcomes.

Methods

Study design

We analyzed retrospective clinical EEGs from children with a genetically confirmed diagnosis of AS and age-matched neurotypical controls. All EEG studies were performed with the approval of institutional review boards (IRBs) at Harvard Medical School and UC San Diego, and consent was given to participate. All EEG data were previously analyzed for spectral content in our prior study [6], which tested the pre-defined hypothesis that delta rhythms are increased in AS. Here, we conducted an exploratory study to identify novel EEG phenotypes that could be measured quantitatively.

Data sources

EEG data from 28 children with AS (14 male, 14 female) were recorded between 2006 and 2014 at the San Diego site (Rady Children's Hospital San Diego) of the AS Natural History Study (ClinicalTrials.gov identifier: NCT00296764). EEG data from 72 neurotypical (NT) children (42 male, 30 female) were recorded at Massachusetts General Hospital between February 1, 2002, and May 1, 2012. All children were aged 4–11 years at the time of EEG recordings (AS 5.8 ± 0.3 years, NT 7.0 ± 0.2 years). Children with AS received EEG recordings as part of the Natural History Study, and neurotypical children were referred to Mass. General for diagnostic EEG evaluation. Only children that were subsequently determined to be non-epileptic and with documented normal neurodevelopment were included for analysis. All EEG data were gathered using the standard clinical method. Subjects were described in greater detail in a prior study [6], including AS molecular diagnosis, seizure history, and medications at the time of recording. An experienced clinical neurophysiologist assessed sleep/wake state in all recordings and categorized data into epochs of clear wakefulness and clear NREM sleep. The following signatures were used to identify NREM sleep: the presence of spindles, vertex waves, K-complexes, the absence of eye blinks, and/or decreased myogenic artifacts. Periods of REM sleep and periods where state was unclear were excluded. Subsequently, we had two separate datasets for analysis: one containing EEG signals during wakefulness (NT: $n = 54$; AS: $n = 26$), and one consisting of periods of NREM sleep (NT: $n = 54$; AS: $n = 13$).

Data acquisition and pre-processing

EEGs were acquired using sampling rates ranging between 200 and 512 Hz using either Bio-Logic or Xltek systems and with standard 10–20 electrode placement. We pre-processed all data prior to this study using methods described in Sidorov et al. [6]. NT and AS EEGs were pre-processed in parallel using identical methods to limit the inherent impact of comparing recordings across two sites. Briefly, pre-processing consisted of re-referencing signals to linked ears, filtering, sleep/wake coding, and artifact removal. We used a second-order Butterworth filter with a high pass of 1 Hz, a low pass of 100 Hz, and a notch at 60 Hz (roll-off 40 dB/decade, attenuation – 0.263 dB at 2 Hz).

Coherence analysis

We made group coherence comparisons (AS versus NT) separately in periods of wakefulness (Fig. 2, Additional file 1: Figure S1) and periods of NREM sleep (Fig. 3, Additional file 2: Figure S2). Within each EEG recording, we calculated the coherence between each of 145 electrode pairs in each of 100 frequency bins (1–50 Hz, 0.5 Hz bin size) by using the "mscohere" function in MATLAB [47–49]. The mscohere function calculates the magnitude-squared coherence, or how well "x" corresponds to "y" at each frequency, for each window (we used 2-s windows with 50% overlap), and averages these windows using Welch's averaged, modified periodogram method. The coherence value of signals x and y, $C_{xy}(f)$, was calculated as a function of the spectral densities of signal x, $P_{xx}(f)$, and y, $P_{yy}(f)$, and the cross spectral density of x and y, $P_{xy}(f)$:

$$C_{xy}(f) = \frac{|P_{xy}(f)|^2}{P_{xx}(f)P_{yy}(f)}$$

Pre-processed EEG signals were non-continuous due to sleep/wake coding and artifact removal. Thus, we calculated coherence separately within each segment of pre-processed data, then averaged coherence from different segments while weighting segment length. We only included continuous data longer than 10 s for coherence analyses.

To simplify interpretation of 14,500 coherence measurements per recording (145 electrode pairs × 100 frequency bins), we grouped data in two ways: (1) by frequency and (2) by electrode location.

Frequency grouping

To assess coherence within frequency bands of interest, we grouped and defined delta as 2–4 Hz, theta as 4–7 Hz, alpha as 8–12 Hz, beta as 12–30 Hz, and gamma as 30–50 Hz (Fig. 2, Fig. 3). To ensure statistical normality, coherence values (R^2) from each 0.5 Hz frequency bin were first z-transformed using Fisher's r to z. Then,

the z-scores were averaged within each of the five frequency bands of interest. These averaged scores were then back-transformed using the Fisher inverse function, to obtain one z'-coherence value per electrode pair per frequency band [48–51].

Location grouping

We grouped electrode pairs according to their distance from each other (short-range and long-range) and their position relative to each other (intra-hemispheric and inter-hemispheric). To group electrode pairs by distance, we arranged electrodes (Fig. 1a) into a grid (Fig. 1b), assigned coordinates to each electrode (e.g., (2,1) for F7), and calculated the Euclidean distance between all coordinate pairs using the MATLAB function pdist [52]. The squared Euclidean distance (d^2) for coordinates "a" and "b" was calculated with the following equation, where x_a is the x-coordinate of "a" and y_a is the y-coordinate of "a":

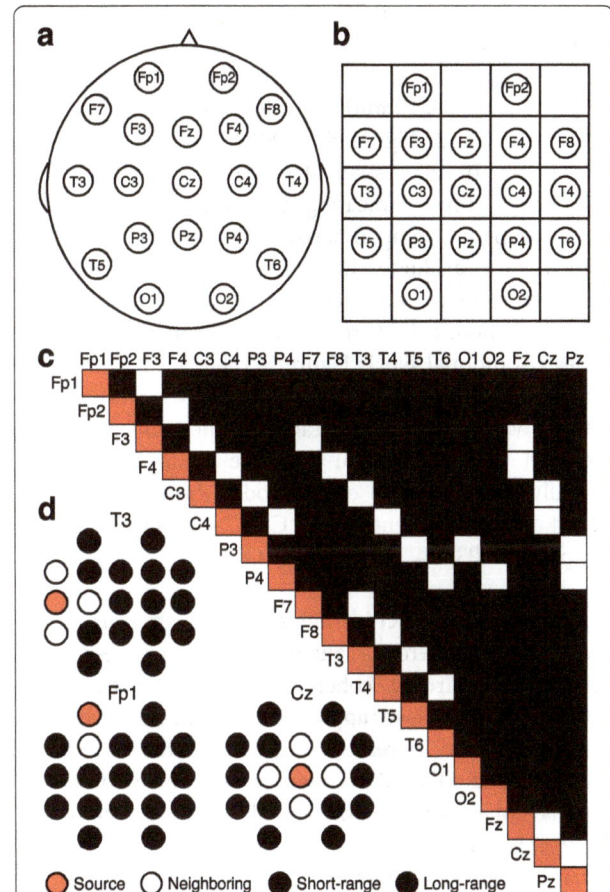

Fig. 1 Defining long-range and short-range electrode pairs for coherence analyses. Standard 10–20 EEG electrode placements **a** on the scalp and **b** on a grid. **c** Grouping of all electrode pairs into short-range (black) and long-range (gray). Neighboring electrode pairs (white) were excluded from analysis. **d** Three examples of source electrodes (red) and their relationships with all other electrodes

$$d^2_{ab} = (x_a - x_b)^2 + (y_a - y_b)^2$$

Based on the Euclidean distance, we divided the electrode pairs into short-range pairs ($d^2 = 2$) and long-range pairs ($d^2 > 2$) (Fig. 1c–d). Directly neighboring electrodes ($d^2 = 1$) were removed from analysis due to the potential confound of volume conduction [52]. We averaged z'-coherence values across all short-range electrode pairs ($n = 24$) and all long-range electrode pairs ($n = 121$) within each of the five frequency bands and overall (from 1 to 50 Hz) (Fig. 2, Fig. 3). When comparing intra-hemispheric coherence and inter-hemispheric coherence (Additional file 1: Figure S1B-G, Additional file 2: Figure S2B-G), we restricted intra-hemispheric analyses to long-range electrode pairs because by definition, all inter-hemispheric pairs were long-range. This approach eliminated the potential confound of short-range pairs in intra- but not inter-hemispheric data. We also excluded all pairs containing one or more midline electrode (Fz, Cz, Pz) from intra-versus-inter-hemispheric analysis. To graphically represent the spatial distribution of coherence, we created topographic coherence maps (Figs. 2e and 3e, Additional file 1: Figure S1D, S1G, Additional file 2: Figure S2A, S2D, S2G). These maps overlay the 10–20 system of electrode placement with color-coded lines indicating coherence between each electrode pair (averaged across all subjects).

To further evaluate the spatial profile of coherence phenotypes in AS, we calculated the coherence through individual nodes (electrodes) and through groups of nodes (Additional file 1: Figure S1H–I, Additional file 2: Figure S2H–I). First, for each electrode, we averaged coherence values for all long-range connections. Next, we averaged these individual-electrode averages for each spatially defined group of electrodes (frontal: Fp1, Fp2, F3, F4, F7, F8, Fz; central: C3, C4, Cz; temporal: T4, T5, T6; parietal: P3, P4, Pz; occipital: O1, O2).

High-frequency artifact identification and removal

We entered coherence analyses with no pre-defined hypothesis regarding coherence in specific frequency bands. This unbiased approach revealed that children with AS showed increased long-range coherence in the gamma band (Fig. 3). However, accurately assessing gamma coherence is complicated by the possibility of electromyogenic (EMG) contamination of temporal signals in this bandwidth [53, 54]. Therefore, in addition to manual artifact removal at the initial stage of data pre-processing, we also conducted a post hoc analysis designed to identify low-amplitude EMG artifacts in sleep EEG data that are difficult to identify visually. Spectral power typically follows a ~ 1/f decay [55]; therefore, we excluded outliers in which the slope of the linear fit of the log power versus frequency (between 30–50 and 65–95 Hz) relationship in temporal electrodes exceeded – 1 [56]. We excluded one AS outlier and one NT outlier, in which muscle artifact likely corrupted interpretation of high-frequency coherence. We restricted these post hoc analyses to sleep EEGs, as altered coherence in wakeful EEGs was not specific to the gamma band and therefore not likely affected by high-frequency EMG artifacts.

Consideration of volume conduction

We removed neighboring electrodes from analysis to minimize the effects of volume conduction [52]. To further assess the possible effects of volume conduction on the remaining electrode pairs, we performed a cross-correlation analysis on each one-second bin of continuous EEG signals and removed all bins in which the maximum cross-correlation between electrodes occurred at zero lag (Additional file 3: Figure S3). The average of all other bins provides a measure of cross-correlation, while robustly and conservatively accounting for the effects of volume conduction [57]. Generally, cross-correlation and coherence measures are expected to result in statistically similar findings [58]. We band-pass-filtered wake data (1–50 Hz) and sleep data (30–50 Hz) prior to cross-correlation analyses and grouped long-range and short-range electrode pairs.

Spectral analysis

We re-analyzed and re-plotted the spectral power of frontal signals during sleep (Fig. 4a–c) using methods identical to our prior study [6], with one exception: here, we normalized power in each 0.5 Hz bin to the total power between 4 and 50 Hz, instead of to the total power between 1 and 50 Hz. We adjusted normalization to account for increased delta power (2–4 Hz) in children with AS. Thus, Fig. 4a represents the same data as Additional file 3: Figure S3J in Sidorov et al. [6].

Spindle detection

We quantified the number and frequency of spindles during epochs of NREM sleep. We automated spindle detection using MATLAB using previously defined analysis parameters [59]. Automated spindle detection can be summarized in four steps (Fig. 4d): (1) To set the impedance levels of electrodes to similar levels, the detector normalized each pre-processed signal to the average power of the 90–100 Hz frequency range of that signal (Fig. 4d, top panel). (2) The data were filtered between 11 and 16 Hz using a 10th order Butterworth band-pass filter (Fig. 4d, middle panel). (3) The instantaneous amplitude was computed using a Hilbert transform and smoothed using a Gaussian kernel of 40 ms (Fig. 4d, bottom panel). (4) A spindle was detected if the instantaneous amplitude of the filtered signal crossed a threshold of 5.5 times the mean amplitude of the signal (red line in Fig. 4, bottom panel). When a spindle was detected, its duration was defined by when the signal crossed a lower threshold, 2.5 times the mean amplitude of the signal (gray line in Fig. 4d, bottom panel). Spindles were only counted if they were between 0.4 and 2.0 s in duration. Analyses of spindle frequency and spindle duration (Fig. 4e–f) represent total spindles across all 19 EEG channels. If two spindles were detected with an initiation interval of < 300 ms, these were considered to be a single event; thus, we did not double-count spindles seen at the same time across more than one channel. Two AS sleep EEGs had zero automatically detected spindles (Fig. 4e, left panel; $n = 13$); therefore, we excluded these recordings from analyses of spindle duration (Fig. 4e, right panel; $n = 11$).

Two trained clinical experts (DJL and ZF) manually analyzed spindle frequency in all sleep EEGs while blind to genotype (Fig. 4f). To ensure that experts remained blind, we filtered out background delta, which is highly prevalent in AS, with a 5 Hz high-pass filter prior to manual coding. Experts noted both the times at which spindles occurred and the confidence level of manually detecting spindles from background activity (high, medium, low).

Statistical analyses
We used Student's t tests to assess overall coherence (grouped across 1–50 Hz) as a function of genotype (Figs. 2b, d, f, and 3b, d, f, Additional file 1: Figure S1C, S1F, Additional file 2: S2C, S2F; "overall"). To assess the contribution of the five different frequency ranges (delta, theta, alpha, beta, gamma) to coherence, we used a two-way ANOVA with genotype and frequency as factors (Figs. 2b, d, f and 3b, d, f, Additional file 1: Figure S1C, S1F, Additional file 2: Figure S2C, S2F). We then used a post hoc test with Bonferroni's correction for multiple comparisons to compare genotypes in individual frequency bands. We used Student's t tests to assess cross-correlation, with volume conduction removed, as a function of genotype (Additional file 3: Fig. S3). We used Student's t tests to compare spectral power, spindle frequency, and spindle duration between groups (Fig. 4c, e, f). We used two-tailed Fisher's exact test to compare confidence in manual spindle detection. Cohen's d effect sizes (Table 1) reflect overall (1–50 Hz) long-range/short-range coherence ratio (Fig. 2f, "overall") during wakefulness, long-range/short-range gamma coherence ratio during sleep (Fig. 3f), spindle rate (Fig. 4e), and delta power averaged across all electrodes (re-analyzed from Sidorov et al. [6]). All statistical analyses were performed using GraphPad Prism 7. In all figures, the

asterisk indicates $p < 0.05$, $**p < 0.01$, and $***p < 0.001$. Where two-way ANOVAs were used, asterisks indicate statistically significant interactions (e.g., Fig. 3d, large brackets) and post hoc tests (e.g., Fig. 3d, gamma, small brackets). Main effects of genotype are noted in text. Error bars indicate SEM.

Results
We calculated coherence between 145 combinations of 19 EEG electrodes for each individual and grouped coherence by short-range and long-range electrode pairs [52] (Fig. 1). To make group comparisons between children with AS and neurotypical (NT) children, we first assessed coherence across all frequency bands between 1 and 50 Hz ("overall coherence") and then assessed coherence within frequency bands of interest (delta, theta, alpha, beta, gamma) while correcting for multiple comparisons, using Bonferroni's multiple comparisons test. We analyzed EEG coherence separately in periods of wakefulness (NT: $n = 54$; AS: $n = 26$) and in periods of NREM sleep (NT: $n = 54$; AS: $n = 13$).

Long-range coherence is increased in Angelman syndrome during wakefulness
During wakefulness, overall (1–50 Hz) short-range coherence (Fig. 2a) was not statistically different between children with AS and neurotypical controls (Fig. 2b, "overall"; $p = 0.1887$, Student's t test). We next tested whether differences in short-range coherence would emerge within specific frequency bands. While two-way ANOVA revealed a statistically significant main effect of genotype (Fig. 2b; $F_{(1, 390)} = 8.32$, $p = 0.0041$), there was no genotype × frequency interaction ($F_{(4, 390)} = 0.0702$, $p = 0.9910$) and short-range coherence was not increased within any specific frequency band (post hoc Bonferroni tests: delta: $p = 0.9113$, theta: $p > 0.9999$, alpha: $p > 0.9999$, beta: $p = 0.7041$, gamma: $p = 0.5514$).

During wakefulness, overall (1–50 Hz) long-range coherence (Fig. 2c) was significantly increased in children with AS (Fig. 2d, "overall"; $p = 0.0207$). Two-way ANOVA revealed a significant main effect of genotype (Fig. 2d; $F_{(1,390)} = 28.11$, $p < 0.0001$) but no genotype × frequency interaction ($F_{(4,390)} = 0.3385$, $p = 0.9224$). While increased long-range coherence was detected statistically within the gamma band (post hoc tests: delta: $p = 0.1258$, theta: $p = 0.3252$, alpha: $p = 0.1769$, beta: $p = 0.0559$, gamma: $p = 0.0105$), the lack of genotype × frequency interaction indicates that this phenotype is not specific to any frequency band.

We next assessed whether increased long-range coherence in AS is expressed broadly across all electrode pairs or in a spatially restricted subset of connections or nodes. First, we created topographic coherence maps to visualize coherence in all electrode pairs (Fig. 2e).

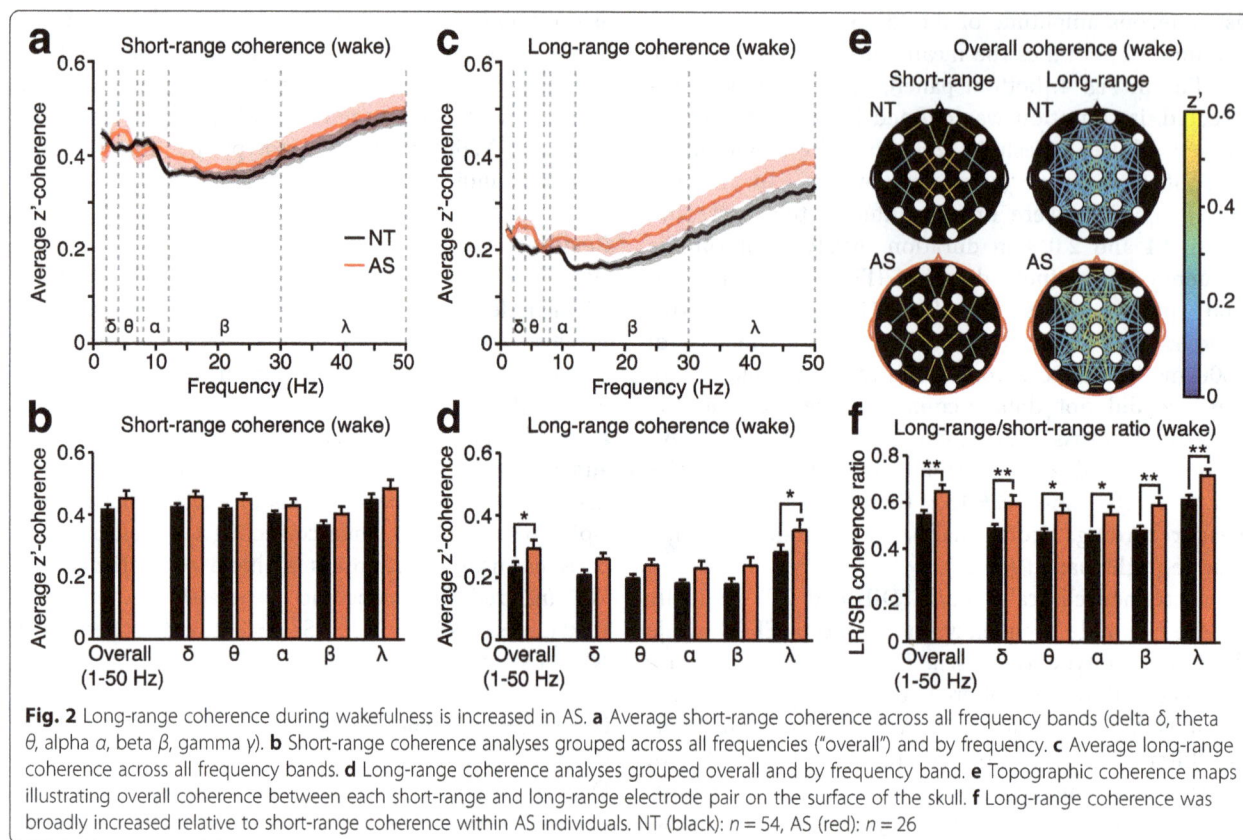

Fig. 2 Long-range coherence during wakefulness is increased in AS. **a** Average short-range coherence across all frequency bands (delta δ, theta θ, alpha α, beta β, gamma γ). **b** Short-range coherence analyses grouped across all frequencies ("overall") and by frequency. **c** Average long-range coherence across all frequency bands. **d** Long-range coherence analyses grouped overall and by frequency band. **e** Topographic coherence maps illustrating overall coherence between each short-range and long-range electrode pair on the surface of the skull. **f** Long-range coherence was broadly increased relative to short-range coherence within AS individuals. NT (black): $n = 54$, AS (red): $n = 26$

Comparison of NT and AS long-range maps suggests that increased long-range coherence is broadly spatially distributed. To quantify this comparison, we spatially grouped long-range electrode pairs: first, as a function of Euclidean distance, and next, by intra-hemispheric versus inter-hemispheric connectivity. Enhanced long-range coherence in AS was evident across a range of electrode distances (Additional file 1: Figure S1A), and in both intra-hemispheric and inter-hemispheric electrode pairs (Additional file 1: Figure S1B–G). We then asked if long-range coherence is selectively increased through specific nodes or groups of nodes. The lack of a significant genotype × region interaction effect demonstrated that increased long-range coherence in AS was not specific for individual electrodes or regions (Additional file 1: Figure S1H–I). Overall, we conclude that enhanced long-range coherence during wakefulness in AS is broadly distributed and is not specific to either certain groups of connections or certain groups of electrodes.

Coherence analyses grouped across individuals revealed that long-range coherence is increased in AS during wakefulness (Fig. 2c–d). Overall short-range coherence (grouped from 1 to 50 Hz) in AS individuals was statistically indistinguishable from NT individuals; therefore, we were surprised to find a significant main

effect of genotype when including multiple comparisons across frequency bands (Fig. 2a–b). Thus, we next tested, within individuals, whether long-range coherence is meaningfully increased relative to short-range coherence. The ratio between long-range and short-range overall coherence (1–50 Hz) was increased in children with AS (Fig. 2f, "overall"; $p = 0.0016$). Two-way ANOVA revealed a significant main effect of genotype ($F_{(1,390)} = 48.39$, $p < 0.0001$), but no genotype × frequency interaction ($F_{(4,390)} = 0.1083$, $p = 0.9796$), and post hoc tests revealed that increased long-range to short-range coherence ratios were detectable in all frequency ranges tested (Fig. 2f; delta: $p = 0.0037$, theta: $p = 0.0401$, alpha: $p = 0.0220$, beta: $p = 0.0040$, gamma: $p = 0.0063$). Thus, we conclude that within individuals, long-range coherence is increased relative to short-range coherence in children with AS during wakefulness. Increased long-range coherence is evident across frequency bands.

Long-range gamma-band coherence is increased in Angelman syndrome during sleep
During periods of sleep, overall (1–50 Hz) short-range coherence (Fig. 3a) was statistically comparable between AS and NT individuals (Fig. 3b, "overall"; $p = 0.3059$). Two-way ANOVA revealed no significant main effect of

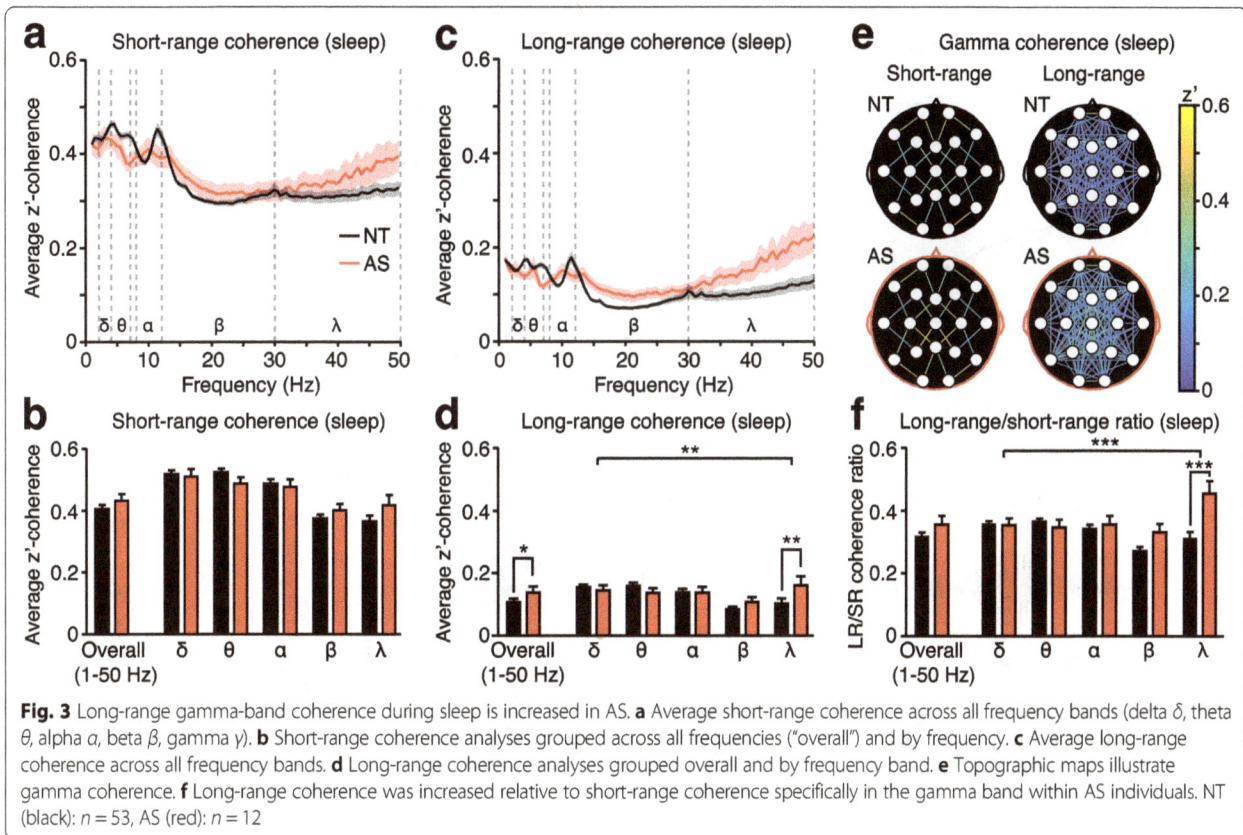

Fig. 3 Long-range gamma-band coherence during sleep is increased in AS. **a** Average short-range coherence across all frequency bands (delta δ, theta θ, alpha α, beta β, gamma γ). **b** Short-range coherence analyses grouped across all frequencies ("overall") and by frequency. **c** Average long-range coherence across all frequency bands. **d** Long-range coherence analyses grouped overall and by frequency band. **e** Topographic maps illustrate gamma coherence. **f** Long-range coherence was increased relative to short-range coherence specifically in the gamma band within AS individuals. NT (black): $n = 53$, AS (red): $n = 12$

genotype (Fig. 3b; $F_{(1,315)} = 0.002$, $p = 0.9672$) and no interaction between genotype and frequency (Fig. 3b; $F_{(4,315)} = 1.958$, $p = 0.1008$). During sleep, overall long-range coherence (Fig. 3c) was increased in AS (Fig. 3d, "overall"; $p = 0.0442$). Increased long-range coherence was driven primarily by increased coherence in the gamma band (Fig. 3d; genotype × frequency interaction: $F_{(4,315)} = 3.758$, $p = 0.0053$; post hoc tests: delta, theta, alpha, beta: $p > 0.75$, gamma: $p = 0.0024$). Topographic coherence maps (Fig. 3e) and analysis (Additional file 2: Figure S2) suggest that increased long-range gamma coherence during sleep is broadly expressed (and not spatially restricted) in AS.

Within individuals, the ratio between long-range and short-range overall (1–50 Hz) coherence was not increased in children with AS (Fig. 3f, "overall"; $p = 0.1824$). Two-way ANOVA revealed a significant genotype × frequency interaction ($F_{(4,315)} = 5.946$, $p = 0.0001$), and post hoc tests revealed that there was an increase in coherence specific to the gamma band (Fig. 3f; delta, theta, alpha: $p > 0.9999$, beta: $p = 0.1796$, gamma: $p < 0.0001$). Gamma coherence is sensitive to electromyogenic (EMG) artifacts [53, 54]; therefore, we identified and excluded recordings in which these artifacts were present, yet were not manually excluded in the initial data preprocessing phase [56] (see the "Methods" section).

These outliers (1 AS, 1 NT) have been excluded from Fig. 3, Additional file 2: Figure S2, and analyses. Overall, long-range coherence is increased in AS during sleep specifically in the gamma band.

Coherence phenotypes in Angelman syndrome are not driven by group differences in volume conduction

Volume conduction of signals propagated from a common source may lead to identification of spuriously coupled scalp EEG signals. We tested whether volume conduction (instantaneous propagation of activity from sources to recording channels) was driving the coherence phenotypes in AS. We calculated cross-correlation and removed all periods where the maximum cross-correlation between electrode pairs occurred at zero lag. This approach is a robust and conservative way of removing potentially spurious electrode pairs [57]. With potential volume conduction excluded, genotype differences in long-range coherence persisted during both periods of wake and sleep (Additional file 3: Figure S3). With conservative removal of volume conduction, short-range gamma coherence was also statistically increased in AS EEGs during sleep. However, the long-range/short-range ratio remained elevated in AS, confirming that long-range coherence gamma coherence is elevated relative to short-range gamma coherence. Overall,

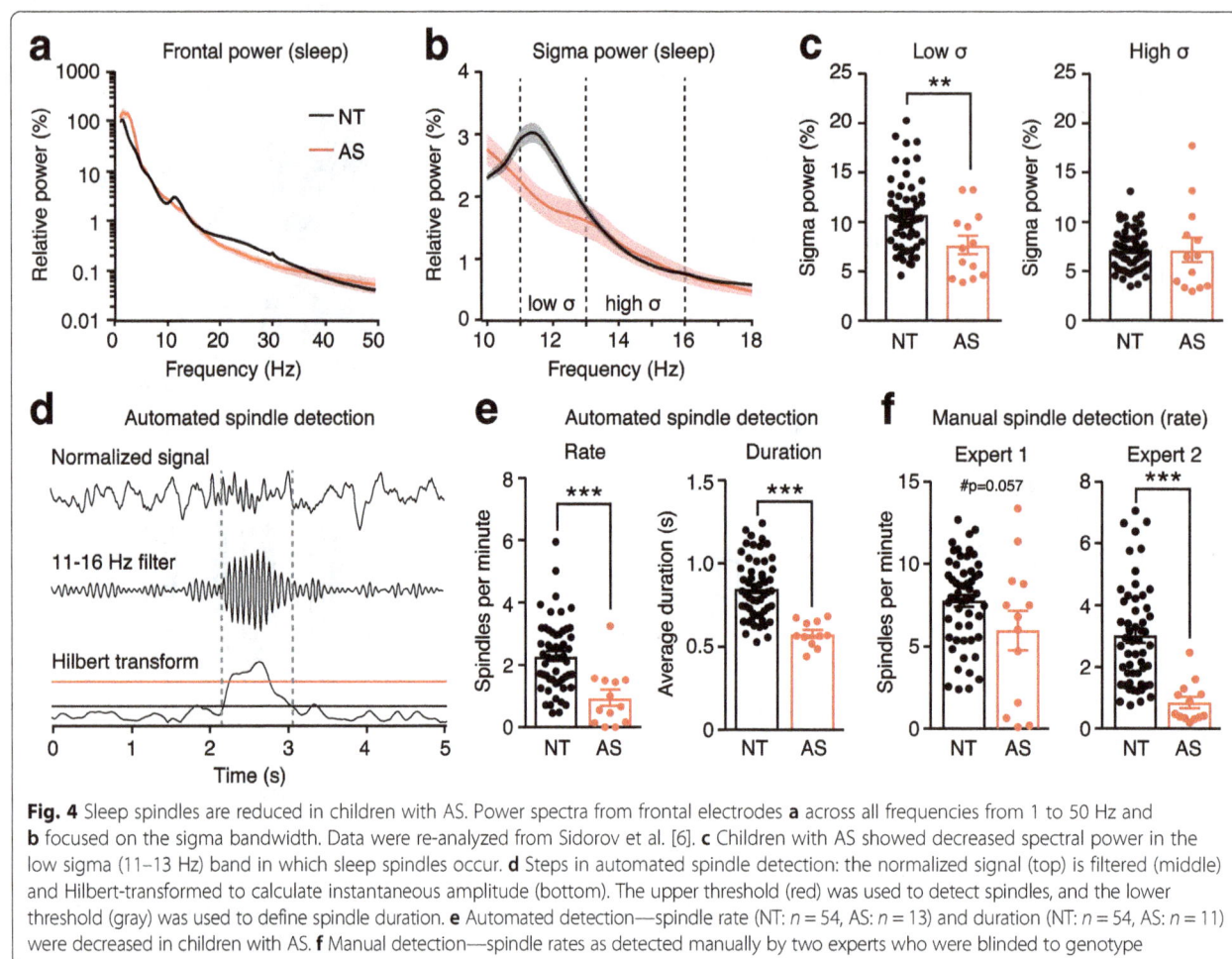

Fig. 4 Sleep spindles are reduced in children with AS. Power spectra from frontal electrodes **a** across all frequencies from 1 to 50 Hz and **b** focused on the sigma bandwidth. Data were re-analyzed from Sidorov et al. [6]. **c** Children with AS showed decreased spectral power in the low sigma (11–13 Hz) band in which sleep spindles occur. **d** Steps in automated spindle detection: the normalized signal (top) is filtered (middle) and Hilbert-transformed to calculate instantaneous amplitude (bottom). The upper threshold (red) was used to detect spindles, and the lower threshold (gray) was used to define spindle duration. **e** Automated detection—spindle rate (NT: $n = 54$, AS: $n = 13$) and duration (NT: $n = 54$, AS: $n = 11$) were decreased in children with AS. **f** Manual detection—spindle rates as detected manually by two experts who were blinded to genotype

differences in coherence between AS and NT groups are not the result of distortion due to volume conduction.

Frequency and duration of sleep spindles is decreased in Angelman syndrome

Sleep spindles are visible in EEGs during NREM sleep as bursts of synchronous activity in the sigma band (11–16 Hz) [60]. In neurotypical children, we observed a local peak in sigma-band coherence during sleep (Fig. 3a, c) but not wakefulness (Fig. 2a, c) that may reflect the presence of sleep spindles [46, 61, 62]. We did not observe a sigma-

band coherence peak in children with AS during sleep (Fig. 3a, c), suggesting that spindles may be decreased in AS. Spindle density also correlates with a peak in spectral power in the sigma band during NREM sleep [46]; therefore, we re-analyzed power spectra from our prior study [6] to focus on the sigma band during sleep. We confirmed that spectral power in the low sigma band (11–13 Hz) was decreased in children with AS (Fig. 4a–c; $p = 0.0071$). Together, decreased sigma coherence and spectral power during sleep provide indirect evidence suggesting that sleep spindles are dysregulated in AS.

We directly tested the hypothesis that sleep spindles are dysregulated in AS by using an automated spindle detection algorithm developed by Kim and colleagues [59] (Fig. 4d). Children with AS had fewer spindles (Fig. 4e; $p = 0.0002$), and the spindles were of shorter duration (Fig. 4e; $p < 0.0001$) than those of neurotypical controls. Although automation provides a fast and objective way to quantify sleep spindles, even established detection methods can be less accurate than human experts [63]. Therefore, we had two clinical experts manually count spindles in all sleep EEGs while

Table 1 Effect sizes of quantitative EEG phenotypes in children with AS. Altered coherence and decreased spindles are less robust than increased delta power

Measure	p value	Cohen's d
Delta power (wake) [6]	< 0.0001	2.198
Overall coherence ratio (wake)	0.0016	0.747
Delta power (sleep) [6]	< 0.0001	2.058
Gamma coherence ratio (sleep)	< 0.0001	1.033
Spindle frequency (sleep)	0.0002	1.290

blind to genotype. Results from expert 1 revealed a trend towards decreased spindle rate in children with AS (Fig. 4f; $p = 0.0570$). Results from expert 2 show a significant decrease in spindle rate in AS children (Fig. 4f; $p < 0.0001$). Expert 1 noted low confidence spindle detection for 11 of 13 AS EEGs and not for a single neurotypical EEG ($n = 54$; $p < 0.0001$, Fisher's exact test). Expert 2 noted medium confidence for all recordings.

Coherence and spindle dysregulation in AS have smaller effect sizes than delta power

Exploratory analyses of retrospective EEGs revealed coherence and spindle phenotypes in children with AS (Figs. 2, 3, and 4). In a prior study, we reported that children with AS also have increased delta power during both wakefulness and sleep [6]. Such quantitative EEG measures may have value as biomarkers or measures of target engagement for future clinical trials in AS. An important factor when considering biomarker viability is the reliability of a measure [64]. Therefore, we compared the Cohen's d effect sizes for each quantitative EEG phenotype in AS (Table 1). Increased delta power was the most robust phenotype we assessed.

Discussion

Quantitative EEG analyses revealed three phenotypes in children with AS that would otherwise be difficult to discern in a routine clinical or research setting: (1) increased long-range coherence during wakefulness, (2) increased long-range gamma-band coherence during sleep, and (3) decreased sleep spindle number and duration.

EEG coherence provides a measure of how neural activity is correlated between brain areas and is widely used as a proxy for functional connectivity [8]. Coherence measures the consistency of the phase and amplitude difference between EEG signals in a given frequency band. Coherence is thus distinct from spectral power, which measures the relative amplitude of electrical activity within a frequency band from a single electrode. Thus, despite robust increases in delta power [5, 6], children with AS have normal delta-band coherence (Figs. 2 and 3). While coherence and delta power phenotypes in AS are both ultimately caused by loss of neuronal UBE3A protein, they likely reflect different proximate circuit-level impairments.

During wakefulness, long-range EEG coherence was increased in children with AS across a broad range of frequencies (Fig. 2). Increased long-range coherence in AS was seen throughout the brain and was not driven by altered coherence in a spatially restricted subset of connections (Fig. 2e, Additional file 1: Figure S1). There is general consensus that functional connectivity is widely disrupted in autism [9–17, 25], and our findings confirm that coherence is also dysregulated in AS, a

disorder with some autistic features. However, increased long-range functional connectivity may be surprising given prior studies of decreased structural connectivity in AS, both in mouse models [65] and patient populations [66, 67]. This suggests that despite reduced structural connectivity, there may be fewer inhibitory constraints on efferent projections in the AS brain.

During sleep, long-range coherence was significantly increased in children with AS, but only in the gamma band (Fig. 3). Gamma-band coherence is an indicator of attentive wakefulness [68], and accordingly, gamma coherence is typically lower during sleep than during wakefulness [69–71]. We confirmed that gamma coherence in neurotypical children is lower during sleep than during wake (compare Figs. 2 and 3). However, the pattern of elevated long-range gamma coherence during sleep in AS children resembles what is typically seen in a wakeful state. A common challenge in analyzing gamma-band coherence is the presence of electromyogenic artifacts, which are visible in EMG spectra and are often seen temporally in the gamma range [53, 54]. Therefore, we used an outlier analysis to exclude recordings in which EMG artifacts exceeded an established threshold [56]. Two additional pieces of evidence confirm that gamma coherence phenotypes in AS are not driven by EMG artifacts: (1) increased gamma coherence is specific to long-range electrode pairs and (2) gamma coherence is not increased specifically in temporal electrodes (Additional file 2: Figure S2I). Overall, long-range functional connectivity was increased in AS EEGs during both wake and sleep states. However, coherence patterns differed as function of state: phenotypes were gamma-specific during sleep and not frequency-specific during wake. Thus, it is critical to control for sleep state when assessing functional connectivity.

We also report that sleep spindles are shorter and less frequent in AS (Fig. 4). This finding is consistent with the decreased spindle frequency seen in autism, intellectual disability, and sleep disorders [39–43]. Despite many clinical studies of Angelman EEGs over the past 30 years, to our knowledge, there have been no reports to date of dysregulated spindles. This is surprising because unlike coherence, sleep spindles may be easily detected by the eye. However, subtle dysregulation of spindles may be difficult to gauge clinically, especially given the pervasive disruptions in background activity in AS [5]. Therefore, automated spindle detection using an unbiased, high-throughput method was used to determine that spindle rate and duration were decreased in AS EEGs. In addition, one of two blinded experts confirmed a statistically significant decrease in spindle rate in AS EEGs, with the other finding a strong trend. To enable blinded data analysis, we filtered out the delta activity that is pervasive in the AS EEG; however, this likely reduced both accuracy and confidence of manual detection. Future studies of sleep spindles in AS must consider and weigh the challenges of manual and automated detection, but we favor an automated approach because it is not subject to the reporter biases that plague qualitative outcome measurements in clinical trials.

More broadly, experimental conditions must be considered when evaluating our exploratory analyses of sleep composition in AS (both spindles and coherence). We used retrospective EEG data, which included periods of sleep and wake and was not designed explicitly as a sleep study. Because children with AS have pervasive sleep problems, it is likely that sleep quality during EEG recordings varied by group. For example, only 46% (13/28) children with AS slept during EEGs, whereas 75% (54/72) of neurotypical children slept. In addition, the nature of sleep during clinical EEG recordings may not be representative of typical overnight sleep. For example, the average length of NREM sleep during EEGs recordings was only ~ 14 min for neurotypical children and ~ 22 min for children with AS [6]. Thus we propose that sleep spindles and gamma coherence phenotypes should be explicitly tested in well-controlled overnight sleep studies.

Clinical trials are on the horizon for AS; therefore, development of biomarkers, outcome measures, and measures of target engagement are especially valuable. Biomarkers for AS need not have diagnostic value, as diagnoses are made genetically. Therefore major considerations in evaluating a biomarker include whether it is quantitative, easily measured, reliable, and linked to clinically meaningful outcomes [64]. Previously, we described enhanced delta rhythmicity in AS, which is quantitative, non-invasive, and reliable, but the link between delta rhythms and behavior has not yet been established. While effect sizes of gamma coherence and sleep spindle phenotypes are less than delta rhythms (Table 1), these phenotypes are likely linked to sleep quality. Therefore, they may be considered as biomarkers, particularly if a study is interested in quantifying sleep as a primary outcome measure. However, delta power is a substantially more robust biomarker, with only slight overlap between AS and neurotypical groups at the level of individuals. Future study of sleep biomarkers in an overnight setting, with AS and neurotypical children studied in parallel at a single site, may have the potential to decrease individual variability and increase robustness.

Quantitative EEG phenotypes may also provide insights into circuit-level biological mechanisms underlying AS. For example, mechanisms governing spindle initiation and propagation have been well characterized [37]. Spindles

are driven by the intrinsic properties of, and interactions between, thalamocortical cells and thalamic reticular cells. Thalamocortical circuits, which also drive cortical delta rhythms [72], may be studied in mouse models to better understand how loss of UBE3A disrupts neural circuits. We hypothesize that loss of UBE3A from a small population of like neurons is sufficient to disrupt sleep spindles in AS. Coherence phenotypes, which are expressed broadly throughout the brain, are likely driven through different processes.

Conclusions

Overall, we identified three novel quantitative EEG phenotypes in an exploratory analysis of retrospective EEGs from children with AS. These results have potential value as biomarkers and in pointing towards underlying neural substrates. Future work is needed to confirm findings in independent samples, particularly under conditions designed to study sleep explicitly.

Additional files

Additional file 1: Figure S1. Spatial analysis of long-range coherence during wakefulness. (A) Overall coherence (1–50 Hz) during wakefulness as a function of Euclidean distance. Dotted line represents the cutoff between short-range and long-range coherence. Two-way ANOVA for long-range coherence: genotype: $F_{(1,774)} = 40.53$, $p < 0.0001$; distance: $F_{(9,774)} = 22.75$, $p < 0.0001$; interaction: $F_{(9,774)} = 0.4326$, $p = 0.9187$. (B) Raw and (C) grouped intra-hemispheric long-range coherence. Overall (1–50 Hz) intra-hemispheric coherence is increased in AS ($p = 0.0145$). Two-way ANOVA: genotype: $F_{(1,390)} = 32.77$, $p < 0.0001$; genotype × frequency interaction: $F_{(4,390)} = 0.1419$, $p = 0.9665$; post hoc tests: delta: $p = 0.0646$, theta: $p = 0.1067$, alpha: $p = 0.1315$, beta: $p = 0.0521$, gamma: $p = 0.0078$. (D) Topographic coherence maps for all intra-hemispheric electrode pairs. (E) Raw and (F) grouped inter-hemispheric long-range coherence. Overall (1–50 Hz) inter-hemispheric coherence was increased in AS ($p = 0.0303$). Two-way ANOVA: genotype: $F_{(1,390)} = 22.49$, $p < 0.0001$; genotype × frequency interaction: $F_{(4,390)} = 0.3383$, $p = 0.8521$; post hoc tests: delta: $p = 0.2771$, theta: $p = 0.8276$, alpha: $p = 0.2657$, beta: $p = 0.0785$, gamma: $p = 0.0180$. (G) Topographic coherence maps for all inter-hemispheric electrode pairs. (H) Overall (1–50 Hz) long-range coherence through individual electrodes and (I) electrodes grouped by region. Two-way ANOVA: genotype: $F_{(1,390)} = 23.11$, $p < 0.0001$; genotype × region interaction: $F_{(4,390)} = 0.8003$, $p = 0.5255$; post hoc tests: frontal: $p = 0.0555$, central: $p = 0.0783$, parietal: $p = 0.0112$, temporal: $p > 0.9999$, occipital: $p = 0.2414$. NT (black): $n = 54$, AS (red): $n = 26$. (PDF 271 kb)

Additional file 2: Figure S2. Spatial analysis of gamma-band coherence during sleep. (A) Gamma-band coherence during sleep as a function of Euclidean distance. Dotted line represents the dividing line between short-range and long-range coherence. Two-way ANOVA for long-range coherence: genotype: $F_{(1,629)} = 30.93$, $p < 0.0001$; distance: $F_{(9,629)} = 15.46$, $p < 0.0001$; interaction: $F_{(9,629)} = 0.8704$, $p = 0.5516$. Asterisk indicates significance by post hoc Bonferroni tests. (B) Raw and (C) grouped intra-hemispheric long-range gamma-band coherence. Overall: $p = 0.0565$; two-way ANOVA: genotype: $F_{(1,315)} = 1.484$, $p = 0.2240$; genotype × frequency interaction: $F_{(4,315)} = 2.943$, $p = 0.0206$; post hoc tests: delta, theta, alpha, beta: $p > 0.9999$, gamma: $p = 0.0070$. (D) Topographic coherence maps for all intra-hemispheric electrode pairs. LR long-range. (E) Raw and (F) grouped inter-hemispheric long-range coherence. Overall: $p = 0.1139$; two-way ANOVA: genotype: $F_{(1,315)} = 0.409$, $p = 0.5230$; genotype × frequency interaction: $F_{(4,315)} = 3.303$, $p = 0.0114$; post hoc tests: delta: $p > 0.9999$, theta: $p = 0.4283$, alpha, beta: $p > 0.9999$, gamma: $p = 0.0140$. (G) Topographic coherence maps for all inter-hemispheric electrode pairs. (H) Gamma coherence through individual electrodes and (I) electrodes grouped by region. Two-way ANOVA for region: genotype: $F_{(1,315)} = 24.86$, $p < 0.0001$; genotype × region interaction: $F_{(4,315)} = 0.9112$, $p = 0.4576$; post hoc tests: frontal: $p = 0.3285$, central: $p = 0.0465$, parietal: $p = 0.0022$, temporal: $p > 0.9999$, occipital: $p = 0.1522$. NT (black): $n = 53$, AS (red): $n = 12$. (PDF 503 kb)

Additional file 3: Figure S3. Coherence phenotypes persist with conservative exclusion of volume conduction. (A) Cross-correlation during wakefulness across all frequencies (1–50 Hz). Left panel: short-range electrode pairs ($p = 0.0549$). Center panel: long-range electrode pairs ($p < 0.0001$). Right panel: long-range/short-range ratio ($p = 0.0027$). (B) Cross-correlation during sleep in the gamma band (30–50 Hz). Left panel: short-range ($p = 0.0004$). Center panel: long-range ($p < 0.0001$). Right panel: long-range/short-range ratio ($p = 0.0016$). (PDF 405 kb)

Abbreviations

AS: Angelman syndrome; EEG: Electroencephalography; EMG: Electromyography; NT: Neurotypical; NREM: Non-rapid eye movement sleep

Acknowledgements

We thank Matt Judson (UNC) and Mark Nespeca (UCSD) for the thoughtful discussion and advice and Gina Deck (Brown University) and Marjan Dolatshahi (Massachusetts General Hospital) for initially coding sleep/wake EEG data.

Funding

This work was supported by NINDS (R56 NS097831), the Angelman Syndrome Alliance, and the Angelman Syndrome Foundation to BDP. MSS was supported by NICHD training fellowship (T32 HD040127).

Authors' contributions

HDB and MSS analyzed the data and prepared all figures. LMB and CJC provided the data. DJL and ZF manually coded the sleep spindles. HDB, MSS, and BDP wrote the manuscript. All authors reviewed the manuscript. All authors read and approved the final manuscript.

Competing interests

The authors declare that they have no competing interests.

Author details

[1]Department of Cell Biology and Physiology, University of North Carolina, Chapel Hill, NC 27599, USA. [2]Carolina Institute for Developmental Disabilities, University of North Carolina, Chapel Hill, NC 27599, USA. [3]Neuroscience Center, University of North Carolina, Chapel Hill, NC 27599, USA. [4]Department of Neurology, University of North Carolina, Chapel Hill, NC 27599, USA. [5]Department of Neurosciences, University of California, San Diego, CA, USA. [6]Department of Pediatrics, University of California, San Diego, CA, USA. [7]Division of Dysmorphology/Genetics, Rady Children's Hospital, San Diego, CA, USA. [8]Department of Neurology, Massachusetts General Hospital, Boston, MA 02114, USA. [9]Harvard Medical School, Boston, MA 02215, USA.

References

1. Thibert RL, Larson AM, Hsieh DT, Raby AR, Thiele EA. Neurologic manifestations of Angelman syndrome. Pediatr Neurol. 2013;48:271–9.

2. Bird LM. Angelman syndrome: review of clinical and molecular aspects. Appl Clin Genet. 2014;7:93–104.

3. Williams CA, Driscoll DJ, Dagli AI. Clinical and genetic aspects of Angelman syndrome. Genet Med. 2010;12:385–95.

4. Korff CM, Kelley KR, Nordli DR. Notched delta, phenotype, and Angelman syndrome. J Clin Neurophysiol. 2005;22:238–43.

5. Vendrame M, Loddenkemper T, Zarowski M, Gregas M, Shuhaiber H, Sarco DP, Morales A, Nespeca M, Sharpe C, Haas K, Barnes G, Glaze D, Kothare SV. Analysis of EEG patterns and genotypes in patients with Angelman syndrome. Epilepsy Behav. 2012;23:261–5.

6. Sidorov MS, Deck GM, Dolatshahi M, Thibert RL, Bird LM, Chu CJ, Philpot BD. Delta rhythmicity is a reliable EEG biomarker in Angelman syndrome: a parallel mouse and human analysis. J Neurodev Disord. 2017;9:17.

7. Uemura M, Matsumoto A, Nakamura M, Watanabe K, Negoro T, Kumagai T, Miura K, Ohki T, Mizuno S, Okumura A, Aso K, Hayakawa F, Kondo Y. Evolution of seizures and electroencephalographical findings in 23 cases of deletion type Angelman syndrome. Brain Dev. 2005;27:383–8.

8. Srinivasan R, Winter WR, Ding J, Nunez PL. EEG and MEG coherence: measures of functional connectivity at distinct spatial scales of neocortical dynamics. J Neurosci Methods. 2007;166:41–52.

9. Murias M, Webb SJ, Greenson J, Dawson G. Resting state cortical connectivity reflected in EEG coherence in individuals with autism. Biol Psychiatry. 2007;62:270–3.

10. Shou G, Mosconi MW, Wang J, Ethridge LE, Sweeney JA, Ding L. Electrophysiological signatures of atypical intrinsic brain connectivity networks in autism. J Neural Eng. 2017;14:046010.

11. Pineda JA, Juavinett A, Datko M. Self-regulation of brain oscillations as a treatment for aberrant brain connections in children with autism. Med Hypotheses. 2012;79:790–8.

12. Barttfeld P, Wicker B, Cukier S, Navarta S, Lew S, Sigman M. A big-world network in ASD: dynamical connectivity analysis reflects a deficit in long-range connections and an excess of short-range connections. Neuropsychologia. 2011;49:254–63.

13. Moseley RL, Ypma RJ, Holt RJ, Floris D, Chura LR, Spencer MD, Baron-Cohen S, Suckling J, Bullmore E, Rubinov M. Whole-brain functional hypoconnectivity as an endophenotype of autism in adolescents. Neuroimage Clin. 2015;9:140–52.

14. Coben R, Clarke AR, Hudspeth W, Barry RJ. EEG power and coherence in autistic spectrum disorder. Clin Neurophysiol. 2008;119:1002–9.

15. Duffy FH, Als H. A stable pattern of EEG spectral coherence distinguishes children with autism from neurotypical controls—a large case control study. BMC Med. 2012;10. https://doi.org/10.1186/1741-7015-10-64.

16. Han YMYC, S A. Disordered cortical connectivity underlies the executive function deficits in children with autism spectrum disorders. Res Dev Disabil. 2017;61:19–31.

17. Schwartz S, Kessler R, Gaughan T, Buckley AW. Electroencephalogram coherence patterns in autism: an updated review. Pediatr Neurol. 2017;67:7–22.

18. Bie Mertz LG, Thaulov P, Trillingsgaard A, Christensen R, Vogel I, Hertz JM, Østergaard JR. Neurodevelopmental outcome in Angelman syndrome: genotype–phenotype correlations. Res Dev Disabil. 2014;35:1742–7.

19. Bonati MT, Russo S, Finelli P, Valsecchi MR, Cogliati F, Cavalleri L, Roberts W, Elia M, Larizza L. Evaluation of autism traits in Angelman syndrome: a resource to unfold autism genes. Neurogenetics. 2007;8:169–78.

20. Peters SU, Horowitz L, Barberi-Welge R, Taylor JL, Hundley RJ. Longitudinal follow-up of autism spectrum features and sensory behaviors in Angelman syndrome by deletion class. J Child Psychol Psychiatry. 2012;53:152–9.

21. Sahoo T, Bacino CA, German JR, Shaw CA, Bird LM, Kimonis V, Anselm I, Waisbren S, Beaudet AL, Peters SU. Identification of novel deletions of 15q11q13 in Angelman syndrome by array-CGH: molecular characterization and genotype–phenotype correlations. Eur J Hum Genet. 2007;15:943–9.

22. Trillingsgaard A, Østergaard JR. Autism in Angelman syndrome: an exploration of comorbidity. Autism. 2004;8:163–74.

23. Moreno-De-Luca D, Sanders SJ, Willsey AJ, Mulle JG, Lowe JK, Geschwind DH, State MW, Martin CL, Ledbetter DH. Using large clinical data sets to infer pathogenicity for rare copy number variants in autism cohorts. Mol Psychiatry. 2013;18:1090–5.

24. Glessner JT, Wang K, Cai G, Korvatska O, Kim CE, Wood S, Hakonarson H. Autism genome-wide copy number variation reveals ubiquitin and neuronal genes. Nature. 2009;459:569–73.

25. Matlis S, Boric K, Chu CJ, Kramer MA. Robust disruptions in electroencephalogram cortical oscillations and large-scale functional networks in autism. BMC Neurol. 2015;15:97.

26. Walz NC, Beebe D, Byars K. Sleep in individuals with Angelman syndrome: parent perceptions of patterns and problems. Am J Ment Retard. 2005;110:243–52.

27. Pelc K, Cheron G, Boyd SG, Dan B. Are there distinctive sleep problems in Angelman syndrome? Sleep Med. 2008;9:434–41.

28. Spruyt K, Braam W, Curfs LM. Sleep in Angelman syndrome: a review of evidence. Sleep Med Rev. 2018;37:69-84.

29. Trickett J, Heald M, Oliver C. Sleep in children with Angelman syndrome: parental concerns and priorities. Res Dev Disabil. 2017;69:105–15.

30. Larson AM, Shinnick JE, Shaaya EA, Thiele EA, Thibert RL. Angelman syndrome in adulthood. Am J Med Genet. 2015;167A:331–44.

31. Goldman SE, Bichell TJ, Surdyka K, Malow BA. Sleep in children and adolescents with Angelman syndrome: association with parent sleep and stress. J Intellect Disabil Res. 2012;56:600–8.

32. Didden R, Korzilius H, Smits MG, Curfs LMG. Sleep problems in individuals with Angelman syndrome. Am J Ment Retard. 2004;109:275–84.

33. Bruni O, Ferri R, D'Agostino G, Miano S, Roccella M, Elia M. Sleep disturbances in Angelman syndrome: a questionnaire study. Brain Dev. 2004;26:233–40.

34. Miano S, Bruni O, Leuzzi V, Elia M, Verrillo E, Ferri R. Sleep polygraphy in Angelman syndrome. Clin Neurophysiol. 2004;115:938–45.

35. Ehlen JC, Jones KA, Pinckney L, Gray CL, Burette S, Weinberg RJ, Evans JA, Brager AJ, Zylka MJ, Paul KN, et al. Maternal Ube3a loss disrupts sleep homeostasis but leaves circadian rhythmicity largely intact. J Neurosci. 2015;35:13587–98.

36. Shi SQ, Bichell TJ, Ihrie RA, Johnson CH. Ube3a imprinting impairs circadian robustness in Angelman syndrome models. Curr Biol. 2015;25:537–45.

37. McCormick DA, Bal T. Sleep and arousal: thalamocortical mechanisms. Annu Rev Neurosci. 1997;20:185–215.

38. Ulrich D. Sleep spindles as facilitators of memory formation and learning. Neural Plast. 2016;2016:1796715.

39. Shibagaki M, Kiyono S, Watanabe K. Spindle evolution in normal and mentally retarded children: a review. Sleep. 1982;5:47–57.

40. Limoges E, Mottron L, Bolduc C, Berthiaume C, Godbout R. Atypical sleep architecture and the autism phenotype. Brain. 2005;128:1049–61.

41. Himanen SL, Virkkala J, Huupponen E, Hasan J. Spindle frequency remains slow in sleep apnea patients throughout the night. Sleep Med. 2003;4:229–34.

42. Espa F, Ondze B, Deglise P, Billiard M, Besset A. Sleep architecture, slow wave activity, and sleep spindles in adult patients with sleepwalking and sleep terrors. Clin Neurophysiol. 2000;111:929–39.

43. Gruber R, Wise MS. Sleep spindle characteristics in children with neurodevelopmental disorders and their relation to cognition. Neural Plast. 2016;2016:4724792.

44. Petit D, Gagnon JF, Fantini ML, Ferini-Strambi L, Montplaisir J. Sleep and quantitative EEG in neurodegenerative disorders. J Psychosom Res. 2004;56:487–96.

45. Myatchin I, Lagae L. Sleep spindle abnormalities in children with generalized spike-wave discharges. Pediatr Neurol. 2007;36:106–11.

46. Wamsley EJ, Tucker MA, Shinn AK, Ono KE, McKinley SK, Ely AV, Goff DC, Stickgold R, Manoach DS. Reduced sleep spindles and spindle coherence in schizophrenia: mechanisms of impaired memory consolidation? Biol Psychiatry. 2012;71:154–61.

47. Takagaki K, Russell J, Lippert MT, Motamedi GK. Development of the posterior basic rhythm in children with autism. Clin Neurophysiol. 2015;126:297–303.

48. Machado C, Estevez M, Leisman G, Melillo R, Rodriguez R, DeFina P, Hernandez A, Perez-Nellar J, Naranjo R, Chinchilla M, et al. QEEG spectral and coherence assessment of autistic children in three different experimental conditions. J Autism Dev Disord. 2015;45:406–24.

49. Machado C, Rodriguez R, Estevez M, Leisman G, Melillo R, Chinchilla M, Portela L. Anatomic and functional connectivity relationship in autistic children during three different experimental conditions. Brain Connect. 2015;5:487–96.

50. Mathewson KJ, Jetha MK, Drmic IE, Bryson SE, Goldberg JO, Schmidt LA. Regional EEG alpha power, coherence, and behavioral symptomatology in autism spectrum disorder. Clin Neurophysiol. 2012;123:1798–809.

51. Han YM, Chan AS. Disordered cortical connectivity underlies the executive function deficits in children with autism spectrum disorders. Res Dev Disabil. 2017;61:19–31.

52. Peters JM, Taquet M, Vega C, Jeste SS, Fernández IS, Tan J, Nelson CA, Sahin M, Warfield SK. Brain functional networks in syndromic and non-syndromic autism: a graph theoretical study of EEG connectivity. BMC Med. 2013;11:54.

53. Buzsaki G, Schomburg EW. What does gamma coherence tell us about inter-regional neural communication? Nat Neurosci. 2015;18:484–9.

54. Hipp JF, Siegel M. Dissociating neuronal gamma-band activity from cranial and ocular muscle activity in EEG. Front Hum Neurosci. 2013;7:338.

55. Buzsaki G, Mizuseki K. The log-dynamic brain: how skewed distributions affect network operations. Nat Rev Neurosci. 2014;15:264–78.

56. Chu CJ, Leahy J, Pathmanathan J, Kramer MA, Cash SS. The maturation of cortical sleep rhythms and networks over early development. Clin Neurophysiol. 2014;125:1360–70.

57. Chu CJ, Kramer MA, Pathmanathan J, Bianchi MT, Westover MB, Wizon L, Cash SS. Emergence of stable functional networks in long-term human electroencephalography. J Neurosci. 2012;32:2703–13.

58. Guevara MA, Corsi-Cabrera M. EEG coherence or EEG correlation? Int J Psychophysiol. 1996;23:145–53.

59. Kim D, Hwang E, Lee M, Sung H, Choi JH. Characterization of topographically specific sleep spindles in mice. Sleep. 2015;38:85–96.

60. 't Wallant DC, Maquet P, Phillips C. Sleep spindles as an electrographic element: description and automatic detection methods. Neural Plast 2016; 2016:6783812.

61. Tarokh L, Carskadon MA, Achermann P. Early adolescent cognitive gains are marked by increased sleep EEG coherence. PLoS One. 2014;9:e106847.

62. Duckrow RBZ, P H. Coherence of the electroencephalogram during the first sleep cycle. Clin Neurophysiol. 2005;116:1088–95.

63. Warby SC, Wendt SL, Welinder P, Munk EG, Carrillo O, Sorensen HB, Jennum P, Peppard PE, Perona P, Mignot E. Sleep-spindle detection: crowdsourcing and evaluating performance of experts, non-experts and automated methods. Nat Methods. 2014;11:385–92.

64. Jeste SS, Frohlich J, Loo SK. Electrophysiological biomarkers of diagnosis and outcome in neurodevelopmental disorders. Curr Opin Neurol. 2015; 28:110–6.

65. Judson MC, Burette AC, Thaxton CL, Pribisko AL, Shen MD, Rumple AM, Del Cid WA, Paniagua B, Styner M, Weinberg RJ, Philpot BD. Decreased axon caliber underlies loss of Fiber tract integrity, disproportional reductions in white matter volume, and microcephaly in Angelman syndrome model mice. J Neurosci. 2017;37:7347–61.

66. Tiwari VN, Jeong J, Wilson BJ, Behen ME, Chugani HT, Sundaram SK. Relationship between aberrant brain connectivity and clinical features in Angelman syndrome: a new method using tract based spatial statistics of DTI color-coded orientation maps. NeuroImage. 2012;59:349–55.

67. Wilson BJ, Sundaram SK, Huq A, Jeong J, Halverson SR, Behen ME, Bui DQ, Chugani HT. Abnormal language pathway in children with Angelman syndrome. Pediatr Neurol. 2011;44:350–6.

68. Lee K, Williams LM, Breakspear M, Gordonc E. Synchronous gamma activity: a review and contribution to an integrative neuroscience model of schizophrenia. Brain Res Rev. 2003;41:57–78.

69. Cavelli M, Castro S, Schwarzkopf N, Chase MH, Falconi A, Torterolo P. Coherent neocortical gamma oscillations decrease during REM sleep in the rat. Behav Brain Res. 2015;281:318–25.

70. Castro S, Cavelli M, Vollono P, Chase MH, Falconi A, Torterolo P. Inter-hemispheric coherence of neocortical gamma oscillations during sleep and wakefulness. Neurosci Lett. 2014;578:197–202.

71. Fell J, Staedtgen M, Burr W, Kockelmann E, Helmstaedter C, Schaller C, Elger CE, Fernández G. Rhinal–hippocampal EEG coherence is reduced during human sleep. Eur J Neurosci. 2003;18:1711–6.

72. Lewis LD, Voigts J, Flores FJ, Schmitt LI, Wilson MA, Halassa MM, Brown EN. Thalamic reticular nucleus induces fast and local modulation of arousal state. Elife. 2015;4:e08760.

The impact of robotic intervention on joint attention in children with autism spectrum disorders

Hirokazu Kumazaki[1]*[iD], Yuichiro Yoshikawa[2], Yuko Yoshimura[1], Takashi Ikeda[1], Chiaki Hasegawa[1], Daisuke N. Saito[1], Sara Tomiyama[1], Kyung-min An[1], Jiro Shimaya[2], Hiroshi Ishiguro[2], Yoshio Matsumoto[3], Yoshio Minabe[1] and Mitsuru Kikuchi[1]

Abstract

Background: A growing body of anecdotal evidence indicates that the use of robots may provide unique opportunities for assisting children with autism spectrum disorders (ASD). However, previous studies investigating the effects of interventions using robots on joint attention (JA) in children with ASD have shown insufficient results. The robots used in these studies could not turn their eyes, which was a limitation preventing the robot from resembling a human agent.

Methods: We compared the behavior of children with ASD with that of children with typical development (TD) during a JA elicitation task while the children interacted with either a human or a robotic agent. We used the robot "CommU," which has clear eyes and can turn its eyes, for the robotic intervention. The age range of the participants was limited to 5–6 years.

Results: Sixty-eight participants participated in this study, including 30 (10 females and 20 males) children with ASD and 38 (13 females and 25 males) children with TD. The participants were randomly assigned to one of the following two groups: the robotic intervention group or the control group. JA in the children with ASD was better during the robotic intervention than during the human agent intervention. These children exhibited improved performance in the JA task with human after interacting with the robot CommU. JA was differentially facilitated by the human and robotic agents between the ASD and TD children.

Conclusions: The findings of this study significantly contribute to the literature on the impact of robots on JA and provide information regarding the suitability of specific robot types for therapeutic use.

Keywords: Autism spectrum disorders, Typical development, Intervention, Joint attention, Robot

Background

Autism spectrum disorders (ASD) are characterized by social communication deficits and a tendency to engage in repetitive behaviors [1]. A core social-communication deficit observed in children with ASD is limited joint attention (JA) behaviors. JA refers to a social exchange in which a child coordinates attention with a social partner or aspect of the environment by the acts of eye-gazing and pointing or other verbal or non-verbal indications. JA serves as a foundation for developing communicative competence and early social and cognitive skills [2–9]. Early interventions that facilitate JA are promising because these strategies increase children's opportunities to learn from their environment and change their developmental trajectories [10, 11].

To engage in JA, children must orient toward their social partners and shift attention rapidly between social and non-social stimuli in their surroundings [12, 13]. Children with ASD require a well-suited interaction partner to develop JA skill [14]. In many cases, children with ASD do not show sustained motivation to interact with an interaction partner. For caregivers and trainers, concentrating on interactions with children with ASD is a difficult task [15, 16].

* Correspondence: kumazaki@tiara.ocn.ne.jp
[1]Research Center for Child Mental Development, Kanazawa University, 13-1, Takaramachi, Kanazawa, Ishikawa 920-8640, Japan
Full list of author information is available at the end of the article

Children with ASD preferentially orient visually toward non-social objects, such as robots, rather than social objects [17–19]. These children prefer non-social objects because they are predictable, simple, and easy to comprehend. The use of robots may provide unique opportunities for assisting children with ASD [20–25]. For example, children with ASD exhibit improved performance in imitation tasks using a robot [22, 26]. However, previous studies [14, 27, 28] investigating the efficacy of interventions using robots on JA in children with ASD have shown insufficient results because these studies used a robot (i.e., "Nao") that cannot turn its eyes. The robot's inability to turn its eyes was a limitation that prevented the robot from resembling a human agent, and eye-gazing is among the primary elements of JA [28, 29].

Thus, we selected the communication robot "CommU" (Fig. 1; Vstone Co., Ltd.) [30, 31] to facilitate JA. CommU has clear eyes and can turn its eyes. Because eye contact is a basic social skill that children with ASD often lack, CommU's clear eyes allow the children to recognize and

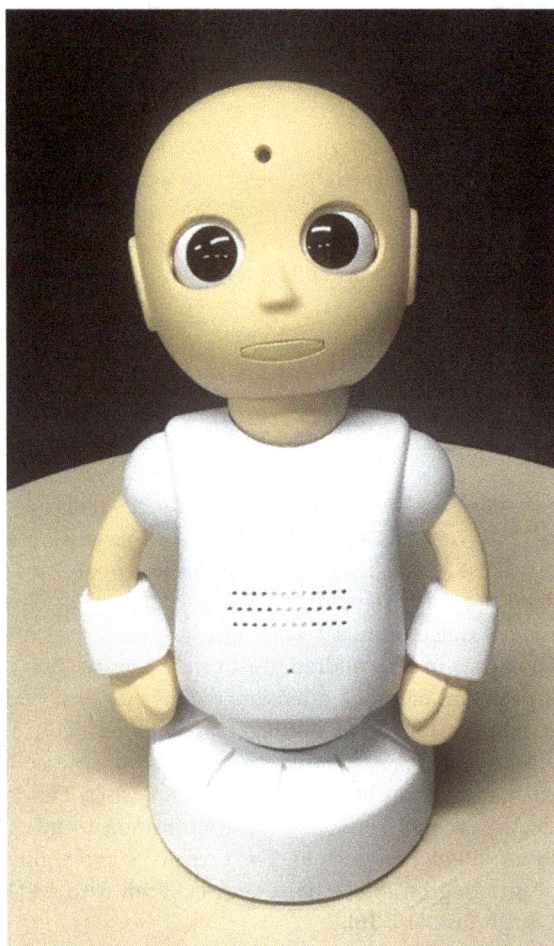

Fig. 1 CommU

interpret the communication signals and are expected to facilitate JA.

We compared the behavior of children with ASD with that of children with typical development (TD) during a JA elicitation task while the children interacted with a human or a robotic agent. The primary objective of this study was to test whether the robot is more useful in facilitating JA than a human agent in children with ASD during an interactive session. Second, we tested whether children with ASD show improvement in JA during human interactions after interacting with the robot CommU. Third, we tested whether the robot is more useful in facilitating JA in children with ASD than children with TD. We hypothesized that (a) children with ASD would demonstrate better JA under the CommU condition than under the human agent condition, (b) children with ASD would show improvement in JA tasks with a human after interacting with CommU, and (c) the facilitative effect of JA due to robot intervention would be larger in children with ASD than in TD children.

The age of the participants naturally affects the outcome of experiments investigating JA. JA performance in older children with ASD (mean age 9.25 ± 1.87 years) is similar to that in TD children during interactions with a human agent [14]. However, these experiments are too difficult for younger children to complete. In fact, in a previous study [28] involving children with ASD under 5 years of age, many participants dropped out of the study. In our preliminary study (unpublished), many children younger than 4 years of age were afraid of CommU and could not participate in the study. This confounding factor should be minimized using subjects within a narrow age range over 5 years. In addition, Vailouli et al. [32] suggested that challenges with JA do not abate, even at the time the child enters elementary school. There are several studies reporting the efficacy of JA intervention in children with ASD older than 5 years of age. For example, Vailouli et al. [32] have shown that JA intervention for children with ASD between the ages of 5 and 7 years was effective in promoting social engagement. Eissa [33] showed that JA intervention for children with ASD between the ages of 5 and 7 years was effective in improving eye contact, gesturing, following instructions, initiating caressing/singing, and communication skills. Therefore, we studied participants whose age range was limited to 5–6 years.

Methods
Participants
The present study was approved by the ethics committee of Kanazawa University. All participants were recruited from the Research Center for Child Mental Development, Kanazawa University. All procedures involving human participants were conducted according to the ethical standards

of the institutional and/or national research committee and the 1964 Helsinki Declaration and its subsequent amendments or comparable ethical standards. After providing a complete explanation of the study, all participants provided written informed consent. All participants and their guardians agreed to participate in the study. The inclusion criteria for the participants were as follows: (1) age 5–6 years, (2) mental processing score on the Kaufman Assessment Battery for Children (K-ABC) [34] ≥ 70, and (3) acquisition score on the K-ABC ≥ 70. The K-ABC was employed to estimate the intelligence levels of the children. The children with ASD were diagnosed using the Autism Diagnostic Observational Schedule-Generic (ADOS-G) [35], the Diagnostic Interview for Social and Communication Disorders (DISCO) [36], and the DSM-5 criteria at the time of recruitment for this study. Children with ASD were included in this study if they met the diagnosis criteria for childhood autism, atypical autism or Asperger's syndrome with DISCO or the ADOS criteria for an autism spectrum disorder.

The parents of the children in the TD group completed the Social Communication Questionnaire (SCQ) [37] to screen for clinically significant ASD symptoms in the TD children. Furthermore, to exclude children with psychiatric diagnoses, the Mini-International Neuropsychiatric Interview for Children and Adolescents (MINI Kids) [38, 39] was administered.

Procedures

Both the children with ASD and the TD children were randomly assigned to one of two groups (see Fig. 2). The participants completed a sequence of three interaction conditions that were done consecutively within the same visit. In the robotic intervention group, the participants interacted with "human A," "CommU," and "human A." In the control group, the participants interacted with "human A," "human B," and "human A." The participants were informed of the interaction order after the group assignments. During each session, the participants interacted with the robot or human agent for approximately 5 min (i.e., the participants in each group had approximately 15 min of total interaction). During each interaction, a human agent or "CommU" followed a specific interview script and protocol. Across the sessions, the scripts were slightly varied to promote engagement but followed the same basic structure. Please refer to the Additional file 1 for examples of the scripts.

During the "CommU" session, the robot was placed on a table in the middle of the room. To elicit the belief that the robot behaved and responded autonomously, we adopted a Wizard-of-Oz scheme similar to the systems conventionally used in robotics studies [40]. Specifically, the robot was operated by the researchers, who sat in front of a terminal computer located against a wall in the experimental room; the researchers were not visible during the trial. The participants were not informed that the robots were controlled by the researchers. The researchers operated the robots according to the prepared scripts.

To capture the relevant information, a simple joint interaction performance was prepared. A child-sized

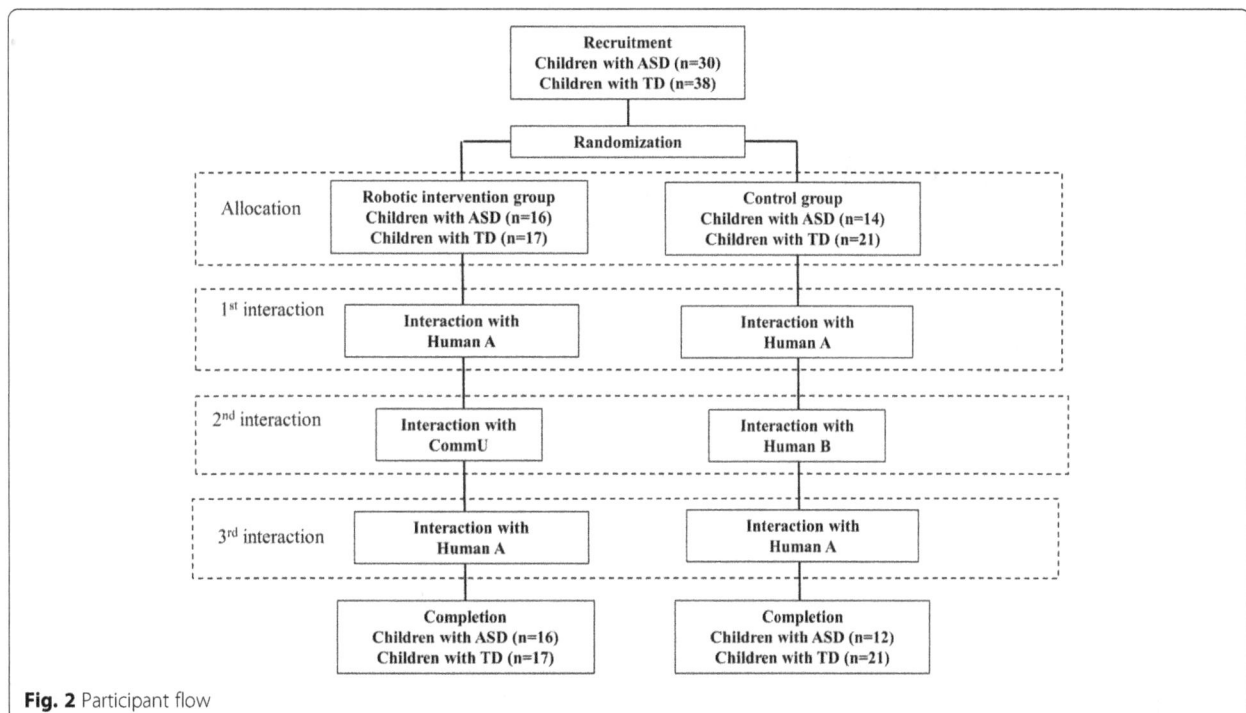

Fig. 2 Participant flow

table with chairs was set up in the middle of the experimental room. The parents were invited to sit 150 cm diagonally behind their child. CommU or a human agent was seated in front of the participant at a distance of 150 cm. We placed CommU on a desk at a height similar to that of a human agent. Two images were placed on the left and right sides of the participant, which were used as the foci of attention by the system. The images were 21 cm × 29.7 cm (width × height). The images were replaced each session. The images were placed at locations 200 cm to the side of the participant. Figures 3 (robotic setting) and Fig. 4 (human agent setting) illustrate the experimental room setup.

During each session, the participants were individually brought to the room by a research assistant and were accompanied by their parents, who remained in the room throughout the entire procedure. Each trial lasted as long as the participants were comfortable in the room and ended immediately if the children indicated that they wanted to stop the interaction or if the prepared content of the interaction had been completed.

During the latter half of each interaction session, after calling "Ne!," which corresponds to the English "Hey!" (we used this syllable because /ne/ is a sentence-ending word in Japanese and conveys prosodic information [41]), the human agent or CommU attempted to induce JA by alternatively gazing toward the child for 1 s and then toward the image on the left side of the participant for 3 s; then, without calling, the agent again gazed toward the child for 1 s and then toward the image for 3 s. Then, the human agent or CommU gazed again toward the child for 1 s and then toward the other image on right side of the participant for 3 s using the same

procedure, first after calling "Ne!," and second without calling "Ne!" (i.e., the human agent or CommU attempted to induce JA four times during each interaction session). Three digital videos were set up to capture any participant response to the social prompts for an off-line analysis. Figure 5 provides an example of how the participants typically interacted with the robots. The person in this manuscript provided written informed consent to publish this picture. He agreed to publish the picture.

"Achievement of JA" was defined as a participant responding (i.e., turning to look at) to the correct target within the 3 s window. Regardless of the participant response, the human agent or robot returned to a neutral position (standing straight and facing the participant) after each prompt. Each "achievement of JA" was measured offline by counting the number of times the child turned his/her head and/or eyes in the direction of the target without fully turning, following the social prompt. Each JA event was rated a 1 (success) or 0 (failure). Each score in each interaction was calculated by simple addition (maximum score = 4). Two trainers who did not know the objective of this study independently rated the scores by watching the videotape. The raters attained a high degree of reliability (intraclass coefficient (ICC) = .98). If their scores differed, they watched the videotape together and determined the score.

Robotic platform

CommU (Vstone Co., Ltd.) is 304 mm tall. CommU has 14 ° of freedom (DoFs) as follows: waist (2), left shoulder (2), right shoulder (2), neck (3), eyes (3), eyelids (1), and

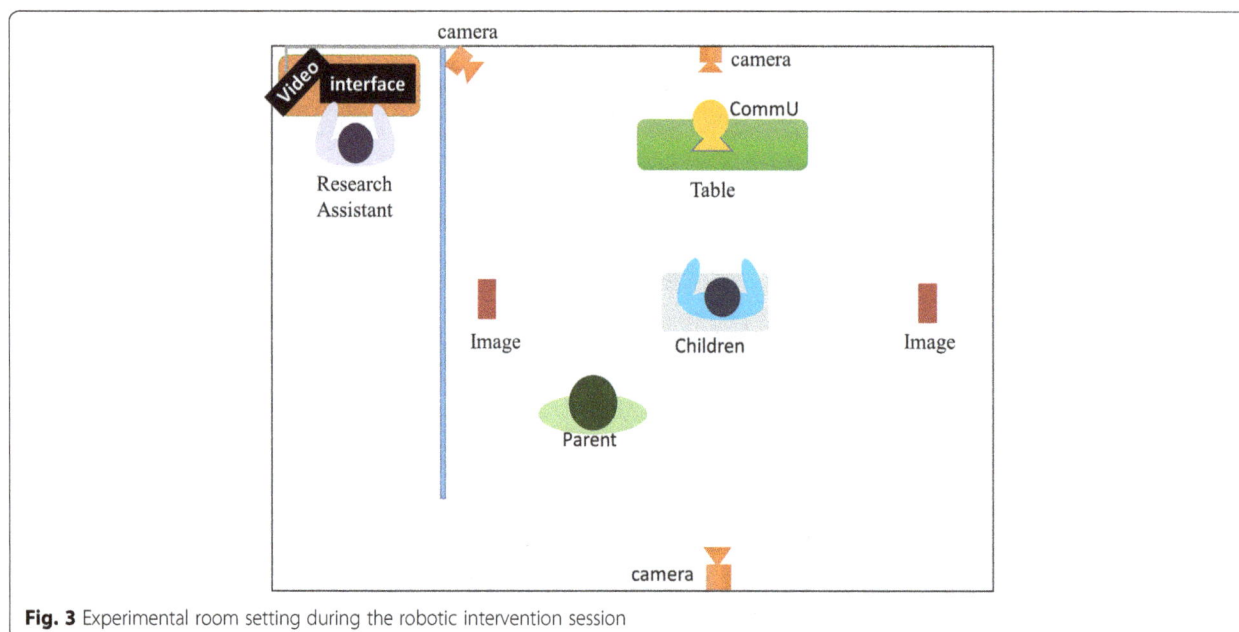

Fig. 3 Experimental room setting during the robotic intervention session

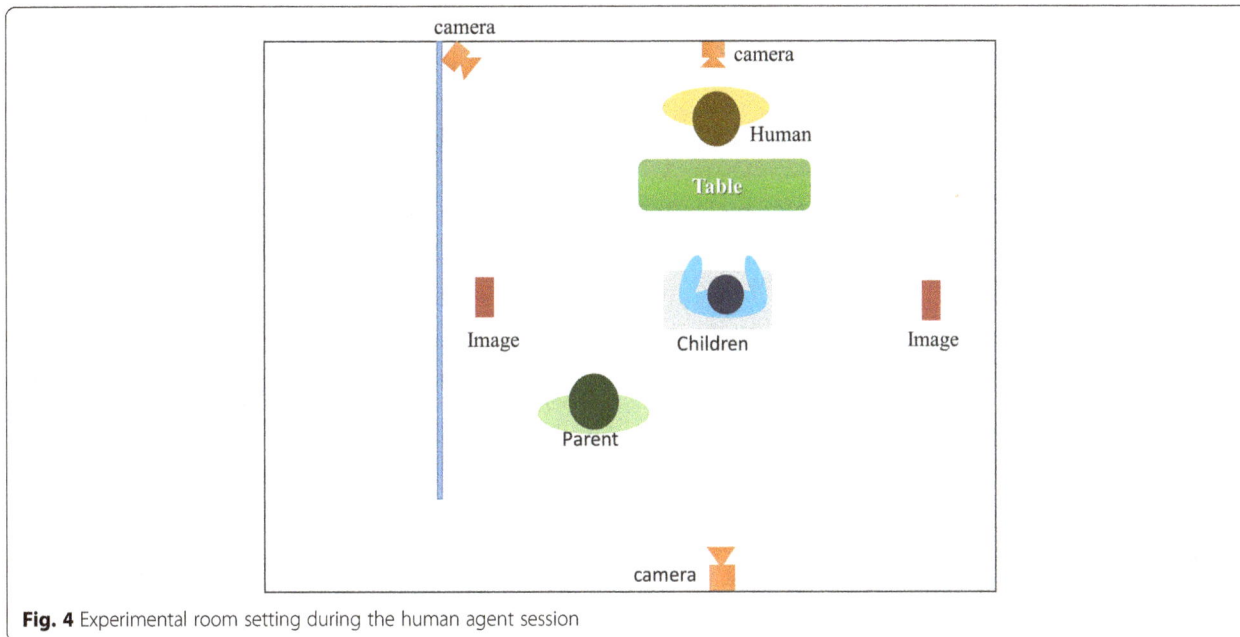

Fig. 4 Experimental room setting during the human agent session

lips (1). The careful design of the eyes and multiple DoFs dedicated to controlling its field of vision contribute to its rich gaze expressions. Its face can show a range of simplified expressions that are less complex than those of a real human face. The robot's cute shape, which resembles a child, is expected to be easy to anthropomorphize. Furthermore, its small and cute appearance is expected to help prevent fearfulness among

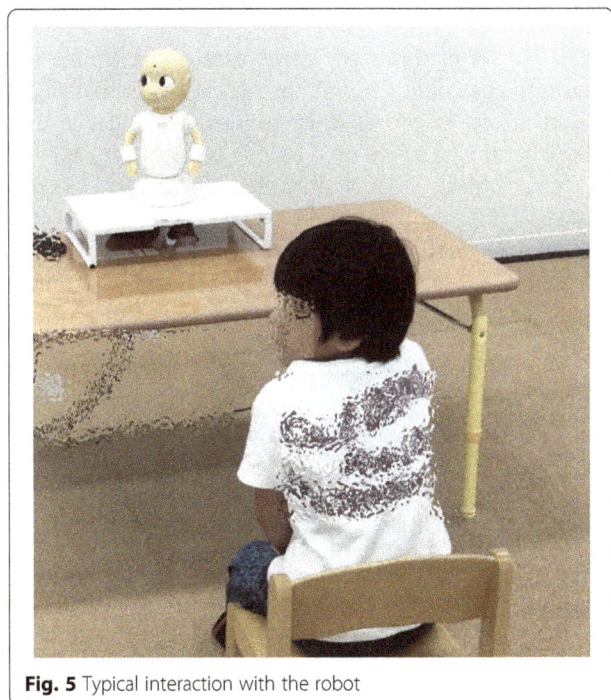

Fig. 5 Typical interaction with the robot

children. In addition, CommU makes very little noise, and its interlocutor is not distressed by its noise.

Statistical analysis

The statistical analyses were performed using SPSS version 24.0 (IBM, Armonk, NY, USA). Descriptive statistics were performed to describe the sample. The differences between the groups in terms of age, K-ABC mental processing score, and K-ABC achievement score were analyzed by performing independent samples t tests. The gender proportion was analyzed by performing a $\chi2$ test. To test the first hypothesis that children with ASD would demonstrate better JA under the CommU condition than under the human agent condition, a two-way mixed ANOVA was performed to analyze the collected data from the children with ASD (JA) with one repeated factor (time; first and second interactive sessions) and one group factor (i.e., robot intervention group vs. control group). To test the second hypothesis that children with ASD would exhibit improved JA tasks with human after interacting with CommU, a two-way mixed ANOVA was performed to analyze the collected data from the children with ASD (JA) with one repeated factor (time; first and third interactive sessions) and one group factor (i.e., robot intervention group vs. control group). To test the third hypothesis that JA was facilitated differently by the human and robot agents between the children with ASD and TD children in the robotic intervention group, a two-way mixed ANOVA was used to analyze the collected data (JA) with one repeated factor (time: first and second interactive sessions) and one group factor (ASD vs. TD). An alpha level of 0.05 was employed for these analyses.

Results

Demographic data

Thirty children with ASD (aged 5–6 years) and 38 children with typical development (TD) (aged 5–6 years) participated in this experiment. Two children with ASD who were assigned to the control group were unable to complete the study due to distress. The ASD robotic intervention group included 16 participants (12 males), with a mean age of 70.56 ± 6.09 months. The ASD control group included 12 participants (7 males), with a mean age of 69.00 ± 4.39 months. The TD robotic intervention group included 17 participants (11 males), with a mean age of 69.88 ± 5.88 months. The TD control intervention group included 21 participants (14 males) with a mean age of 67.62 ± 6.03 months. No significant differences were observed among the groups in terms of the mean age, gender proportion, K-ABC mental processing score, or K-ABC achievement score. The SCQ total score of all participants was under 10. The participant details are presented in Table 1.

Performance of the children during the JA task

Regarding the differences in the ratings of JA between the robotic interaction and human agent groups in the children with ASD, the results of a two-way mixed ANOVA with one repeated factor (time; first and second interactive sessions) and one group factor (i.e., robot intervention group vs. control group) showed a significant interaction between the time and group effect ($F_{(1, 26)} = 11.45$; $p < 0.01$; see Fig. 6). This result supported our first hypothesis that children with ASD would demonstrate better JA under the CommU condition than under the human agent condition. In addition, the results of a two-way mixed ANOVA with one repeated factor (time; first and third interactive sessions) and one group factor (i.e., robot intervention group vs. control group) showed a significant interaction between the time and group effect ($F_{(1, 26)} = 8.90$; $p < 0.01$; see Fig. 6). This result supported our second hypothesis that children with ASD would exhibit improvement in JA tasks with human after interacting with CommU.

Regarding the differences in the ratings of the JA under the robotic condition between the ASD and TD children, the results of a two-way mixed ANOVA with one repeated factor (time; first and second interactive sessions) and one group factor (i.e., ASD vs. TD) showed a significant interaction between the time and group effect ($F_{(1, 31)} = 8.00$; $p < 0.01$; see Fig. 7). This result supported our third hypothesis that the facilitative effect of JA due to robot intervention would be larger in children with ASD than in TD children. The details are presented in Table 2.

Among the children with ASD in the robotic interaction group, 8 of 16 participants (50.0% of total sample) had improved JA responses, and no participants had worsened JA responses under the human agent condition before vs. after interaction with CommU (i.e., first and third interactive sessions).

Discussion

In the current study, we examined the differences between children with ASD and TD children in their responses to induction of JA by either a human or robotic agent with clear eyes that can turn its eyes. The children with ASD who interacted with the robot had better outcomes in terms of JA than the children who interacted with a human agent during all sessions and exhibited improved performance in a JA task with human after interacting with the robot. In addition, the facilitative effect of JA due to robot intervention was larger in children with ASD than in TD children. While we used a simple design, our aim was to provide preliminary data regarding which agent better elicits JA from children with ASD and TD children with the goal of designing appropriate and tailored robotic intervention paradigms in the future.

The results of this study demonstrate that simple exposure to the robot CommU increased JA. Interestingly, this occurred in the absence of specific guidance and special settings (i.e., we used simple pictures on paper as the target objects.). Thus, utilizing this robot could contribute to improvements in JA.

Many interventions using non-social objects are available for children with ASD; however, humanoid robot-assisted interventions could be more interesting to the

Table 1 Descriptive characteristics of the participants in the ASD robot intervention group, ASD control group, TD robot intervention group, and TD control group

Characteristics	ASD robot intervention group (n = 16) (M, SD)	ASD control group (n = 12) (M, SD)	TD robot intervention group (n = 17) (M, SD)	TD control group (n = 21) (M, SD)
Age in months	70.56 (6.09)	69.00 (4.39)	69.88 (5.88)	67.62 (6.03)
Sex (male:female)	12:4	7:5	11:6	14:7
K-ABC mental score	97.75 (13.42)	99.83 (17.69)	108.59 (12.54)	103.86 (13.79)
K-ABC achievement score	97.88 (19.04)	104.17 (13.29)	105.47 (13.15)	103.10 (15.79)
SCQ			1.94 (1.30)	3.33 (2.31)

M mean, *SD* standard deviation, *K-ABC mental* K-ABC mental processing scale, *K-ABC achievement* K-ABC achievement scale, *SRS-2*: Social Responsiveness Scale—Second Edition, T-score, *SCQ* Social Communication Questionnaire Lifetime Total Score

1st and 2nd Interactive session: Interaction $F(1,26)=11.45$ $p < 0.01$
1st and 3rd Interactive session: Interaction $F(1,26)=8.90$ $p < 0.01$

Rating of
Joint attention

Group

—— Robotic intervention group in the children with ASD

------ Control group in the children with ASD

Interactive session

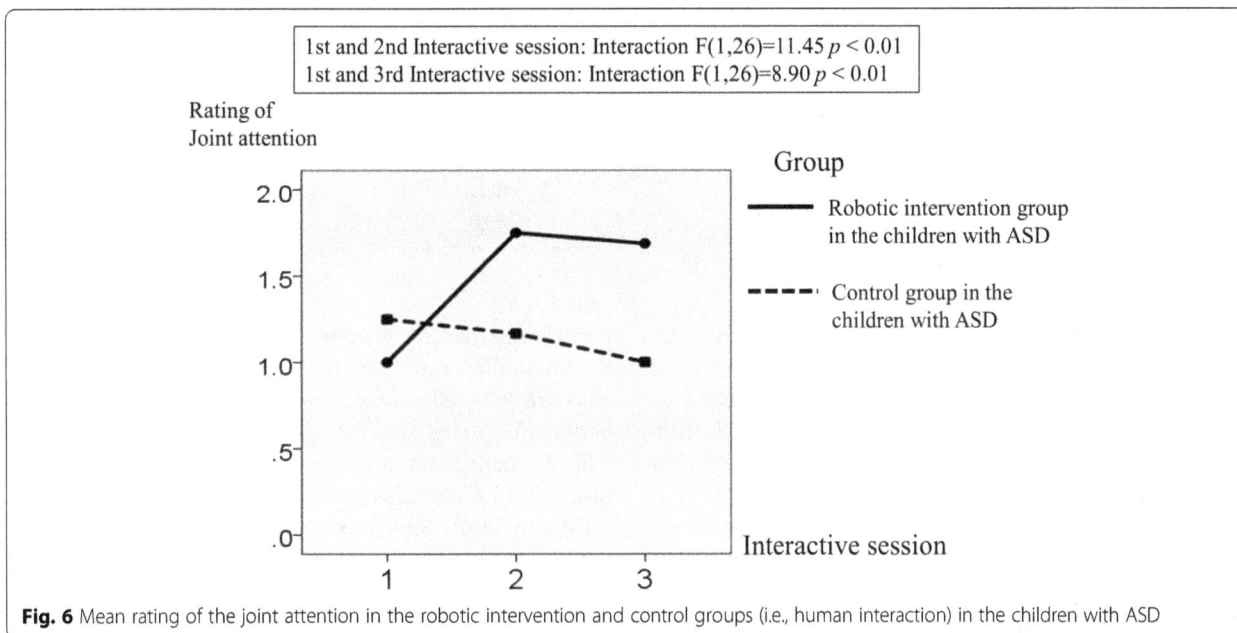

Fig. 6 Mean rating of the joint attention in the robotic intervention and control groups (i.e., human interaction) in the children with ASD

children than two-dimensional programs (i.e., virtual reality) [42] because the physical presence of a robot allows for a more engaging and enjoyable interaction than the use of virtual agents [43, 44]. In this study, many children with ASD showed sustained motivation to interact with the robot, which is an important factor in facilitating JA.

Madipakkam et al. [45] suggested that children with ASD exhibit an atypical response to eye contact due to their unconscious avoidance of eye contact. Thus, CommU's clear eyes likely urged the children with ASD to pay attention to the existence of its eyes. In previous studies using Flobi, which has clear eyes and can turn its eyes, the children with ASD paid attention to the robot's

eyes [46]. In contrast, in previous studies using Nao, whose eyes are relatively small, although the children with ASD appeared to be absorbed by the robot, they could not pay attention to its eyes [14, 27, 28]. Notably, Nao is a strong attractor for children with ASD. Nao does not highly resemble a human; thus, children with ASD do not feel threatened. However, Nao's body parts may not lead to the best results, as the attractive body parts can prevent the children from attending to a third object [29]. While brightly colored body parts attract attention, they must not be so bright as to over-stimulate the child in order to prompt JA. The color of the body parts of CommU is quiet and may contribute to the facilitation of JA in this study.

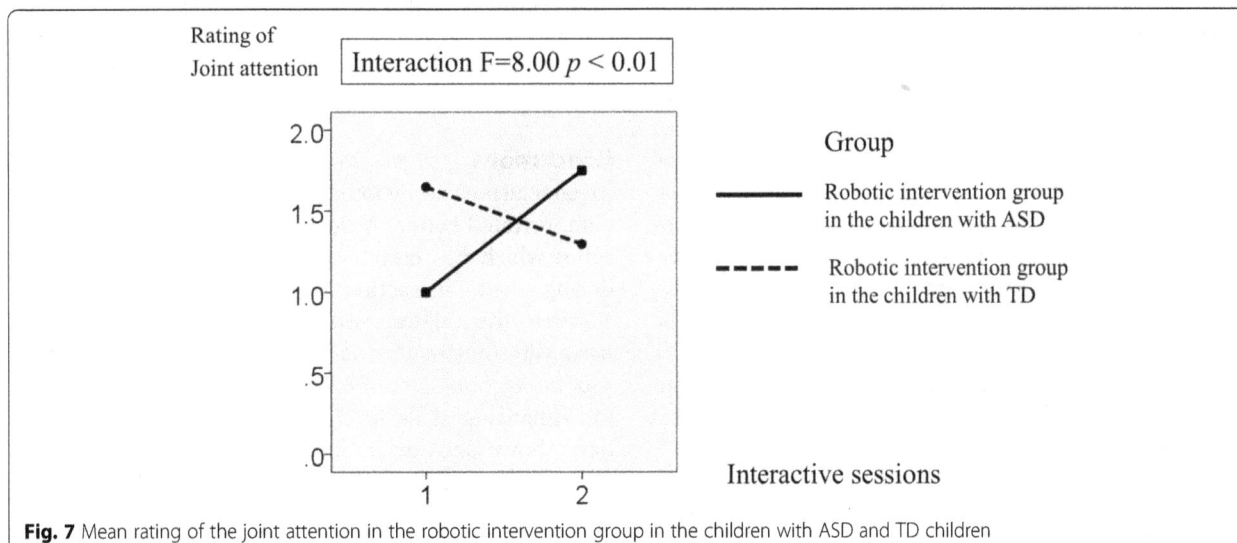

Rating of
Joint attention | Interaction $F=8.00$ $p < 0.01$

Group

—— Robotic intervention group in the children with ASD

------ Robotic intervention group in the children with TD

Interactive sessions

Fig. 7 Mean rating of the joint attention in the robotic intervention group in the children with ASD and TD children

Table 2 Performance of the participants in the ASD robot intervention group, ASD control group, TD robot intervention group, and TD control group during the JA task

Group	First interaction (M, SEM)	Second interaction (M, SEM)	Third interaction (M, SEM)
ASD robot intervention group (n = 16)	1.00 (0.27)	1.75 (0.27)	1.69(0.29)
ASD control group (n = 12)	1.25 (0.31)	1.17 (0.35)	1.00 (0.33)
TD robot intervention group (n = 17)	1.65 (0.32)	1.29 (0.29)	1.82 (0.35)
TD control group (n = 21)	1.81 (0.31)	1.76 (0.22)	1.57 (0.27)

M mean, SEM standard error of the mean

Pierno et al. [22] showed that during an imitation task, facilitation effects were only observed under the human agent condition in the TD children and only under the robot condition in ASD children. Our results are consistent with these findings in terms of the behaviors of the ASD children toward the robots and the behaviors of the TD children toward the human agents. One plausible theory might be that the complexity of the tasks completed by the robot and the human partner differ considerably. That is, variables in human behaviors include body pose, head pose, facial expression, head rotation during the experiment, and special unintentional gestures not present in the robotic experiment. The much larger number of potential uncontrolled variables in the experiments with the human partner makes it difficult to improve performance for children with ASD. Using a more complex robot like iCub [47] which has many other variables, it may be impossible to improve performance in children with ASD. Future studies using robots with different degrees of social complexity for children with various social abilities would help clarify an important factor in facilitating JA in children with ASD.

Although the changes observed in children with ASD in the robotic intervention group were statistically significant, we must consider whether they are also clinically significant. On average, the total JA score improved by 0.69 following interaction with CommU (i.e., first vs. third interactive sessions). This comprises an increase of 69% when compared to the pre-test score. In contrast, the total JA score was reduced by 0.25 in children with ASD in the control group following interaction with "human B" (i.e., first vs. third interactive sessions). This indicates that JA can improve in children with ASD in a quite limited number of sessions over a short period. Although the children in this sample demonstrated variable baseline JA skills under the human agent condition (i.e., first interactive session), 8 of 16 participants (50.0% of total sample) had improved JA responses, and no participants had worsened JA responses following interaction with CommU. Collectively, these findings suggest that robotic intervention successfully improved JA. Therefore, we believe that this increase is clinically relevant.

The strength of this study is its simple setting (i.e., we used simple pictures on paper as the target objects.) compared to that in previous studies [14, 28, 48]. The participants had no previous experience interacting with an unfamiliar robot. Notably, the children with ASD, who are generally weak in novel settings, demonstrated better JA during the interactions with the robot than with humans, and they exhibited improvement in JA tasks with human after interacting with the robot.

Certain limitations must be acknowledged. First, this study was a single session study and did not provide any indication of whether the children respond similarly over multiple sessions. Multiple sessions may offer a more extensive understanding of habituation to the robotic agent over time. While the current study did not test habituation effects in any way, it represents one of the first systematic investigations of JA using robots in children with ASD. Future studies should evaluate habituation effects with the robots by observing JA over an extended period. In addition, we do not have evidence supporting the generalizability of acquired JA to daily life. Therefore, we cannot comment on the social utility of our intervention program. The ultimate goal of the program is to enhance communication skills in daily life. In order to examine whether our program can attain this goal, future studies with a long-term longitudinal design are needed to confirm the generalized effect of this intervention in daily life (e.g., in kindergarten and at home). Third, the studied group had average cognitive skills. Clearly, future studies involving a broader range of functioning individuals are necessary to obtain a richer understanding of the potential use and impact of robotic interventions.

Conclusions

In conclusion, as hypothesized, the children with ASD demonstrated better JA during their interaction with the robot which has clear eyes and can turn its eyes than during their interaction with the human agents. In addition, the children with ASD exhibited improved JA tasks with human after interacting with the robot. While robotic technologies are considered potential vehicles for enhancing skills in children with ASD, few studies have shown such an impact using experimental designs relevant to core challenging areas. It is both unrealistic and unlikely that robotic technology will constitute a sufficient intervention paradigm addressing all areas of impairment for all individuals with the disorder in the immediate future. Given the current state of robotic technologies, we recommend that robots be used as adjunctive tools for short-term training in individuals with ASD. The findings of this study represent a meaningful contribution to the literature on the impact of robots on JA and provide information regarding the suitability of specific robot types for therapeutic use.

Abbreviations
ASD: Autism spectrum disorders; DSM-5: Diagnostic and Statistical Manual of Mental Disorders; JA: Joint attention; K-ABC: Kaufman Assessment Battery for Children; MINI Kids: Mini-International Neuropsychiatric Interview for Children and Adolescents; SCQ: Social Communication Questionnaire; TD: Typical development

Acknowledgements
We sincerely thank the participants and all the families who participated in this study. We thank M. Ozawa, Y. Morita, S. Kitagawa, and Y. Saotome for assisting with the data collection.

Funding
This study was partially supported by Grants-in-Aid for Scientific Research from the Japan Society for the Promotion of Science (17H05857), ERATO ISHI-GURO Symbiotic Human-Robot Interaction Project and the Center of Innovation Program from the Japan Science and Technology Agency, JST, Japan.

Authors' contributions
HK designed the study, conducted the experiment, performed the statistical analyses, analyzed and interpreted the data, and drafted the manuscript. YuiY, YukY, TI, CH, DS, ST, AK, JS, HI, YMa, YMi, and MK conceived the study, participated in its design, assisted with the data collection and scoring of the behavioral measures, analyzed and interpreted the data, were involved in drafting the manuscript, and revised the manuscript critically for important intellectual content. MK was involved in the final approval of the version to be published. All authors read and approved the final manuscript.

Competing interests
Yuichiro Yoshikawa and Hiroshi Ishiguro serve as consultants for Vstone Co. Ltd. Hiroshi Ishiguro owns stock in the same company. This involvement does not alter our adherence to the *Molecular Autism* policies regarding sharing data and materials.

Author details
[1]Research Center for Child Mental Development, Kanazawa University, 13-1, Takaramachi, Kanazawa, Ishikawa 920-8640, Japan. [2]Department of Systems Innovation, Graduate School of Engineering Science, Osaka University, 1-3, Machikaneryamachou, Toyonaka, Osaka 560-0043, Japan. [3]Service Robotics Research Group, Intelligent Systems Institute, National Institute of Advanced Industrial Science and Technology, Ibaraki 305-8560, Japan.

References
1. American Psychiatric Association. Diagnostic and statistical manual of mental disorders. 5th ed. Arlington, VA: American Psychiatric Publishing; 2013.
2. Charman T, Baron-Cohen S, Swettenham J, Baird G, Drew A, Cox A. Predicting language outcome in infants with autism and pervasive developmental disorder. Int J Lang Commun Disord. 2003;38:265–85.
3. Delinicolas EK, Young RL. Joint attention, language, social relating, and stereotypical behaviours in children with autistic disorder. Autism. 2007;11: 425–36.
4. Mundy P, Block J, Delgado C, Pomares Y, Van Hecke AV, Parlade MV. Individual differences and the development of joint attention in infancy. Child Dev. 2007;78:938–54.
5. Schertz HH, Odom SL, Baggett KM, Sideris JH. Effects of joint attention mediated learning for toddlers with autism spectrum disorders: an initial randomized controlled study. Early Child Res Q. 2013;28:249–58.
6. Schietecatte I, Roeyers H, Warreyn P. Exploring the nature of joint attention impairments in young children with autism spectrum disorder: associated social and cognitive skills. J Autism Dev Disord. 2012;42:1–12.
7. Mundy P, Sigman M, Kasari C. A longitudinal study of joint attention and language development in autistic children. J Autism Dev Disord. 1990;20: 115–28.
8. Murza KA, Schwartz JB, Hahs-Vaughn DL, Nye C. Joint attention interventions for children with autism spectrum disorder: a systematic review and meta-analysis. Int J Lang Commun Disord. 2016;51:236–51.
9. Mundy P, Kim K, McIntyre N, Lerro L, Jarrold W. Brief report: joint attention and information processing in children with higher functioning autism spectrum disorders. J Autism Dev Disord. 2016;46:2555–60.
10. Kasari C, Gulsrud AC, Wong C, Kwon S, Locke J. Randomized controlled caregiver mediated joint engagement intervention for toddlers with autism. J Autism Dev Disord. 2010;40:1045–56.
11. Poon KK, Watson LR, Baranek GT, Poe MD. To what extent do joint attention, imitation, and object play behaviors in infancy predict later communication and intellectual functioning in ASD? J Autism Dev Disord. 2012;42:1064–74.
12. Dawson G, Meltzoff AN, Osterling J, Rinaldi J, Brown E. Children with autism fail to orient to naturally occurring social stimuli. J Autism Dev Disord. 1998; 28:479–85.
13. Courchesne E, Chisum H, Townsend J. Neural activity-dependent brain changes in development: implications for psychopathology. Dev Psychopathol. 1994;6:697–722. https://doi.org/10.1017/S0954579400004740.
14. Anzalone SM, Tilmont E, Boucenna S, Xavier J, Jouen A-L, Bodeau N, et al. How children with autism spectrum disorder behave and explore the 4-dimensional (spatial 3D+time) environment during a joint attention induction task with a robot. Res Autism Spec Disord. 2014;8:814–26.
15. Scott JG, Saint-Georges C, Mahdhaoui A, Chetouani M, Cassel RS, Laznik M-C, et al. Do parents recognize autistic deviant behavior long before diagnosis? Taking into account interaction using computational methods. PLoS One. 2011;6:e22393.
16. White SA, Cohen D, Cassel RS, Saint-Georges C, Mahdhaoui A, Laznik M-C, et al. Do parentese prosody and fathers' involvement in interacting facilitate social interaction in infants who later develop autism? PLoS One. 2013;8: e61402.
17. Klin A, Lin DJ, Gorrindo P, Ramsay G, Jones W. Two-year-olds with autism orient to non-social contingencies rather than biological motion. Nature. 2009;459:257–61.
18. Baron-Cohen S. The hyper-systemizing, assortative mating theory of autism. Prog Neuro-Psychopharmacol Biol Psychiatry. 2006;30:865–72.
19. Baron-Cohen S. The extreme male brain theory of autism. Trends Cogn Sci. 2002;6:248–54.
20. Kumazaki H, Muramatsu T, Yoshikawa Y, Matsumoto Y, Miyao M, Ishiguro H, et al. Tele-operating an android robot to promote the understanding of facial expressions and to increase facial expressivity in individuals with autism spectrum disorder. Am J Psychiatry. 2017;174:904–5.
21. Cook J, Swapp D, Pan X, Bianchi-Berthouze N, Blakemore SJ. Atypical interference effect of action observation in autism spectrum conditions. Psychol Med. 2014;44:731–40.

22. Pierno AC, Mari M, Lusher D, Castiello U. Robotic movement elicits visuomotor priming in children with autism. Neuropsychologia. 2008;46:448–54.

23. Yun SS, Choi J, Park SK, Bong GY, Yoo H. Social skills training for children with autism spectrum disorder using a robotic behavioral intervention system. Autism Res. 2017;10:1306–23.

24. Huskens B, Palmen A, Van der Werff M, Lourens T, Barakova E. Improving collaborative play between children with autism spectrum disorders and their siblings: the effectiveness of a robot-mediated intervention based on Lego® therapy. J Autism Dev Disord. 2015;45:3746–55.

25. Diehl JJ, Schmitt LM, Villano M, Crowell CR. The clinical use of robots for individuals with autism spectrum disorders: a critical review. Res Autism Spectr Disord. 2012;6:249–62.

26. Bird G, Leighton J, Press C, Heyes C. Intact automatic imitation of human and robot actions in autism spectrum disorders. Proc Biol Sci. 2007;274: 3027–31.

27. Warren ZE, Zheng Z, Swanson AR, Bekele E, Zhang L, Crittendon JA, et al. Can robotic interaction improve joint attention skills? J Autism Dev Disord. 2015;45:3726–34.

28. Bekele E, Crittendon JA, Swanson A, Sarkar N, Warren ZE. Pilot clinical application of an adaptive robotic system for young children with autism. Autism. 2014;18:598–608.

29. Pennisi P, Tonacci A, Tartarisco G, Billeci L, Ruta L, Gangemi S, et al. Autism and social robotics: a systematic review. Autism Res. 2016;9:165–83.

30. Shimaya J, Yoshikawa Y, Matsumoto Y, Kumazaki H, Ishiguro H, Mimura M, et al. Advantages of indirect conversation via a desktop humanoid robot: case study on daily life guidance for adolescents with autism spectrum disorders. 25th IEEE Int Symp Robot Hum Interact Commun. 2016:831–6.

31. Kumazaki H, Warren Z, Swanson A, Yoshikawa Y, Matsumoto Y, Takahashi H, et al. Can robotic systems promote self-disclosure in adolescents with autism spectrum disorder? A pilot study. Front Psychiatry. 2018;9:36.

32. Vaiouli P, Grimmet K, Ruich LJ. "Bill is now singing": joint engagement and the emergence of social communication of three young children with autism. Autism. 2013;19:73–83.

33. Eissa MA. The effectiveness of a joint attention training program on improving communication skills of children with autism spectrum disorder. Int J Psycho-Educational Sci. 2015;4:3–12.

34. Kaufman A, Kaufman N. Kaufman assessment battery for children: administration and scoring manual. Circle Pines, MN: American Guidance Service; 1983.

35. Lord C, Risi S, Lambrecht L, Cook EH Jr, Leventhal BL, DiLavore PC, et al. The autism diagnostic observation schedule-generic: a standard measure of social and communication deficits associated with the spectrum of autism. J Autism Dev Disord. 2000;30:205–23.

36. Wing L, Leekam SR, Libby SJ, Gould J, Larcombe M. The diagnostic interview for social and communication disorders: background, inter-rater reliability and clinical use. J Child Psychol Psychiatry. 2002;43:307–25.

37. Rutter M, Bailey A, Lord C. The social communication questionnaire. Los Angeles, CA: Western Psychological Services; 2010.

38. Sheehan DV, Lecrubier Y, Sheehan KH, Amorim P, Janavs J, Weiller E, et al. The Mini-International Neuropsychiatric Interview (M.I.N.I.): the development and validation of a structured diagnostic psychiatric interview for DSM-IV and ICD-10. J Clin Psychiatry. 1998;59(Suppl 20):22–33. quiz 34

39. Otsubo T, Tanaka K, Koda R, Shinoda J, Sano N, Tanaka S, et al. Reliability and validity of Japanese version of the Mini-International Neuropsychiatric Interview. Psychiatry Clin Neurosci. 2005;59:517–26.

40. Nishio S, Taura K, Sumioka H, Ishiguro H. Teleoperated android robot as emotion regulation media. Int J Soc Rob. 2013;5:563–73.

41. Anderson V, Hiramoto M, Wong A. Prosodic analysis of the interactional particle ne in Japanese gendered speech. Japanese/Korean Linguis. 2007;15:43–54.

42. Pan Y, Steed A. A comparison of avatar-, video-, and robot-mediated interaction on users' trust in expertise. Front Robot AI. 2016;3. https://doi.org/10.3389/frobt.2016.00012.

43. Lee KM, Jung Y, Kim J, Kim SR. Are physically embodied social agents better than disembodied social agents? The effects of physical embodiment, tactile interaction, and people's loneliness in human–robot interaction. Int J Hum Comput Stud. 2006;64:962–73.

44. Wainer J, Feil-seifer D, Shell D, Mataric M. The role of physical embodiment in human-robot interaction. 15th IEEE Int Symp Robot Hum Interactive Commun. 2006:117–22.

45. Madipakkam AR, Rothkirch M, Dziobek I, Sterzer P. Unconscious avoidance of eye contact in autism spectrum disorder. Sci Rep. 2017;7:13378.

46. Damm O, Malchus K, Jaecks P, Krach S, Paulus F, Naber M, et al. Different gaze behavior in human-robot interaction in Asperger's syndrome: an eye-tracking study. IEEE RO-MAN. 2013:368–9.

47. Metta G, Natale L, Nori F, Sandini G, Vernon D, Fadiga L, et al. The iCub humanoid robot: an open-systems platform for research in cognitive development. Neural Netw. 2010;23:1125–34.

48. Warren Z, Zheng Z, Das S, Young EM, Swanson A, Weitlauf A, et al. Brief report: development of a robotic intervention platform for young children with ASD. J Autism Dev Disord. 2015;45:3870–6.

Sleep disturbances are associated with specific sensory sensitivities in children with autism

Orna Tzischinsky[1*†], Gal Meiri[2†], Liora Manelis[2,3], Asif Bar-Sinai[2,3], Hagit Flusser[4], Analya Michaelovski[4], Orit Zivan[2], Michal Ilan[2,3], Michal Faroy[4], Idan Menashe[5] and Ilan Dinstein[3,6†]

Abstract

Background: Sensory abnormalities and sleep disturbances are highly prevalent in children with autism, but the potential relationship between these two domains has rarely been explored. Understanding such relationships is important for identifying children with autism who exhibit more homogeneous symptoms.

Methods: Here, we examined this relationship using the Caregiver Sensory Profile and the Children's Sleep Habits Questionnaire, which were completed by parents of 69 children with autism and 62 age-matched controls.

Results: In line with previous studies, children with autism exhibited more severe sensory abnormalities and sleep disturbances than age-matched controls. The sleep disturbance scores were moderately associated with touch and oral sensitivities in the autism group and with touch and vestibular sensitivities in the control group. Hypersensitivity towards touch, in particular, exhibited the strongest relationship with sleep disturbances in the autism group and single-handedly explained 24% of the variance in total sleep disturbance scores. In contrast, sensitivity in other sensory domains such as vision and audition was not associated with sleep quality in either group.

Conclusions: While it is often assumed that sensitivities in all sensory domains are similarly associated with sleep problems, our results suggest that hypersensitivity towards touch exhibits the strongest relationship with sleep disturbances when examining children autism. We speculate that hypersensitivity towards touch interferes with sleep onset and maintenance in a considerable number of children with autism who exhibit severe sleep disturbances. This may indicate the existence of a specific sleep disturbance mechanism that is associated with sensitivity to touch, which may be important to consider in future scientific and clinical studies.

Keywords: Autism, Children, Sensory abnormalities, Sleep disturbances, Hypersensitivity towards touch

Background

Autism is a remarkably heterogeneous disorder where different individuals exhibit distinct behavioral symptoms. This heterogeneity is apparent in the core symptoms that define the disorder (i.e., impaired social communication/interaction, repetitive behaviors, restricted interests, and sensory abnormalities) [1] and in additional symptoms that are prevalent in individuals with autism (e.g., sleep disturbances). A major goal of contemporary autism research is to identify individuals who share more homogeneous

symptoms and who may benefit from targeted interventions [2, 3]. Understanding potential relationships across symptom domains is an important step in characterizing individuals with more homogenous symptoms.

A large body of literature has shown that sensory problems are apparent in 60–90% of individuals with autism [4–9]. This has motivated the addition of sensory problems as a diagnostic criterion of autism in the DSM-5 [1]. However, sensory problems in autism can vary widely and include both hypo- and hypersensitivities in multiple sensory modalities [4, 6, 10–14]. Indeed, both hypo- and hypersensitivity can appear within the same individuals with autism at different times and in different contexts/situations [15]. Previous studies have shown that sensory

* Correspondence: orna3007@gmail.com
†Equal contributors
[1]Behavioral Science Department, Emek Yesreel College, Emek Yesreel, Israel
Full list of author information is available at the end of the article

abnormalities are positively correlated with autism severity in adults [16] and may [7] or may not [8] be correlated with adaptive behaviors in children with autism.

Sleep disturbances are another common symptom that is apparent in 40–80% of individuals with autism [17–20]. Disturbances include difficulty falling asleep, frequent wakings during the night, shorter sleep duration, and restlessness during sleep. Previous studies have reported that sleep disturbances are more prevalent in regressive autism [19], increase with autism severity [18, 21], and may [22, 23] or may not [17, 20] be associated with cognitive levels. In addition, the severity of sleep disturbances in children with autism seems to scale with their level of anxiety, attention deficits, impulsivity, challenging behaviors, and the use of medication [18, 21, 24–26].

Several studies have hypothesized that sleep disturbances may be associated with or even caused by sensory sensitivities in autism [19, 27], but this potential relationship has rarely been examined empirically. With this in mind, two recent studies used Autism Speaks' Autism Treatment Network (ATN) to examine the potential relationship between sensory abnormalities and sleep disturbances in autism. The ATN is a large national database [28] containing a wide variety of behavioral information from children with autism, which includes the Child Behavior Checklist (CBCL) [29], Short Sensory Profile [30], and a short, 23 item version, of the Children's Sleep Habits Questionnaire (CSHQ) [31].

Both studies reported that sleep disturbances were significantly associated with children's anxiety levels as measured by the CBCL. In addition, one study reported that adding the under-responsive/sensory-seeking and auditory filtering scores of the Short Sensory Profile to a hierarchical regression model significantly improved the ability to predict total sleep disturbance scores from the CSHQ by 1% [21]. The second study computed a sensory over-responsivity score for each child (equivalent to sensory hypersensitivity), by summing the scores of several questions in the Short Sensory Profile that pertain to sensory hypersensitivity in multiple domains (i.e., touch, vision, taste/smell, and audition). This study reported significant correlations between sensory over-responsivity and several CSHQ subscales, which explained 1–6% of the variance in CSHQ scores [25]. Taken together, these studies suggest that Short Sensory Profile scores offer significant, but limited utility in explaining sleep disturbance scores of individuals with autism.

The goal of the current study was to perform a more in-depth examination of the relationship between sleep disturbances and sensory sensitivities by using the complete Caregiver Sensory Profile [32]. Unlike the Short Sensory Profile, which integrates scores across multiple sensory domains [30], the complete Caregiver Sensory Profile contains a larger number of questions that allow one to compute separate hypo- and hypersensitivity scores for each of five sensory domains (audition, vision, taste/smell, vestibular, and touch). This allowed us to determine whether sleep disturbances are more strongly associated with some sensory sensitivities than others. Determining such specificity has value for elucidating the physiological mechanisms that may generate sleep disturbances in autism and for guiding future clinical trials with sensory therapies and aids.

Methods

Participants

A total of 131 children participated in the study (Table 1): 69 children with autism (age 3–7, mean age 4.94 ± 1.23, 56 male) and 62 age-matched controls (age 3–7, mean age 4.82 ± 1.15, 41 males). There was no significant difference in the age of participating children across groups ($t(129)$) $= 0.64$, $p = 0.57$, two-tailed t test). Children with autism were recruited through the Negev Autism Center [33]. Control children of the same age were recruited from the community through an online forum at Ben Gurion University. Parents of all control children reported that their children were never suspected of having any developmental problems. Both the Helsinki committee at Soroka Medical Center and ethics committee at Ben Gurion University approved this study, and parents of all participating children signed an informed consent form.

Diagnosis

All children with autism met the DSM-5 criteria for autism as determined by both a physician (child psychiatrist or neurologist) and a developmental psychologist. Forty-nine of the 69 children with autism also completed an Autism Diagnostic Observation Schedule (ADOS) assessment to confirm the diagnosis [34]. Twenty-two of the 69 children with autism were taking medications that included Melatonin, Risperdal, Ritalin, and Neuleptil.

Table 1 Sample characteristics

	Autism $n = 69$	Typically developing $n = 62$
Gender	56 males, 13 females	41 males, 21 females
Age (years)	4.94 (1.23)	4.82 (1.15)
ADOS social*	12.4 (5.2)	
ADOS repetitive behaviors*	4.02 (1.8)	
ADOS total*	16.4 (6.5)	
ADOS comparison score*	6.9 (1.92)	

Gender and age of autism and control children as well as ADOS scores from the 49 children with autism who completed the assessment
*$n = 49$

Sensory profile

We used the Hebrew version of the Caregiver Sensory Profile questionnaire to assess sensory sensitivities in all children [35]. This questionnaire contains 125 questions that quantify the frequency of abnormal behavioral responses to various sensory experiences [32]. In the current study, we focused only on the five sensory sub-scales of the Sensory Profile, which include questions about auditory, visual, vestibular, touch, and oral sensory processing. These questions are split into high-threshold and low-threshold items, which measure hypo- and hyper-sensitivities respectively, with lower scores indicating more severe symptoms. We examined differences across groups for each of these scores separately and also for their total raw score, which combines both low- and high-threshold items, while keeping in mind that some children exhibit both hypo- and hypersensitivity to different sensory experiences (Tables 2 and 3).

CSHQ

Parents of all participants scored their child's sleep behaviors using the Hebrew version of the CSHQ [31, 36]. This caregiver questionnaire includes 33 items which are divided into eight subscales representing different sleep disturbances: bedtime resistance, sleep anxiety, sleep onset delay, sleep duration, night wakings, daytime sleepiness, sleep-disordered breathing, and parasomnias. The scores of these eight domains are summed to generate a total score of sleep disturbances for each child. The internal consistency values of the CSHQ subscales in our study were $\alpha = 0.533$–0.758, and their consistency with the total sleep score was $\alpha = 0.838$.

Statistical analyses

All statistical analyses were performed with Matlab (Mathworks, USA). We performed two-tailed t tests with unequal variance to compare the five sensory measures (visual, auditory, vestibular, touch, and oral) of the Sensory Profile across the autism and control groups. Equivalent tests were performed for the sleep measures (bedtime resistance, sleep onset delay, sleep duration, sleep anxiety, night wakings,

Table 2 Sensory Profile scores

Sensory Profile					
	Autism	Control	T stat	p value	Cohen's d
Auditory	24.30 (0.76)	33.4 (0.6)	$t(129) = -9.37$	$p < 0.001$	2.02
Visual	33.97 (0.78)	39.58 (0.57)	$t(129) = -5.78$	$p < 0.001$	1.00
Vestibular	42.54 (0.75)	51.34 (0.47)	$t(129) = -9.97$	$p < 0.001$	1.72
Touch	64.48 (1.54)	81.81 (0.82)	$t(129) = -9.95$	$p < 0.001$	1.71
Oral	40.29 (1.28)	52.84 (0.91)	$t(129) = -7.97$	$p < 0.001$	1.39

The mean and standard error (in parentheses) are presented for the autism (left column) and control (second column) groups along with the statistics of two-sample t tests with unequal variances (right hand column). Italicized p values were significant after Bonferroni correction ($p < 0.01$)

Table 3 Correlations across sensory domains

	Visual	Vestibular	Touch	Oral
Autism ($n = 69$)				
Auditory score	$P = 0.5*$	$P = 0.46*$	$P = 0.46*$	$P = 0.44*$
	$S = 0.49*$	$S = 0.41*$	$S = 0.45*$	$S = 0.44*$
Visual score		$P = 0.47*$	$P = 0.46*$	$P = 0.5*$
		$S = 0.45*$	$S = 0.49*$	$S = 0.52*$
Vestibular score			$P = 0.67*$	$P = 0.52*$
			$S = 0.68*$	$S = 0.53*$
Touch score				$P = 0.63*$
				$S = 0.64*$
Control ($n = 62$)				
Auditory score	$P = 0.6*$	$P = 0.61*$	$P = 0.57*$	$P = 0.32$
	$S = 0.59*$	$S = 0.63*$	$S = 0.61*$	$S = 0.38*$
Visual score		$P = 0.53*$	$P = 0.55*$	$P = 0.38*$
		$S = 0.57*$	$S = 0.63*$	$S = 0.55*$
Vestibular score			$P = 0.75*$	$P = 0.51*$
			$S = 0.71*$	$S = 0.53*$
Touch score				$P = 0.47*$
				$S = 0.50*$

Pearson's (P) and Spearman's (S) correlation coefficients are presented for each pair of sensory domains in the Sensory Profile for the autism (top) and control (bottom) groups. Asterisks indicate significant correlation coefficients after Bonferroni correction ($p < 0.005$)

parasomnias, sleep-disordered breathing, daytime sleepiness, and total sleep score). All tests were corrected for multiple comparisons using the Bonferroni method (i.e., five subscales of the Sensory Profile and eight subscales in the CSHQ). All sensory and sleep measures were close to normal distributions as demonstrated by their skewness and kurtosis values, which were all between -1 and 1, except for the visual and vestibular scores in the control group (skewness $= -1.48$ and -1.23, kurtosis $= 4.38$ and 1.59, respectively). Potential relationships between scores from each of the sensory modalities and the total sleep score were examined using both Pearson's and Spearman's correlations. This ensured that our conclusions were not based on the assumption that the distributions of the variables were normal or that the relationships were linear.

In a final set of analyses, we performed several regression analyses, separately for children with autism and controls, and separately for the total raw scores, low-threshold items, and high-threshold items of the Sensory Profile. In each case, we examined the ability of the sensory profile scores to explain the total sleep disturbance scores. Initial regression models contained a single predictor containing the scores from each of the five sensory domains (i.e., visual, auditory, vestibular, touch, or oral), and in a sixth model we included all five predictors together. This enabled us to examine the contribution of scores from each sensory modality, when attempting to explain the severity of sleep disturbances in individual children. In a final regression analysis, we also added age, gender, medication-use, and ADOS scores to determine whether these variables had an effect on the variance explained.

Results

Sensory sensitivities in autism

Children with autism exhibited abnormal sensory sensitivities that were evident in the Sensory Profile scores of all five sensory modalities (Fig. 1 and Table 2). The total raw scores from the Sensory Profile were significantly lower in children with autism as compared to the control children in the auditory, visual, vestibular, touch, and oral domains (Table 2). Similar results were also evident in all five sensory domains when comparing only male children in the two groups ($t(95) < -4.7$, $p < 0.001$), when including only children with autism who completed an ADOS assessment ($t(109) < -4.1$, $p < 0.001$), or when excluding children with autism who were taking medications ($t(107) < -5.5$, $p < 0.001$). Furthermore, sensory sensitivity scores from all five sensory modalities were not significantly different between children with autism who were or were not taking medication ($t(41) < 0.9$, $p > 0.34$), nor between male and female children with autism ($t(20) > -1$, $p > 0.29$).

The total raw scores of the Sensory Profile are the sum of scores from both low- and high-threshold items on the questionnaire, which measure hyper and hyposensitivities respectively (Fig. 2). Note that children can be hypersensitive to some stimuli and hyposensitive to other stimuli even within the same sensory domain. Children with autism exhibited significantly lower scores on the low-threshold (hypersensitivity) items as compared with controls in all five sensory modalities ($t(129) < -4.55$, $p < 0.005$). The same was also true for high-threshold items ($t(129) < -5.75$, $p < 0.005$).

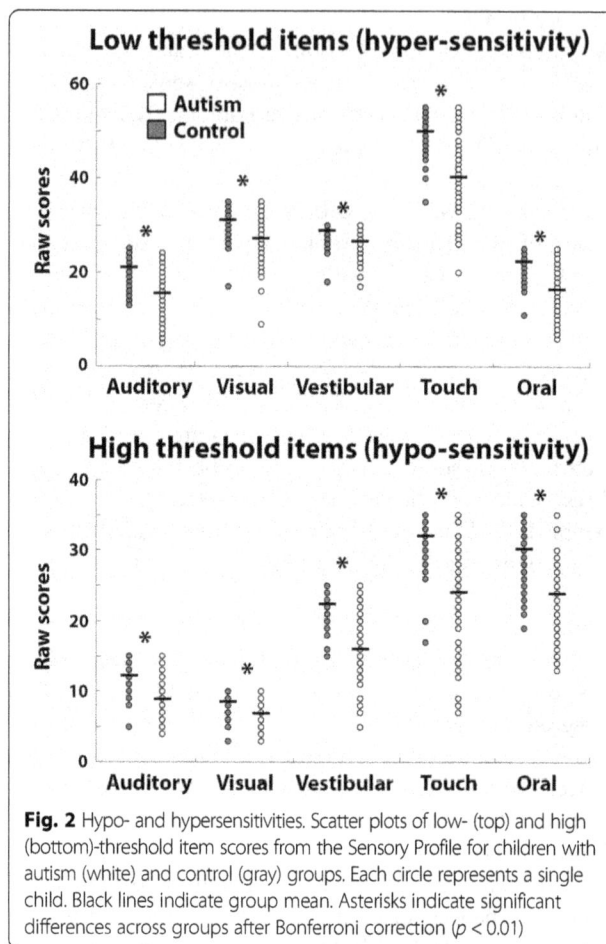

Fig. 2 Hypo- and hypersensitivities. Scatter plots of low- (top) and high (bottom)-threshold item scores from the Sensory Profile for children with autism (white) and control (gray) groups. Each circle represents a single child. Black lines indicate group mean. Asterisks indicate significant differences across groups after Bonferroni correction ($p < 0.01$)

Equivalent results were found when including only male children, for both low- ($t(95) < -4.1$, $p < 0.001$) and high-threshold items ($t(95) < -4.6$, $p < 0.005$), when including only children who had ADOS scores, for both low-

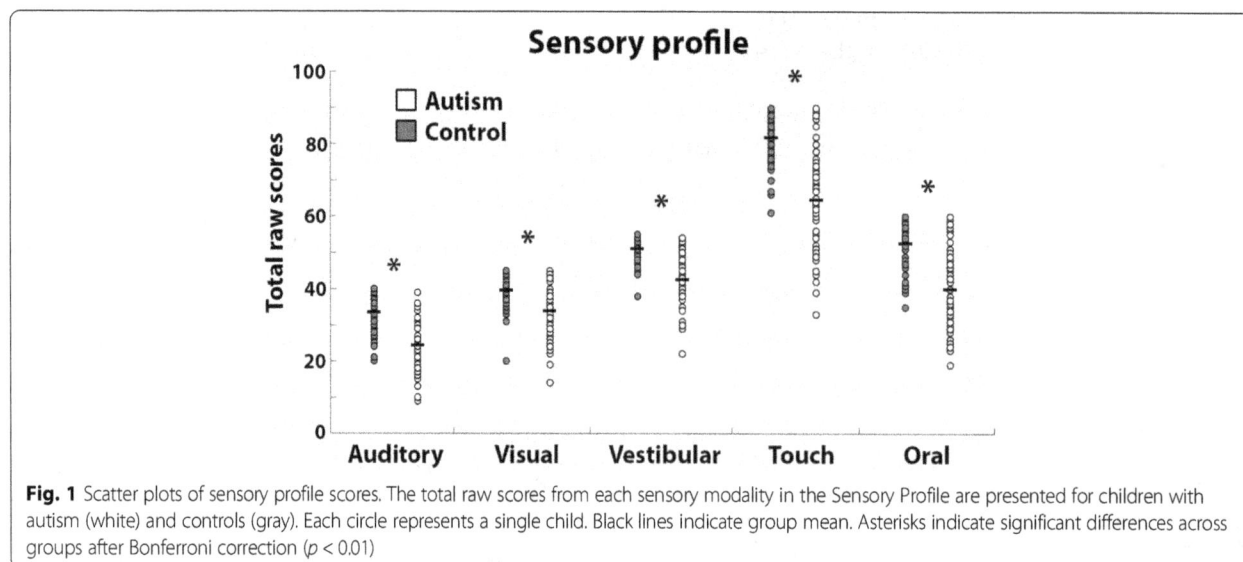

Fig. 1 Scatter plots of sensory profile scores. The total raw scores from each sensory modality in the Sensory Profile are presented for children with autism (white) and controls (gray). Each circle represents a single child. Black lines indicate group mean. Asterisks indicate significant differences across groups after Bonferroni correction ($p < 0.01$)

$(t(109) < -3.65, p < 0.01)$ and high-threshold items $(t(109) < -4.5, p < 0.001)$, and when excluding children with autism who were taking medication, for both low- $(t(107) < -4.8, p < 0.001)$ and high-threshold items $(t(107) < -5.2, p < 0.001)$.

Strong and significant correlations were found between Sensory Profile scores of different sensory domains in both the autism and control groups (Table 3), demonstrating that sensory sensitivities of individual children were similar across most sensory domains in both groups.

Sleep problems in autism

Children with autism exhibited significantly larger sleep disturbance scores than control children in the total score and in all CSHQ subscales, except for sleep-disordered breathing, night wakings, and day time sleepiness (Table 4 and Fig. 3). A total sleep disturbances score of 41 is considered to be a useful clinical cutoff when screening children for sleep problems [27]. Significantly more children with autism (85.5%) had scores higher than this cutoff in comparison to control children (54.8%) $(X^2(1) = 14.91, p < 0.001)$.

Performing the same analysis while including different subsets of children with autism yielded similar results. Total sleep disturbance scores were significantly larger in the autism group when excluding children with autism who were taking medication $(t(107) = 3.23, p = 0.001)$, when including only male children in both groups $(t(95) = 5.09, p < 0.001)$, and when including only children who completed the ADOS in the autism group $(t(109) = 4.3, p < 0.001)$.

The relationship between sleep disturbances and sensory sensitivities

We examined the relationship between the total sleep disturbance scores and sensory sensitivity scores in each of the five sensory domains (Table 5). Significant negative correlations were apparent between the touch or oral sensitivity scores and total sleep disturbance scores of children with autism when computing Pearson's or Spearman's correlations. Control children exhibited significant negative correlations between the vestibular or touch sensitivity scores and total sleep disturbance scores when computing Pearson's correlations, and similar trends were apparent when computing Spearman's correlations. All other correlations were not statistically significant.

Despite the strong correlations across sensory scores of the different modalities assessed by the Sensory Profile (Table 3), only *some* of the sensory scores were significantly correlated with the total sleep disturbance scores (Table 5). Furthermore, while significant negative correlations were apparent in the touch domain of both groups, scores of children with autism were distributed over a much wider range of values than control children as demonstrated in a scatter plot (Fig. 4). This means that the correlations in the autism group represented a tight relationship, which was apparent also in cases of severe sleep disturbances and sensory problems (i.e., correlation was robust throughout a larger range).

In additional analyses, we examined whether the total sleep disturbance scores were more strongly associated with low- or high-threshold items from the Sensory Profile (Table 6). Significant negative correlations were apparent between low item scores (i.e., hypersensitivity) in the touch and oral domains of children with autism and in the touch and vestibular domains of controls. Low item scores in all other sensory domains were not significantly correlated with sleep disturbance scores. Significant negative correlations were also apparent between high item scores (hyposensitivity) in the touch and oral domains of children with autism. High item scores in all other sensory domains of children with autism and all sensory domains in control children were not significantly correlated with sleep scores.

Table 4 CSHQ scores

CSHQ scores					
	Autism	Control	T stats	p value	Cohen's d
Bedtimes resistance	10.26 (0.39)	7.66 (0.29)	$t(129) = 5.35$	$p < 0.001$	0.93
Sleep onset delay	1.97 (0.10)	1.26 (0 .06)	$t(129) = 6.03$	$p < 0.001$	1.04
Sleep duration	4.38 (0.20)	3.31 (0.08)	$t(129) = 4.88$	$p < 0.005$	0.84
Sleep anxiety	6.73 (0.25)	5.24 (0.21)	$t(129) = 4.54$	$p < 0.005$	0.79
Parasomnia	9.49 (0.27)	7.92 (0.15)	$t(129) = 5.13$	$p < 0.001$	0.88
Night wakings	4.86 (0.20)	4.0 (0.16)	$t(129) = 3.27$	$p < 0.01$	0.57
Sleep-disordered breathings	3.64 (0.15)	3.23 (0.07)	$t(129) = 2.48$	$p = 0.12$	0.43
Day time sleepiness	13.1 (0.40)	13.05 (0.34)	$t(129) = 0.1$	$p = 0.92$	0.02
Total sleep disturbances	50.74 (1.13)	42.86 (0.73)	$t(129) = 5.87$	$p < 0.001$	1.02

The mean and standard error (in parentheses) are presented for the autism (left column) and control (middle column) groups along with the statistics of a two-sample t tests with unequal variances (right hand columns). Italicized p values were significant after Bonferroni correction ($p < 0.006$)

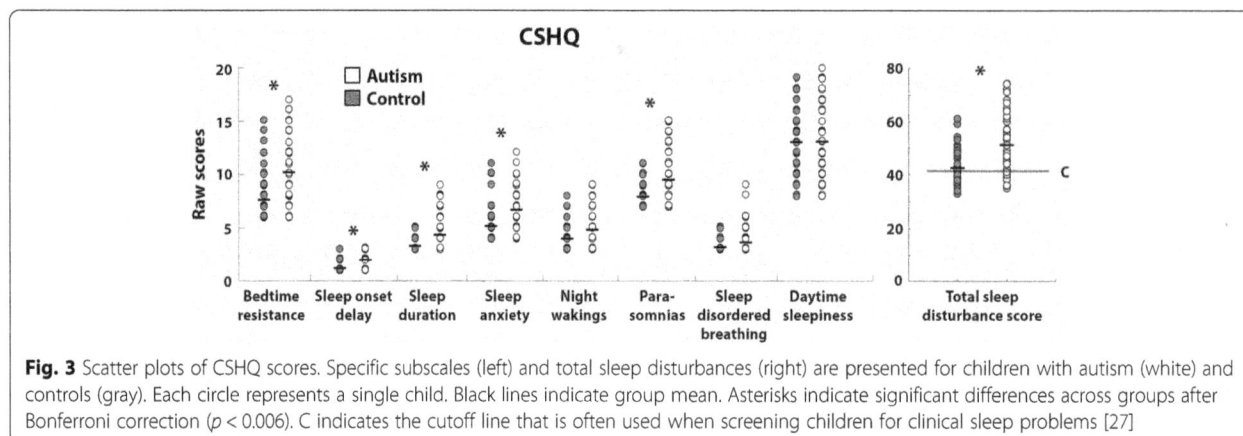

Fig. 3 Scatter plots of CSHQ scores. Specific subscales (left) and total sleep disturbances (right) are presented for children with autism (white) and controls (gray). Each circle represents a single child. Black lines indicate group mean. Asterisks indicate significant differences across groups after Bonferroni correction (p < 0.006). C indicates the cutoff line that is often used when screening children for clinical sleep problems [27]

Explaining sleep disturbances with sensory sensitivity scores

In a final set of regression analyses, we quantified how much of the variance in total sleep disturbance scores could be explained by the total raw scores from each of the five sensory domains separately and also when including all of them together. Incorporating the total raw scores from all of the sensory domains into a single regression model yielded an adjusted R^2 value of 0.29 in the autism group and 0.20 in the control group (Table 7).

When performing the regression with a single predictor from each sensory modality separately, the touch scores stood out in their ability to explain sleep disturbance scores in children with autism (adjusted R^2 = 0.29). This suggests that the touch scores could single-handedly explain as much of the variance in sleep scores as the integrated model, which contained all five predictors. In the control group, the vestibular and touch scores yielded adjusted R^2 of 0.20 and 0.16 respectively, thereby demonstrating their ability to explain large portions of the variability in sleep scores in the control group.

We performed equivalent analyses while separating the scores from the low-threshold (hypersensitivity) and high-threshold (hyposensitivity) items. The full low-threshold regression model (containing five predictors/modalities) yielded adjusted R^2 values of 0.24 and 0.21 in the autism

and control groups respectively while the full high-threshold model yielded adjusted R^2 values of 0.20 and 0.07. This demonstrates that low-threshold items that measure sensory hypersensitivity can explain sleep disturbance scores better than high-threshold items that measure hyposensitivity.

When examining low-threshold items in each sensory modality separately, the touch domain again stood out in its ability to explain sleep disturbance scores in children with autism (adjusted R^2 = 0.24). This result demonstrates that low-threshold touch scores could single-handedly explain most of the variance that was explained by the full

Table 5 Relationship between total sleep disturbance scores and total sensory scores in each of the sensory domains

	Autism (n = 69)		Control (n = 62)	
	Pearson	Spearman	Pearson	Spearman
Auditory	−0.19	−0.17	−0.22	−0.19
Visual	−0.18	−0.23	−0.16	−0.16
Vestibular	−0.26	−0.28	−0.47*	−0.33
Touch	−0.54*	−0.53*	−0.42*	−0.31
Oral	−0.42*	−0.41*	−0.29	−0.29

Pearson's and Spearman's correlations were computed for the autism (left) and control (right) groups. Asterisks indicate significant correlation coefficients after Bonferroni correction (p < 0.01)

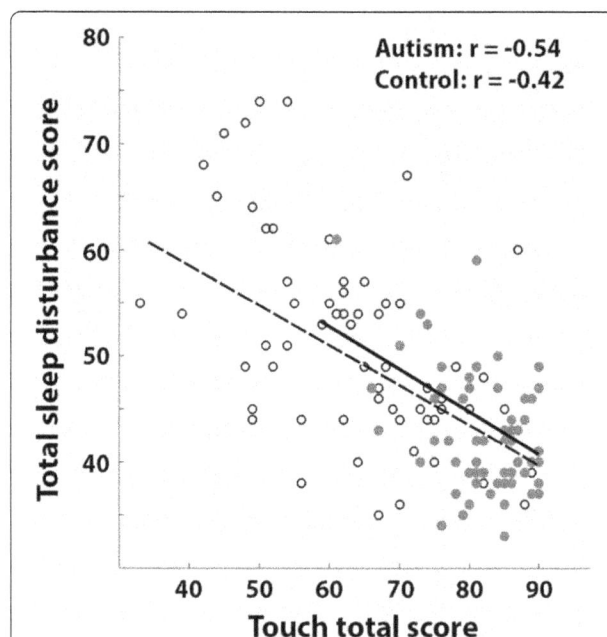

Fig. 4 Relationship between total sleep disturbance scores and touch total scores. Scatter plot of autism (white) and control (gray) children. Pearson's correlations are noted for each group. Each circle represents a single child. Dashed line indicates the linear fit for autism group. Solid line indicates the linear fit for the control group

Table 6 Relationship between total sleep disturbance scores and hyper- or hyposensitivity scores in each of the sensory domains

		Autism ($n = 69$)		Control ($n = 62$)	
		Pearson	Spearman	Pearson	Spearman
Auditory	Hypersensitivity	− 0.13	− 0.13	− 0.30	− 0.24
	Hyposensitivity	− 0.21	− 0.14	− 0.05	− 0.12
Visual	Hypersensitivity	− 0.13	− 0.18	− 0.15	− 0.17
	Hyposensitivity	− 0.27	− 0.29	− 0.16	− 0.07
Vestibular	Hypersensitivity	− 0.08	− 0.14	− 0.46*	− 0.34
	Hyposensitivity	− 0.26	− 0.18	− 0.29	− 0.24
Touch	Hypersensitivity	− 0.50*	− 0.50*	− 0.42*	− 0.25
	Hyposensitivity	− 0.41*	− 0.36*	− 0.25	− 0.26
Oral	Hypersensitivity	− 0.35*	− 0.33*	− 0.31	− 0.32
	Hyposensitivity	−0.43*	− 0.44*	− 0.26	− 0.26

Pearson's and Spearman's correlations are presented for the autism (left) and control (right) groups. Asterisks indicate significant correlation coefficients after Bonferroni correction ($p < 0.01$)

Table 7 Variance explained by Sensory Profile scores

		Visual	Auditory	Vestibular	Touch	Oral	All
Raw scores (all items)							
Autism	F stat	2.61	2.22	4.67	28.3	14.2	6.64
	p value	0.11	0.14	0.03	< 0.001	< 0.001	< 0.001
	adj. R^2	0.02	0.02	0.05	0.29	0.16	0.29
Control	F stat	2.93	1.81	15.8	12.8	5.67	3.96
	p value	0.45	0.18	< 0.001	< 0.001	0.1	0.015
	adj. R^2	0.03	0.01	0.2	0.16	0.07	0.18
Low-threshold items only (hypersensitivity)							
Autism	F stat	1.22	1.1	0.4	22.2	9.2	5.38
	p value	0.27	0.3	0.53	< 0.001	0.003	< 0.001
	adj. R^2	0.03	0	0	0.24	0.11	0.24
Control	F stat	5.87	1.4	16.2	12.8	6.46	4.12
	p value	0.5	0.24	< 0.001	< 0.001	0.05	0.015
	adj. R^2	0.07	0	0.2	0.16	0.08	0.21
High-threshold items only (hyposensitivity)							
Autism	F stat	3.01	5.1	5.1	13.8	14.9	4.35
	p value	0.45	0.15	0.15	< 0.001	< 0.001	0.01
	adj. R^2	0.03	0.06	0.06	0.16	0.17	0.2
Control	F stat	0.03	2.03	4.76	3.87	4.5	1.99
	p value	0.86	0.64	0.15	0.25	0.2	0.45
	adj. R^2	0	0.02	0.06	0.04	0.05	0.07

Results of regression analyses using six different models: one model with a single predictor for each of the sensory modalities and a sixth model containing all five predictors together. This analysis was performed once with the total raw scores (i.e., sum of low- and high-threshold items) and again with the low- and high-threshold items separately. F stats, p values, and adjusted R^2 are presented for each model. Italics indicate significant after Bonferroni correction ($p < 0.01$)

model with the total raw scores from all sensory modalities.

Adding age, gender, medication usage, and ADOS scores as additional predictors to the full models that contained all five predictors had negligible effects on the results. The adjusted R^2 value improved from 0.29 to 0.30, demonstrating that these additional predictors explained only 0.2% of the variance in the sleep disturbance scores.

Taken together, these results suggest that total sleep disturbances in children with autism are most strongly associated with hypersensitivity towards touch. In contrast, sleep disturbances in control children are most strongly associated with vestibular hypersensitivity. Notably, scores in the visual and auditory sensory domains were remarkably weak in explaining sleep disturbances in both groups.

Discussion

Our results reveal that sensory hyper- and hyposensitivity measures estimated using the complete Caregiver Sensory Profile can explain a considerable amount (29%) of the variance in sleep disturbance scores of children with autism (Tables 5, 6, and 7). In particular, hypersensitivity towards touch exhibited the strongest relationship with sleep disturbances and single-handedly explained 24% of the variability in sleep disturbance scores (Table 7). Similar, yet somewhat weaker relationships were also evident in the control group where touch and vestibular hypersensitivity scores explained up to 20% of the variance in sleep disturbance scores (Table 7). Interestingly, only hypersensitivity scores were significantly associated with sleep disturbance scores in the control group, but both hyper- and hyposensitivity scores were significantly associated with sleep disturbance scores in the autism group. This demonstrates the paradoxical overlap of sensory hyper- and hyposensitivity problems within the same children in the autism group (Fig. 2).

While one cannot infer causality from correlations, we speculate that hypersensitivity towards touch may interfere with sleep onset and sleep maintenance in children with autism, thereby generating severe sleep disturbances in children with touch sensitivities (Fig. 4). With this in mind, future studies examining sleep in autism may benefit from stratifying individuals with autism based on their sensitivity to touch as this measure may indicate the presence of a specific sleep disturbance mechanism.

Specificity of sensory abnormalities associated with sleep disturbances

Are sleep disturbances associated with a general multi-modal sensory problem in autism, or with hyper- or hypo-sensitivity in particular sensory domains? Recent studies using the Short Sensory Profile have suggested that sleep disturbances are weakly associated with general sensory abnormalities, which explain 1–6% of the variance in sleep disturbance scores [21, 25]. The Short Sensory Profile, however, does not allow one to separate hypo- and hypersensitivity scores in individual sensory modalities.

Our in-depth assessment using the complete Sensory Profile reveals that sleep disturbances are not equally associated with sensitivities in all sensory modalities. In contrast to the moderate relationship between sleep disturbances and sensory problems in the touch domain, sensory problems in the visual and auditory domains were not associated with sleep problems in either the autism or the control groups (Tables 5, 6, and 7). Furthermore, sleep disturbances were more strongly associated with hypersensitivity towards touch than hyposensitivity (Tables 5, 6, and 7). Our results, therefore, clearly demonstrate that sleep disturbances are associated with sensory abnormalities in specific sensory modalities and cannot be generalized across all sensory domains. This highlights the need to use modality-specific measures of sensory sensitivity when studying autism.

Sensory sensitivities, anxiety, and arousal

Sleep disturbances can be generated by a wide variety of interacting physiological and behavioral causes, which lead to hyper-arousal and insomnia [37]. Previous studies about sleep disturbances in autism have mostly highlighted the potential roles of anxiety [21, 25], poor sleep hygiene [20, 38], and a variety of physiological factors such as low endogenous levels of melatonin [39, 40]. These factors and others may create hyper-arousal and cortical over-reactivity to sensory stimuli, which in many cases can be ameliorated by behavioral and pharmacological interventions [41].

Our results suggest that hypersensitivity to touch may be an important factor in generating or exacerbating sleep disturbances in at least some children with autism. Further examination of the relationship between this specific sensory problem and the level of anxiety or arousal in individual children with autism is highly warranted. Furthermore, future studies could examine whether children with sleep disturbances and hypersensitivity to touch also exhibit excessive EEG responses to tactile stimuli, indicating cortical over-reactivity. Previous studies have revealed that EEG responses to auditory stimuli right before sleep onset and during different stages of sleep were abnormally strong in insomnia patients without autism [42–44]. Interestingly, it has been hypothesized that autism may be caused by the abnormal development of hyper-aroused and over-responsive neural circuits [45, 46].

The relationship between sensory problems and sleep disturbances in typical development

Our findings are in line with several previous studies, which have also reported significant relationships between hypersensitivity on the Sensory Profile and sleep disturbances in infants [47] children [48] and adults [49] with typical development. Two of these studies examined sensitivity scores

separately in each of the sensory modalities and reported that tactile hypersensitivity scores explained the largest amount of variability in sleep disturbance scores (~ 25%), while scores in other sensory domains, such as vision and audition, explained a considerably smaller portion of the variability [48, 49]. In our study, both vestibular hypersensitivity and hypersensitivity towards touch scores single-handedly explained a considerable amount of the variability in sleep disturbance scores of control children (20 and 16% respectively). Taken together, accumulating evidence suggests that hypersensitivity towards tactile and vestibular modalities is particularly useful for explaining sleep disturbances in children with typical development.

Limitations of the study

This study has several limitations. First, our estimates of sleep quality and sensory sensitivities were based only on parental report. Previous research has shown that there is good agreement between parental report and objective techniques (i.e., actigraph and polysomnography) on some measures of sleep, but not all [50, 51]. For example, previous studies have shown that parental reports underestimate wakings during the night and overestimate sleep duration in typically developing children [52]. Second, control children in our study were not precisely matched to children with autism in terms of gender and we did not measure IQ in any of our participants. Third, while all of the children were diagnosed with autism by a child psychiatrist based on DSM V criteria, some of the children with autism did not complete a formal ADOS assessment. We addressed these issues by demonstrating that equivalent results were apparent in comparisons of specific subsets of the children (e.g., when including only male children or when including only the children with autism who had completed an ADOS assessment).

Conclusions

The current study revealed that hypersensitivity to touch is likely to be an important factor in generating and/or exacerbating sleep disturbances in children with autism. This finding motivates further studies to examine this relationship with objective and more direct techniques such as psychometric and neuroimaging measures for tactile sensitivity as well as actigraph and polysomnography for sleep disturbances.

Characterizing the heterogeneity of autism and identifying individuals with shared symptoms and etiologies is a major goal of contemporary autism research [3, 53, 54]. With this in mind, we believe that stratifying children based on their hypersensitivity to touch may be important for elucidating the physiological mechanisms that generate sleep disturbances in autism and for determining the therapeutic effects of existing and new interventions and sensory aids.

Abbreviations

ADOS: Autism Diagnostic Observation Schedule; ATN: Autism Treatment Network; CSHQ: Child Sleep Habits Questionnaire

Funding

Not applicable.

Authors' contributions

MI, LM, and ABS, collected the data in Soroka Medical Center, and GM, HF, AM, and MF diagnosed the ASD children. ID, IM, LM, OZ, and OT analyzed the data, GM, LM, IM, ID, and OT wrote the manuscript. All authors read, commented, and approved the manuscript.

Competing interests

The authors declare that they have no competing interests.

Author details

[1]Behavioral Science Department, Emek Yesreel College, Emek Yesreel, Israel. [2]Pre-School Psychiatry Unit, Soroka University Medical Center, Beer Sheva, Israel. [3]Psychology Department, Ben Gurion University, Beer Sheva, Israel. [4]Zusman Child Development Center, Soroka University Medical Center, Beer Sheva, Israel. [5]Public Health Department, Ben Gurion University, Beer Sheva, Israel. [6]Cognitive and Brain Sciences Department, Ben Gurion University, Beer Sheva, Israel.

References

1. American Psychiatric Association, Association AP. Diagnostic and statistical manual of mental disorders. 5th ed. Arlington: American Psychiatric Publishing; 2013.
2. Grzadzinski R, Huerta M, Lord C. DSM-5 and autism spectrum disorders (ASDs): an opportunity for identifying ASD subtypes. Mol Autism. 2013;4:12.
3. Jeste SS, Geschwind DH. Disentangling the heterogeneity of autism spectrum disorder through genetic findings. Nat Rev Neurol. 2014;10:74–81.
4. Baranek GT, David FJ, Poe MD, Stone WL, Watson LR. Sensory Experiences Questionnaire: discriminating sensory features in young children with autism, developmental delays, and typical development. J Child Psychol Psychiatry Allied Discip. 2006;47:591–601.
5. Klintwall L, Holm A, Eriksson M, Carlsson LH, Olsson MB, Hedvall Å, et al. Sensory abnormalities in autism. A brief report. Res Dev Disabil. 2011;32:795–800.
6. Leekam SR, Nieto C, Libby SJ, Wing L, Gould J. Describing the sensory abnormalities of children and adults with autism. J Autism Dev Disord. 2007;37:894–910.
7. Rogers SJ, Hepburn S, Wehner E. Parent reports of sensory symptoms in toddlers with autism and those with other developmental disorders. J Autism Dev Disord. 2003;33:631–42.
8. McCormick C, Hepburn S, Young GS, Rogers SJ. Sensory symptoms in children with autism spectrum disorder, other developmental disorders and typical development: a longitudinal study. Autism. 2015;20:572–9.
9. Rogers SJ, Ozonoff S. Annotation: what do we know about sensory dysfunction in autism? A critical review of the empirical evidence. J Child Psychol Psychiatry. 2005;46:1255–68.
10. Kern JK, Trivedi MH, Garver CR, Grannemann BD, Andrews AA, Savla JS, et al. The pattern of sensory processing abnormalities in autism. Autism. 2006;10:480–94.
11. Zwaigenbaum L, Bryson S, Rogers T, Roberts W, Brian J, Szatmari P. Behavioral manifestations of autism in the first year of life. Int J Dev Neurosci. 2005;23:143–52.
12. Ben-Sasson A, Hen L, Fluss R, Cermak SA, Engel-Yeger B, Gal E. A meta-analysis of sensory modulation symptoms in individuals with autism spectrum disorders. J Autism Dev Disord. 2009;39:1–11.
13. Heaton P, Davis RE, Happé FGE. Research note: exceptional absolute pitch perception for spoken words in an able adult with autism. Neuropsychologia. 2008;46:2095–8.
14. Tavassoli T, Bellesheim K, Tommerdahl M, Holden JM, Kolevzon A, Buxbaum JD. Altered tactile processing in children with autism spectrum disorder. Autism Res. 2015;9:1–5.
15. Brown NB, Dunn W. Relationship between context and sensory processing in children with autism. Am J Occup Ther. 2010;64:474–83.
16. Tavassoli T, Miller LJ, Schoen SA, Nielsen DM, Baron-Cohen S. Sensory over-responsivity in adults with autism spectrum conditions. Autism. 2014;18:428–32.
17. Krakowiak P, Goodlin-Jones B, Hertz-Picciotto I, Croen LA, Hansen RL. Sleep problems in children with autism spectrum disorders, developmental delays, and typical development: a population-based study. J Sleep Res. 2008;17:197–206.
18. Mayes SD, Calhoun SL. Variables related to sleep problems in children with autism. Res Autism Spectr Disord. 2009;3:931–41.
19. Cortesi F, Giannotti F, Ivanenko A, Johnson K. Sleep in children with autistic spectrum disorder. Sleep Med. 2010;11:659–64.
20. Souders MC, Mason TBA, Valladares O, Bucan M, Levy SE, Mandell DS, et al. Sleep behaviors and sleep quality in children with autism spectrum disorders. Sleep. 2009;32:1566–78.
21. Hollway JA, Aman MG, Butter E. Correlates and risk markers for sleep disturbance in participants of the autism treatment network. J Autism Dev Disord. 2013;43:2830–43.
22. Williams GP, Sears LL, Allard A. Sleep problems in children with autism. J Sleep Res. 2004;13:265–8.
23. Taylor MA, Schreck KA, Mulick JA. Sleep disruption as a correlate to cognitive and adaptive behavior problems in autism spectrum disorders. Res Dev Disabil. 2012;33:1408–17.
24. Goldman SE, McGrew S, Johnson KP, Richdale AL, Clemons T, Malow BA. Sleep is associated with problem behaviors in children and adolescents with autism spectrum disorders. Res Autism Spectr Disord. 2011;5:1223–9.
25. Mazurek MO, Petroski GF. Sleep problems in children with autism spectrum disorder: examining the contributions of sensory over-responsivity and anxiety. Sleep Med. 2015;16:270–9.
26. Hirata I, Mohri I, Kato-Nishimura K, Tachibana M, Kuwada A, Kagitani-Shimono K, et al. Sleep problems are more frequent and associated with problematic behaviors in preschoolers with autism spectrum disorder. Res Dev Disabil. 2016;49–50:86–99.
27. Reynolds AM, Malow BA. Sleep and autism spectrum disorders. Pediatr Clin N Am. 2011;58:685–98.
28. Murray DS, Fedele A, Shui A, Coury DL. The autism speaks autism treatment network registry data: opportunities for investigators. Pediatrics. 2016;137:S72–8.
29. Achenbach TM, Ruffle TM. The child behavior checklist and related forms for assessing behavioral/emotional problems and competencies. Pediatrics in Rev. 2000;21:265–71.
30. Tomchek SD, Dunn W. Sensory processing in children with and without autism: a comparative study using the short sensory profile. Am J Occup Ther. 2007;61:190–200.
31. Owens JA, Spirito A, McGuinn M. The Children's Sleep Habits Questionnaire (CSHQ): psychometric properties of a survey instrument for school-aged children. Sleep. 2000;23:1043–51.
32. Kientz MA, Dunn WA. Comparison of the performance of children with and without autism on the sensory profile. Am J Occup Ther. 1997;51:530–7.
33. Meiri G, Dinstein I, Michaelowski A, Flusser H, Ilan M, Faroy M, et al. The Negev hospital-university-based (HUB) autism database. J Autism Dev Disord. 2017;47:2918–26.
34. Lord C1, Risi S, Lambrecht L, Cook EH Jr, Leventhal BL, DiLavore PC, Pickles A, Rutter M. The autism diagnostic observation schedule-generic: a standard measure of social and communication deficits associated with the spectrum of autism. J Autism Dev Disord. 2000;30(3):205–23.

35. Neuman A, Greenberg DF, Labovitz DR, Suzuki LA. Cross-cultural adaptation of the sensory profile: establishing linguistic equivalency of the Hebrew version. Occup Ther Int. 2004;11:112–30.

36. Tzchishinsky O, Lufi D, Shochat T. Reliability of the Children's sleep habits questionnaire Hebrew translation and cross cultural comparison of the psychometric properties. Sleep Diagnosis Ther. 2008;3:30–4.

37. Riemann D, Spiegelhalder K, Feige B, Voderholzer U, Berger M, Perlis M, et al. The hyperarousal model of insomnia: a review of the concept and its evidence. Sleep Med Rev. 2010;14:19–31.

38. Jan JE, Owens JA, Weiss MD, Johnson KP, Wasdell MB, Freeman RD, et al. Sleep hygiene for children with neurodevelopmental disabilities. Pediatrics. 2008;122:1343–50.

39. Melke J, Goubran Botros H, Chaste P, Betancur C, Nygren G, Anckarsäter H, et al. Abnormal melatonin synthesis in autism spectrum disorders. Mol Psychiatry. 2008;13:90–8.

40. Leu RM, Beyderman L, Botzolakis EJ, Surdyka K, Wang L, Malow BA. Relation of melatonin to sleep architecture in children with autism. J Autism Dev Disord. 2011;41:427–33.

41. Miano S, Ferri R. Epidemiology and management of insomnia in children with autistic spectrum disorders. Paediatr Drugs. 2010;12:75–84.

42. Milner CE, Cuthbert BP, Kertesz RS, Cote KA. Sensory gating impairments in poor sleepers during presleep wakefulness. Neuroreport. 2009;20:331–6.

43. Hairston IS, Talbot LS, Eidelman P, Gruber J, Harvey AG. Sensory gating in primary insomnia. Eur J Neurosci. 2010;31:2112–21.

44. Yang C-M, Lo H-S. ERP evidence of enhanced excitatory and reduced inhibitory processes of auditory stimuli during sleep in patients with primary insomnia. Sleep. 2007;30:585–92.

45. Markram H, Rinaldi T, Markram K. The intense world syndrome—an alternative hypothesis for autism. Front Neurosci. 2007;1:77–96.

46. Rubenstein JLR, Merzenich MM. Model of autism: increased ratio of excitation/inhibition in key neural systems. Genes Brain Behav. 2003;2:255–67.

47. Vasak M, Williamson J, Garden J, Zwicker JG, et al. Sensory processing and sleep in typically developing infants and toddlers. Am J Occup Ther. 2015; 69:6904220040p1.

48. Shochat T, Tzischinsky O, Engel-Yeger B. Sensory hypersensitivity as a contributing factor in the relation between sleep and behavioral disorders in normal schoolchildren. Behav Sleep Med. 2009;7:53–62.

49. Engel-Yeger B, Shochat T. The relationship between sensory processing patterns and sleep quality in healthy adults. Can J Occup Ther Rev. 2012;79:134–41.

50. Sadeh A. Assessment of intervention for infant night waking: parental reports and activity-based home monitoring. J Consult Clin Psychol. 1994;62:63–8.

51. Malow BA, Marzec ML, McGrew SG, Wang L, Henderson LM, Stone WL. Characterizing sleep in children with autism spectrum disorders: a multidimensional approach. Sleep. 2006;29:1563–71.

52. Goodwin JL, Silva GE, Kaemingk KL, Sherrill DL, Morgan WJ, Quan SF. Comparison between reported and recorded total sleep time and sleep latency in 6- to 11-year-old children: the Tucson Children's Assessment of Sleep Apnea Study (TuCASA). Sleep Breath. 2007;11:85–92.

53. State MW, Šestan N, Jamain S, Sebat J, Szatmari P, State MW, et al. Neuroscience. The emerging biology of autism spectrum disorders. Science. 2012;337:1301–3.

54. Happé F, Ronald A, Plomin R. Time to give up on a single explanation for autism. Nat Neurosci. 2006;9:1218–20.

Oscillatory rhythm of reward: anticipation and processing of rewards in children with and without autism

Katherine Kuhl-Meltzoff Stavropoulos[1*] and Leslie J. Carver[2]

Abstract

Background: Autism spectrum disorder (ASD) is a complex neurodevelopmental condition, and multiple theories have emerged concerning core social deficits. While the social motivation hypothesis proposes that deficits in the social reward system cause individuals with ASD to engage less in social interaction, the overly intense world hypothesis (sensory over-responsivity) proposes that individuals with ASD find stimuli to be too intense and may have hypersensitivity to social interaction, leading them to avoid these interactions.

Methods: EEG was recorded during reward anticipation and reward processing. Reward anticipation was measured using alpha asymmetry, and post-feedback theta was utilized to measure reward processing. Additionally, we calculated post-feedback alpha suppression to measure attention and salience. Participants were 6- to 8-year-olds with ($N = 20$) and without ($N = 23$) ASD.

Results: Children with ASD showed more left-dominant alpha suppression when anticipating rewards accompanied by nonsocial stimuli compared to social stimuli. During reward processing, children with ASD had less theta activity than typically developing (TD) children. Alpha activity after feedback showed the opposite pattern: children with ASD had greater alpha suppression than TD children. Significant correlations were observed between behavioral measures of autism severity and EEG activity in both the reward anticipation and reward processing time periods.

Conclusions: The findings provide evidence that children with ASD have greater approach motivation prior to nonsocial (compared to social) stimuli. Results after feedback suggest that children with ASD evidence less robust activity thought to reflect evaluation and processing of rewards (e.g., theta) compared to TD children. However, children with ASD evidence greater alpha suppression after feedback compared to TD children. We hypothesize that post-feedback alpha suppression reflects general cognitive engagement—which suggests that children with ASD may experience feedback as overly intense. Taken together, these results suggest that aspects of both the social motivation hypothesis and the overly intense world hypothesis may be occurring simultaneously.

Keywords: Autism spectrum disorder, Alpha asymmetry, Theta, Reward processing, Social stimuli

Background

Autism spectrum disorders (ASD) are characterized by impairments in two broad categories: social communication (including both verbal and non-verbal communication), and presence of restricted interests and/or repetitive behaviors [1]. Given that autism is hypothesized to be neurologically based [2, 3], it is not surprising that theories have attempted to identify underlying neural systems that account for this complex condition. In order to accurately identify neural systems that might be of interest, researchers turn to hypotheses concerning the underlying causes of symptoms of ASD. Although many theories of ASD have been proposed, of particular relevance to the current investigation are two alternative theories: the social motivation hypothesis [4–6] and sensory over-responsivity [7–9] as described by the overly intense world hypothesis [10, 11].

* Correspondence: katherine.stavropoulos@ucr.edu
[1]Riverside Graduate School of Education, University of California, 9500 University Avenue, Riverside, CA 92521, USA
Full list of author information is available at the end of the article

The social motivation hypothesis (SMH) proposes that individuals with ASD are not driven to seek out or engage in social interaction because those interactions are not as rewarding for them as they are to their typically developing (TD) peers. The hypothesis states that less social interaction during critical periods of development leads to abnormal neural specialization, which can affect cognitive development and lead to fewer social interactions over time.

Given that a central assumption of the SMH is that social interactions are not as rewarding for children with ASD as they are for TD children, previous investigations of the hypothesis have measured neural responses to social versus nonsocial stimuli in children and adolescents with and without ASD. Whereas the SMH supposes *hypo*activation of the reward system for social stimuli, the intense world hypothesis (IWH) posits that individuals with ASD experience neural *hyper*reactivity, which leads to the inability to "gate" information flow and selectively attend to information. Overall, the IWH argues that individuals with ASD perceive the world as presenting overwhelming multisensory stimulation. With regard to social deficits, the IWH notes that because social situations are particularly complex and difficult to predict, individuals with ASD find them particularly intense and unpleasant, which leads to withdrawal or self-soothing behaviors [10]. Thus, while the SMH implicates the reward system as a critical neural mechanism underlying social deficits in ASD, the IWH implicates sensory and/or attentional systems underlying behavioral patterns in ASD.

Although the SMH and IWH appear quite different (and potentially contradictory insofar as they hypothesize different neural mechanisms in ASD), the current investigation attempts to explore whether these theories could exist in tandem. In this view, both reduced social rewards and overwhelming responses to social stimuli could co-exist. The approach we take utilizes a reward-related paradigm that allows us to separate the effects of reward *anticipation* from reward *processing* [12].

Specifically, we hypothesize that the SMH will hold true for periods of reward anticipation—when individuals with ASD are waiting for a social reward. According to the SMH account, individuals with ASD will evidence less anticipatory reward-related brain activity compared to TD individuals when anticipating social rewards. We hypothesize *hypoactivation* of social reward anticipation as this appears concordant with behavioral observations of ASD symptoms. That is, individuals with ASD are less likely to initiate social engagement with others, which we hypothesize may be due to aberrant reward anticipation for social information. In contrast to typically developing individuals, people with ASD may not expect social interactions to be inherently rewarding and

therefore may be less likely to initiate such interactions. However, we simultaneously hypothesize that after rewards are delivered (e.g., during reward *processing*), individuals with ASD will show signs of neural *hyperreactivity*, providing evidence for the IWH. In line with the IWH, we hypothesize that individuals with ASD may be overwhelmed by the social stimuli provided in the feedback phase. If social stimuli are aversive to individuals with ASD, then in addition to evidencing reduced reward-related anticipation, individuals with ASD may overreact to them when they are presented.

Previous neuroscience research on reward anticipation and processing in ASD has utilized both electrophysiology and functional magnetic resonance (fMRI) imaging. As the current manuscript focuses on electrophysiology, we will not review the fMRI literature in detail. Note, however, that there have been a number of manuscripts exploring social and nonsocial reward anticipation and processing in ASD using fMRI. Findings of these studies are mixed, with some finding evidence of global deficits in reward responsiveness for individuals with ASD [13–15], and others suggesting that responses to social rewards are diminished [16–18].

Our previous research has used event-related potentials (ERP), which measure time-locked neural activity averaged over multiple trials. However, the published reward-related literature demonstrates that interesting information can also be gained from exploring event-related spectral perturbations (ERSP). ERSP measures can provide information about brain activity patterns in single trials rather than averaging activity over multiple trials, which is necessary to observe patterns of activity that are not both time and phase-locked. In this way, ERSP measures can provide information beyond what can be observed using more traditional ERP measures. ERSP measures stimulus-related modulation of power in the EEG signal relative to baseline. Differences in EEG power are of interest in ASD, as this oscillatory electrical activity is hypothesized to involve inhibitory processes and activity of GABAergic interneurons [19]. Disruption of inhibitory activity has been proposed as an explanation for symptoms commonly observed in ASD (for a review, see [20]).

Reward anticipation

Previous research suggests that anticipation of feedback is related to the suppression of activity in the alpha band (8–12 Hz). Studies of both visual and auditory modalities have found alpha power suppression prior to feedback on a time-estimation task [21, 22]. However, of particular relevance to motivation and reward anticipation is alpha band asymmetry. Decades of research have focused on asymmetry in EEG activity between the right and left hemispheres (particularly increased left versus right hemisphere activity) to indicate reward sensitivity and approach motivation [23–26]. Over two decades ago, researchers found evidence that left-dominant alpha suppression occurred more robustly during anticipation of reward versus punishment trials [23]. Conversely, right-dominant alpha suppression was observed during anticipation of punishment relative to reward trials. The authors hypothesized that left-dominant alpha suppression was an accurate marker for approach motivation in healthy adults.

Reward anticipation and autism spectrum disorder

Although much of the previous research concerning alpha asymmetry in individuals with psychiatric diagnoses has focused on depression and schizophrenia, recent attention has been given to the reward system in autism spectrum disorder (ASD). Of the studies that have directly measured reward anticipation in ASD, none have measured stimulus-locked alpha asymmetry. Rather, research has used event-related-potential (ERP) measures of reward anticipation. Two ERP components have been studied: the stimulus preceding negativity (SPN) and P300. The SPN is a negative slow-wave component thought to reflect reward expectation and activity in the dopaminergic reward system [27]. The P300 is thought to index attentional orienting and stimulus salience [28, 29].

Of the previous studies measuring reward anticipation in ASD, one found that both children with ASD and attention-deficit hyperactivity disorder (ADHD) evidenced a larger stimulus preceding negativity (SPN) component compared to their TD peers when anticipating positive outcomes, but equivalent activity when anticipating negative outcomes [30]. A second group found that TD children had greater P300 activity when anticipating reward versus nonreward conditions, whereas children with ASD did not [31]. Our own previous results measured the SPN component during anticipation of social versus nonsocial rewards and found that children with ASD evidenced a smaller SPN when anticipating social rewards compared to their TD peers [12].

Studies of reward anticipation in ASD have not utilized stimulus-locked measures of oscillatory activity (e.g., event-related spectral perturbations, ERSP). To our knowledge, no studies have been conducted on alpha asymmetry in ASD during social reward anticipation. We note, however, that there have been previous EEG studies of resting asymmetry in ASD (e.g., brain activity measured "at rest," while the subject is not watching or listening to specific stimuli). For example, [32] explored the relationship between resting frontal asymmetry and social symptoms of ASD. The authors found that children with ASD with left dominant frontal asymmetry displayed less severe social impairments compared to

children with right frontal asymmetry. The authors interpreted this finding as consistent with the hypothesis that left asymmetry is related to approach motivation whereas right asymmetry appears related to withdrawal. More recently, [33] also studied resting EEG asymmetry in ASD. The authors found children with ASD with left asymmetry had less severe social deficits, but this effect was mediated by verbal IQ. The authors also found that parents of children who demonstrated left dominant asymmetry reported later age of symptom onset compared to the age of onset reported by parents whose children had right dominant asymmetry.

Reward processing

Whereas the suppression and asymmetry of alpha-band activity is thought to reflect anticipation of rewards, another important consideration in research related to reward is reward processing. Reward processing occurs after feedback and has been measured using both EEG and event-related potentials (ERP). Previous ERP research suggests that the feedback-related negativity (FRN) relates to reward processing and may reflect processes related to expected versus actual rewards [34]. Less research has been done on neural oscillations related to reward processing, but extant studies point to enhancement of theta band (4–8 Hz) activity as a likely candidate to reflect reward processing. Post-stimulus theta appears sensitive to reward evaluation [35], and previous studies have measured both the FRN and theta as they are hypothesized to reflect similar neural processes [36]. Finally, as has been observed in the FRN component, theta appears to be stronger for negative feedback compared to positive feedback [37, 38] and is stronger when feedback reflects a higher magnitude of reward [39].

Reward processing and autism spectrum disorder

Studies of reward processing in ASD are more plentiful than those of reward anticipation, although few studies have explored reward processing in ASD using *social* stimuli. Two previous ERP studies comparing the feedback-related negativity (FRN) component of individuals with and without ASD suggest that individuals with ASD do not demonstrate significant differences in feedback processing for nonsocial rewards [40, 41]. However, most studies of the FRN utilize nonsocial reward paradigms (i.e., paradigms with monetary rewards). In our previous work comparing social versus nonsocial rewards in ASD, we found differences in how children with and without ASD respond to feedback indicating correct or incorrect performance on a guessing task, compared to their TD peers [12]. Importantly, no studies to our knowledge have measured ERSPs during social reward processing in children with and without ASD.

Although not directly related to reward processing, there is a body of literature on oscillatory activity and ASD in response to social stimuli (e.g., after stimuli have been presented). Although these tasks were not designed to elicit activity of the reward system, they are relevant to the current investigation as they provide information about oscillatory activity in ASD in response to faces and will be reviewed briefly. Dawson and colleagues [42] measured both alpha and theta-band activity after a 2-year behavioral intervention (early start Denver model; ESDM) designed to improve social skills of toddlers with ASD. The authors interpreted oscillatory activity in these two bands as a marker of general cognitive engagement and cortical activity, arguing that greater alpha suppression and enhanced theta-band activity suggest enhanced cortical activation. Findings suggested that toddlers with ASD who participated in ESDM "normalized" their degree of theta and alpha band EEG activity in response to repeated images of faces. In a study of adults with Asperger syndrome (AS), researchers observed lower delta/theta synchronization in temporal and occipital-parietal regions in the AS versus control groups in response to emotional faces [43]. The authors interpreted these differences to reflect difficulty of individuals with AS with implicit emotional face recognition, as previous literature suggests both delta and theta are involved with limbic-cortical connections. This is particularly interesting due to findings suggesting delta/theta synchronization is associated with nonconscious versus conscious face recognition [44]. Therefore, the authors conclude that this pattern of oscillatory activity underscores difficulties individuals with AS experience when identifying emotional faces (e.g., individuals with AS must rely on cognitive, rather than implicit, processes to correctly identify facial expressions). In a different study of adults with AS, results suggested less theta activity, but increased activity in the beta2 range (16–20 Hz) after viewing faces compared to a control group [45]. The authors interpreted enhanced beta2 in the AS to reflect greater reliance on voluntary attention and cognitive processes during facial recognition compared to controls, and decreased theta activity to reflect abnormalities in thalamic-cortical and hippocampal-cortical circuits, as well as potential abnormalities in amygdala activity in response to faces in AS. These studies underscore the utility of measuring oscillatory activity in individuals with ASD and provide information about potential differences between typically developing individuals and those with ASD in response to emotional faces.

Current study

The current study was conducted to gain understanding of event-related spectral perturbations (ERSP) in children with and without ASD for social reward anticipation and reward processing. We are unaware of any previous investigations that have measured ERSP in this population during both reward anticipation and reward processing. In addition, the current study will add to the literature comparing brain activity of children with and without ASD in response to social versus nonsocial rewards.

Consistent with the SMH, we hypothesized that children with ASD would evidence less left-dominant alpha suppression when anticipating social rewards compared to their TD peers, as this would reflect less approach motivation. Similarly, we expected that children with ASD would evidence less theta-band activity in response to social rewards compared to their TD peers, as activity in the theta band after feedback is thought to reflect reward processing. However, we also hypothesized that we would observe enhanced alpha-band suppression in children with ASD during reward processing and argue that this would provide evidence in favor of the IWH as alpha band suppression after stimulus presentation is thought to reflect cortical activity and cognitive engagement [42]. We postulate that if theta-band activity was *hypo*active in ASD during reward processing, but alpha band suppression was *hyper*active, it would provide initial evidence that reward-related activity in ASD is under-active while attentional processes are over-active. Finally, we hypothesized that measures of social behavior would be correlated with alpha asymmetry (during reward anticipation), and both theta and alpha activity (during reward processing).

We previously reported the results of event-related potential (ERP) brain activity from the cohort of children with ASD in the current investigation [12]. The current manuscript reports the results of a novel analysis designed to address the specific predictions of the SMH and the IWH theories regarding the reward system in ASD.

Methods
Stimuli and task

The stimuli and task are described in detail in [12, 46]. Briefly, the task was a guessing game that presented blocks of trials that used left and right visual stimuli (question marks). Participants were asked to indicate their guess via button press whether the left or right stimulus was "correct." After this choice, the left and right question marks were replaced with an arrow in the middle pointing towards whichever question mark the participant chose. This was done to reinforce the idea that participants had control over the task and their responses were being recorded.

There were two blocked feedback conditions: social versus nonsocial. Incidental stimuli in the social condition were faces obtained from the NimStim database

[47] that were smiling for "correct" answers and frowning for "incorrect" answers. To avoid confounds resulting from use of a single face or gender, 33 faces (18 female, 15 male) from the database were utilized. Incidental stimuli in the nonsocial condition were composed of scrambled face elements from the social condition formed into an arrow that pointed upwards for "correct" answers and downwards for "incorrect" answers. The use of scrambled faces to construct the arrow controlled for low-level visual features of the stimuli. Images were scrambled using the Adobe Photoshop "scramble" filter. This filter breaks images into square blocks and rearranges them randomly. The scrambled face images were then made into the shape of an arrow using Photoshop.

Both faces and arrows were presented in pseudorandom order, with no image repeating on consecutive trials (e.g., participants never saw the same face or arrow as "correct" or "incorrect" more than once in a row). Presented stimuli had a horizontal visual angle of 14.5° and a vertical visual angle of 10.67°. Each participant viewed identical stimuli in the same order for each condition (e.g., the social feedback block was the same for each participant), but whether individuals viewed the social versus nonsocial block first was counterbalanced between participants.

Participants were told that the reward for each correct answer was a goldfish cracker, or if they preferred, fruit snacks. Participants were told there was no penalty for incorrect answers. Participants were told that if they guessed correctly, they would see a ring of intact goldfish crackers, and the goldfish would be crossed out for incorrect answers. Importantly, in both the social and nonsocial feedback trials, the face/arrow information

was incidental. Figure 1 depicts the stimuli and timeline in the social and nonsocial conditions. A computer program predetermined correct versus incorrect answers in pseudorandom order such that children got 50% "correct" and 50% "incorrect," with no more than three of the same answer in a row.

The two feedback conditions (face/"social" trials and arrow/"nonsocial" trials) were tested in separate blocks, each composed of 80 trials. Within each block of 80 trials, there were 30-s breaks every 15 trials. During breaks, participants were asked to relax or move if they felt restless. Between blocks, a longer break (5–10 min) was taken. To control for attentional effects, children were observed via webcam, and trials in which they were not attending to the stimulus were marked and discarded during analysis. Of the final sample, three children had trials excluded for this reason, and of those three, none had more than 10 trials excluded in this way.

Participants

We tested TD children ($N = 23$) and children with ASD ($N = 20$). Exclusionary criteria for participants with ASD included history of seizures, brain injury, neurological disorders, or any concurrent psychiatric condition (other than ASD), based on parent report. Exclusionary criteria for TD participants included all of the above criteria, plus an immediate family history of ASD. None of the children in the TD group were taking psychoactive medications. Three children in the ASD group were taking medication in order to improve concentration, but one of the three did not take his medication on the day he came in for the current study. Participants were recruited from a UC San Diego subject pool and through

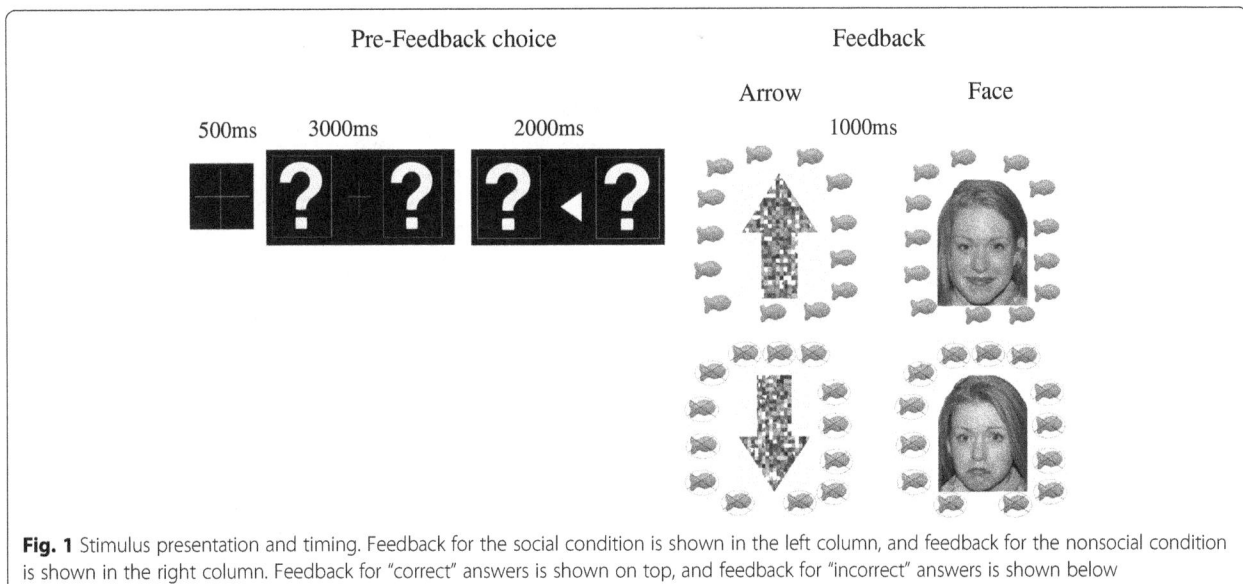

Fig. 1 Stimulus presentation and timing. Feedback for the social condition is shown in the left column, and feedback for the nonsocial condition is shown in the right column. Feedback for "correct" answers is shown on top, and feedback for "incorrect" answers is shown below

postings on websites for parents of children on the autism spectrum. All participants had normal hearing and normal or corrected to normal vision. Procedures were approved by the institutional review board, and written consent was obtained from caregivers. All children over 7 years of age signed an assent form.

IQ scores [48] were available for all 20 children with ASD, and 22 of 23 TD children (one TD child was unable to complete the WASI due to time constraints). Of the final sample of 43 children, no significant differences were found between groups on full scale IQ scores, $F(1,40) = .36$. There were differences between the TD and ASD groups in chronological age, $F(1,41) = 5.86$, $p = .02$. Children in the ASD group had been previously diagnosed with ASD through various sources (e.g., formal evaluations through an autism center or school diagnosis). Diagnosis was confirmed for the current study with module 3 of the ADOS-2 [49]. The ADOS-2 was administered by an individual trained to research reliability on administration, scoring, and interpretation of the measure. Participant information can be found in Table 1.

Behavioral measures

Participants' caregivers completed the Social Responsiveness Scales (SRS-2) [50], which measures social responsiveness and behavior. We also tested for overt motivational or affective differences between groups for each condition. To accomplish this, children ($N = 21$ TD, 19 ASD) completed a 1–7 Likert rating scale of how much they enjoyed the game (1 = "I do not like this game," and 7 = "I love this game") after each block. Participants also completed a 1–7 Likert scale about their perception of getting correct answers (1 = "I never got correct answers," and 7 = "I always got correct answers"). In reality, the ratio of correct versus incorrect answers was predetermined and controlled by experimental design, and the rating was used to verify that the groups did not differ in their perception that they were obtaining correct answers.

EEG recording

Participants wore a standard, fitted cap (Electrocap International) with 33 silver/silver-chloride (Ag/AgCl)

electrodes placed according to the extended international 10–20 system. Continuous EEG was recorded with a NeuroScan 4.5 System with a reference electrode at Cz and re-referenced offline to the average activity at left and right mastoids. Electrode resistance was kept under 10 kΩ. Continuous EEG was amplified with a low pass filter (70 Hz), a directly coupled high-pass filter (DC), and a notch filter (60 Hz). The signal was digitized at a rate of 250 samples per second via an Analog-to-Digital converter. Eye movement artifacts and blinks were monitored via horizontal electrooculogram (EOG) placed at the outer canthi of each eye and vertical EOG placed above and below the left eye. Trials were time locked to the onset of the feedback stimulus. To measure reward anticipation, the baseline period was – 2200 to – 2000 ms, and the data were epoched from – 2200 to 100 ms. To measure reward processing, the baseline period was – 200 to 0 ms, and the data were epoched from – 200 to 800 ms. The interval between trials was varied between 1800 and 2000 ms. Trials with no behavioral response, or containing electrophysiological artifacts, were excluded from the averages.

Artifacts were removed via a four-step process. Data were visually inspected for drift exceeding +/– 200 mV in all electrodes, high frequency noise visible in all electrodes larger than 100 mV, and flatlined data. Following inspection, data were epoched and eyeblink artifacts were identified using independent component analysis (ICA). Individual components were inspected alongside epoched data, and blink components were removed. To remove additional artifacts, we utilized a moving window peak-to-peak procedure in ERPlab [51], with a 200-ms moving window, a 100-ms window step, and a 150-mV voltage threshold. Our final analyses for reward anticipation included 20 children with ASD and 23 TD children, and our final analyses for the reward processing included 19 children with ASD and 23 TD children.

Time-frequency decomposition was performed to compute event-related spectral perturbations (ERSP). ERSP measures changes in EEG power from the baseline period at a specific frequency (or frequency band) and time [52]. ERSPs were calculated using the "newtimef" plugin in EEGlab (version 12.0.2.6b) and MATLab (version R2014a). Standard settings within EEGlab

Table 1 Participant characteristics including: IQ (WASI), age, gender, SRS-2T-score, and ADOS-2 severity scores for the ASD group. Reprinted from [12]

Group	Participants	WASI (full scale)	Age	Gender	SRS-2 SCI T score	SRS-2 RBB T score	ADOS-2 Severity score
ASD	20	$M = 107.35$ SD = 16.27	$M = 27.56^a$ SD = 7.20	19 M 1 F	$M = 71.26^b$ SD = 12.25	$M = 69.63^b$ SD = 11.40	$M = 6.88$ SD = 2.05
TD	23	$M = 111.60$ SD = 15.50	$M = 21.68^a$ SD = 6.65	22 M 1 F	$M = 48.52^b$ SD = 6.97	$M = 50.69^b$ SD = 9.38	N/A

[a] $p = .02$
[b] $p = < .0001$

newtimef were used (cycles set at 1.4, .5). This procedure yields a time × frequency transform with numbers for each time point, frequency, and trial. We utilized a linear space for frequency (1 Hz for reward processing and 2 Hz for reward anticipation). Alpha-band activity was operationalized as the average activity between 8 and 12 Hz, and theta-band activity was operationalized as the average activity between 4 and 6 Hz. Note that the theta-band was operationalized in this way (e.g., 4–6 Hz) to avoid overlap with the alpha band.

Results

Data were analyzed using JMP (version 11.0). We used repeated measures analysis of variance (ANOVA) to test for differences between conditions and caudality (anterior-posterior scalp locations). Greenhouse-Geisser-corrected degrees of freedom are reported to account for violations of sphericity.

Behavior

As reported in [12], no significant differences were found between groups on children's Likert ratings of liking the game, $F(1,39) = .72$ ns, or perception of generating correct answers, $F(1,39) = .95$ ns. As expected, significant differences were found between groups on the SRS-2 social subscale, $F(1,41) = 64.27$ $p < .001$, and the repetitive behavior subscale, $F(1,41) = 38.23$ $p < .001$, with children with ASD scoring significantly higher on both subscales compared to TD children.

ERSP

Reward anticipation

ERSP data during the feedback anticipation period were measured as the mean activation during the time period prior to feedback onset (e.g., – 2200 to 100 ms) with the time period from – 2200 to 2000 ms as the baseline. Alpha-band activity (8–12 Hz) was measured for the following electrodes: F3/F4, C3/C4, P3/P4, and T5/T6. For analysis concerning alpha asymmetry, log power in the left hemisphere was subtracted from the right hemisphere. Therefore, positive values indicate more right-hemisphere activity, whereas negative values indicate more left-hemisphere activity. Electrodes were chosen due to our and other groups' previous research on event-related potential (ERP) measures of reward anticipation [12, 53].

Alpha band A 2 (group) × 2 (condition) × 4 (electrode position) ANOVA was conducted. A marginal main effect of electrode, $F(3,120) = 2.61$, $p = .059$ was observed. No other interactions or effects were observed. Although the effect of electrode position was marginal, we conducted exploratory analysis of each electrode position (e.g., frontal, central, parietal, temporal). Therefore, these results should be interpreted cautiously. An interaction was observed between group × condition in the temporal electrodes, $F(1,40) = 3.96$, $p = .05$. Follow-up tests revealed a marginal effect of condition for children with ASD, $F(1,40) = 3.78$, $p = .058$, such that more left-hemisphere suppression was observed for the arrow (versus face) condition. Follow-up tests also revealed a marginal effect of the face condition, $F(1,40) = 3.55$, $p = .06$, such that TD children had greater left-hemisphere suppression in the face condition compared to children with ASD. No effects or interactions were observed in the other electrode positions. ERSPs for reward anticipation in the alpha band are shown in Fig. 2.

Brain and behavior correlations In order to explore whether EEG activity was related to behavioral and parent report measures of social responsiveness and severity of ASD symptoms, correlations were conducted. For the alpha band, correlations were conducted using EEG asymmetry (left to right) in the temporal electrodes (as the other positions did not reveal any significant effects or interactions) and continuous measures of autism symptoms. For individuals diagnosed with ASD, correlations were run using alpha asymmetry and severity score on the Autism Diagnostic Observation Schedule, second edition [49]. A significant correlation was observed between alpha asymmetry prior to nonsocial stimuli and severity score on the ADOS-2, $F(1,16) = 7.49$, $p = .014$, $\underline{R}^2 = .27$, such that individuals with more severe ASD evidenced greater left-dominant alpha band suppression and those with less severe ASD evidenced less left-dominant alpha band suppression prior to viewing nonsocial stimuli. Bonferroni-corrected threshold probability for statistical significance was .025 for these correlations. Correlations are shown in Fig. 3.

Feedback/reward processing

ERSP data during the feedback/reward processing period was measured as the mean activation during the time period immediately after feedback onset (i.e., – 200 to 800 ms) with the time period from – 200 to 0 ms as the baseline. Two separate bands of activation were measured: alpha-band activity (8–12 Hz) and theta-band activity (4–6 Hz). Mean activation was measured for the midline electrodes Fz, Cz, and Pz and was averaged across electrodes. These electrodes were chosen based on previous investigations on the FRN and theta band [38]. Trials were separated by whether participants received "correct" versus "incorrect" feedback (e.g., whether they were rewarded or not). However, it is important to note that our task was set up such that whether or not participants got a reward or not was pre-programmed and thus did not actually depend on participant response.

Arrow   Face

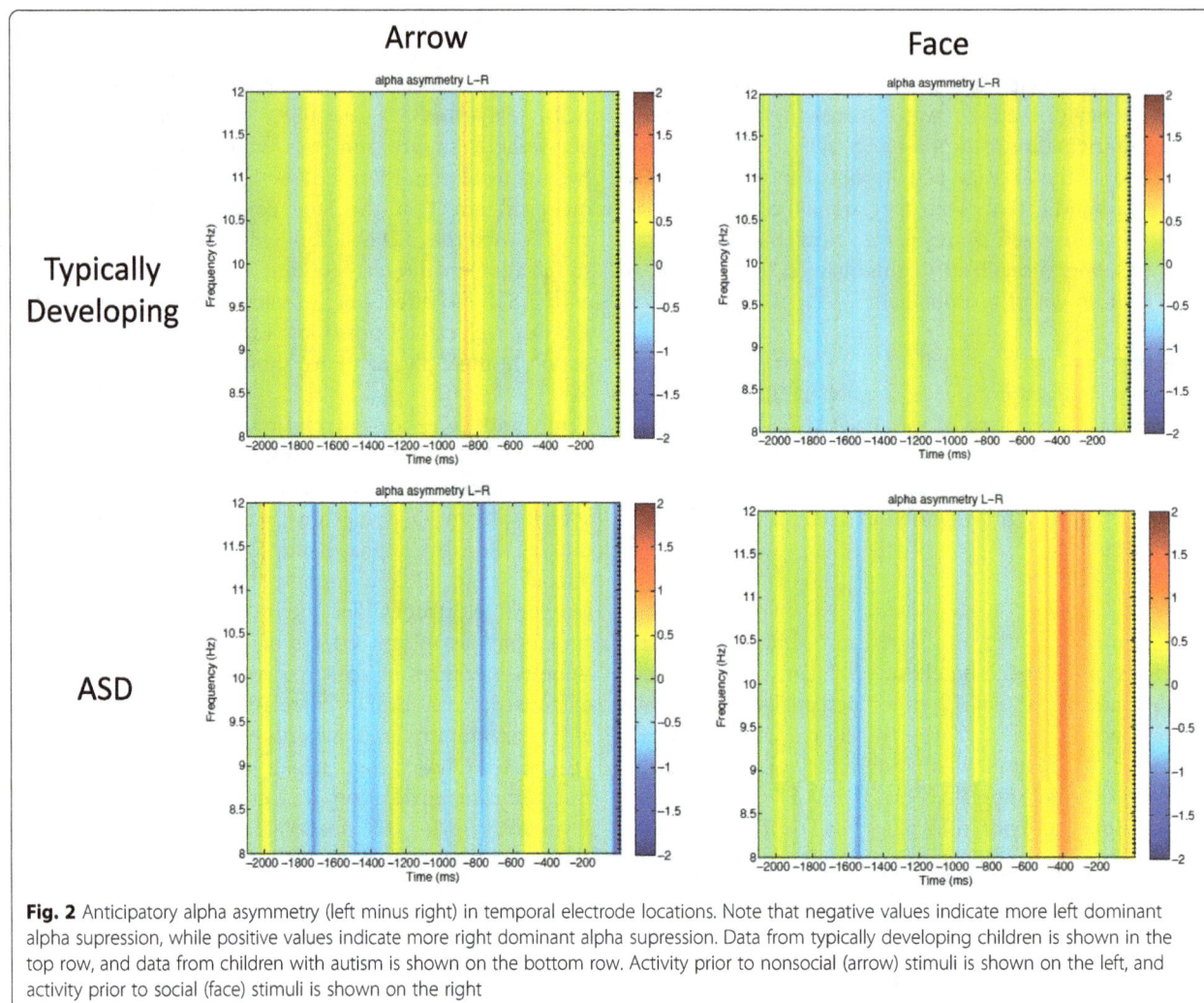

Fig. 2 Anticipatory alpha asymmetry (left minus right) in temporal electrode locations. Note that negative values indicate more left dominant alpha supression, while positive values indicate more right dominant alpha supression. Data from typically developing children is shown in the top row, and data from children with autism is shown on the bottom row. Activity prior to nonsocial (arrow) stimuli is shown on the left, and activity prior to social (face) stimuli is shown on the right

Alpha band A 2 (group) × 2 (feedback) × 2 (condition) ANOVA was conducted. A main effect of group was observed, $F(1,40) = 6.5$, $p = .01$, such that children with ASD had more alpha suppression (8–12 Hz) during reward processing than TD children regardless of condition or feedback type. No other main effects or interactions were observed. ERSPs for post-feedback alpha are shown in Fig. 4.

Theta band A 2 (group) × 2 (feedback) × 2 (condition) ANOVA was conducted. A main effect of group was observed, $F(1,46.28) = 5.4$, $p = .02$ such that TD children had more activity in the theta band (4–6 Hz) during reward processing than children diagnosed with ASD. No other main effects or interactions were observed. ERSPs for post-feedback theta are shown in Fig. 4.

Brain and behavior correlations Correlations were conducted for reward processing for both the alpha and

theta bands and measures of autism severity for the ASD group (ADOS-2).

Alpha band For activity in the alpha band, a negative correlation was observed between alpha suppression in response to "correct" responses in the face condition and ADOS-2 severity score, $F(1,16) = 5.64$, $p = .03$, $R^2 = .21$. Individuals with more severe ASD had less alpha suppression after "correct" feedback in the face condition, and those with less severe ASD had more alpha suppression after "correct" feedback in the face condition. However, as four conditions (correct/incorrect for both social and nonsocial conditions) were analyzed, and this correlation did not reach significance under the Bonferroni-corrected threshold for statistical significance level of .0125.

Theta band For activity in the theta band, a significant positive correlation was observed between ADOS-2 severity score and theta-band activity for "correct"

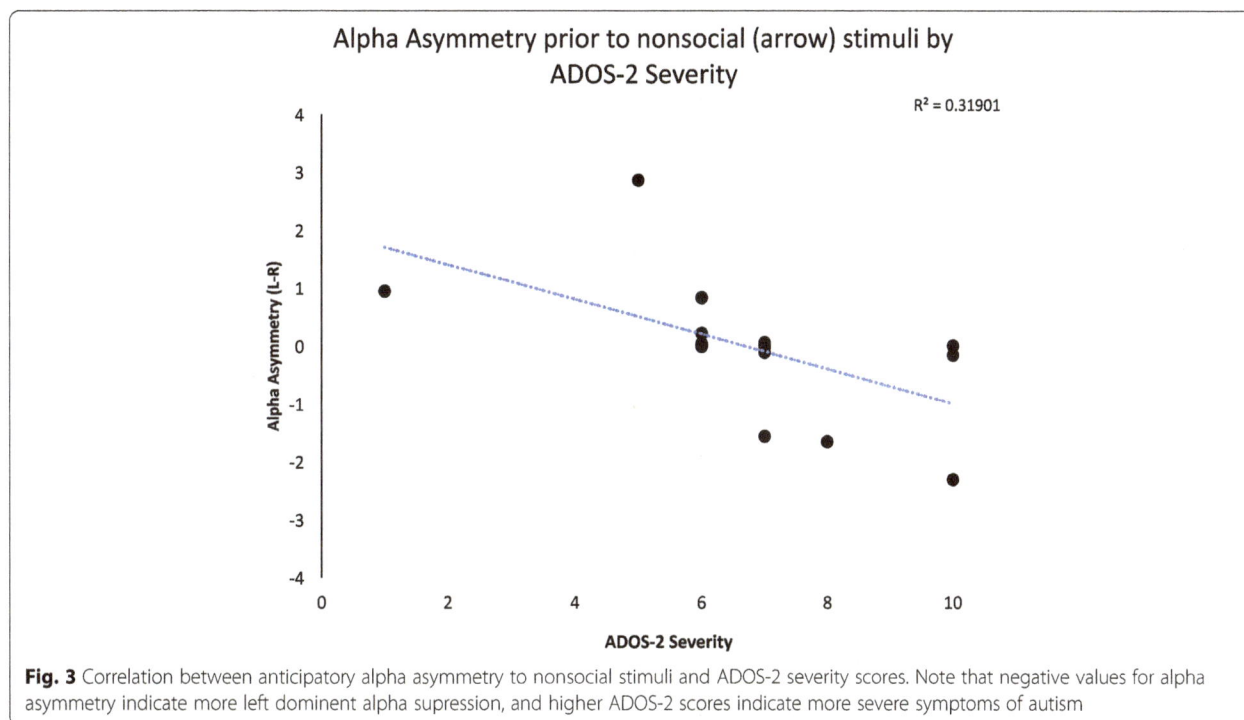

Fig. 3 Correlation between anticipatory alpha asymmetry to nonsocial stimuli and ADOS-2 severity scores. Note that negative values for alpha asymmetry indicate more left dominent alpha supression, and higher ADOS-2 scores indicate more severe symptoms of autism

feedback in the face condition, $F(1,16) = 9.7$, $p = .006$, $R^2 = .33$. Individuals with more severe ASD evidenced more theta activity after "correct" feedback in the face condition, and those with less severe ASD evidenced less theta activity. Correlations for post-feedback theta are shown in Fig. 5.

Anticipatory and feedback correlations

To better understand whether individuals with ASD in the current study might be experiencing both reduced reward anticipation and sensory/attentional hypoactivation during reward processing, correlations between pre-stimulus alpha and post-stimulus alpha were conducted. Note that the threshold for significance was set at .00625 (.05/8), as correlations were run between pre-stimulus alpha in two conditions and post-stimulus alpha in four conditions—leading to eight independent correlations. A significant negative correlation was observed between pre-stimulus alpha in the face condition and post-stimulus alpha in the correct arrows condition, ($F = 16.85$, $p = .0007$, $R^2 = .45$). That is, children with ASD with *greater* left-hemisphere alpha suppression when anticipating faces had *less* alpha suppression in response to correct arrows after feedback. No other significant correlations were observed.

Discussion

Results of the current investigation have implications for neural mechanisms in ASD and increase our understanding of how different theoretical perspectives may be simultaneously accurate. We analyzed event-related spectral perturbations (ERSPs) during a reward task designed to explore both reward anticipation and processing for social and nonsocial rewards. We focused on activity in the alpha (8–12 Hz) and theta (4–6 Hz) bands, due to their hypothesized role in reward anticipation, reward processing, and general cognitive engagement.

Reward anticipation

We analyzed alpha asymmetry during reward anticipation, as alpha asymmetry has been thought to reflect approach motivation and anticipation of upcoming rewards [23–25]. Our findings largely agree with previous literature, although the topographic distribution of our findings differs from previous reports. Previous literature has related increased approach motivation with alpha asymmetry in frontal regions (e.g., [23, 54]), whereas the current investigation found significant results only in temporal electrode locations. These differences may be largely attributable to the stimuli used in the current study. Previous work investigating alpha asymmetry has utilized reward paradigms with monetary incentives (e.g., [23, 54]), whereas the current paradigm used social (face) versus nonsocial (scrambled face) reward information. Given that face stimuli are thought to be processed in temporal locations [55], our topographic findings are consistent with literature on face processing.

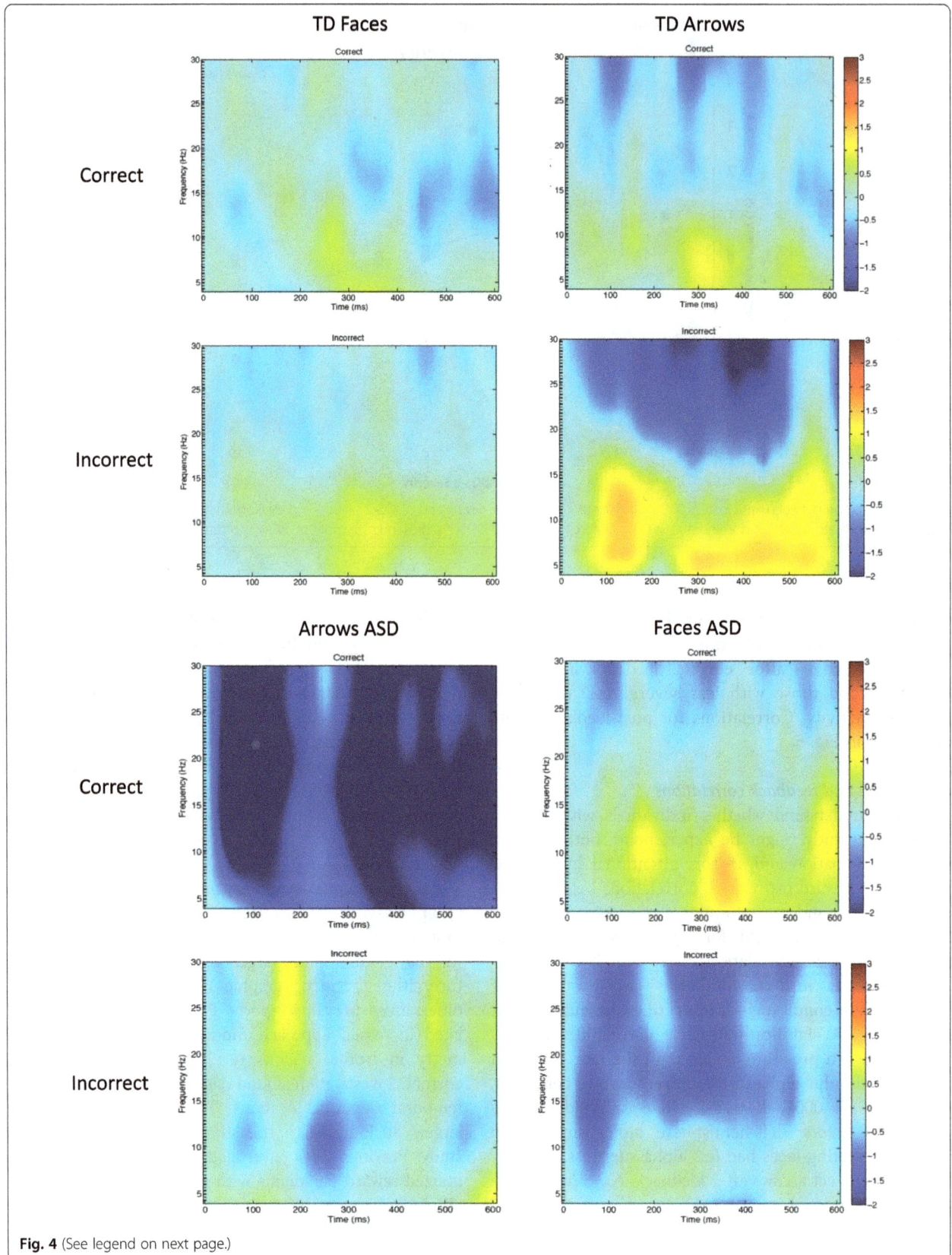

Fig. 4 (See legend on next page.)

Fig. 4 a Post-feedback ERSP for typically developing (TD) children in the theta (4–6 Hz) and alpha band (8–12 Hz). Activity after social (face) stimuli is shown on the left, and activity after nonsocial (arrow) stimuli is shown on the right. Activity after "correct" feedback is shown in the top row, and activity after "incorrect" feedback is shown in the bottom row. **b**. Post-feedback ERSP for children with ASD children in the theta (4–6 Hz) and alpha band (8–12 Hz). Activity after social (face) stimuli is shown on the left, and activity after nonsocial (arrow) stimuli is shown on the right. Activity after "correct" feedback is shown in the top row, and activity after "incorrect" feedback is shown in the bottom row

Though exploratory, our findings provide evidence in favor of the social motivation hypothesis of ASD during reward anticipation. That is, children with ASD had marginally less left-dominant alpha activity when anticipating faces compared to their TD peers. Further, children with ASD-evidenced greater left-dominant alpha activity when anticipating arrows versus faces. Interestingly, these findings not only suggest that children with ASD have less anticipatory activity (compared to their TD peers) prior to viewing faces but also suggests that children with ASD have greater approach motivation prior to viewing non-face versus face stimuli.

It may be the case that, compared to their TD peers, children with ASD have over-active reward anticipation prior to nonface stimuli. It is possible that reward value is placed on nonsocial stimuli at the expense of social information. This view is further corroborated by correlations between ASD severity and alpha asymmetry. Children with ASD who scored higher on the ADOS-2 severity score algorithm (indicating more severe ASD) had more left-dominant alpha suppression prior to viewing nonsocial stimuli (arrows), and those who had less left-dominant alpha suppression prior to nonsocial stimuli had lower ADOS-2 severity scores. Taken together, these findings are in line with what would be expected given the social motivation hypothesis, but extend the hypothesis with evidence that perhaps social deficits in

ASD are due to both *hypo*active reward anticipation for social information and *hyper*active anticipation for non-social stimuli.

Reward processing
Theta band
We analyzed reward processing by looking at activity in the theta band (4–6 Hz) after feedback was provided. We separated trials based on whether participants got "correct" versus "incorrect" feedback. It is important to note that we did not observe significant effects of feedback type (e.g., "correct" versus "incorrect"), which differs from previous investigations of reward processing in ASD [40, 41]. However, one explanation for this may be that in the current paradigm, "incorrect" feedback did not lead to participants losing rewards but rather meant that participants did not get a reward on that trial. So, rather than having "win" versus "loss" conditions, it is more accurate to conceptualize our paradigm as containing "win" versus "no-win" conditions. Further, previous studies have utilized monetary rewards [40, 41] rather than contrasting social versus nonsocial reward. Taken together, it seems likely that these differences in paradigm design may contribute to why we did not observe significant effects of feedback type in the current study.

Although we hypothesized a group by condition interaction, we observed a main effect of group such that TD children evidenced more theta activity compared to children with ASD regardless of whether rewards contained social or nonsocial information. This suggests that during reward processing, TD children have more reward-related oscillatory brain activity than children with ASD. This is particularly interesting given that we observed a different pattern during reward anticipation (e.g., children with ASD evidenced less reward-related activity when anticipating social versus nonsocial reward feedback). However, we believe this may illuminate an important aspect of neural functioning in ASD. It is possible that children with ASD experience less anticipation for social rewards than TD children, but less overall reward-related activity once rewards are presented.

Interestingly, we observed a significant positive correlation between theta activity and severity of ASD (via ADOS-2 severity scores) in the group with ASD. Specifically, we found that children who evidenced less theta activity after correct feedback in the social condition had less severe symptoms of ASD than those who had more

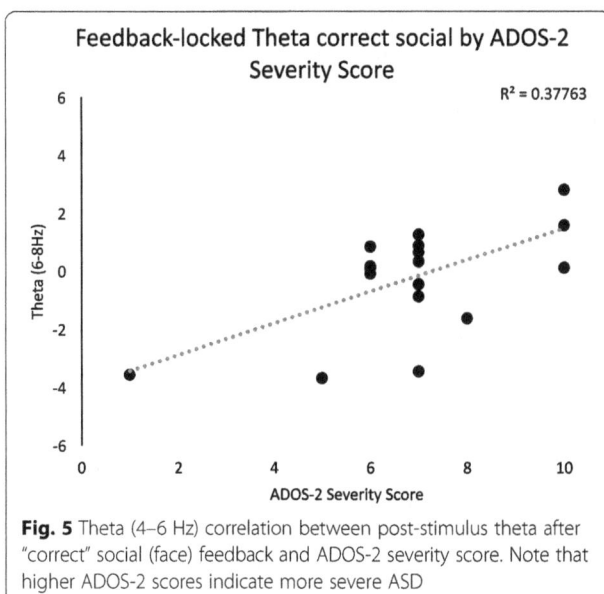
Fig. 5 Theta (4–6 Hz) correlation between post-stimulus theta after "correct" social (face) feedback and ADOS-2 severity score. Note that higher ADOS-2 scores indicate more severe ASD

theta activity in response to correct feedback in the social condition. This suggests that children who are more responsive to positive social feedback have more severe ASD symptoms compared to those who are less responsive to this feedback, which may provide preliminary evidence in favor of the IWH.

Thus, although we did not observe differences in reward processing for social versus nonsocial conditions between groups, correlations involving individual scores may provide a more detailed picture of what is occurring on an individual subject level. Within the ASD group, participants who were more responsive to correct social feedback had more ASD symptomology. Given that previous investigations of theta-band activity after rewards have found greater activity in response to "incorrect" versus "correct" feedback, it is possible that these results point to a dysfunction in how children with ASD process rewards. It is possible that children with ASD who experience greater theta activity in response to "correct" social feedback are experiencing hyperreactivity or are overwhelmed by the "correct" social feedback. We hypothesize that perhaps children with more severe ASD symptoms may be overwhelmed by social and/or emotional feedback (e.g., the feedback involved a smiling face and was thus both social and emotional). However, the current study was not designed to assess children's subjective experiences of the reward feedback, but future studies may consider adding a child interview in order to help shed light on these types of findings.

Alpha band

We also analyzed activity in the alpha (8–12 Hz) band after feedback. However, we note that activity in the alpha band is not typically thought to reflect reward processing but rather to reflect general cognitive engagement. Therefore, we hypothesized that if children with ASD tend to experience stimuli as overly intense, we might observe greater suppression in the alpha band for children with ASD during feedback. As expected, we found that children with ASD evidence greater suppression in the alpha band after feedback compared to TD children regardless of condition. This is particularly interesting given that results in the theta band held the opposite pattern (e.g., greater activity for TD children compared to those with ASD). Taken together, these findings provide novel evidence that simultaneously supports both the social motivation hypothesis and the overly intense world hypothesis.

Anticipation and processing

To explore the potential relationship between reward anticipation and over-responsivity in ASD, correlations between pre-stimulus alpha asymmetry and post-stimulus alpha were conducted. We found that children

with ASD who evidenced *greater* left-hemisphere alpha suppression when anticipating faces had *less* alpha suppression in response to correct arrows after feedback. This provides preliminary evidence for an important relationship between reward anticipation and hyperresponsivity in ASD. That is, children with ASD who evidenced greater approach motivation prior to face stimuli had less evidence of hyperresponsivity after correct feedback for nonsocial stimuli, and conversely, children with ASD with less approach motivation prior to face stimuli had more evidence of hyperresponsivity after correct feedback for nonsocial stimuli. These findings provide preliminary evidence that individuals with ASD may experience both the SMH and IWH.

Limitations

There are limitations to the current study, which must be taken into account when interpreting the results. Children with ASD who took part in the current study all had cognitive abilities within the average range and can therefore be considered relatively high functioning. Therefore, our results may not be generalizable to other children with ASD who experience greater impairment. Further, although we hypothesize that activity in the alpha band after reward feedback reflects cognitive engagement, and a global increase in alpha band activation may reflect over-reactivity of attentional systems in ASD, the current study did not ask children about their subjective experiences. Therefore, results concerning the alpha band after reward feedback may be considered exploratory rather than confirmatory and should be replicated in future studies. Finally, although we utilized ERSP in order to measure changes in spectral power that are both phase-locked and nonphase-locked, the current study cannot rule out contributions of large-amplitude brain activity (e.g., P300) to our post-stimulus alpha and theta results. That is, we cannot claim that post-stimulus changes in alpha or theta-band spectral power are not due, in part, to attentional processes related to the P300. However, even if our post-stimulus findings are related to attentional processes, it does not negate the importance of our results for understanding neural processes in children with ASD.

Conclusions

To our knowledge, this is the first study to measure ERSP activity in children with and without ASD in response to social versus nonsocial rewards. Our results provide further evidence that children with ASD have anticipatory reward deficits for social information and may anticipate nonsocial rewards more than social rewards. This is an intriguing possibility and has implications for neural mechanisms of ASD and potential targets for early intervention. That is, if social motivation deficits in ASD can be traced back to over-active anticipation of nonsocial rewards, it will be particularly important to deliver early interventions designed to increase the reward value of social information. Increasing the reward value of social information and social interactions can be done using a variety of methods, including taking the perspective of the child with ASD (e.g., [56]) and setting up the environment to reward social initiation (e.g., [57]).

Along with considerations related to intervention for children with ASD, it is important to investigate how it has come to be that children with ASD appear to be less rewarded by social information. Although the current study represents a developmental snapshot and thus cannot empirically address this question, it is important to consider the origins of the brain responses we report here to promote understanding of social perception development in ASD.

As detailed by de Haan, Humphreys, and Johnson in the "interactive specialization" hypothesis [58], typically developing infants' preference for faces may be driven by subcortical biases which, in turn, cause infants to frequently look at faces. As a product of looking at faces so frequently, cortical systems develop to be "specialized" for faces. Retrospective studies of infants who do versus do not go on to develop ASD found that looking time to faces does not differ between groups at 2 months of age, but does differ at 6 months of age such that infants who go on to develop ASD initially look at faces less than their TD peers [59]. Connecting these findings to our own, we hypothesize that although the initial subcortical systems which cause infants to be biased towards faces exist in infants with ASD, neural pathways that are involved in the latter stages of "interactive specialization" are not functioning appropriately, which causes individuals with ASD to not connect face stimuli with the reward system or preferential attention during development.

We hypothesize that is attributable to either (a) infants with ASD not connecting positive emotions to faces, which for TD children turns the initial subcortical bias into something more cortically based for TD children, and causes TD children (and adults) to be rewarded by social stimuli, or (b) initial cortical bias to attend towards faces is overwhelming or aversive for infants with ASD, causing them to begin avoiding face stimuli, which in turn causes a developmental cascade of missed social opportunities and thus lack of neural specialization and reward anticipation.

It is important for future investigations to shed light on the developmental processes in ASD that lead social information to be less rewarding, as understanding when and how developmental processes deviate from TD children will assist in developing both behavioral and medical interventions. Brain measures in response to faces in young infants and children who are at risk for ASD versus those not at risk may provide experimental data that inform theory.

The design of the current study allowed us to investigate neural activation both during reward anticipation and reward processing. Reward processing results in the theta band indicate a global *hypo*activation for children with ASD regardless of whether rewards are social versus nonsocial. Results of activity in the alpha band during reward processing provide preliminary evidence that children with ASD may experience *hyper*activation of cognitive engagement during reward processing. It is possible that the attentional or sensory processing systems are over-active in ASD during reward processing at the expense of more typical reward processing systems. However, the current investigation was not designed to directly parse the relative contribution of attention, reward, and sensory processing. Future investigations may consider combining temporally sensitive techniques with spatially sensitive measures (e.g., combined EEG and fMRI) in order to maximize our understanding of both temporal activation and responses from discrete brain areas.

Acknowledgments

We are grateful to all participants who took part in this study. This work was supported by the Bezos Family Foundation (PI: Stavropoulos).

Authors' contributions

The study was designed by KKMS and LJC. KKMS collected the data under the supervision and mentorship of LJC. KKMS and LJC analyzed the data. All authors read and approved the final manuscript.

Competing interests

The authors declare that they have no competing interests.

Author details

[1]Riverside Graduate School of Education, University of California, 9500 University Avenue, Riverside, CA 92521, USA. [2]University of California, San Diego, USA.

References

1. Association P: Diagnostic and statistical manual of mental disorders: DSM 5. Washington, DC; 2013.
2. Mundy P. Annotation: the neural basis of social impairments in autism: the role of the dorsal medial-frontal cortex and anterior cingulate system. J Child Psychol Psychiatry. 2003;44(6):793–809.
3. Neuhaus E, Beauchaine TP, Bernier R. Neurobiological correlates of social functioning in autism. Clin Psychol Rev. 2010;30(6):733–48.
4. Dawson G, Webb SJ, McPartland J. Understanding the nature of face processing impairment in autism: insights from behavioral and electrophysiological studies. Dev Neuropsychol. 2005;27(3):403–24.
5. Grelotti DJ, Gauthier I, Schultz RT. Social interest and the development of cortical face specialization: what autism teaches us about face processing. Dev Psychobiol. 2002;40(3):213–25.

6. Schultz RT. Developmental deficits in social perception in autism: the role of the amygdala and fusiform face area. Int J Dev Neurosci. 2005;23(2–3):125–41.

7. Liss M, Saulnier C, Fein D, Kinsbourne M. Sensory and attention abnormalities in autistic spectrum disorders. Autism. 2006;10(2):155–72.

8. Baranek GT, David FJ, Poe MD, Stone WL, Watson LR. Sensory Experiences Questionnaire: discriminating sensory features in young children with autism, developmental delays, and typical development. J Child Psychol Psychiatry. 2006;47(6):591–601.

9. Ben-Sasson A, Cermak SA, Orsmond GI, Tager-Flusberg H, Carver AC, Kadlec M, Dunn W. Extreme sensory modulation behaviors in toddlers with autism spectrum disorders. Am J Occup Ther. 2007;61:584–92.

10. Markram H, Rinaldi T, Markram K. The intense world syndrome—an alternative hypothesis for autism. Front Neurosci. 2007;1(1):77–96.

11. Markram K, Markram H. The intense world theory—a unifying theory of the neurobiology of autism. Front Hum Neurosci. 2010;4:224.

12. Stavropoulos KK, Carver LJ. Reward anticipation and processing of social versus nonsocial stimuli in children with and without autism spectrum disorders. J Child Psychol Psychiatry. 2014;55(12):1398–408.

13. Scott-Van Zeeland AA, Dapretto M, Ghahremani DG, Poldrack RA, Bookheimer SY. Reward processing in autism. Autism Res. 2010;3(2):53–67.

14. Mikita N, Simonoff E, Pine DS, Goodman R, Artiges E, Banaschewski T, Bokde AL, Bromberg U, Buchel C, Cattrell A, et al. Disentangling the autism-anxiety overlap: fMRI of reward processing in a community-based longitudinal study. Transl Psychiatry. 2016;6(6):e845.

15. Kohls G, Schulte-Ruther M, Nehrkorn B, Muller K, Fink GR, Kamp-Becker I, Herpertz-Dahlmann B, Schultz RT, Konrad K. Reward system dysfunction in autism spectrum disorders. Soc Cogn Affect Neurosci. 2013;8(5):565–72.

16. Dichter GS, Richey A, Rittenberg AM, Sabatino A, Bodfish JW. Reward circuitry function in autism during face anticipation and outcomes. J Autism Dev Disord. 2012;42:147–60.

17. Richey JA, Rittenberg A, Hughes L, Damiano CR, Sabatino A, Miller S, Hanna E, Bodfish JW, Dichter GS. Common and distinct neural features of social and non-social reward processing in autism and social anxiety disorder. Soc Cogn Affect Neurosci. 2014;9(3):367–77.

18. Delmonte S, Balsters JH, McGrath J, Fitzgerald J, Brennan S, Fagan AJ, Gallagher L. Social and monetary reward processing in autism spectrum disorders. Molecular Autism. 2012;3:1–13.

19. Uhlhaas PJ, Singer W. Neural synchrony in brain disorders: relevance for cognitive dysfunctions and pathophysiology. Neuron. 2006;52(1):155–68.

20. Uzunova G, Pallanti S, Hollander E. Excitatory/inhibitory imbalance in autism spectrum disorders: implications for interventions and therapeutics. World J Biol Psychiatry. 2016;17(3):174–86.

21. Bastiaansen MC, Brunia CH. Anticipatory attention: an event-related desynchronization approach. Int J Psychophysiol. 2001;43(1):91–107.

22. Bastiaansen MC, Posthuma D, Groot PF, de Geus EJ. Event-related alpha and theta responses in a visuo-spatial working memory task. Clin Neurophysiol. 2002;113(12):1882–93.

23. Sobotka SS, Davidson RJ, Senulis JA. Anterior brain electrical asymmetries in response to reward and punishment. Electroencephalogr Clin Neurophysiol. 1992;83(4):236–47.

24. Davidson RJ. Asymmetric brain function, affective style, and psychopathology: the role of early experience and plasticity. Dev Psychopathol. 1994;6(4):741–58.

25. Davidson RJ. Anterior electrophysiological asymmetries, emotion, and depression: conceptual and methodological conundrums. Psychophysiology. 1998;35(5):607–14.

26. Shankman SA, Nelson BD, Sarapas C, Robison-Andrew EJ, Campbell ML, Altman SE, SK MG, Katz AC, Gorka SM. A psychophysiological investigation of threat and reward sensitivity in individuals with panic disorder and/or major depressive disorder. J Abnorm Psychol. 2013;122(2):322–38.

27. GJM v B, KBE B. Cortical measures of anticipation. J Psychophysiol. 2004;18:61–76.

28. Nieuwenhuis S, Aston-Jones G, Cohen JD. Decision making, the P3, and the locus coeruleus-norepinephrine system. Psychol Bull. 2005;131(4):510–32.

29. Nieuwenhuis S, de Geus EJ, Aston-Jones G. The anatomical and functional relationship between the P3 and autonomic components of the orienting response. Psychophysiology. 2011;48:162–75.

30. Groen Y, Wijers AA, Mulder LJ, Waggeveld B, Minderaa RB, Althaus M. Error and feedback processing in children with ADHD and children with autistic spectrum disorder: an EEG event-related potential study. Clin Neurophysiol. 2008;119(11):2476–93.

31. Kohls G, Peltzer J, Schulte-Ruther M, Kamp-Becker I, Remschmidt H, Herpertz-Dahlmann B, Konrad K. Atypical brain responses to reward cues in autism as revealed by event-related potentials. J Autism Dev Disord. 2011;41(11):1523–33.

32. Sutton SK, Burnette CP, Mundy PC, Meyer J, Vaughan A, Sanders C, Yale M. Resting cortical brain activity and social behavior in higher functioning children with autism. J Child Psychol Psychiatry. 2005;46(2):211–22.

33. Burnette CP, Henderson HA, Inge AP, Zahka NE, Schwartz CB, Mundy PC. Anterior EEG asymmetry and the modifier model of autism. J Autism Dev Disord. 2011;41(8):1113–24.

34. Hajcak G, Moser JS, Holroyd CB, Simons RF. The feedback-related negativity reflects the binary evaluation of good versus bad outcomes. Biol Psychol. 2006;71(2):148–54.

35. Luft CD. Learning from feedback: the neural mechanisms of feedback processing facilitating better performance. Behav Brain Res. 2014;261:356–68.

36. Van den Berg I, Shaul L, Van der Veen FM, Franken IHA: The role of monetary incentives in feedback processing: why we should pay our participants. Neuroreport 2012, 23(6):347-353.

37. Pornpattananangkul N, Nusslock R. Willing to wait: elevated reward-processing EEG activity associated with a greater preference for larger-but-delayed rewards. Neuropsychologia. 2016;91:141–62.

38. Cohen MX, Krohn-Grimberghe A, Elger CE, Weber B. Dopamine gene predicts the brain's response to dopaminergic drug. Eur J Neurosci. 2007;26(12):3652–60.

39. Leicht G, Troschutz S, Andreou C, Karamatskos E, Ertl M, Naber D, Mulert C. Relationship between oscillatory neuronal activity during reward processing and trait impulsivity and sensation seeking. PLoS One. 2013;8(12):e83414.

40. Larson MJ, South M, Krauskopf E, Clawson A, Crowley MJ. Feedback and reward processing in high-functioning autism. Psychiatry Res. 2011;187(1–2):198–203.

41. JC MP, Crowley MJ, Perszyk DR, Mukerji CE, Naples AJ, Wu J, Mayes LC. Preserved reward outcome processing in ASD as revealed by event-related potentials. J Neurodev Disord. 2012;4(1):16.

42. Dawson G, Jones EJ, Merkle K, Venema K, Lowy R, Faja S, Kamara D, Murias M, Greenson J, Winter J, et al. Early behavioral intervention is associated with normalized brain activity in young children with autism. J Am Acad Child Adolesc Psychiatry. 2012;51(11):1150–9.

43. Tseng Y-L, Yang HH, Savostyanov AN, Chien VSC, Liou M. Voluntary attention in Asperger's syndrome: brain electrical oscillation and phase-synchronization during facial emotion recognition. Research in Autism Spectrum Disorders. 2015;13–14:32–51.

44. Basar E, Guntekin B, Oniz A. Principles of oscillatory brain dynamics and a treatise of recognition of faces and facial expressions. Prog Brain Res. 2006;159:43–62.

45. Yang HH, Savostyanov AN, Tsai AC, Liou M. Face recognition in Asperger syndrome: a study on EEG spectral power changes. Neurosci Lett. 2011; 492(2):84–8.

46. Stavropoulos KK, Carver LJ. Reward sensitivity to faces versus objects in children: an ERP study. Soc Cogn Affect Neurosci. 2014;9(10):1569–75.

47. Tottenham N, Tanaka JW, Leon AC, McCarry T, Nurse M, Hare TA, Marcus DJ, Westerlund A, Casey BJ, Nelson C. The NimStim set of facial expressions: judgments from untrained research participants. Psychiatry Res. 2009;168(3): 242–9.

48. Wachsler D. Wechsler abbreviated scale of intelligence (WASI). New York: NY: The Psychological Corporation; 1999.

49. Lord C, PC DL, Gotham K, Guthrie W, Luyster RJ, Risi S, Rutter M. Autism diagnostic observation schedule: ADOS-2. Los Angeles, CA: Western Psychological Services; 2012.

50. Constantino JN, Gruber CP. Social responsiveness scale (2nd edition). Los Angeles, CA: Western Psychological Services; 2012.

51. Lopez-Calderon J, Luck SJ. ERPLAB: an open-source toolbox for the analysis of event-related potentials. Front Hum Neurosci. 2014;8:213.

52. Makeig S, Debener S, Onton J, Delorme A. Mining event-related brain dynamics. Trends Cogn Sci. 2004;8(5):204–10.

53. Kotani Y, Kishida S, Hiraku S, Suda K, Ishii M, Aihara Y. Effects of information and reward on stimulus-preceding negativity prior to feedback stimuli. Psychophysiology. 2003;40(5):818–26.

54. Gorka SM, Phan KL, Shankman SA. Convergence of EEG and fMRI measures of reward anticipation. Biol Psychol. 2015;112:12–9.

55. Puce A, Allison T, Bentin S, Gore JC, McCarthy G. Temporal cortex activation in humans viewing eye and mouth movements. J Neurosci. 1998;18(6): 2188–99.

56. Wieder S, Greenspan S. Can children with autism master the core deficits and become epathetic, creative, and reflective? The Journal of Developmental and Learning Disorders. 2005;9

57. Koegel RL, Schreibman L, Good A, Cerniglia L, Murphey C, Koegel LK. How to teach pivotal behaviors to children with autism: a training manual. Santa Barbara: University of California, Santa Barbara; 1989.

58. de Haan M, Humphreys K, Johnson MH. Developing a brain specialized for face perception: a converging methods approach. Dev Psychobiol. 2002; 40(3):200–12.

59. Jones W, Klin A. Attention to eyes is present but in decline in 2–6-month-old infants later diagnosed with autism. Nature. 2013;504(7480):427–31.

The effect of age on vertex-based measures of the grey-white matter tissue contrast in autism spectrum disorder

Caroline Mann[1*] , Anke Bletsch[1], Derek Andrews[2], Eileen Daly[3], Clodagh Murphy[3], MRC AIMS Consortium, Declan Murphy[3] and Christine Ecker[1,3]

Abstract

Background: Histological evidence suggests that autism spectrum disorder (ASD) is accompanied by a reduced integrity of the grey-white matter boundary. This has also recently been confirmed by a structural neuroimaging study in vivo reporting significantly reduced grey-white matter tissue contrast (GWC) in adult individuals (18–42 years of age) with ASD relative to typically developing (TD) controls. However, it remains unknown whether the neuroanatomical differences in ASD at the grey-white matter boundary are stable across development or are age-dependent.

Methods: Here, we examined differences in the neurodevelopmental trajectories of GWC in a cross-sectional sample of 77 male ASD individuals and 76 typically developing (TD) controls across childhood and early adulthood (from 7 to 25 years).

Results: Using nested model comparisons, we first established that the developmental trajectory of GWC is complex in many regions across the cortex and includes linear and non-linear effects of age. Second, while ASD individuals have significantly reduced GWC overall, these differences are age-dependent and are most prominent during childhood (< 15 years).

Conclusions: Taken together, our findings suggest that differences in GWC in ASD are unlikely to reflect atypical grey matter cytoarchitecture alone, but may also represent other aspects of the cortical architecture such as age-dependent variability in myelin integrity.

Keywords: Autism spectrum disorder, Neurodevelopment, Structural MRI, Neuroimaging, Brain anatomy

Background

Autism spectrum disorder (ASD) is a complex neurodevelopmental condition characterized by deficits in social communication, social reciprocity, and repetitive/stereotypic behaviour [1]. There is strong evidence to suggest that these core symptoms are accompanied by differences in grey matter (GM) neuroanatomy and white matter (WM) connectivity [2], which typically manifest during early infancy [3, 4]. Despite the large number of existing neuroimaging studies, however, the neurobiological

mechanisms that drive the atypical development of the brain in ASD remain poorly understood.

To date, most neuroimaging studies examining atypical brain development in ASD have focused on measures of brain volume [5–7] and its two constituent components cortical thickness [8] and surface area [9, 10]. More recently, however, the attention of structural neuroimaging studies is shifting towards examining the grey-white matter boundary, as histological evidence suggests that the grey-white matter tissue contrast may be regionally less well defined (i.e. less distinct) in ASD [11]. Such 'blurring' of the grey-white matter transition zone seems to be caused by the presence of supernumerary neurons beneath the cortical plate, which—in turn—may result from migration deficits or failed apoptosis in the subplate region [12]. This finding also agrees with genetic investigations linking the

* Correspondence: caroline.mann@kgu.de
[1]Department of Child and Adolescent Psychiatry, Psychosomatics and Psychotherapy, University Hospital, Goethe University Frankfurt am Main, Deutschordenstrasse 50, 60528 Frankfurt am Main, Germany
Full list of author information is available at the end of the article

aetiology of ASD to atypical neuronal proliferation, migration, and maturation [13, 14]. For stratification purposes, and to capture aspects of ASD neuropathology that may be more closely linked to aetiological factors, it is therefore important to also investigate neuroimaging measures that map onto these particular characteristics of the cortical microstructure in vivo.

With this aim in mind, we recently examined the contrast between grey and white matter (GWC) across different cortical layers in a sample of males and females with ASD and typically developing (TD) controls [15]. We found that the GWC was significantly reduced in ASD, particularly at the grey-white matter boundary, and in many brain regions that have previously been linked to autistic symptoms and traits [16]. Our in vivo finding of a reduced GWC is also consistent with prior *postmortem* reports of a less well-defined grey-white matter boundary in ASD [11, 12]. However, based on tissue contrast alone, it is not possible to disentangle whether the observed between-group effects are driven by (1) differences in grey matter cytoarchitecture, as suggested by the above histological studies, or by (2) local variations in myelin content. For instance, a recent neuroimaging study of typical ageing, examining a sample of healthy adults (with an age range of 20–84 years), suggests that the GWC typically declines with increasing age and most likely reflects local (i.e. region-dependent) age-related changes of myelin integrity in the superficial WM [17]. Thus, by studying the GWC in ASD across different developmental stages, it may be possible to gain in vivo insights into neurobiological processes that (1) should be completed around birth (e.g. migration deficits), (2) end during early childhood (e.g. apoptosis), and (3) that are ongoing (e.g. myelination). Here, we examined age-related changes in GWC in ASD individuals compared to TD controls during childhood and adolescence. In addition to between-group differences in GWC, the present study investigated age-by-group interactions in a cross-sectional sample of male individuals with ASD and matched TD controls using a spatially unbiased 'vertex-wise' approach (i.e. not restricted to regions of interest). We expected the differences in the contrast to be age-dependent (i.e. there are significant age × group interactions), which would suggest that differences observed during postnatal brain development are not exclusively driven by atypical grey matter cytoarchitecture.

Furthermore, it has previously been shown that the trajectory of brain maturation for different morphological features is complex and cannot adequately be captured by linear effects alone. For example, the trajectory of total brain volume seems to be U-shaped with an increase in volume during early childhood, a peak during adolescence, and a subsequent decline in volume [18]. There are also studies to suggest that

there is considerable regional variation in the complexity of the normal developmental trajectory of cortical thickness, for example, which includes cubic, quadratic, and linear effects [19]. When examining age effects, it is therefore important to establish linear as well as non-linear effects, in order to adequately model the neurodevelopmental trajectory. While the typical neurodevelopmental trajectories are well established for measures of brain volume or cortical thickness, there is currently no comparable data for vertex-based measures of GWC. In the present study, we therefore examined linear, quadratic, and cubic effects of age in order to model the complex trajectory of the GWC in children and young adults between 7 and 25 years of age.

Methods

Participants

Eighty-two (82) right-handed males with ASD and eighty-two (82) TD controls, aged 7 to 25 years were recruited and assessed at the Institute of Psychiatry, Psychology, and Neuroscience, King's College, London. Both groups were matched for age, handedness (all right-handed), and full-scale IQ. Exclusion criteria for all participants included (1) history of major psychiatric disorder, (2) head injury, (3) genetic disorder associated with autism (e.g. fragile X syndrome and tuberous sclerosis), or (4) any other medical condition affecting the brain function (e.g. epilepsy). Furthermore, individuals with a history of substance abuse (including alcohol) and individuals taking antipsychotic medication, mood stabilizers, or benzodiazepines were excluded from the study. A diagnosis of ASD was based on the International Statistical Classification of Diseases, 10th Revision (ICD-10) [20] research criteria, and subsequently confirmed using the Autism Diagnostic Interview-Revised (ADI-R) [21] to ensure that all participants with ASD met the criteria for childhood autism. All individuals with ASD had to reach ADI-R algorithm cutoffs in the three domains of impaired reciprocal social interaction, communication, and repetitive behaviours and stereotyped patterns, although failure to reach cutoff in one of the domains by one point was permitted (see Table 1). The Autism Diagnostic Observation Schedule (ADOS) [22] was used to assess current symptoms, but was not used as inclusion criterion. Overall intellectual ability was assessed using the Wechsler Abbreviated Scale of Intelligence (WASI) [23]. All participants had a full-scale IQ (FSIQ) greater than 70 and gave informed written consent in accordance with the ethics approval by the National Research Ethics Committee, Suffolk, England. The participants over 18 years of age ($n = 37$ individuals with ASD and $n = 22$ TD controls) were also part of a recent study by our group examining the GWC during adulthood [15].

Table 1 Participant demographics

	ASD (n = 77)	TD controls (n = 76)
Age (years)	17 ± 4 (7–25)	16 ± 4 (8–25)
FSIQ	107 ± 14 (70–140)	111 ± 10 (84–134)
ADI-R social	20 ± 5 (9–28)	–
ADI-R communication	15 ± 5 (7–24)	–
ADI-R repetitive behaviour	6 ± 3 (2–20)	–
ADOS total	9 ± 3 (3–19)	–
Total grey matter volume [cm^3]	716.99 ± 58.12	726.57 ± 66.99
Total white matter volume [cm^3]	473.66 ± 55.87	478.71 ± 54.49
Total brain volume [cm^3]	1190.65 ± 113.99	1205.28 ± 121.48

Note. FSIQ, full-scale IQ; *ADI-R*, Autism Diagnostic Interview-Revised; *ADOS*, Autism Diagnostic Observation Schedule. Data expressed as mean ± standard deviation (range). There were no significant between-group differences in age, FSIQ, or global brain measures at $p < 0.05$ (two-tailed)

Structural MRI data acquisition

For all 164 participants, high-resolution structural T1-weighted volumetric images were acquired at the Centre of Neuroimaging Sciences, Institute of Psychiatry, Psychology, and Neuroscience, London, UK. Images were obtained using a 3-Tesla GE Signa System (General-Electric, Milwaukee, WI) with full-head coverage, 196 contiguous slices (1.1-millimetre (mm) thickness, with 1.09 × 1.09 mm in-plane resolution), a 256 × 256 × 196 matrix, and a repetition time/echo time (TR/TE) of 7/2.8 milliseconds (ms) (flip angle = 20°, FOV = 28 cm). A (birdcage) head coil was used for radiofrequency transmission and reception.

Cortical reconstruction using FreeSurfer

Each T1-weighted scan was initially screened for clinical abnormalities or large-scale motion artifacts by a radiologist. Two percent of scans (n = 3 participants) had to be excluded from the analysis due to insufficient quality. Models of the inner (i.e. white matter) surface and outer (i.e. pial or grey matter) surface were derived using FreeSurfer v5.3.0 (http://surfer.nmr.mgh.harvard.edu/). These well-validated and fully automated procedures have been extensively described elsewhere [24–26]. In brief, a single filled white matter volume was generated for each hemisphere after intensity normalization, skull stripping, and image segmentation using a connected components algorithm. Then, a triangular surface tessellation was generated for each white matter volume by fitting a deformable template. This resulted in a triangular cortical mesh for grey and white matter surfaces consisting of approximately 150.000 vertices (i.e. points) per hemisphere. The resulting surface models were visually inspected for reconstruction errors. Surface reconstructions with visible inaccuracies were further excluded and are not described in this study. Dropout rates due to surface reconstruction errors represented approximately 5% of the total sample (n = 8 participants) and were approximately equal between groups. This procedure resulted in a final sample size of 153 participants (n = 77 individuals with ASD and n = 76 TD controls).

Grey-to-white matter tissue contrast and absolute tissue intensities

At each cerebral vertex (i), the grey-to-white matter tissue contrast (GWC) was calculated as the percentage of grey matter intensity (GMI) sampled at 30% cortical thickness (CT) relative to the white matter intensity (WMI) at 1 mm below the grey-white matter boundary (see Fig. 1), i.e.

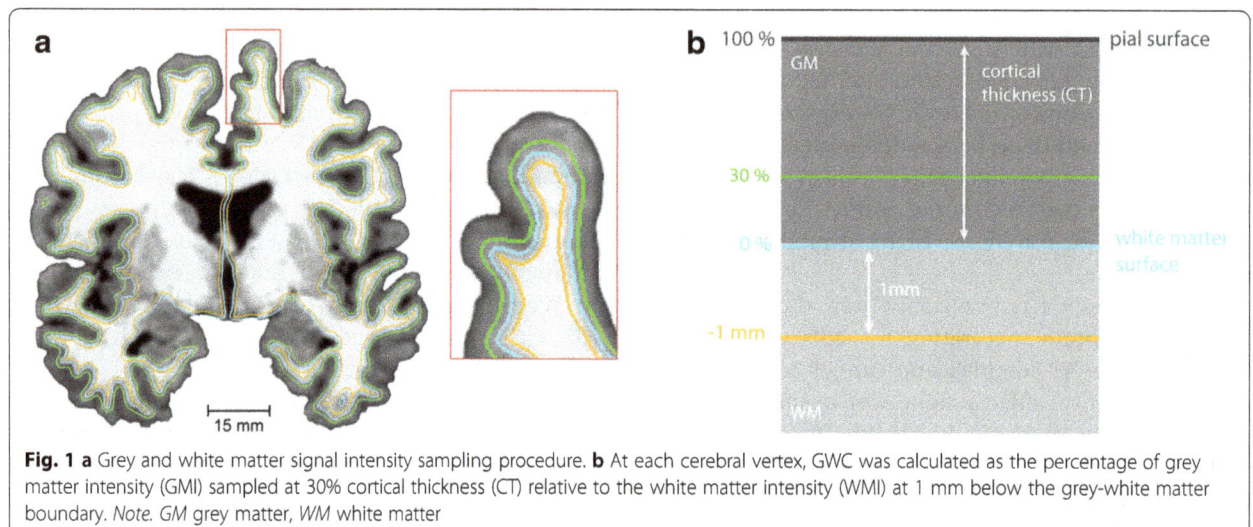

Fig. 1 a Grey and white matter signal intensity sampling procedure. **b** At each cerebral vertex, GWC was calculated as the percentage of grey matter intensity (GMI) sampled at 30% cortical thickness (CT) relative to the white matter intensity (WMI) at 1 mm below the grey-white matter boundary. *Note. GM* grey matter, *WM* white matter

$$GWC_i = \frac{100 \times \left(WMI_{i,1mm} - GMI_{i,0.3}\right)}{0.5 \times \left(WMI_{i,1mm} + GMI_{i,0.3}\right)}$$

In a next analysis step, to determine the influence of grey and white matter intensity on the GWC, we also extracted the absolute grey (GMI) and white matter intensities (WMI) at each cerebral vertex following non-uniform (NU) intensity correction and normalization (i.e. scaling of mean intensity of the white matter to 110) of the images in FreeSurfer. Grey matter tissue intensities were sampled at a projection fraction of 0% CT (i.e. at the grey-white matter boundary), as well as at 30% CT. White matter tissue intensities were sampled at 1 mm into the white matter from the grey-white matter boundary (the FreeSurfer 'default' for the computation of the GWC). To improve the ability to detect population changes, the resulting GWC, GMI, and WMI overlays were smoothed using a 10-mm full-width at half-maximum (FWHM) surface-based Gaussian kernel prior to statistical analyses.

Statistical analysis

Statistical analysis was conducted using the SurfStat toolbox (http://www.math.mcgill.ca/keith/surfstat/) for Matlab (R2016a; www.mathworks.com). To determine developmental trajectories for the GWC, we initially tested for linear, quadratic, and cubic effects of age, in addition to the main effect of group in a vertex-wise fashion. Here, an F-test for nested model comparisons was performed at each vertex, employing a step-up model selection procedure. Initially, the linear (i.e. most reduced) model was compared to a more complex (i.e. quadratic) model in order to determine if the addition of a quadratic age effect significantly improved the goodness-of-fit. If the quadratic model performed significantly better, it was then compared to the most complex (i.e. cubic) model, which contained a linear, quadratic, and cubic age term. Corrections for multiple comparisons across the whole brain were performed using random-field theory (RFT)-based cluster-corrected analysis for non-isotropic images using a $p < 0.05$ (two-tailed) cluster-significance threshold [27]. This procedure allowed us to identify the most parsimonious model at each vertex, i.e. the most simple plausible model that explained age-related variability in measures of GWC with the smallest set of predictors. All nested model comparisons were performed based on the combined sample of ASD and TD individuals.

Next, we examined between-group differences and age-by-group interactions by applying a general linear regression model (GLM) at each vertex i for subject j, with (1) group (G) as categorical fixed-effects factor and (2) linear, quadratic, or cubic terms for age, as well as their interactions with group. Based on

previous reports suggesting that there is a significant negative association between the GWC and general cognitive abilities [28–31], FSIQ was included as continuous covariate, so that $GWC_i = \beta_0 + \beta_1 G_j + \beta_2$ $age_j + \beta_3 \, age_j^2 + \beta_4 \, age_j^3 + \beta_5 \, (age_j \times group_j) + \beta_6$ $(age_j^2 \times group_j) + \beta_7 \, (age_j^3 \times group_j) + \beta_8 \, IQ_j + \varepsilon_i$, where ε denotes the residual error. Corrections for multiple comparisons across the whole brain were performed as outlined above (i.e. using random-field theory (RFT)-based cluster-corrected analysis for non-isotropic images). All statistical effects (i.e. between-group differences and age-by-group interactions) were mapped onto the FreeSurfer high-resolution common-group template in standard space (i.e. 'fsaverage' with ~ 300.000 vertices). For reasons of completeness, we also performed the analysis using total brain volume (TBV) as a continuous covariate in the statistical model. The results of this analysis are presented in an additional file (see Additional file 1).

Results

Demographics

There were no significant between-group differences in age [t (151) = 1.32, $p = 0.19$], FSIQ [t (151) = − 1.76, $p = 0.08$], total grey matter volume [t (151) = − 0.94, $p = 0.35$], or total white matter volume [t (151) = − 0.57, $p = 0.57$] (see Table 1). We therefore did not covary for total brain measures in the statistical analysis of GWC, GMI, or WMI.

Nested model comparison

Based on the nested model comparison, we established that the quadratic model provided a significantly better fit than the linear model in several clusters across the cortex when modelling neurodevelopmental trajectories in GWC (see Fig. 2a). There were no brain regions which showed a significant improvement in fit when also including a cubic term for age (RFT-based, cluster-corrected, $p < 0.05$) (see Fig. 2b). Thus, the quadratic model was chosen as the most parsimonious model for the examination of age-related differences in GWC between ASD individuals and TD controls.

Between-group differences in grey-to-white matter tissue contrast

Overall, we found that the GWC was significantly reduced in ASD individuals relative to controls in seven large clusters following correction for multiple comparisons (RFT-based, cluster-corrected, $p < 0.05$, two-tailed). These clusters predominantly included (1) bilateral prefrontal cortices (approximate Brodmann area [BA] 6/10), (2) the right inferior parietal cortex (BA 39), (3) the right postcentral gyrus (BA 1/2), (4) the right precuneus (BA 7), and (5) the left supramarginal gyrus (BA 40, see Fig. 3a; for detailed statistical values see Table 2). There

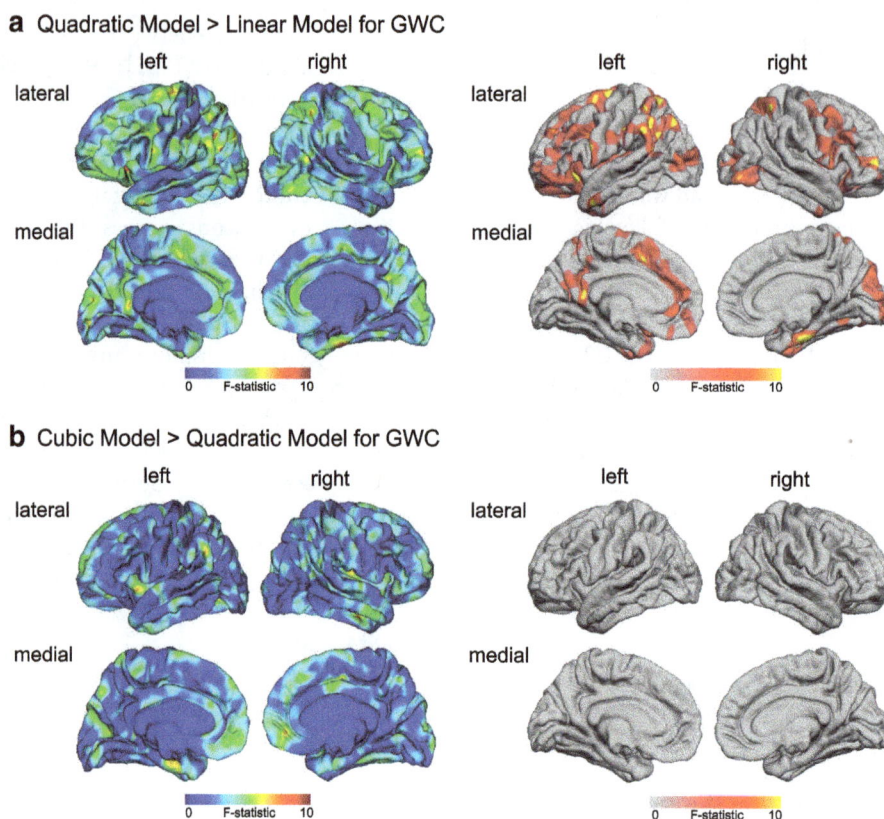

Fig. 2 Nested model comparisons of GWC age effects mapped onto FreeSurfer default common group template ('fsaverage'). **a** Comparison of the linear vs. quadratic model including all age effects and age-by-group interactions. **b** Comparison of the quadratic vs. cubic model including all age effects and age-by-group interactions. *Left panel* shows the difference map resulting from the model comparison. *F*-values (blue to red) indicate voxels where the more complex model provided a better fit than the more reduced model (*F*-statistic, unthresholded). *Right panel* indicates random-field theory (RFT)-based, cluster-corrected (*p* < 0.05) difference maps in goodness of fit (based on *F*-statistic). Here, the colourscale relates to *F*-statistic within significant clusters where the quadratic model provided a significantly better fit than the linear model

were no brain regions where ASD individuals showed a significant increase in GWC compared to TD controls.

Significant age-by-group interactions in grey-to-white matter tissue contrast

In four of the seven clusters with a significant between-group difference in GWC, we also observed significant age-by-group interactions in addition to the main effect of group. Linear age-by-group interactions were observed in (1) the right inferior parietal cortex (BA 39), (2) the right prefrontal cortex (BA 10), (3) the right postcentral gyrus (BA 1/2; see Fig. 3b), and (4) the left supramarginal gyrus (BA 40). In addition, three clusters in the right hemisphere that included frontal, parietal, and temporal regions displayed a significant quadratic interaction (i.e. age^2-by-group) (see Fig. 3c). In brain regions with significant age-by-group interactions, individuals with ASD tended to have the most prominent decrease in GWC during childhood and early adolescence (i.e. between 7 and 15 years of age) as compared to TD controls, but showed no differences (or enhanced GWC)

during early adulthood (see Fig. 4). There were no clusters with significant linear or quadratic age-by-group interactions that did not also have a significant main effect of group, i.e. all clusters with significant age-by-group interactions also displayed a significant main effect of group.

Between-group differences in grey matter intensities and white matter intensities

In addition to the GWC, we also examined between-group differences in absolute grey and white matter tissue intensities (i.e. GMI and WMI) in order to identify whether the between-group differences in GWC were driven by variability within the cortical grey or white matter or a combination of both. We did not observe any significant between-group differences in absolute tissue intensities when sampling at 0% (i.e. at the grey-white matter boundary) or at 30% into the grey matter (*p* > 0.05, two-tailed). However, individuals with ASD had significantly decreased WMI relative to controls in many brain regions that also showed decreases

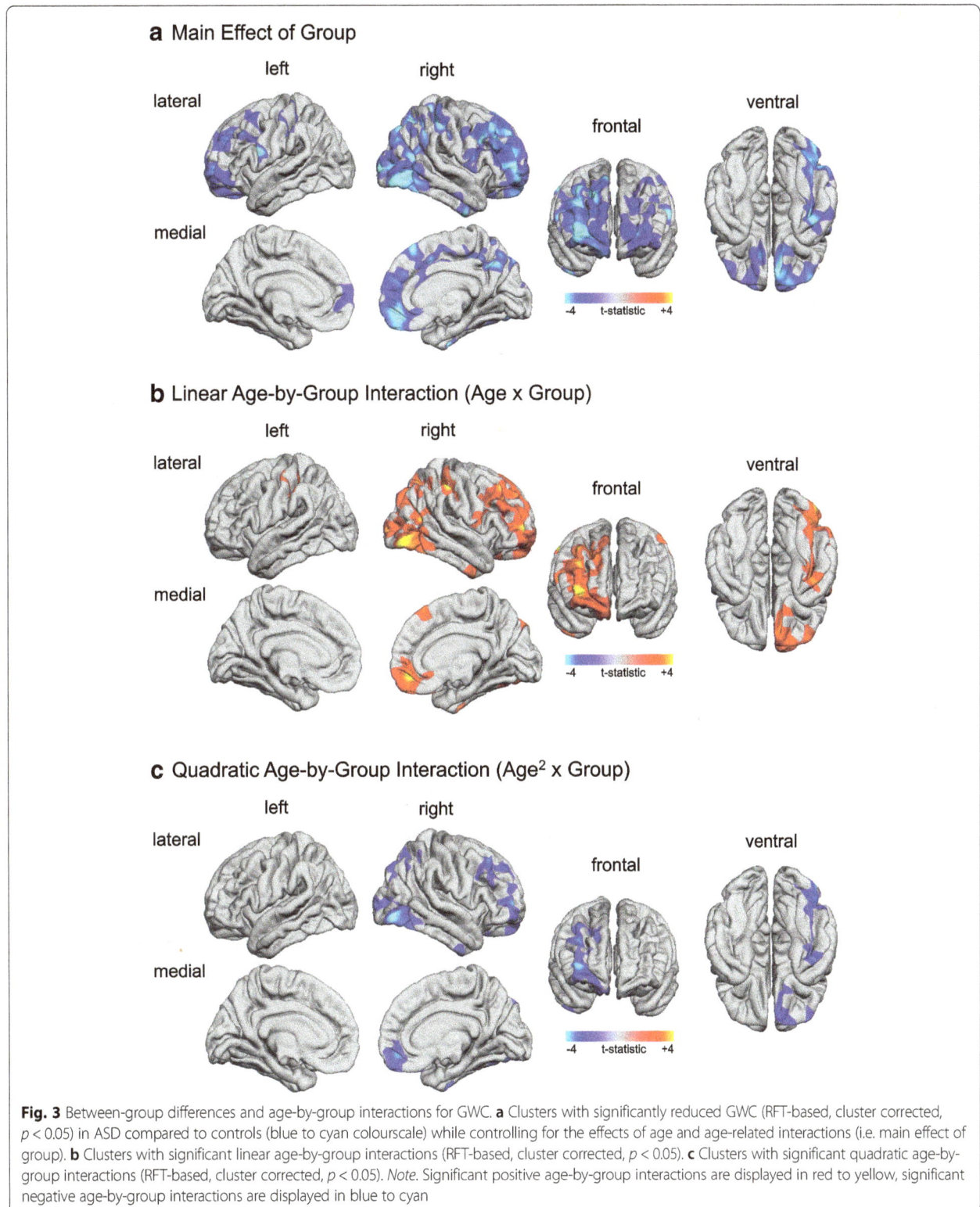

Fig. 3 Between-group differences and age-by-group interactions for GWC. **a** Clusters with significantly reduced GWC (RFT-based, cluster corrected, $p < 0.05$) in ASD compared to controls (blue to cyan colourscale) while controlling for the effects of age and age-related interactions (i.e. main effect of group). **b** Clusters with significant linear age-by-group interactions (RFT-based, cluster corrected, $p < 0.05$). **c** Clusters with significant quadratic age-by-group interactions (RFT-based, cluster corrected, $p < 0.05$). *Note*. Significant positive age-by-group interactions are displayed in red to yellow, significant negative age-by-group interactions are displayed in blue to cyan

in GWC. These regions included (1) bilateral lateral occipital cortices (approximate Brodmann area [BA] 37/19), (2) the right prefrontal cortex (BA 9/47), (3) the right inferior parietal cortex (BA 39), (4) the right fusiform gyrus (BA 37), (5) the left supramarginal gyrus (BA 40), and (6) the left precuneus (BA 7; see Fig. 5; for detailed statistical values, see Table 2). There were no brain regions where ASD individuals showed a

Table 2 Clusters of significant reductions in GWC and WMI in ASD relative to controls

	Cluster	Region labels	Side	BA	Vertices	t_{max}	p	Age (age^2)-by-group interactions
GWC	1	Rostral middle frontal gyrus, superior frontal gyrus, precentral gyrus	R	10	24,950	−3.96	3.17×10^{-6}	Age (age^2)
	2	Inferior parietal cortex, lateral occipital cortex, superior parietal cortex	R	39	20,502	−4.10	3.17×10^{-6}	Age (age^2)
	3	Postcentral gyrus, superior parietal cortex, supramarginal gyrus	R	1/2	6528	−4.22	3.49×10^{-5}	Age (age^2)
	4	Supramarginal gyrus, postcentral gyrus, inferior parietal cortex	L	40	4828	−3.84	.00026	Age
	5	Caudal middle frontal gyrus, superior frontal gyrus, rostral middle frontal gyrus	L	6	5778	−3.78	.00046	–
	6	Rostral middle frontal gyrus, superior frontal gyrus, lateral orbital frontal cortex	L	10	5243	−3.18	.0036	–
	7	Precuneus cortex, paracentral lobule	R	7	3448	−3.14	.037	–
WMI	1	Inferior parietal cortex, precuneus cortex, superior parietal cortex	R	39	7320	−3.77	2.27×10^{-6}	Age (age^2)
	2	Rostral middle frontal gyrus, caudal middle frontal gyrus, pars orbitalis	R	9	5219	−3.48	2.95×10^{-5}	Age (age^2)
	3	Supramarginal gyrus, inferior parietal cortex, superior temporal gyrus	L	40	7096	−3.75	.0003	Age (age^2)
	4	Lateral occipital cortex, inferior temporal gyrus, lingual gyrus	L	37	5296	−3.91	.0005	Age (age^2)
	5	Precuneus cortex, isthmus-cingulate cortex	L	7	1656	−3.82	.0018	Age
	6	Lateral orbital frontal cortex	R	47	1052	−4.25	.022	–
	7	Lateral occipital cortex, inferior temporal cortex, middle temporal gyrus	R	19	2907	−3.07	.04	–
	8	Fusiform gyrus	R	37	1568	−3.27	.048	–

Note. GWC, Grey-white matter contrast; *WMI,* white matter intensity; *BA,* approximate Brodmann area at t_{max} within cluster; *L,* left; *R,* right; t_{max} test statistic within cluster; *p,* cluster-corrected *p* value. Vertices: the number of vertices within the cluster; age/age^2 indicates existence of significant age-by-group interaction for linear and/or quadratic terms. For each cluster, the three most significant regions are reported

significant increase in WMI compared to TD controls. Thus, our data suggests that in children and adolescents with ASD, between-group differences in WMI underneath the cortical mantle contribute more to differences in the GWC than do differences in GMI.

Discussion

In the present study, we examined between-group differences in cross-sectional age-related trajectories of GWC in ASD and neurotypical controls across childhood and early adulthood (from 7 to 25 years) using a spatially unbiased vertex-wise approach. We first established that the developmental trajectory of GWC is complex in many areas of the brain and included linear as well as non-linear (i.e. quadratic) effects of age. Moreover, we found that while ASD individuals had significantly reduced GWC overall, these differences were age-dependent, with the most prominent decreases in GWC occurring during childhood. This is of importance as our findings suggest that differences in GWC in ASD are unlikely to reflect atypical grey matter cytoarchitecture alone, which is typically set around birth, but may

also represent age-related variability in the white matter architecture (i.e. differences in myelination, axonal density, and diameter, etc.). Measures of GWC might thus be considered an age-sensitive in vivo marker for atypical neurodevelopment in ASD. Our finding of significantly reduced GWC in children and adolescents with ASD extends our previous neuroimaging study examining the GWC in adults with the condition, which concluded in suggesting that the tissue contrast between cortical grey and white matter may be less well defined in ASD [15].

Moreover, our study agrees with previous post-mortem reports suggesting that the boundary between cortical layer VI and the underlying white matter may be more 'indistinct' in ASD. This indistinct boundary may be due to increased 'dispersion' of neuronal cells across the grey-white matter interface [11, 12]. In turn, supernumerary neurons beneath the cortical plate may then arise as a consequence of disrupted migratory processes during prenatal brain development and/or atypical development and resolution of the cortical subplate (e.g. overproduction of subplate neurons or reduced apoptosis) [32]. Additionally, the cortical suplate plays a crucial role in the

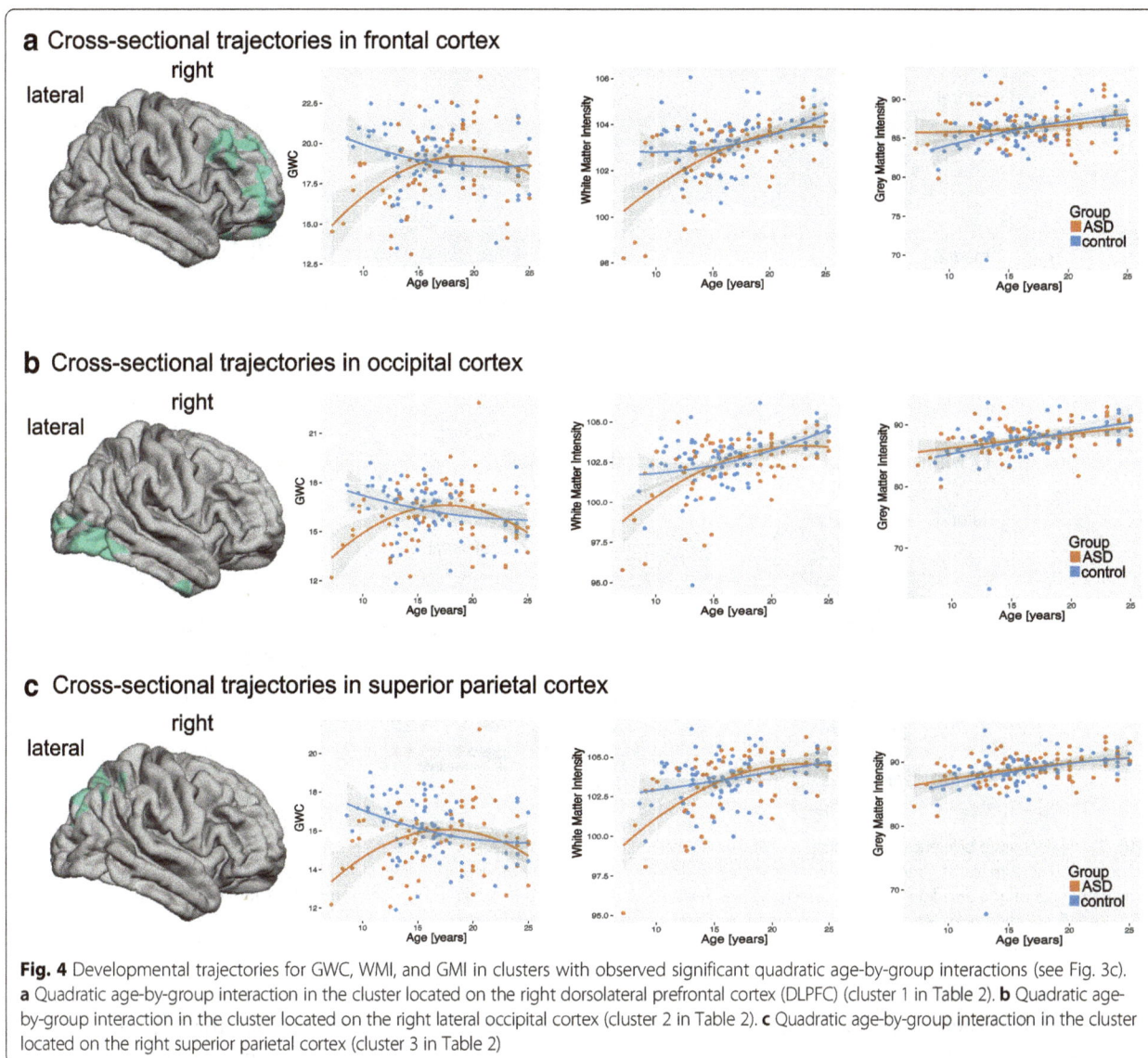

Fig. 4 Developmental trajectories for GWC, WMI, and GMI in clusters with observed significant quadratic age-by-group interactions (see Fig. 3c). **a** Quadratic age-by-group interaction in the cluster located on the right dorsolateral prefrontal cortex (DLPFC) (cluster 1 in Table 2). **b** Quadratic age-by-group interaction in the cluster located on the right lateral occipital cortex (cluster 2 in Table 2). **c** Quadratic age-by-group interaction in the cluster located on the right superior parietal cortex (cluster 3 in Table 2)

formation of the early intra- and extra-cortical neurocircuitry and contributes to the guidance and targeting of thalamocortical axons [33].

Significant reductions in GWC were found in several regions across the cortex, most of which have previously been associated with symptoms characteristic for ASD. More specifically, the medial and dorsolateral prefrontal cortices (mPFC and DLPFC) are integral parts of the so-called social and emotional brain, which encompasses a set of brain regions involved in wider aspects of social cognition and emotional processing [34, 35]. ASD-related neuroanatomical variation in these regions has also been linked to deficits in theory of mind [36], face processing [37], and various other aspects of impaired social cognition, for example, self-referential cognition and empathy [38]. In addition, some of our identified clusters (mPFC and precuneus) are also an integral component of

the so-called default mode network (DMN), which characterizes a wider network of brain regions showing decreased activity during cognitive tasks and increased activity when the brain is 'at rest' [39]. In ASD, the DMN has been reported to be among the most disrupted functional networks, and this disrupted intrinsic DMN organization (e.g. in terms of functional connectivity patterns) seems to be associated with social deficits in children and adults with ASD [40]. Further significant reductions in GWC were found in occipital regions, which on a functional level have been associated with communication deficits and social reciprocity [2].

In many brain regions where we found a significant main effect of group in GWC, we also observed significant linear and quadratic age-by-group interactions. This implies that the between-group differences in these regions are age-dependent and caused by an atypical

a Main Effect of Group on White Matter Intensity

b Main Effect of Group on Grey Matter Intensity

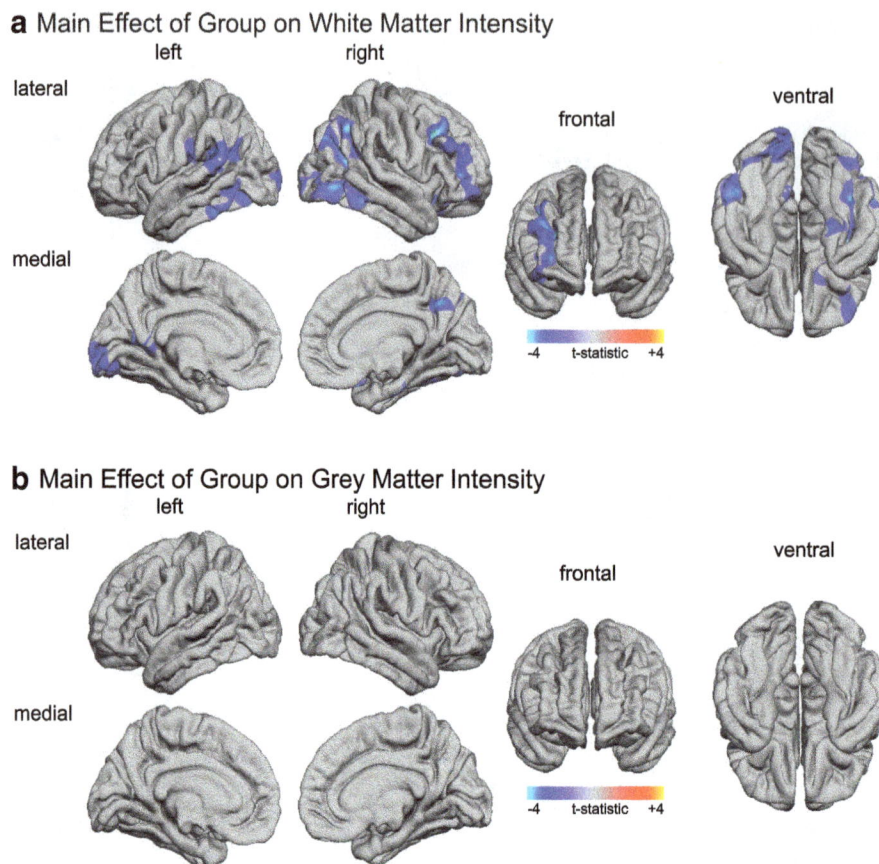

Fig. 5 Between-group differences for absolute grey and white matter tissue intensities (GMI, WMI respectively). **a** Clusters with significantly reduced WMI (blue to cyan colourscale) at 1 mm below the white matter surface (RFT-based, cluster-corrected, $p < 0.05$) in ASD compared to controls while controlling for the effects of age and age-related interactions (i.e. main effect of group). **b** Between-group differences for GMI at 30% cortical thickness (RFT-based, cluster corrected, $p < 0.05$). The colourbar shows t-statistics resulting from the main effect of group. Significant positive age-by-group interactions are displayed in red to yellow, and significant negative age-by-group interactions are displayed in blue to cyan

developmental trajectory of GWC in the ASD individuals. More specifically, while the GWC in TD controls declined consistently from 7 to 25 years of age, the cross-sectional age-related trajectory in ASD was significantly decreased relative to the normative trajectory during early childhood, followed by a period of no, or small, differences between the ages of 15 and 23 years. This early age-related reduction in tissue contrast was most prominent in temporal and prefrontal regions, which are also the latest ones to mature during typical development [41]. Given previous evidence to suggest that the GWC declines significantly as part of the typical ageing process [17, 42], and based on our previous results of a reduced GWC in adults with ASD [15], it is likely that the GWC also declines more rapidly across the remaining life-span (i.e. after the age of 23 years). However, future research is needed to test this hypothesis directly, using samples with a wider age range (i.e. 25 years plus). Taken together, our study suggests that the developmental trajectory of GWC in the ASD brain not

only differs quantitatively from the trajectory in TD controls, but also qualitatively (i.e. in terms of its shape), and particularly during childhood. In turn, this implies that the GWC in ASD may be mediated via different neurobiological mechanisms as compared to TD controls.

Notably, our results show a lateralization towards the right hemisphere, i.e. group differences in GWC were mostly located in the right hemisphere while the left hemisphere seems to be relatively unimpaired. Previous studies have yielded highly heterogeneous findings concerning the lateralization of structural and functional abnormalities in the brain in ASD (e.g. [43]). On the functional level, studies demonstrate that the right hemisphere in particular seems to play a crucial role in mediating several autistic core symptoms, such as communication [44] and theory of mind deficits [45]. Furthermore, in a study by Dapretto et al. [46], ASD individuals showed no activation of the right hemisphere mirror neuron system (MNS) during an emotion recognition and imitation task, i.e. the right pars opercularis showed significantly greater activation in typically developing children than in children with ASD. Activity in the right pars opercularis was also negatively correlated with symptom severity measured by ADOS and ADI-R. These previous reports of a right hemispheric involvement of the brain in mediating ASD symptomatology are thus in line with our findings of more significant reductions in GWC predominantly in the right hemisphere.

Little is, however, currently known about the neurobiological mechanisms that underpin variability in GWC. In general, the T1-weighted signal, which constitutes the basis of the GWC, is heavily influenced by the structure and density of axonal myelin [47, 48], as well as non-architectural components such as iron deposition and water content [49, 50]. Out of these potential candidates, studies examining cortical ageing in the TD brain show that the age-related decline in GWC is foremost related to reduced signal intensities in the superficial white matter [17] and reduced intracortical myelin content as measured by the ratio between T1w/T2w image contrast [51]. Thus, the most prominent biological candidate influencing the GWC may be the degree of myelin in the superficial WM under the cortical mantle, which mostly contains short association and U-shaped fibers [17, 42, 52]. Deficits of short association fibers have been reported previously [53] and may hence contribute to the atypical GWC observed in our study.

In addition, we examined whether the differences in GWC were driven by differences in absolute tissue intensities within the grey or white matter. In many regions with significantly reduced GWC, ASD individuals also showed significantly decreased WMI sampled at 1 mm below the grey-white matter boundary. However, there were no differences in GMI (sampled at 30% CT and at the grey-white matter boundary) compared to TD controls. Analogue to the trajectories of GWC, differences in WMI seem to be most prominent during childhood and become less pronounced during adolescence and early adulthood. This finding is in agreement with previous voxel-based-morphometry (VBM) studies in ASD that compare white matter intensity using a whole-volume approach [5, 6, 54]. Evidence for general white matter abnormalities in ASD is further supported by DTI studies applying techniques such as tract-based spatial statistics (TBSS) [55]. For example, a study by Shukla et al. [56] examined atypicalities in the trajectories of white matter development in a sample of 9- to 20-year-old ASD individuals and TD controls. Here, ASD individuals showed less orientational coherence (i.e. fractional anisotropy) and stronger water diffusion (i.e. mean diffusivity) in many of the most prominent

white matter fiber tracts in the brain compared to controls [56]. These maturational differences, however, diminished from childhood to adolescence and are thus in agreement with our finding of a delayed white matter maturation (based on tissue intensities) during early childhood. Our results are thus consistent with previous publications examining cortical white matter employing different methodological frameworks and spatial scales.

Last, our findings should be interpreted in the light of a number of limitations given the data and methods presented. First, we employed a cross-sectional study design to examine age-related differences in GWC associated with ASD. Thus, the resulting age-related trajectories were based on inter- rather than intra-individual variability in GWC. Future studies are required to replicate our findings in longitudinal samples, which would provide a more accurate characterization of developmental trajectories based on repeated measures acquired in the same set of individuals. Second, our sample only included right-handed males with ASD in the high-functioning range of the spectrum. It therefore remains to be established whether our findings generalize to other (sub)groups on the autism spectrum (e.g. left-handed individuals, females with ASD, or individuals with intellectual disability). Furthermore, our study examined age-related changes in GWC by sampling tissue intensities around the grey-white matter boundary, even though this boundary may be 'blurred' (i.e. less well distinct) in ASD as suggested by histological evidence [12]. In this histological study, however, such microstructural blurring occured up to 500 micrometers underneath the grey-white matter transition zone [12], which would result in a maximal displacement of the boundary of 0.5 mm. As we are sampling GMI at 30% CT, which roughly equals between 0.56 and 1.5 mm into the cortical mantle depending on CT variability across the cortex (see Additional file 2), and WMI at 1 mm into the white matter, we can be certain that our sampling points remain located within the grey or white matter even in case of a maximal boundary displacement. However, while our model can accommodate such potential displacements in terms of intensity sampling, we are unable to unambiguously allocate sampling points to specific cortical layers given the restraints with regard to the current resolution of structural MRI images (see also [17]). Similarly, while surface-based mapping allows for morphometric inferences on a sub-millimeter scale, the derived grey-white matter tissue intensity values, and hence the GWC, remain dependent on the native spatial resolution of the T1-weighted images (i.e. 1 mm isotropic). Thus, partial volume effects and/or the ability to clearly delineate the grey-white matter boundary may affect GWC values. However, both of these factors are expected to affect both groups equally, and our findings of significant between-group differences and age-by-group interactions cannot be fully explained by these limitations.

Conclusions

Using 3-Tesla structural MRI, we provide evidence that the tissue contrast at the grey-white matter boundary is regionally reduced in the brain of individuals with autism spectrum disorder. Compared to healthy controls, this neuroanatomical difference seems to be most prominent during childhood and early adolescence. Taken together, while future research is required to identify the specific neurobiological mechanisms underpinning the atypical development of tissue contrast in ASD, the findings presented in the present study suggest that the differences in GWC previously reported in adults with the condition [15] do not reflect differences in the grey matter cytoarchitecture alone. Instead, our study suggests that the differences in GWC are dynamic (i.e. ongoing) across the human life-span and are thus most likely caused by a combination of factors that include many of the grey matter atypicalities highlighted by the histological studies above [11, 12], but also by perturbations to the formation of the axonal neurocircuitry and subsequent myelination within the superficial white matter.

Additional files

Additional file 1: Between-group differences and age-by-group interactions for GWC when including total brain volume (TBV) as a covariate. (A) Clusters with significantly reduced GWC (RFT-based, cluster corrected, $p < 0.05$) in ASD compared to controls (blue to cyan colourscale) while controlling for the effects of age and age-related interactions (i.e. main effect of group). (B) Clusters with significant linear age-by-group interactions (RFT-based, cluster corrected, $p < 0.05$). (C) Clusters with significant quadratic age-by-group interactions (RFT-based, cluster corrected, $p < 0.05$). Note. Significant positive age-by-group interactions are displayed in red to yellow, significant negative age-by-group interactions are displayed in blue to cyan. (PDF 1284 kb)

Additional file 2: Cumulative distribution for measures of cortical thickness (CT) across all vertices and participants. The horizontal bar shows the upper 90% of the distribution, corresponding to a CT value of 1.85 mm. (PDF 38 kb)

Abbreviations

ADI-R: Autism Diagnostic Interview-Revised; ADOS: Autism Diagnostic Observation Schedule; ASD: Autism spectrum disorder; BA: Brodmann area; CT: Cortical thickness; DLPFC: Dorsolateral prefrontal cortex; DMN: Default mode network; DTI: Diffusion tensor imaging; FOV: Field of view; FSIQ: Full-scale intelligence quotient; FWHM: Full-width at half-maximum; GLM: General linear model; GM: Grey matter; GMI: Grey matter intensity; GWC: Grey-white matter tissue contrast; ICD: International statistical classification of diseases; IQ: Intelligence quotient; MNS: Mirror neuron system; mPFC: Medial prefrontal cortex; NU: Non-uniform; RFT: Random-field theory; TBSS: Tract-based spatial statistics; TD: Typically developing; TE: Echo time; TR: Repetition time; VBM: Voxel-based morphometry; WASI: Wechsler Abbreviated Scale of Intelligence; WM: White matter; WMI: White matter intensity

Acknowledgements

CE, CM, and AB gratefully acknowledge support from the German Research Foundation (DFG) under the Heisenberg programme (grant number EC480/1-1 and EC480/2-1). Furthermore, we would like to thank the National Institute for Health Research Biomedical Research Centre (BRC) for Mental Health, and the Dr. Mortimer and Theresa Sackler Foundation.

Funding

This work was supported by the Autism Imaging Multicentre Study Consortium funded by Medical Research Council UK Grant (G0400061), by the EU-AIMS Consortium receiving support from the Innovative Medicines Initiative Joint Undertaking under grant agreement no. 115300, which includes financial contributions from the EU Seventh Framework Programme (FP7/2007-2013), from the EFPIA companies in kind, and from Autism Speaks.

Authors' contributions

CM prepared and analyzed the data and drafted and revised the manuscript. DA provided analytical tools for the calculation of GWC in FreeSurfer and revised the manuscript. AB revised the manuscript. ED acquired the data, carried out neuropsychological testing, and revised the manuscript. CM carried out the clinical assessments and revised the manuscript. DM helped to design the study and revised the manuscript. CE designed the research, analyzed the data, and revised the manuscript. All authors read and approved the final manuscript.

Authors' information

CM, MSc and AB, Dipl.-Psych., Department of Child and Adolescent Psychiatry, Psychosomatics and Psychotherapy, University Hospital, Goethe-University Frankfurt am Main, Deutschordenstrasse 50, 60528 Frankfurt, Germany; DA, PhD, The Medical Investigation of Neurodevelopmental Disorders (MIND) Institute and Department of Psychiatry and Behavioural Sciences, UC Davis School of Medicine, University of California Davis, Sacramento, CA, USA; ED, PhD and CM, PhD, Department of Forensic and Neurodevelopmental Sciences, and the Sackler Institute for Translational Neurodevelopmental Sciences, Institute of Psychiatry, Psychology & Neuroscience (IoPPN), King's College London, London SE5 8AF, United Kingdom; DM, Professor, Head of Department of Forensic and Neurodevelopmental Sciences, and the Sackler Institute for Translational Neurodevelopmental Sciences, Institute of Psychiatry, Psychology & Neuroscience (IoPPN), King's College London, London SE5 8AF, United Kingdom; CE, Professor, Department of Child and Adolescent Psychiatry, Psychosomatics and Psychotherapy, University Hospital, Goethe-University Frankfurt am Main, Deutschordenstrasse 50, 60528 Frankfurt, Germany and Department of Forensic and Neurodevelopmental Sciences, and the Sackler Institute for Translational Neurodevelopmental Sciences, Institute of Psychiatry, Psychology & Neuroscience (IoPPN), King's College London, London SE5 8AF, United Kingdom.

Competing interests

The authors declare that they have no competing interests.

Author details

[1]Department of Child and Adolescent Psychiatry, Psychosomatics and Psychotherapy, University Hospital, Goethe University Frankfurt am Main, Deutschordenstrasse 50, 60528 Frankfurt am Main, Germany. [2]Department of Psychiatry and Behavioural Sciences, The Medical Investigation of Neurodevelopmental Disorders (MIND) Institute, UC Davis School of Medicine, University of California Davis, Sacramento, CA, USA. [3]Department of Forensic and Neurodevelopmental Sciences, and the Sackler Institute for Translational Neurodevelopmental Sciences, Institute of Psychiatry, Psychology & Neuroscience (IoPPN), King's College London, London SE5 8AF, UK.

References

1. Wing L. The autistic spectrum. Lancet. 1997;350:1761–6.
2. Amaral DG, Schumann CM, Nordahl CW. Neuroanatomy of autism. Trends Neurosci. 2008;31:137–45.
3. Wolff JJ, Gu H, Gehrig G, et al. Differences in white matter fiber tract development present from 6 to 24 months in infants with autism. Am J Psychiatry. 2012;169:589–600.
4. Wolff JJ, Gehrig G, Lewis JD, et al. Altered corpus callosum morphology associated with autism over the first 2 years of life. Brain. 2015;138:2046–58.
5. Ecker C, Suckling J, Deoni SC, et al. Brain anatomy and its relationship to behavior in adults with autism spectrum disorder. Arch Gen Psychiatry. 2012;69:195–209.
6. McAlonan GM, Cheung V, Cheung C, et al. Mapping the brain in autism. A voxel-based MRI study of volumetric differences and intercorrelations in autism. Brain. 2005;128:268–76.
7. Lange N, Travers BG, Bigler ED, et al. Longitudinal volumetric brain changes in autism spectrum disorder ages 6-35 years. Autism Res. 2015;8:82–93.
8. Wallace GL, Dankner N, Kenworthy L, Giedd JN, Martin A. Age-related temporal and parietal cortical thinning in autism spectrum disorders. Brain. 2010;133:3745–54.
9. Ecker C, Ginestet C, Feng Y, et al. Brain surface anatomy in adults with autism: the relationship between surface area, cortical thickness, and autistic symptoms. JAMA Psychiatry. 2013;70:59–70.
10. Ecker C, Shahidiani A, Feng Y, et al. The effect of age, diagnosis, and their interaction on vertex-based measures of cortical thickness and surface area in autism spectrum disorder. J Neural Transm. 2014;121:1157–70.
11. Hutsler JJ, Avino TA. Sigmoid fits to locate and characterize cortical boundaries in human cerebral cortex. J Neurosci Methods. 2013;212:242–6.
12. Avino TA, Hutsler JJ. Abnormal cell patterning at the cortical gray-white matter boundary in autism spectrum disorders. Brain Res. 2010;1360:138–46.
13. Pinto D, Delaby E, Merico D, et al. Convergence of genes and cellular pathways dysregulated in autism spectrum disorders. Am J Hum Genet. 2014;94:677–94.
14. Huguet G, Ey E, Bourgeron T. The genetic landscapes of autism spectrum disorders. Annu Rev Genomics Hum Genet. 2013;14:191–213.
15. Andrews DS, Avino TA, Gudbrandsen M, et al. In vivo evidence of reduced integrity of the gray-white matter boundary in autism spectrum disorder. Cereb Cortex. 2017;27:877–87.
16. Ecker C, Bookheimer SY, Murphy DG. Neuroimaging in autism spectrum disorder: brain structure and function across the lifespan. Lancet Neurol. 2015;14:1121–34.
17. Vidal-Piñeiro D, KKB W, ABA S, Grydeland H, Rohani DA, Fjell AM. Accelerated longitudinal gray/white matter contrast decline in aging in lightly myelinated cortical regions. Hum Brain Mapp. 2016;37:3669–84.
18. JN G, Blumenthal J, Jeffries NO, et al. Brain development during childhood and adolescence: a longitudinal MRI study. Nat Neurosci. 1999;2:861–3.
19. Shaw P, Lerch J, Greenstein D, et al. Longitudinal mapping of cortical thickness and clinical outcome in children and adolescents with attention-deficit/hyperactivity disorder. Arch Gen Psychiatry. 2006;63:540–9.
20. World Health Organization (WHO). Clinical descriptions and diagnostic guidelines. In WHO (Ed.), The ICD-10 classification of mental and behavioural disorders. Geneva; 2010.
21. Lord C, Rutter M, Le Couteur A. Autism Diagnostic Interview-Revised: a revised version of a diagnostic interview for caregivers of individuals with possible pervasive developmental disorders. J Autism Dev Disord. 1994;24: 659–85.
22. Lord C, Rutter M, Goode S, et al. Austism diagnostic observation schedule: a standardized observation of communicative and social behavior. J Autism Dev Disord. 1989;19:185–212.
23. Wechsler D. Wechsler abbreviated scale of intelligence. San Antonio: Psychological Corporation; 1999.
24. Fischl B, Sereno M, Dale A. Cortical surface-based analysis II: inflation, flattening, and a surface-based coordinate system. Neuroimage. 1999;9: 195–207.
25. Dale AM, Fischl B, Sereno MI. Cortical surface-based analysis I: segmentation and surface reconstruction. Neuroimage. 1999;194:179–94.
26. Ségonne F, Dale AM, Busa E, et al. A hybrid approach to the skull stripping problem in MRI. Neuroimage. 2004;22:1060–75.
27. Worsley KJ, Andermann M, Koulis T, Macdonald D, Evans AC. Detecting changes in non-isotropic images. Hum Brain Mapp. 1999;8:98–101.
28. Grydeland H, Westlye LT, Walhovd KB, Fjell AM. Improved prediction of Alzheimer's disease with longitudinal white matter/gray matter contrast changes. Hum Brain Mapp. 2013;34:2775–85.
29. Jefferson AL, Gifford KA, Damon S, et al. Gray & white matter tissue contrast differentiates Mild Cognitive Impairment converters from non-converters. Brain Imaging Behav. 2015;9:141–8.
30. Salat DH, Chen JJ, van der Kouwe AJ, et al. Hippocampal degeneration is associated with temporal limbic gray matter/white matter tissue contrast in Alzheimer's disease. Neuroimage. 2011;54:1795–802.
31. Bletsch A, Mann C, Andrews DS, et al. Down syndrome is accompanied by significantly reduced cortical grey–white matter tissue contrast. Hum Brain Mapp. 2018;39:1–12.
32. Hutsler JJ, Casanova MF. Cortical construction in autism spectrum disorder: columns, connectivity and the subplate. Neuropathol Appl Neurobiol. 2016; 42:115–34.
33. Hoerder-Suabedissen A, Molnár Z. Development, evolution and pathology of neocortical subplate neurons. Nat Rev Neurosci. 2015;16:133–46.
34. Blakemore SJ. The social brain in adolescence. Nat Rev Neurosci. 2008;9: 267–77.
35. Pessoa L. On the relationship between emotion and cognition. Nat Rev Neurosci. 2008;9:148–58.
36. Castelli F, Frith C, Happé F, Frith U. Autism, Asperger syndrome and brain mechanisms for the attribution of mental states to animated shapes. Brain. 2002;125:1839–49.
37. Golarai G, Grill-Spector K, Reiss AL. Autism and the development of face processing. Clin Neurosci Res. 2006;6:145–60.
38. Lombardo MV, Chakrabarti B, Bullmore ET, et al. Shared neural circuits for mentalizing about the self and others. J Cog Neurosci. 2010;22:1623–35.
39. Raichle ME, MacLeod AM, Snyder AZ, Powers WJ, Gusnard DA, Shulman GL. A default mode of brain function. PNAS. 2001;98:676–82.
40. Padmanabhan A, Lynch CJ, Schaer M, Menon V. The default mode network in autism. Biol Psy CNNI. 2017;2:476–86.
41. Gogtay N, Giedd JN, Lusk L, et al. Dynamic mapping of human cortical development during childhood through early adulthood. PNAS. 2004;101: 8174–9.
42. Salat D, Lee S, Van Der Kouwe A, Greve D, Fischl B, Rosas H. Age-associated alterations in cortical gray and white matter signal intensity and gray to white matter contrast. Neuroimage. 2009;48:21–8.
43. Ecker C, Marquand A, Mourão-Miranda J, et al. Describing the brain in autism in five dimensions--magnetic resonance imaging-assisted diagnosis of autism spectrum disorder using a multiparameter classification approach. J Neurosci. 2010;30:10612–23.
44. Ozonoff S, Miller JN. An exploration of right-hemisphere contributions to the pragmatic impairments of autism. Brain Lang. 1996;52:411–34.
45. Mason RA, Williams DL, Kana RK, Minshwe N, Just MA. Theory of mind disruption and recruitment of the right hemisphere during narrative comprehension in autism. Neuropsychologica. 2008;46:269–80.
46. Dapretto M, Davies MS, Pfeifer JH, et al. Understanding emotions in others: mirror neuron dysfunction in children with autism spectrum disorders. Nat Neuroscience. 2006;9:28–30.
47. Clark VP, Courchesne E, Grafe M. In vivo myeloarchitectonic analysis of human striate and extrastriate cortex using magnetic resonance imaging. Cereb Cortex. 1992;2:417–24.
48. Koenig SH. Cholesterol of myelin is the determinant of gray-white contrast in MRI of brain. Magn Reson Med. 1991;20:285–91.
49. Bansal R, Hao X, Liu F, Xu D, Liu J, Peterson BS. The effects of changing water content, relaxation times, and tissue contrast on tissue segmentation and measures of cortical anatomy in MR images. Magn Reson Imaging. 2013;31:1709–30.
50. Eickhoff S, Walters NB, Schleicher A, et al. High-resolution MRI reflects myeloarchitecture and cytoarchitecture of human cerebral cortex. Hum Brain Mapp. 2005;24:206–15.
51. Glasser MF, Van Essen DC. Mapping human cortical areas in vivo based on myelin content as revealed by T1-and T2-weighted MRI. J Neurosci. 2011;31: 11597–616.
52. Westlye LT, Walhovd KB, Dale AM, et al. Increased sensitivity to effects of normal aging and Alzheimer's disease on cortical thickness by adjustment for local variability in gray/white contrast: a multi-sample MRI study. Neuroimage. 2009;47:1545–57.

53.	Thompson A, Murphy DG, Dell'Acqua F, et al. Impaired communication between the motor and somatosensory homunculus is associated with poor manual dexterity in autism spectrum disorder. Biol Psychiatry. 2017;81: 211–9.

54.	Waiter GD, Williams JHG, Murray AD, Gilchrist A, Perret DI, Whiten A. Structural white matter deficits in high-functioning individuals with autistic spectrum disorder: a voxel-based investigation. Neuroimage. 2004;24:455–61.

55.	Smith SM, Jenkinson M, Johansen-Berg H, et al. Tract-based spatial statistics: voxelwise analysis of multi-subject diffusion data. Neuroimage. 2006;31: 1487–505.

56.	Shukla DK, Kheen B, Müller R-A. Tract-specific analyses of diffusion tensor imaging show widespread white matter compromise in autism spectrum disorder. J Child Psychol Psychiatry. 2011;52:286–95.

Analysis of neuroanatomical differences in mice with genetically modified serotonin transporters assessed by structural magnetic resonance imaging

Jacob Ellegood[1][*] [iD], Yohan Yee[1,4], Travis M. Kerr[3], Christopher L. Muller[3], Randy D. Blakely[2,3,5], R. Mark Henkelman[1,4], Jeremy Veenstra-VanderWeele[2,6] and Jason P. Lerch[1,4]

Abstract

Background: The serotonin (5-HT) system has long been implicated in autism spectrum disorder (ASD) as indicated by elevated whole blood and platelet 5-HT, altered platelet and brain receptor and transporter binding, and genetic linkage and association findings. Based upon work in genetically modified mice, 5-HT is known to influence several aspects of brain development, but systematic neuroimaging studies have not previously been reported. In particular, the 5-HT transporter (serotonin transporter, SERT; 5-HTT) gene, *Slc6a4*, has been extensively studied.

Methods: Using a 7-T MRI and deformation-based morphometry, we assessed neuroanatomical differences in an *Slc6a4* knockout mouse on a C57BL/6 genetic background, along with an *Slc6a4* Ala56 knockin mouse on two different genetic backgrounds (129S and C57BL/6).

Results: Individually (same sex, same background, same genotype), the only differences found were in the female *Slc6a4* knockout mouse; all the others had no significant differences. However, an analysis of variance across the whole study sample revealed a significant effect of *Slc6a4* on the amygdala, thalamus, dorsal raphe nucleus, and lateral and frontal cortices.

Conclusions: This work shows that an increase or decrease in SERT function has a significant effect on the neuroanatomy in 5-HT relevant regions, particularly the raphe nuclei. Notably, the *Slc6a4* Ala56 knockin alone appears to have an insignificant, but suggestive, effect compared to the KO, which is consistent with *Slc6a4* function. Despite the small number of 5-HT neurons and their localization to the brainstem, it is clear that 5-HT plays an important role in neuroanatomical organization.

Keywords: Serotonin, Slc6a4, 5-HT, 5HTT, Magnetic resonance imaging, Neurodevelopment, Brain, Dorsal raphe

Background

The brain serotonergic system influences multiple processes during development and throughout life, including neurogenesis, programmed cell death, cell migration, dendritic and axonal development, synaptogenesis, and synaptic plasticity [1–4]. Serotonergic neurons are among the earliest in the brain to be specified for neurotransmitter phenotype and project from the raphe

nuclei, which flank the midline along the rostral-caudal extension of the midbrain and brainstem [1–4]. Based on the distribution of the main projections from the raphe, two clusters of raphe nuclei can be defined, a rostral and a caudal group [1, 5–8]. The rostral group projects mainly to the forebrain and is composed of the caudal linear, the dorsal raphe, and median raphe nuclei. This rostral group accounts for 85% of all the serotonergic neurons in the brain [1]. The caudal group primarily projects to the brainstem, cerebellum, and spinal cord [1]. Relative to the rest of the cell bodies in the brain, which number in the billions, serotonin (5-HT) neurons

* Correspondence: jacob.ellegood@sickkids.ca
[1]Mouse Imaging Centre (MICe), Hospital for Sick Children, 25 Orde Street, Toronto, Ontario M5T 3H7, Canada
Full list of author information is available at the end of the article

account for approximately 1/1,000,000 of all neurons in the brain [9]. While this is a small portion of the overall brain neurons, the serotonergic neurons project throughout the brain, touching multiple systems.

The 5-HT system has been linked to several disorders, including, but not limited to, obsessive compulsive disorder (OCD), anxiety, depression, schizophrenia, Down syndrome, and autism spectrum disorder (ASD) [10]. In ASD, the disruption of the serotonergic system is one of the more consistent and well-replicated findings [11–13]. In fact, elevated blood 5-HT levels in a group of 50 children with autism was first reported in 1961 [14], and this hyperserotonemia in ~ 25% of autistic patients has been consistently reported [11, 15]. Of the 800+ genes that have been associated with autism [16, 17], there are several related to 5-HT signaling, including the antidepressant-sensitive 5-HT transporter (serotonin transporter, SERT; 5-HTT) gene (*SLC6A4*) [18] and the integrin β3 gene (*ITGβ3*) [19], a SERT-interacting protein that influences 5-HT levels in the periphery and in the brain [20–22]. SERT is the primary mechanism of 5-HT inactivation, responsible for reuptake of the neurotransmitter into the presynaptic 5-HT neuron, where it can be repackaged or metabolized [23]. Therefore, changes in SERT expression and function alter extracellular 5-HT levels and signaling at 5-HT receptors.

The SERT gene has been extensively studied in the human population, and over 20 different gene variants have been found [24], the most studied of which is the functional promoter length polymorphic repeat (5-HTTLPR) [18], which has also been linked recently in a study of amygdala cortex connections [25]. An additional functional variant includes a variable number of tandem repeats (VNTR) in intron 2 (STin2) [26]. Overall results of those gene variants have been inconclusive; however, there appears to be mounting evidence for a linkage in the 17q11.2 region, which includes the SERT gene [27]. Regardless, it had been speculated that optimal *Slc6a4* activity may need to be highly regulated [28], i.e., both high and low *Slc6a4* activity could correlate with illness susceptibility. We would hypothesize, however, that changes in *Slc6a4* function may lead to disparate or even opposing morphological changes throughout the brain. For instance, the loss of SERT causes disruptions in the organization of the barrel fields in the somatosensory cortex of the mouse [29].

In 1998, the first *Slc6a4* knockout (KO) mouse was created [30], and in that study the authors confirmed that 5-HT levels were 60–80% decreased in the brainstem, frontal cortex, hippocampus, and striatum, likely due to diminished synthesis and recycling of 5-HT. Further, these mice demonstrate a 50% reduction in serotonergic cell number in the dorsal raphe nucleus [31]. *Slc6a4* KO mice display increased anxiety-like behaviors, reduced aggression, and

exaggerated stress responses [32]. Despite adult brain expression being limited to 5-HT neurons, SERT is transiently expressed in a number of sensory regions as well as in the prefrontal cortex. Accordingly, disruption of SERT function during development has been linked to changes in the architecture and function of the somatosensory cortex and the medial prefrontal cortex [29, 33–35].

Linkage findings in autism spectrum disorder pointed to the chromosome 17q11 region that contains the SERT gene, and multiple amino acid variants in the SERT gene, including Gly56Ala, which increase 5-HT uptake, have been identified in the families with the strongest evidence of linkage [27]. A *Slc6a4* Ala56 knockin (KI) mouse was created and initially found hyperserotonemia, altered CNS 5-HT system function, and changes in social and repetitive behaviors [36] To examine the effects of genetic background, these animals were backcrossed from the initial 129S6 inbred strain to the C57BL/6 inbred strain frequently used for behavioral experiments [37]. Multiple phenotypes were sensitive to different backgrounds. Additionally, neuroanatomy has also been found to be sensitive across inbred strains [38].

With the long-standing association between 5-HT and autism and the well-described effects of 5-HT on neurodevelopment, it is perhaps surprising that the direct relationship between 5-HT and mesoscopic morphological changes throughout the brain has not been systematically investigated. Volume differences in several mouse models related to both autism and the 5-HT system have been examined previously, including an *Itgb3* KO, which encodes a SERT-binding partner [39]. Also, a recent investigation of 26 mouse models related to autism revealed that the neuroanatomical differences clustered into three distinct groups with similar neuroanatomical phenotypes [40]. While that study includes the male animals from the *Slc6a4* KO and *Slc6a4* Ala56 KI models, that paper did not examine the individual models in detail but only the similarities and differences across multiple autism-related mouse models. Given the effect these genetic manipulations on 5-HT levels in the two different models, we hypothesize that changes in brain structure may occur as a direct result of differing levels of serotonin fiber projections brought about by the manipulation. Therefore, the purpose of the current study is to examine, in detail, the specific neuroanatomical differences caused by the different *Slc6a4* mutations.

Methods
Mice

Three different mouse lines were used in this study: (1) homozygous *Slc6a4* knockout mice (*Slc6a4* KO) and control animals (C57Bl6/J) were purchased directly from The Jackson Laboratory (JAX #008355, B6.129(Cg)-*Slc6a4*^{tm1Kpl}/J and JAX #000664, C57Bl6/J), (2) and (3)

Slc6a4 Ala56 knockin (KI) mice on different inbred strain backgrounds, namely C57BL6/J (B6) and 129S6/SvEvTac (129). *Slc6a4* Ala56 KI mice were created as previously described [28, 36], and their colony was maintained in Vanderbilt University in Nashville, TN, USA. In total 121 mice were examined in this study. Thirty-nine were in the *Slc6a4* KO group, 19 wild-type (WT, 9M and 10 F) and 20 *Slc6a4* KO (10M, 10F); 40 were in the *Slc6a4* Ala56 KI (B6) group, 20 WT (10M and 10F) and 20 *Slc6a4* Ala56 KI (10M and 10F); and 42 were in the *Slc6a4* Ala 56 KI (129) group, 21 WT (11M and 10F) and 21 *Slc6a4* Ala56 KI (11M and 10F). All experimental mice were 60 ± 2 days old.

Perfusions

Perfusions were either performed on site at the Mouse Imaging Centre (MICe) in Toronto, ON, Canada, for the *Slc6a4* KO mice, or at Vanderbilt University prior to being shipped overnight to MICe. The details of the perfusion protocol have been previously discussed at length [41, 42]. Briefly, mice are anesthetized with a ketamine/xylazine mix or pentobarbital and then intercardially perfused with 30 mL of 0.1 M PBS containing 10 U/mL heparin and 2 mM Prohance (Bracco Diagnostics Inc., a gadolinium contrast agent) followed by 30 mL of 4% paraformaldehyde (PFA) also containing 2 mM Prohance. After perfusion the mouse was decapitated and the skin, ears, and lower jaw were removed. The brain is left within the skull to minimize any deformations and is first incubated in the 4% PFA/Prohance solution overnight. Then, prior to scanning, the brain was incubated for an additional 7 days, at a minimum, in a solution of PBS, 2 mM ProHance, and 0.02% sodium azide, in order to equalize the contrast agent.

Magnetic resonance imaging

A 7.0-T MRI scanner (Agilent Inc.) was used to acquire all images. For the anatomical scan, a 40-cm inner bore diameter gradient was used (max gradient 30 G/cm) in conjunction with a custom-built solenoid coil array to image 16 samples in parallel [42, 43].

Anatomical scan

In order to assess the volume differences throughout the brain, a T2-weighted 3D fast spin echo (FSE) sequence was used and is designed for optimized gray/white matter contrast. The sequence parameters for this scan are as follows: TR = 2000 ms, echo train length = 6, echo spacing = 10 ms, with the center of k-space acquired on the fourth echo, TE_{eff} = 42 ms, field of view (FOV) 14 mm × 28 mm × 25 mm, and a matrix size of 250 × 504 × 450, which yields an isotropic (3D) resolution of 56 μm. In the first phase encode dimension, consecutive lines of k-space were assigned to alternating echoes to move discontinuity-related ghosting artifacts to the edges of the FOV [44]. This sequence, therefore, involves an oversampling of k-space in the phase encode direction by a factor of 2 to avoid the interference of ghosting artifacts in the main image, which yields a FOV of 28 mm that is subsequently cropped to 14 mm after reconstruction. Total imaging time for this sequence was 11.7 h.

Registration and analysis

Deformation-based morphometry (DBM) was used to analyze the volume differences throughout the brain. DBM was performed by registering the mouse brains together through a series of linear (6 parameter fit followed by a 12 parameter fit) and nonlinear fits. After the registration pipeline, all scans are then resampled with the appropriate transform and averaged to create a population atlas representing the average anatomy of the study sample. All registrations were performed with a combination of mni_autoreg tools [45] and advanced normalization tools (ANTs) [46, 47]. The result of the registration is to have all the scans deformed into alignment with each other in an unbiased fashion. This allows for the analysis of the deformations required to take each individual mouse's anatomy into the final atlas space. The goal is to model how the deformation fields relate to the genotype [48, 49]. The Jacobian determinants of the deformation fields are then used as measures of volume at each voxel. The quantification of the absolute and relative DBM changes are measured from these Jacobians, including the diffeomorphic alignment plus the affine changes for the absolute volume calculation and the diffeomorphic warp alone for the relative volumes. Regional volume differences are then calculated by warping a pre-existing classified MRI atlas onto the population atlas, which allows the calculation of regional volumes across the brain. The classified MRI atlas includes 159 different structures and incorporates three separate pre-existing atlases: (1) delineates 62 different structures throughout the brain including subcortical white and gray matter structures, corpus callosum, striatum, and thalamus [50]; (2) further divides the cerebellum into its various regions, individual lobules, white and gray matter, and the deep cerebellar nuclei [51]; and (3) divides the cortex into 64 different regions, including areas of the cingulate cortex and primary motor and somatosensory cortices [52]. The total brain volume and seven summary regions are also assessed including the cortex (as a whole), cerebellum, ventricles, brainstem, olfactory bulbs, cerebral white matter, and cerebral gray matter. Multiple comparisons were controlled for using the false discovery rate (FDR) [53].

Additional Slc6a4 comparisons

As the *Slc6a4* Ala56 KI mice and *Slc6a4* KO mice were acquired from different colonies (Jackson Labs for the

Slc6a4 KO mice and Vanderbilt University for the *Slc6a4* Ala56 KI mice), in order to assess the effect of *Slc6a4* across all the mice in this study, we needed to normalize one of the studies to the other using the WT C57Bl6/J mice, since this would account for colony effects between groups. This was done by calculating the differences in the C57Bl6/J WT from the *Slc6a4* Ala56 KI (B6) group acquired from Vanderbilt and the C57Bl6/J WT from Jackson Labs. After the standardization (beta) coefficient was calculated between the two WT groups during the registration process, the calculated 3D scalar value was applied to the full *Slc6a4* KO group (WT and *Slc6a4* KO mice) used in this study to normalize that group to the *Slc6a4* Ala56 KI groups. That normalization applied to the *Slc6a4* KO mice takes into account colony effects between sites and allows a comparison across all mice in this study to determine the variance caused by the *Slc6a4* gene. Variance in the *Slc6a4* gene was assessed across groups using an ANOVA and co-varying for sex and background (~Background + Sex + Genotype).

Assessment of the dorsal raphe nucleus (DRN) connectivity

To determine whether the *Slc6a4* neuroanatomical phenotype is consistent or related to specific fiber tracts projecting out of the DRN, we compared the absolute *F*-statistic map with neuronal projection data from the Allen Institute [54, 55] after aligning our dataset to the Allen Institute's Common Coordinate Framework (CCFv3) reference atlas (http://mouse.brain-map.org/static/atlas).

Projection density data derived from 3D, high resolution, whole-brain two-photon microscopy images of neuronal tracers injected into a variety of brain regions were obtained from the Allen Institute's publicly available API. Specifically, this data is from mouse brains injected with a recombinant adeno-associated viral anterograde tracer that expresses EGFP. Original resolution data is gridded at 50 μm and summarized as the number of voxels within the 50-μm grid that contained a tracer signal ("projection density"). Since data from the connectivity experiments are obtained by injecting only in the right hemisphere, whereas volume changes are bilateral, bilateral fiber tract connectivity is estimated by reflecting each 3D tracer dataset across the sagittal midline plane and merging the data with its mirrored pair by taking the maximum projection density value at each voxel. Of the connectivity experiment datasets downloaded, five consisted of the DRN as the primary injection structure. These five experiments are further merged together by taking the maximum projection density value at each voxel. To determine the association between volume differences and DRN-related connectivity, the absolute *F*-statistic map, taken from the

assessment of the variance in the *Slc6a4* gene, is thresholded at an FDR of $q < 0.05$ ($F > 4.56$) and compared with the merged DRN projection density image that was thresholded at 0.1. All voxelwise analyses were carried out within a mask of the whole brain but excluded voxels in the seed region to avoid selection bias.

Results

The first assessment for differences in neuroanatomy was the total brain volume, in which no differences were found in the *Slc6a4* Ala56 KI mice. This was true for the full group, males or females separately, and on both backgrounds (B6 or 129). On the other hand, the *Slc6a4* KOs had a smaller total brain volume for the full group (448 ± 17 mm^3 for KO versus 462 ± 15 mm^3 for the WT B6, $q = 0.04$, where q is the FDR-corrected *p* value), largely driven by the female mice (439 ± 10 mm^3 for KO versus 459 ± 19 mm^3 for WT, $q = 0.03$), whereas the male-only group had no significant difference in total brain volume (457 ± 18 mm^3 for KO versus 466 ± 10 mm^3 for WT, $q = 0.66$) (see Fig. 1). Assessment of the seven summary regions revealed that the total brain volume difference that we were seeing in the full group of *Slc6a4* KO mice was driven largely by the cortex (-3.8%, $q = 0.02$) and cerebellum (-3.5%, $q = 0.01$). While the whole brain volume of the female mice was found to be significantly smaller, the female *Slc6a4* KO mice had additional differences in the olfactory (-4.3%, $q < 0.05$) cerebral gray (-4.1%, $q < 0.05$) and white matter (-4.5%, $q = 0.04$) regions. Figure 1 highlights the differences in these summary regions across groups, which includes the normalized *Slc6a4* KO group for comparison. When the relative volume of the summary regions is examined (i.e., each region is measured as a percentage of total brain volume), no significant differences were found. Therefore, the differences we observed in the female *Slc6a4* KO mice indicate that the brains are *almost* uniformly smaller.

Of the 159 regions examined, no significant differences were found in the *Slc6a4* Ala56 KI mice (Fig. 2). This was seen in the full group or individually in the males and females and was measured with either absolute or relative volume and compared to their corresponding WT. There were, however, some regions within the cerebellum, specifically in the gray matter of the cerebellar vermis, that had trends towards an increase compared to WT with *p* values less than 0.05, but these results did not survive the correction for multiple comparisons (Fig. 2). In the *Slc6a4* KO mice, we see 47 out of the 159 regions have absolute volume differences compared to WT in the full group; again, this is driven primarily by the females, which have 69 regional differences while the males have 0. The smaller regions in the female mice are located in the cortex, specifically in the piriform, auditory, temporal association, and entorhinal cortices, as well as large scale

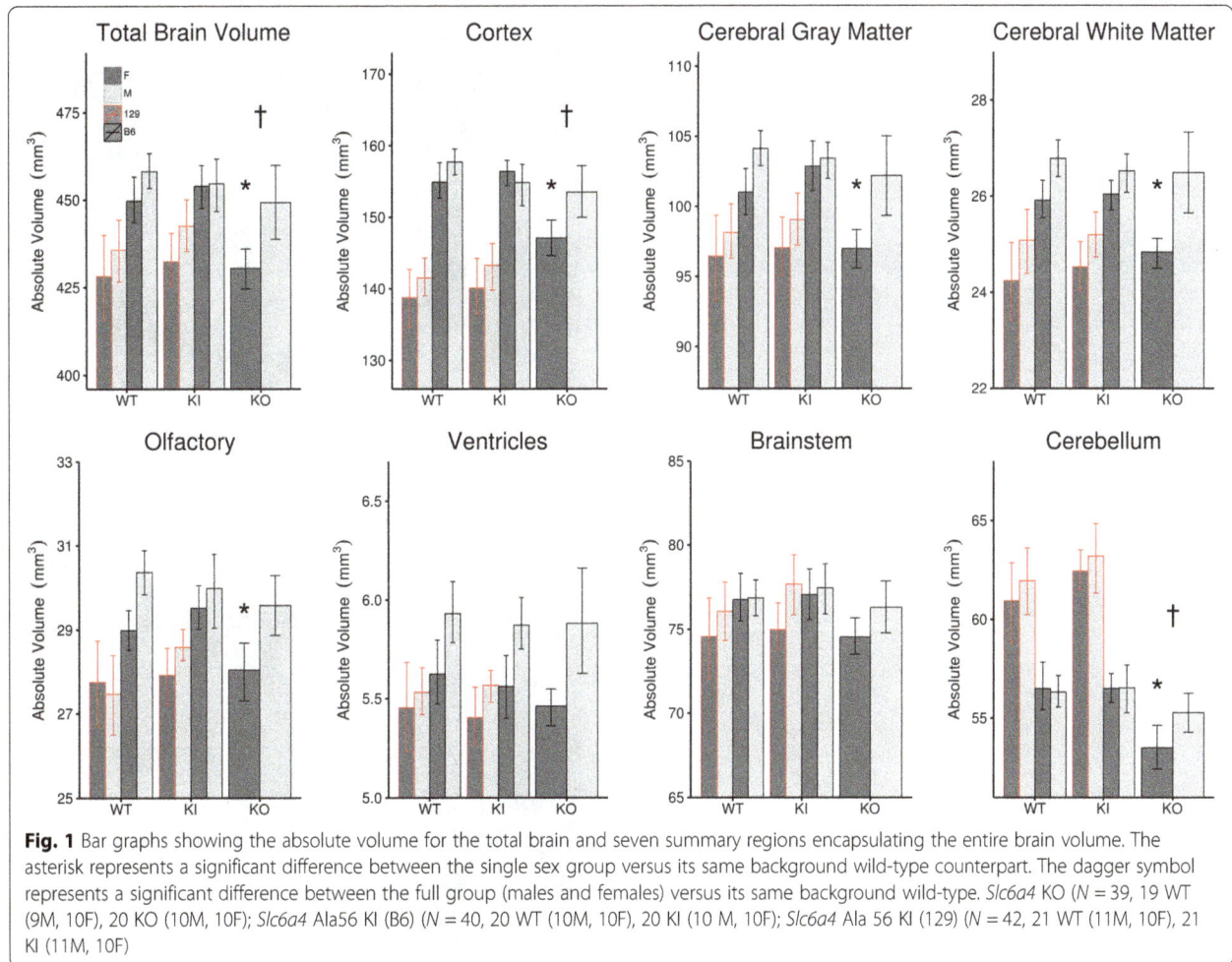

Fig. 1 Bar graphs showing the absolute volume for the total brain and seven summary regions encapsulating the entire brain volume. The asterisk represents a significant difference between the single sex group versus its same background wild-type counterpart. The dagger symbol represents a significant difference between the full group (males and females) versus its same background wild-type. *Slc6a4* KO (N = 39, 19 WT (9M, 10F), 20 KO (10M, 10F); *Slc6a4* Ala56 KI (B6) (N = 40, 20 WT (10M, 10F), 20 KI (10 M, 10F); *Slc6a4* Ala 56 KI (129) (N = 42, 21 WT (11M, 10F), 21 KI (11M, 10F)

decreases throughout the cerebellum (Fig. 2). Despite the lack of findings for the female *Slc6a4* KO mice with relative volume in the summary regions, there were specific areas where differences were found, including the auditory, ectorhinal, and entorhinal cortices as well as the cortical amygdaloid area (Fig. 2). Furthermore, increases in relative volume were found in the cerebral peduncle and lateral septum.

Voxelwise analysis also found no significant differences between the two *Slc6a4* Ala56 KI mice and their WT counterparts on either background. This was true for both absolute and relative volume measures. Similar to the regional findings, the full group of *Slc6a4* KO mice on the B6 background highlighted several areas of significance. Figure 3 shows the significant voxelwise differences in both absolute and relative volume in the *Slc6a4* KO. Absolute volume decreases were seen in the lateral cortex, amygdala, and areas of the thalamus, and relative volume increases were seen in the lateral septum and thalamus.

Further assessment of the variance across all groups, after normalization of the *Slc6a4* KO group (see the

"Methods" section), revealed several areas affected both voxelwise and regionally. Figure 4 shows the significant differences due to the *Slc6a4* gene assessed by an ANOVA while factoring in both the background strain and sex. Four different example voxels are shown on the left (Fig. 4a–d): lobule X, the dorsal raphe, temporal association cortex, and the amygdala. The voxelwise differences recapitulate the differences seen in Fig. 3 but also add a number of new areas of interest, particularly in the colliculi and more widespread differences in the orbital frontal cortex, thalamus, and hypothalamus (see Additional file 1: Table S1 for a full listing of the absolute and relative volume differences seen in Fig. 4). A specific region of interest, relevant to the serotonin system, is the dorsal raphe nuclei, not included in our regional atlas but clearly highlighted.

Figure 5 shows comparisons between the volume differences assessed in Fig. 4 and the neuronal projection data for the DRN from the Allen Institute. A comparison of the *F*-statistic map showing *Slc6a4* volume differences and projections from the DRN (Fig. 5a, columns ii and iii) shows that anterograde

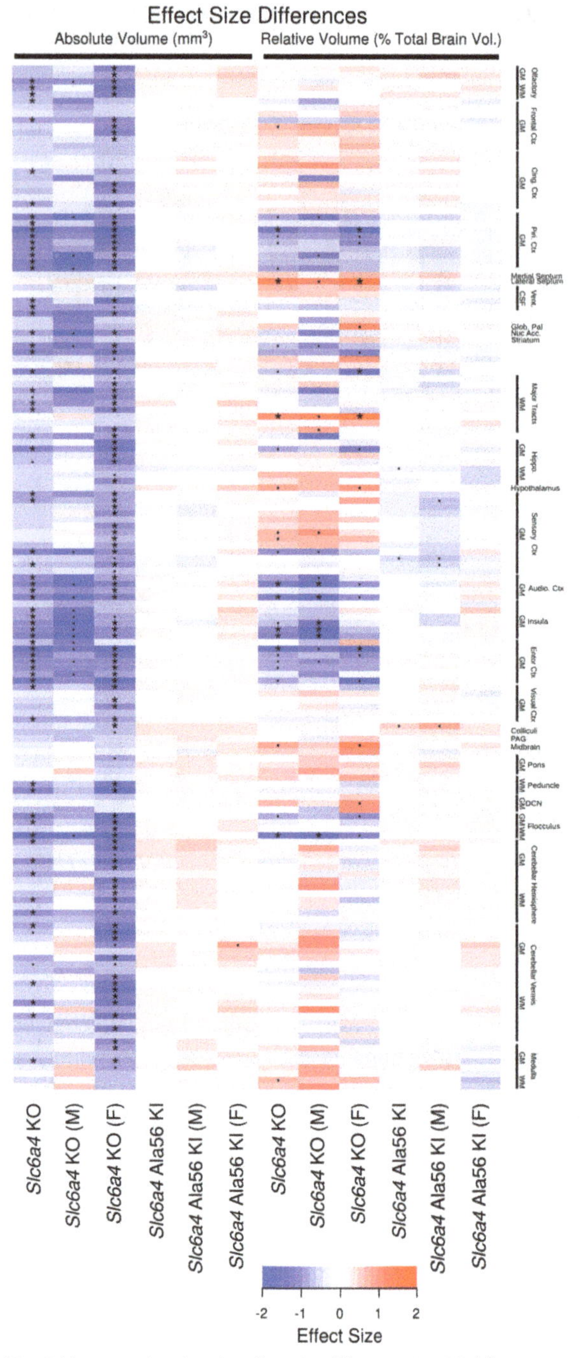

Fig. 2 Heatmap showing the effect size differences in 159 different regions throughout the brain for the Slc6a4 KO group and the full Slc6a4 Ala56 KI group regardless of background. The effect size is calculated as the difference in means divided by the standard deviation of the WT group (Effect Size = $(\mu_{MUT} - \mu_{WT})/\sigma_{WT}$); it is measured in units of standard deviation. The heatmap is organized from the anterior of the brain at the top to the posterior at the bottom. Any region in blue is smaller in the mutant versus wild-type and any in red are larger. The asterisk indicates significance at a $q < 0.05$, The dot indicates a trend at $p < 0.05$. Slc6a4 KO ($N = 39$, 19 WT (9M, 10F), 20 KO (10M, 10F); Slc6a4 Ala56 KI (B6) ($N = 40$, 20 WT (10M, 10F), 20 KI (10M, 10F); Slc6a4 Ala 56 KI (129) ($N = 42$, 21 WT (11M, 10F), 21 KI (11M, 10F)

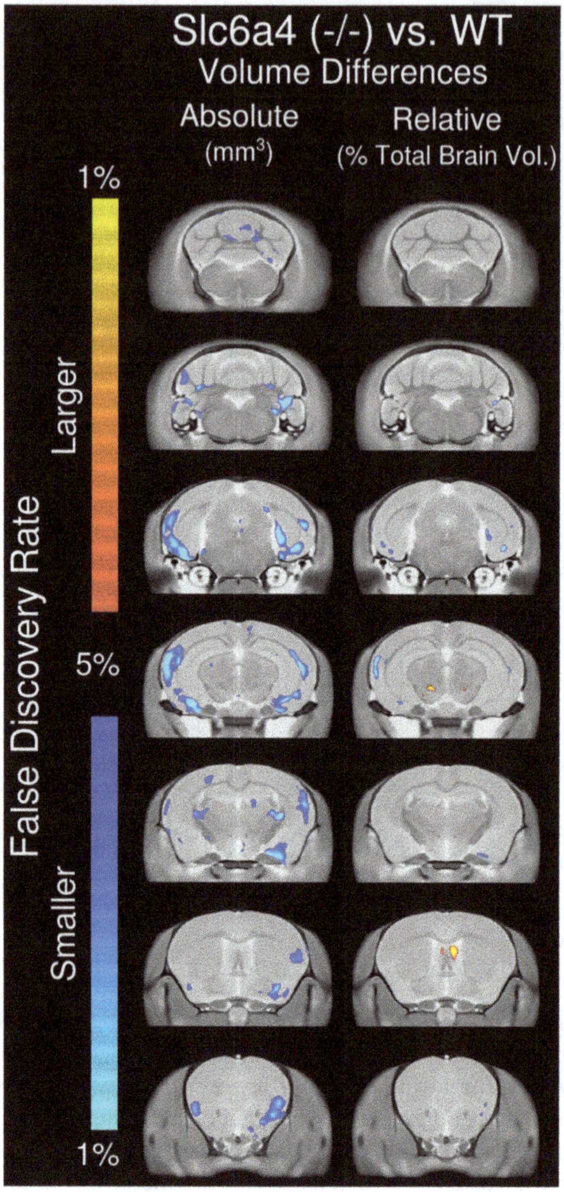

Fig. 3 This figure shows the significant voxelwise differences between the Slc6a4 KO and its corresponding WT. Anything shown in blue/cyan is significantly smaller than the WT and anything in red/orange is significantly larger. Slc6a4 KO ($N = 39$, 19 WT (9M, 10F), 20 KO (10M, 10F)

projections overlap significant *F*-statistic voxels for some frontal cortex areas; however, for most other regions, projections come near to, but do not overlap with regions that show significant differences in volumes (Fig. 5 column iv). Specifically, the amygdala, anterior hypothalamus, and auditory areas of the temporal cortex, along with the superior colliculus, contain significant volumetric differences and have projections from the DRN nearby but do not overlap.

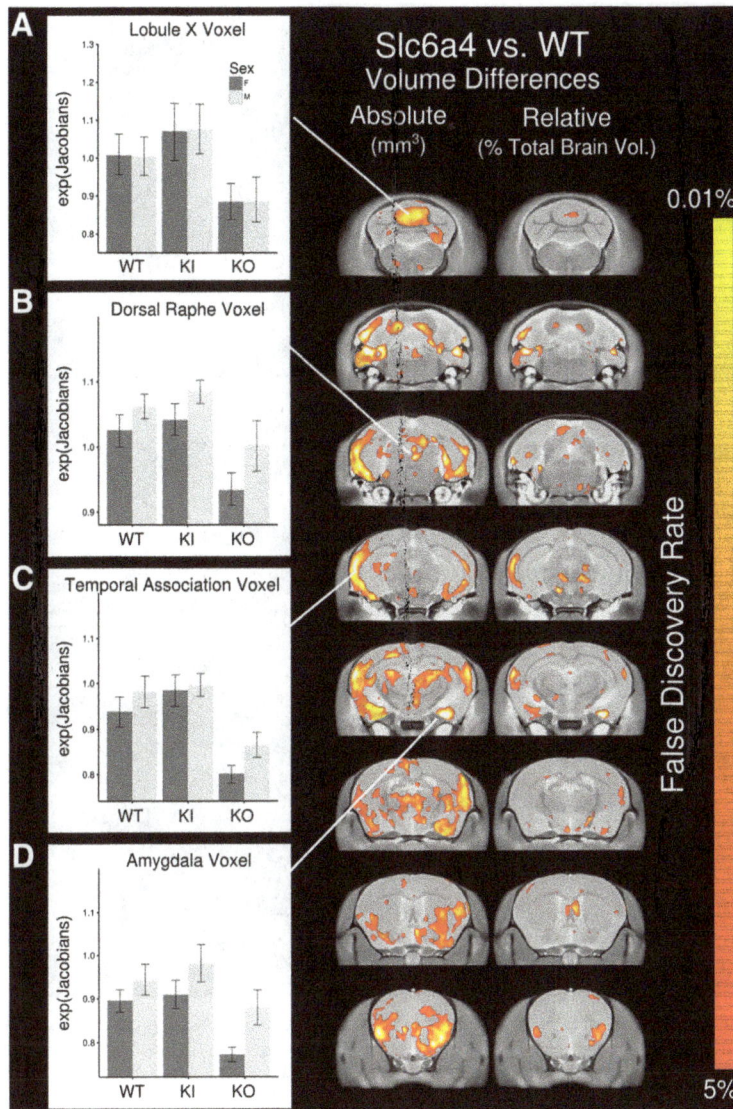

Fig. 4 a–d This figure shows significant voxelwise differences as measured using an ANOVA while factoring in both the sex and background of the mice. All 121 mice were used in this comparison. The panel on the right displays a coronal flythrough highlighting the location of volume differences found due to the *Slc6a4* gene in both absolute and relative volume. For this figure, the C57Bl6/J mice from the Slc6a4 KO group were normalized to the C57Bl6/J mice from the Slc6a4 Ala56 KI group (see the "Methods" section). *Slc6a4* KO (*N* = 39, 19 WT (9M, 10F), 20 KO (10M, 10F); *Slc6a4* Ala56 KI (B6) (*N* = 40, 20 WT (10M, 10F), 20 KI (10M, 10F); *Slc6a4* Ala 56 KI (129) (*N* = 42, 21 WT (11M, 10F), 21 KI (11M, 10F)

Discussion

Gain of function SERT manipulations is thought to have a minimal effect on the anatomy of the brain [56]. It has, however, been shown previously that mice with behavioral phenotypes also feature neuroanatomical phenotypes in 87% of cases [57]. Therefore, there is often an expectation that known behavioral findings will be matched by a mesoscopic anatomical difference. The Slc6a4 Ala56 KI mice have differences in ultrasonic vocalizations (increased for B6 background, decreased for 129) and social interaction, as assessed by the three chamber tests (129S6)

[36, 37]. The *Slc6a4* KO mice have increased anxiety, increased stress, decreased aggression, increased acoustic startle, decreased exploratory behavior, and decreased motor agility [32, 58]. Due to the known behavioral phenotypes, robust neuroanatomical findings were expected across the models. Additionally, as MRI findings tend to be very sensitive, with several studies showing replications across labs (BTBR [59, 60], Neuroligin3 R451C knockin [61, 62]), and differentially created models (16p11.2 CNV [63, 64]), the relatively modest neuroanatomical findings due to modifications in the SERT gene were unexpected.

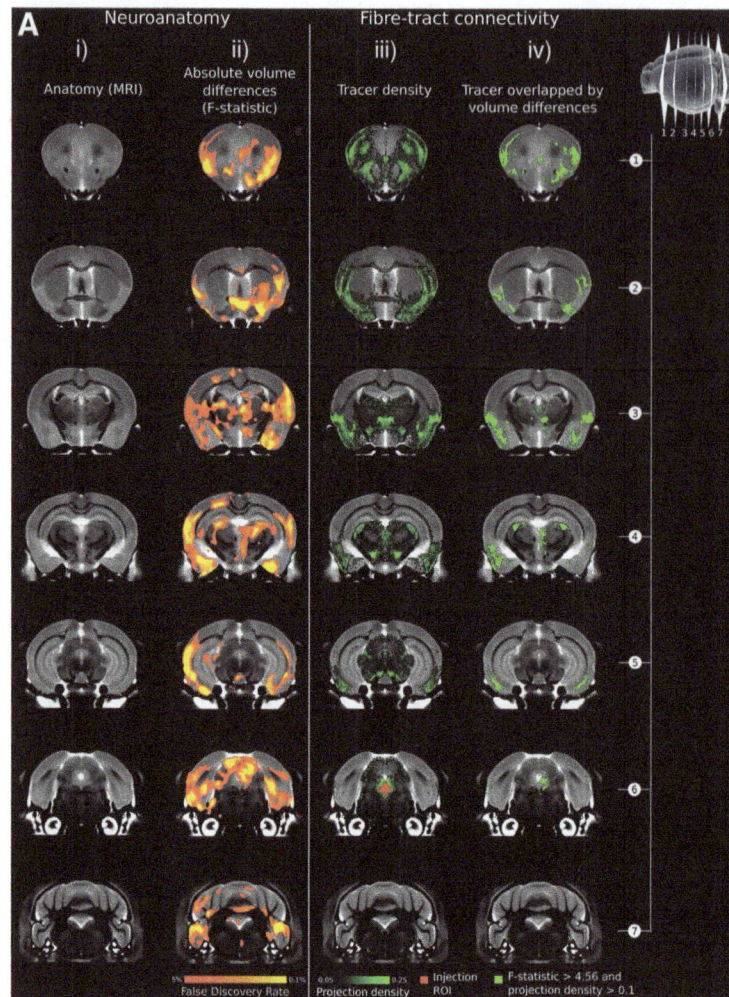

Fig. 5 Association between the dorsal raphe nucleus (DRN) fiber-tract connectivity and SERT volume differences. **a** Shown in vertical panels are coronal slices through the mouse brain from anterior (top row) to posterior (bottom row), see top right of figure for location of slices relative to brain. Vertical panel columns correspond to **i)** anatomy (via MRI), **ii)** absolute volume differences between groups (*F*-statistic), **iii)** neuronal tracers projecting anterograde from the dorsal raphe nucleus, and **iv)** voxels which show significant differences at a FDR *q* < 0.05 (*F* > 4.56) that also express a tracer signal

A recent examination of 26 different mouse models of autism, which included gene deletions, modifications, and duplications, noted that 70%, or 18 of the 26 models examined, were found to have either a significant relative or absolute volume difference [40]. While it should be noted that the data from the male mice used in this study were the same as the *Slc6a4* KO and *Slc6a4* Ala56 KI mice used in that study, none of the female mice used here were included. With 800+ genes associated with autism [16, 17], there are bound to be some null results or undetectable differences at the mesoscopic scale used in this work. The MRI analysis performed here is not at cellular resolution; therefore, any differences at a microscopic scale or the cellular level would be undetectable at the 56-μm isotropic voxel size used. This includes the known deficits in the organization and differentiation of

the *Slc6a4* KO somatosensory whisker barrel cortex [65]; no differences were found in the somatosensory cortex in any sex, measure, or model, which highlights a known functional/organizational difference that is undetectable by volume at the mesoscopic scale of the MRI.

The *Slc6a4* Ala56 KI mutation by itself has no effect on the mesoscopic neuroanatomy, only trends, since no significant differences were found on either background in either absolute or relative volume when compared to its own wild-type. The *Slc6a4* Ala56 KI mutation is a gain of function mutation that causes hyperserotonemia, more so on the 129 backgrounds than B6 [36]. It was also noted that the 5-HT levels in the *Slc6a4* Ala56 KI (129) midbrain and forebrain were unchanged [36], which was not true in the *Slc6a4* KO where there was a reduction in intracellular tissue 5-HT level throughout the brain and in serotonergic cell number in the dorsal raphe nucleus [31]. Therefore, it is likely that the Ala56 KI alone does not produce an *Slc6a4* difference large enough to modify neuroanatomy to a detectable degree with the current methodology. As 5-HT is necessary for early brain development [29], there is also the possibility that at postnatal day 60 we are missing early brain developmental differences. Therefore, a longitudinal investigation would be beneficial to track brain development to see if the developmental trajectories are modified by the changes in *Slc6a4* function. Importantly, it was recently shown that maternal Ala56 genotype impacts forebrain 5-HT levels and thalamocortical projections during midgestation [66], with no observed differences driven by embryo genotype. The *Slc6a4* Ala56 KI animals studied here derive from heterozygous dams and sires so that WT and *Slc6a4* Ala56 KI animals could be generated from mothers of the same genotype. This suggests that future studies should examine the impact of the maternal 5-HT system, which was held constant in this study by the use of heterozygous crosses to generate homozygous *Slc6a4* Ala56 KI mice and wild-type littermate controls.

Regardless of the lack of findings individually for the *Slc6a4* Ala56 KI, Fig. 4 clearly shows there is a significant effect of modifying the *Slc6a4* gene on neuroanatomy across all models used here. The *Slc6a4* Ala56 KI model, which is a gain of function mutation, has the opposite effect of the *Slc6a4* KO mutation in several areas throughout the brain (Fig. 4). For example, the dorsal raphe nucleus, the heart of serotonin function in the brain, trends towards an increase in size for the *Slc6a4* Ala56 KI and decreased for the *Slc6a4* KO (Fig. 4b) but is significant across the entire study. Therefore, we would speculate that a gain or loss in function of SERT corresponds to a gain or loss in volume in several regions in brain, likely originating with the dorsal raphe. In rats and non-human primates, it has been shown that the efferent projections from the rostral group of the raphe nuclei, which includes the dorsal raphe nucleus, ascend through the internal capsule to the lateral cortex and additionally travel through the medial forebrain bundle to the hypothalamus, basal forebrain, and amygdala [1, 5–8]. The internal capsule is also significantly affected by genotype ($F = 6.55$, $q < 0.01$), as well as a large area in the lateral cortex (Fig. 4). Similarly, the hypothalamus ($F = 4.05$, $q = 0.04$), basal forebrain ($F = 6.37$, $q = 0.01$), and amygdala ($F = 9.54$, $q = 0.001$) are also significantly affected by genotype. This indicates that the changes to the *Slc6a4* gene have an impact on the targets of projections from the rostral group of the raphe nuclei. The differences seen here in opposing directions for the *Slc6a4* Ala56 KI versus the *Slc6a4* KO in several

regions (Fig. 4), additionally, are consistent with recently published work showing that these genotypes have opposing functional and developmental effects in the gut [67].

These findings were examined further by comparing our volumetric findings with neuronal projection data from the DRN. It was expected that there would be an overlap between the volume differences seen (Figs. 4 and 5ii) with the projection density images of the neuronal tracer seen in Fig. 5iii. While some areas did show overlap, particularly in the frontal cortical regions, for most areas, the tracer appears to come near to the volumetric differences but does not overlap directly, potentially reflecting the role of 5-HT as a morphogen acting via broader diffusion or volume transmission during development [68, 69]. The DRN projections do, however, project towards several of the affected regions albeit not within them, as visualized by the Allen Brain Atlas data. It is possible, therefore, that the differences in SERT in the DRN in both the *Slc6a4* KO and *Slc6a4* Ala56 KI are in fact causing these volumetric differences in the adjacent regions through this projection.

Of additional interest was the finding of a stronger neuroanatomical phenotype in the female *Slc6a4* KO mice, and to a lesser insignificant extent in the *Slc6a4* Ala56 KI mice, compared to the males. The stronger phenotype in the females is intriguing, and it seems to match up well with a study that reported an increase in 5-HT levels in female rats compared to their male counterparts [70]. This higher level of 5-HT in the females could possibly make them more susceptible to the knockout or knockin of SERT function. This highlights the necessity for investigation of both male and female mice in these types of studies and also lends additional weight to the recent NIH insistence of inclusion of both sexes in biomedical research [71]. Our volumetric findings in females contrast with a previous report that heterozygous male and female *Slc6a4* KO mice (+/−) have increased brain mass, normalized to body mass, compared to controls at 8–12 weeks [72]. It is difficult to compare such different methodological approaches, since the disparity could be driven by genotype differences (+/− versus −/−), differences in age, differences driven by body mass, weight versus volumetric analyses, or removal of the brain from the skull versus in skull neuroimaging.

Future work could benefit from the examination of neuroanatomical differences at earlier timepoints, whether done longitudinally or as a cross-sectional study. Further, examination of the effects of maternal genotype, or maternal-offspring genotype interactions, could reveal broader effects on neurodevelopment due to in utero effects. It would also be worth examining additional genetic modifications of the *Slc6a4* gene to see if they follow a similar pattern to what is shown here with increasing brain volume with increase 5-HT uptake.

The *Slc6a4* Ala56 KI variant was found to have a ~ 30% increase in 5-HT uptake, but there are additional variants that have up to ~ 70% increases [28, 73]. Therefore, it may be beneficial to see if further increases in the areas mentioned here could be found in these other variants. Similarly, one could also examine the heterozygous *Slc6a4* KO, which may show an intermediate loss of volume compared to WT.

There were a few limitations to this study: (1) It has been shown previously in the literature that there are differential effects of the SERT manipulation on the behavior in these different models. Therefore, this implies that there is likely no correlation between the behavior deficits and the neuroanatomical differences seen here. However, since behavior was not tested in these individual mice, this was beyond the scope of this current work. (2) The control animals used for the *Slc6a4* KO mice were not the ideal controls for this work. The *Slc6a4* KO mice were purchased directly from Jackson Laboratory (JAX #008355), and at that time they were bred either homozygote × homozygote or heterozygous × homozygous, both of which do not allow wild-type littermates. Therefore, for controls, C57Bl6/J mice were used as suggested from Jackson Labs. Ideally, one would want to breed heterozygote × heterozygote in order to get WT littermates for comparison. However, the differences, only seen in females, do seem to indicate that C57BL/6J is a reasonable control neuroanatomically.

Conclusions

As suggested previously, this work shows that the SERT activity does contribute to adult neuroanatomy. An increase or decrease in the *Slc6a4* function can cause a differential effect on the neuroanatomy in 5-HT relevant regions, particularly in the raphe nuclei. Considering the small number of 5-HT neurons found within the brain and the localization of those neurons, it is clear that serotonin function can be an integral part of the neuroanatomical organization.

Acknowledgements
We thank the Allen Institute for Brain Science for providing connectivity (©2011 Allen Institute for Brain Science. Allen Mouse Brain Connectivity Atlas. Available from: connectivity.brain-map.org) data used in this study.

Funding
This work was funded by the Canadian Institute for Health Research (CIHR), the Ontario Brain Institute (OBI), and the U.S. National Institutes of Health (MH094604 to JV). JE received salary support from the Ontario Mental Health Foundation (OMHF).

Authors' contributions
JE, TMK, and CLM perfused and prepared all the tissue for MRI scanning. JE imaged and analyzed all the MRI data. YY performed the connectivity analysis using data from the Allen Brain Institute. JE, JPL, RMH, JV, and RB conceived and designed the study. JE wrote the manuscript with contributions from all authors. All authors have read and approved the final manuscript.

Competing interests
JV has received research funding from Seaside Therapeutics, Novartis, Roche Pharmaceuticals, Forest, Sunovion, and SynapDx and has consulted for or served on advisory boards for Novartis, Roche, and SynapDx. The remaining authors declare no conflicts of interest.

Author details
[1]Mouse Imaging Centre (MICe), Hospital for Sick Children, 25 Orde Street, Toronto, Ontario M5T 3H7, Canada. [2]Department of Pharmacology, Vanderbilt University, Nashville, TN 37235, USA. [3]Department of Psychiatry, Vanderbilt University, Nashville, TN 37235, USA. [4]Department of Medical Biophysics, University of Toronto, Toronto, ON M5S, Canada. [5]Department of Biomedical Science and Brain Institute, Florida Atlantic University, Jupiter, FL 33431, USA. [6]Department of Psychiatry, Columbia University, New York, NY 10027, USA.

Abbreviations
5-HT: Serotonin; 5-HTTLPR: Serotonin transporter functional length polymorphic repeat; Ala56: Knockin of an alanine at codon 56; ANTs: Advanced normalization tools; ASD: Autism spectrum disorder; CNV: Copy number variant; DRN: Dorsal raphe nucleus; FDR: False discovery rate; FOV: Field of view; FSE: Fast spin echo; ItgB3: Integrin beta 3; KI: Knockin; KO: Knockout; MRI: Magnetic resonance imaging; OCD: Obsessive compulsive disorder; PBS: Phosphate buffer solution; PFA: Paraformaldehyde; SERT: Serotonin transporter; Slc6a4: Solute carrier family 6 member 4, serotonin transporter gene; T2: Transverse relaxation time; TE: Echo time; TR: Repetition time; VNTR: Variable number of tandem repeats; WT: Wild-type

References
1. Hornung J-P. The human raphe nuclei and the serotonergic system. J Chem Neuroanat. 2003;26:331–43.
2. Lauder JM, Krebs H. Serotonin as a differentiation signal in early neurogenesis. Dev Neurosci. 1978;1:15–30.
3. Chubakov AR, Gromova EA, Konovalov GV, Sarkisova EF, Chumasov EI. The effects of serotonin on the morpho-functional development of rat cerebral neocortex in tissue culture. Brain Res. 1986;369:285–97.
4. Chubakov AR, Tsyganova VG, Sarkisova EF. The stimulating influence of the raphé nuclei on the morphofunctional development of the hippocampus during their combined cultivation. Neurosci Behav Physiol. 1993;23:271–6.

5. Steinbusch HW, van der Kooy D, Verhofstad AA, Pellegrino A. Serotonergic and non-serotonergic projections from the nucleus raphe dorsalis to the caudate-putamen complex in the rat, studied by a combined immunofluorescence and fluorescent retrograde axonal labeling technique. Neurosci Lett. 1980;19:137–42.

6. van der Kooy D, Kuypers HG. Fluorescent retrograde double labeling: axonal branching in the ascending raphe and nigral projections. Science. 1979;204:873–5.

7. van der Kooy D, Hattori T. Dorsal raphe cells with collateral projections to the caudate-putamen and substantia nigra: a fluorescent retrograde double labeling study in the rat. Brain Res. 1980;186:1–7.

8. Kievit J, Kuypers HG. Subcortical afferents to the frontal lobe in the rhesus monkey studied by means of retrograde horseradish peroxidase transport. Brain Res. 1975;85:261–6.

9. Jacobs BL, Azmitia EC. Structure and function of the brain serotonin system. Physiol Rev. 1992;72:165–229.

10. Sodhi MSK, Sanders-Bush E. Serotonin and brain development. Int Rev Neurobiol. 2004;59:111–74.

11. Muller CL, Anacker AMJ, Veenstra-VanderWeele J. The serotonin system in autism spectrum disorder: from biomarker to animal models. Neuroscience. 2016;321:24–41.

12. Yang C-J, Tan H-P, Du Y-J. The developmental disruptions of serotonin signaling may involved in autism during early brain development. Neuroscience. 2014;267:1–10.

13. Whitaker-Azmitia PM. Behavioral and cellular consequences of increasing serotonergic activity during brain development: a role in autism? Int J Dev Neurosci. 2005;23:75–83.

14. SCHAIN RJ, FREEDMAN DX. Studies on 5-hydroxyindole metabolism in autistic and other mentally retarded children. J Pediatr. 1961;58:315–20.

15. Cook EH, Leventhal BL. The serotonin system in autism. Curr Opin Pediatr. 1996;8:348–54.

16. Banerjee-Basu S, Packer A. SFARI gene: an evolving database for the autism research community. Dis Model Mech. 2010;3(3-4):133–5. https://doi.org/10.1242/dmm.005439.

17. Abrahams BS, Arking DE, Campbell DB, Mefford HC, Morrow EM, Weiss LA, et al. SFARI Gene 2.0: a community-driven knowledgebase for the autism spectrum disorders (ASDs). Mol. Autism. 2013;4:36.

18. Cook EH, Courchesne R, Lord C, Cox NJ, Yan S, Lincoln A, et al. Evidence of linkage between the serotonin transporter and autistic disorder. Mol Psychiatry. 1997;2:247–50.

19. Weiss LA, Kosova G, Delahanty RJ, Jiang L, Cook EH, Ober C, et al. Variation in ITGB3 is associated with whole-blood serotonin level and autism susceptibility. Eur J Hum Genet. 2006;14:923–31.

20. Carneiro AMD, Blakely RD. Serotonin-, protein kinase C-, and Hic-5-associated redistribution of the platelet serotonin transporter. J Biol Chem. 2006;281:24769–80.

21. Herrmann MJ, Huter T, Müller F, Mühlberger A, Pauli P, Reif A, et al. Additive effects of serotonin transporter and tryptophan hydroxylase-2 gene variation on emotional processing. Cereb Cortex. 2007;17:1160–3.

22. Weiss LA, Ober C, Cook EH. ITGB3 shows genetic and expression interaction with SLC6A4. Hum Genet. 2006;120:93–100.

23. Murphy DL, Fox MA, Timpano KR, Moya PR, Ren-Patterson R, Andrews AM, et al. How the serotonin story is being rewritten by new gene-based discoveries principally related to SLC6A4, the serotonin transporter gene, which functions to influence all cellular serotonin systems. Neuropharmacology. 2008;55:932–60.

24. Huang CH, Santangelo SL. Autism and serotonin transporter gene polymorphisms: a systematic review and meta-analysis. Am J Med Genet B Neuropsychiatr Genet. 2008;147B:903–13.

25. Velasquez F, Wiggins JL, Mattson WI, Martin DM, Lord C, Monk CS. The influence of 5-HTTLPR transporter genotype on amygdala-subgenual anterior cingulate cortex connectivity in autism spectrum disorder. Dev Cogn Neurosci. 2017;24:12–20.

26. Lesch KP, Bengel D, Heils A, Sabol SZ, Greenberg BD, Petri S, et al. Association of anxiety-related traits with a polymorphism in the serotonin transporter gene regulatory region. Science. 1996;274:1527–31.

27. Sutcliffe JS, Delahanty RJ, Prasad HC, McCauley JL, Han Q, Jiang L, et al. Allelic heterogeneity at the serotonin transporter locus (SLC6A4) confers susceptibility to autism and rigid-compulsive behaviors. Am J Hum Genet. 2005;77:265–79.

28. Veenstra-VanderWeele J, Jessen TN, Thompson BJ, Carter M, Prasad HC, Steiner JA, et al. Modeling rare gene variation to gain insight into the oldest

biomarker in autism: construction of the serotonin transporter Gly56Ala knock-in mouse. J Neurodev Disord. 2009;1:158–71.

29. Chen X, Ye R, Gargus JJ, Blakely RD, Dobrenis K, Sze JY. Disruption of transient serotonin accumulation by non-serotonin-producing neurons impairs cortical map development. Cell Rep. 2015. https://doi.org/10.1016/j.celrep.2014.12.033. [Epub ahead of print]

30. Bengel D, Murphy DL, Andrews AM, Wichems CH, Feltner D, Heils A, et al. Altered brain serotonin homeostasis and locomotor insensitivity to 3, 4-methylenedioxymethamphetamine ("ecstasy") in serotonin transporter-deficient mice. Mol Pharmacol. 1998;53:649–55.

31. Lira A, Zhou M, Castanon N, Ansorge MS, Gordon JA, Francis JH, et al. Altered depression-related behaviors and functional changes in the dorsal raphe nucleus of serotonin transporter-deficient mice. BPS. 2003;54:960–71.

32. Holmes A, Lit Q, Murphy DL, Gold E, Crawley JN. Abnormal anxiety-related behavior in serotonin transporter null mutant mice: the influence of genetic background. Genes Brain Behav. 2003;2:365–80.

33. Rebello TJ, Yu Q, Goodfellow NM, Caffrey Cagliostro MK, Teissier A, Morelli E, et al. Postnatal day 2 to 11 constitutes a 5-HT-sensitive period impacting adult mPFC function. J Neurosci. 2014;34:12379–93.

34. Dawson N, Ferrington L, Olverman HJ, Harmar AJ, Kelly PAT. Sex influences the effect of a lifelong increase in serotonin transporter function on cerebral metabolism. J Neurosci Res. 2009;87:2375–85.

35. Esaki T, Cook M, Shimoji K, Murphy DL, Sokoloff L, Holmes A. Developmental disruption of serotonin transporter function impairs cerebral responses to whisker stimulation in mice. Proc Natl Acad Sci U S A. 2005;102:5582–7.

36. Veenstra-VanderWeele J, Muller CL, Iwamoto H, Sauer JE, Owens WA, Shah CR, et al. Autism gene variant causes hyperserotonemia, serotonin receptor hypersensitivity, social impairment and repetitive behavior. Proc Natl Acad Sci U S A. 2012;109:5469–74.

37. Kerr TM, Muller CL, Miah M, Jetter CS, Pfeiffer R, Shah C, et al. Genetic background modulates phenotypes of serotonin transporter Ala56 knock-in mice. Mol Autism. 2013;4:35.

38. Scholz J, Laliberté C, van Eede M, Lerch JP, Henkelman M. Variability of brain anatomy for three common mouse strains. NeuroImage. 2016;142:656–62.

39. Ellegood J, Henkelman RM, Lerch JP. Neuroanatomical assessment of the integrin β3 mouse model related to autism and the serotonin system using high resolution MRI. Front Psychiatry. 2012;3:37.

40. Ellegood J, Anagnostou E, Babineau BA, Crawley JN, Lin L, Genestine M, et al. Clustering autism: using neuroanatomical differences in 26 mouse models to gain insight into the heterogeneity. Mol Psychiatry. 2015;20(1):118–25. https://doi.org/10.1038/mp.2014.98. Epub 2014 Sep 9

41. Cahill LS, Laliberté CL, Ellegood J, Spring S, Gleave JA, Eede MCV, et al. Preparation of fixed mouse brains for MRI. NeuroImage. 2012;60:933–9.

42. Lerch JP, Sled JG, Henkelman RM. MRI phenotyping of genetically altered mice. Methods Mol Biol. 2011;711:349–61.

43. Dazai J, Spring S, Cahill LS, Henkelman RM. Multiple-mouse neuroanatomical magnetic resonance imaging. J Vis Exp. 2011;(48). https://doi.org/10.3791/2497.

44. Thomas DL, De Vita E, Roberts S, Turner R, Yousry TA, Ordidge RJ. High-resolution fast spin echo imaging of the human brain at 4.7 T: implementation and sequence characteristics. Magn Reson Med. 2004;51:1254–64.

45. Collins DL, Neelin P, Peters TM, Evans AC. Automatic 3D intersubject registration of MR volumetric data in standardized Talairach space. J Comput Assist Tomogr. 1994;18:192–205.

46. Avants BB, Epstein CL, Grossman M, Gee JC. Symmetric diffeomorphic image registration with cross-correlation: evaluating automated labeling of elderly and neurodegenerative brain. Med Image Anal. 2008;12:26–41.

47. Avants BB, Tustison NJ, Song G, Cook PA, Klein A, Gee JC. A reproducible evaluation of ANTs similarity metric performance in brain image registration. NeuroImage. 2011;54:2033–44.

48. Lau JC, Lerch JP, Sled JG, Henkelman RM, Evans AC, Bedell BJ. Longitudinal neuroanatomical changes determined by deformation-based morphometry in a mouse model of Alzheimer's disease. NeuroImage. 2008;42:19–27.

49. Nieman BJ, Flenniken AM, Adamson SL, Henkelman RM, Sled JG. Anatomical phenotyping in the brain and skull of a mutant mouse by magnetic resonance imaging and computed tomography. Physiol Genomics. 2006;24:154–62.

50. Dorr AE, Lerch JP, Spring S, Kabani N, Henkelman RM. High resolution three-dimensional brain atlas using an average magnetic resonance image of 40 adult C57Bl/6J mice. NeuroImage. 2008;42:60–9.

51. Steadman PE, Ellegood J, Szulc KU, Turnbull DH, Joyner AL, Henkelman RM, et al. Genetic effects on cerebellar structure across mouse models of autism using a magnetic resonance imaging atlas. Autism Res. 2014;7:124–37.

52. Ullmann JFP, Watson C, Janke AL, Kurniawan ND, Reutens DC. A segmentation protocol and MRI atlas of the C57BL/6J mouse neocortex. NeuroImage. 2013;78:196–203.

53. Genovese CR, Lazar NA, Nichols T. Thresholding of statistical maps in functional neuroimaging using the false discovery rate. NeuroImage. 2002;15:870–8.

54. Kuan L, Li Y, Lau C, Feng D, Bernard A, Sunkin SM, et al. Neuroinformatics of the Allen Mouse Brain Connectivity Atlas. Methods. 2015;73:4–17.

55. Oh SW, Harris JA, Ng L, Winslow B, Cain N, Mihalas S, et al. A mesoscale connectome of the mouse brain. Nature. 2014;508:207–14.

56. van Kleef ESB, Gaspar P, Bonnin A. Insights into the complex influence of 5-HT signaling on thalamocortical axonal system development. Eur J Neurosci. 2012;35:1563–72.

57. Nieman BJ, Lerch JP, Bock NA, Chen XJ, Sled JG, Henkelman RM. Mouse behavioral mutants have neuroimaging abnormalities. Hum Brain Mapp. 2007;28:567–75.

58. Murphy DL, Lesch K-P. Targeting the murine serotonin transporter: insights into human neurobiology. Nat Rev Neurosci. 2008;9:85–96.

59. Ellegood J, Babineau BA, Henkelman RM, Lerch JP, Crawley JN. Neuroanatomical analysis of the BTBR mouse model of autism using magnetic resonance imaging and diffusion tensor imaging. NeuroImage. 2013;70:288–300.

60. Dodero L, Damiano M, Galbusera A, Bifone A, Tsaftsaris SA, Scattoni ML, et al. Neuroimaging evidence of major morpho-anatomical and functional abnormalities in the BTBR T+TF/J mouse model of autism. PLoS One. 2013;8:e76655.

61. Ellegood J, Lerch JP, Henkelman RM. Brain abnormalities in a Neuroligin3 R451C knockin mouse model associated with autism. Autism Res. 2011;4:368–76.

62. Kumar M, Duda JT, Hwang W-T, Kenworthy C, Ittyerah R, Pickup S, et al. High resolution magnetic resonance imaging for characterization of the neuroligin-3 knock-in mouse model associated with autism spectrum disorder. PLoS One. 2014;9:e109872.

63. Horev G, Ellegood J, Lerch JP, Son Y-EE, Muthuswamy L, Vogel H, et al. Dosage-dependent phenotypes in models of 16p11.2 lesions found in autism. Proc Natl Acad Sci U S A. 2011;108:17076–81.

64. Portmann T, Yang M, Mao R, Panagiotakos G, Ellegood J, Dolen G, et al. Behavioral abnormalities and circuit defects in the basal ganglia of a mouse model of 16p11.2 deletion syndrome. Cell Rep. 2014;7(4):1077–1092. https://doi.org/10.1016/j.celrep.2014.03.036. Epub 2014 May 1

65. Persico AM, Mengual E, Moessner R, Hall FS, Revay RS, Sora I, et al. Barrel pattern formation requires serotonin uptake by thalamocortical afferents, and not vesicular monoamine release. J Neurosci. 2001;21:6862–73.

66. Muller CL, Anacker AM, Rogers TD, Goeden N, Keller EH, Forsberg CG, et al. Impact of maternal serotonin transporter genotype on placental serotonin, fetal forebrain serotonin, and neurodevelopment. Neuropsychopharmacology. 2017;42:427–36.

67. Margolis KG, Li Z, Stevanovic K, Saurman V, Israelyan N, Anderson GM, et al. Serotonin transporter variant drives preventable gastrointestinal abnormalities in development and function. J Clin Invest. 2016;126:2221–35.

68. Suri D, Teixeira CM, Cagliostro MKC, Mahadevia D, Ansorge MS. Monoamine-sensitive developmental periods impacting adult emotional and cognitive behaviors. Neuropsychopharmacology. 2015;40:88–112.

69. Brummelte S, Mc Glanaghy E, Bonnin A, Oberlander TF. Developmental changes in serotonin signaling: implications for early brain function, behavior and adaptation. Neuroscience. 2017;342:212–31.

70. Carlsson M, Carlsson A. A regional study of sex differences in rat brain serotonin. Prog Neuro-Psychopharmacol Biol Psychiatry. 1988;12:53–61.

71. Clayton JA, Collins FS. NIH to balance sex in cell and animal studies. Nature. 2014;509(7500):282–3.

72. Page DT, Kuti OJ, Prestia C, Sur M. Haploinsufficiency for Pten and serotonin transporter cooperatively influences brain size and social behavior. Proc Natl Acad Sci U S A. 2009;106:1989–94.

73. Prasad HC, Steiner JA, Sutcliffe JS, Blakely RD. Enhanced activity of human serotonin transporter variants associated with autism. Philos Trans R Soc Lond Ser B Biol Sci. 2009;364:163–73.

17-β estradiol increases parvalbumin levels in *Pvalb* heterozygous mice and attenuates behavioral phenotypes with relevance to autism core symptoms

Federica Filice[1], Emanuel Lauber[1], Karl Jakob Vörckel[2], Markus Wöhr[2,3] and Beat Schwaller[1]* (iD)

Abstract

Background: Autism spectrum disorder (ASD) is a group of neurodevelopmental disorders characterized by two core symptoms: impaired social interaction and communication, and restricted, repetitive behaviors and interests. The pathophysiology of ASD is not yet fully understood, due to a plethora of genetic and environmental risk factors that might be associated with or causal for ASD. Recent findings suggest that one putative convergent pathway for some forms of ASD might be the downregulation of the calcium-binding protein parvalbumin (PV). PV-deficient mice (PV−/−, PV+/−), as well as Shank1−/−, Shank3−/−, and VPA mice, which show behavioral deficits relevant to all human ASD core symptoms, are all characterized by lower PV expression levels.

Methods: Based on the hypothesis that PV expression might be increased by 17-β estradiol (E2), PV+/− mice were treated with E2 from postnatal days 5–15 and ASD-related behavior was tested between postnatal days 25 and 31.

Results: PV expression levels were significantly increased after E2 treatment and, concomitantly, sociability deficits in PV+/− mice in the direct reciprocal social interaction and the 3-chamber social approach assay, as well as repetitive behaviors, were attenuated. E2 treatment of PV+/+ mice did not increase PV levels and had detrimental effects on sociability and repetitive behavior. In PV−/− mice, E2 obviously did not affect PV levels; tested behaviors were not different from the ones in vehicle-treated PV−/− mice.

Conclusion: Our results suggest that the E2-linked amelioration of ASD-like behaviors is specifically occurring in PV+/− mice, indicating that PV upregulation is required for the E2-mediated rescue of ASD-relevant behavioral impairments.

Keywords: ASD, Parvalbumin, 17-β estradiol, Estradiol treatment, Excitation/inhibition balance, Social behavior, Ultrasonic vocalizations

Background

Autism spectrum disorder (ASD) core symptoms include impaired sociability, communication problems, and restricted or repetitive behaviors. The etiology of ASD remains still unclear, but recent advances in genetics and genomics have provided powerful tools to unraveling how mutations in certain genes might result in ASD [1].

Although a plethora of genetic and environmental risk factors are associated with ASD [2], therapeutic approaches of treating ASD subjects are rather limited and moreover, most often do not target all core symptoms [3, 4].

Recent studies suggest that the calcium-binding protein parvalbumin (PV) is downregulated in some forms of ASD. Most notably, *Shank1−/−* and *Shank3−/−* mice and offspring from mice exposed to valproic acid in utero (VPA mice), all validated mouse models for ASD, are characterized by a prominent PV reduction in ASD-associated brain regions [5, 6]. Genetically modified mice deficient for PV (PV+/− and PV−/−) display behavioral

* Correspondence: beat.schwaller@unifr.ch
Federica Filice and Emanuel Lauber are shared first authorship.
Markus Wöhr and Beat Schwaller are shared last authorship.
[1]Anatomy Unit, Section of Medicine, University of Fribourg, Route Albert-Gockel 1, CH-1700 Fribourg, Switzerland
Full list of author information is available at the end of the article

deficits relevant to all human ASD core symptoms [7]. Moreover, the number of PV-immunoreactive (PV⁺) GABAergic interneurons (hereafter termed Pvalb neurons) was reported to be decreased in several cortical areas in postmortem brains of ASD subjects [8]. However, since no other marker than PV had been used to identify the Pvalb neurons in that study, the decreased number of PV⁺ neurons might equally well be the result of a decreased number of Pvalb neurons or of a decrease in PV expression levels, as also acknowledged by the authors. Preliminary results on two ASD brains also did not allow to unequivocally ascribing the observed decrease of PV⁺ neurons to either mechanism [9]. Recently, RNA-seq and qRT-PCR analyses of postmortem samples of frontal and temporal cortex and cerebellum from 48 ASD individuals and 49 controls revealed that the *PVALB* and *SYT2* (synaptotagmin 2) genes were among the most strongly downregulated ones in the ASD group [10]. In the absence of clear evidence of Pvalb neuron loss in human ASD, but of confirmed decreased *PVALB* mRNA levels in human ASD individuals and additionally of PV protein levels in mouse ASD models with construct and face validity, we hypothesize that a decrease in PV levels might represent a converging pathway of ASD pathophysiology, at least in a subgroup of ASD cases.

Estrogen receptors β (ERβ) are strongly co-localized with cortical Pvalb neurons [11], and several lines of indirect evidence (reported as an increase in the number of PV⁺ neurons) indicate that PV expression might be positively modulated by 17-β estradiol (E2) [11–13]. Moreover, in the rat pituitary cell line GH3 shown to be E2 responsive, *Pvalb* was found to be one of the most E2-responsive genes [14]. E2 administration was also found to significantly increase *Pvalb* mRNA expression resulting in an augmentation in the number of PV⁺ neurons in the CA1 pyramidal cell layer of rat hippocampus [15].

In this study, we aimed to increase PV expression in PV+/− mice to possibly re-establish the state prevailing in PV+/+ mice, both with respect to PV protein levels and also behavior, for the latter applying assays with relevance to all human ASD core symptoms [16, 17]. Our approach consisted in supplementing PV+/+, PV+/−, and PV−/− pups with E2 during the early postnatal period from postnatal day (PND) 5 to 15. This time period was chosen in order to cover the critical period of sexual differentiation of neuronal circuits in rodents [18] and the previously reported developmental onset of PV expression in the rodent brain [19, 20]. Moreover, Pvalb neurons are implicated in the maturation of the cortical GABA inhibitory circuitry, including the modulation (initiation, termination) of critical developmental periods. A maturation index of Pvalb neurons proposed by Gandal et al. [21] shows a highly significant correlation between Pvalb neuron maturation status and PV expression levels. Whether this is only correlative in nature or possibly causal, i.e., PV "driving" Pvalb neuron maturation to some extent, is currently unknown. It has been shown before that E2 induces a "significant increase of parvalbumin immunoreactive neurons" in both the deep and superficial cortical layers in rat organotypic slice cultures in vitro [12]. Moreover, in vivo, estrogens have been shown to have a potential compensatory effect at behavioral levels in animal models carrying mutations in genes associated with ASD, such as the reeler heterozygous mice (rl+/−) or the *CNTNAP2−/−* zebrafish ASD model [22, 23]. However, none of these studies directly proved whether E2 treatment leads to an upregulation of PV at the transcript and/or protein levels.

In the present study, we found that E2 treatment of PV+/− mouse pups increased PV protein levels and consequently ameliorated ASD-associated social behavioral deficits and decreased repetitive behavior in later life. Thus, we provide a rationale for the positive effects of E2 on ASD-linked behavior and propose that E2 treatment should be given further attention as a potential therapeutic strategy in ASD.

Methods
Mouse colonies and genotyping
Mice were group-housed and maintained as described before [7]. PV-deficient mice (PV−/−; B6.Pvalb^tm1Swal) [24] congenic with C57Bl/6J [25] were mated with C57Bl/6J wild-type mice. Heterozygous breedings were set up in order to be able to compare littermates. Day of birth was defined as PND0; genotyping and paw marking was carried out at PND2-3. Only male animals were used in this study. All experiments were performed with permission of the local animal care committee (Canton of Fribourg, Switzerland) and according to the present Swiss law and the European Communities Council Directive of 24 November 1986 (86/609/EEC).

Estradiol treatment and determination of PV protein and *Pvalb* mRNA levels
Litters, including all genotypes, were randomly assigned to one of two experimental groups. In the first group, pups were administered with vehicle (sesame oil; 10 μl/day/pup), while the second group received 17-β estradiol (E2; Sigma-Aldrich, Buchs, Switzerland) at a dose of either 10 μg E2/day/pup (modified from [26]) or 50 μg E2/day/pup (modified from [27]) in 10 μl vehicle between PND5-15. Thus, mice of all genotypes from the same litter either received E2 or vehicle. Additional details on mouse husbandry, mouse handling, and E2 administration are reported in Additional file 1. Pups were weaned at PND22 and tested at (I) PND25 ± 1 for reciprocal social interaction and communication, (II) PND26 ± 1 for social approach in the three-chamber

assay, and (III) PND31 ± 1 for repetitive, ritualistic behavior in the marble-burying test, following our previously established protocols [7, 28]. In all behavioral assays, littermate controls were included and for all experiments and analyses, experimenters were blinded with respect to genotype and treatment. For the determination of PV protein and *Pvalb* mRNA levels, PND25 was chosen, the identical time point as for the start of behavioral experiments; mice were sacrificed by cervical dislocation; and brains were collected for Western blot analyses and qRT-PCR analyses as described before [5].

Direct reciprocal social interaction and ultrasonic vocalizations

Prior to testing, mice were socially isolated for 24 h in order to enhance the level of social motivation. To measure reciprocal social interaction behavior, pairs of juvenile mice were allowed to socially interact at PND25 ± 1 for 5 min after one mouse of the pair was habituated to the test environment for 1 min. Same-treatment/same-genotype pairs consisting of non-littermates were used. Experimental details, including measurement of ultrasonic vocalizations and behavioral analysis, have been reported before [7]. Specifically, reciprocal social interactions were recorded using a video camera. Direct reciprocal social interactions were scored and analyzed offline by an experienced observer with high reliability (inter-rater correlation coefficient: $r = 0.902$; $p < 0.001$; Pearson) using the Noldus The Observer XT 10.0 software (Noldus Information Technology, Wageningen, The Netherlands). Parameters of social behaviors included facial sniffing (sniffing the nose and snout region of the partner), anogenital sniffing (sniffing the anogenital region of the partner), following (walking straight behind the partner, keeping pace with the one ahead), push past (squeezing between the wall and the partner), crawling under/over (pushing the head underneath the partner's body or crawling over or under the partner's body), social grooming (grooming the partner), and being socially inactive while having social contact (lying flat or standing motionless, while maintaining close physical contact with the partner). In addition to social behaviors, non-social behaviors were measured and included rearing (number of times an animal reared on its hind legs), grooming (number of bouts of face, body, and genital grooming movements) and digging (number of bouts of digging in the bedding, pushing, and kicking it around). Parameters of social behaviors, such as anogenital sniffing, nose-to-nose sniffing, or following, were grouped together, and a mouse was scored as "engaging in a social interaction" any time those behaviors were observed. Results from reciprocal social interaction and ultrasonic vocalization assays reflect the cumulative performance of the two animals in the assay.

Social approach behavior in the three-chamber assay

Sociability in PV+/+, PV+/−, and PV−/− mice treated or not with E2 was determined by the well-described three-chamber social approach task for each individual mouse [29]. The apparatus consisted of an open rectangular box (60 × 40 × 40 cm) divided into three chambers by retractable doors. Stranger stimulus mice were C57Bl/6J mice of the same sex and age as the test subjects. The test session began with a 10-min habituation period, with the subject mouse free to move in all the empty compartments of the chamber; in the meanwhile, a new unfamiliar stranger mouse was habituated (10 min) to a wire cup; an identical empty wire cup was used as novel object. After the 10-min habituation period, the test subject was briefly confined to the center chamber and the novel object was placed in one of the side chambers, while the novel mouse was placed on the other side. The location of the novel object and the novel mouse were alternated between the left and right chambers across test subjects to avoid a side preference bias. After both stimuli were positioned, the two side doors were simultaneously lifted and the subject mouse had access to all three compartments for 10 min. The time spent in each compartment and entries into each one and the time spent exploring the novel mouse or the empty cup were manually scored by an observer blinded to the mouse genotype/treatment using two stopwatches. Exploration of an enclosed mouse or of the empty wire cup was scored positive, when the test mouse was oriented with the head towards the cup within a 2-cm distance between the head of the mouse and the cup, or when climbing on the cup. Between tests, the apparatus was cleaned with 0.1% acetic acid and water.

Marble-burying test

The marble-burying test consisted of introducing items that a mouse can bury during a set period of time; mice with an ASD-associated behavior often tend to engage in a higher degree of digging (burying) than what is observed in controls [28]. Mice were individually placed in Plexiglas type III cages containing 5-cm deep clean bedding with 20 ceramic marbles (14 mm diameter) arranged in 5 × 4 evenly spaced rows as described before [30]. Test duration was 30 min. Marbles were considered buried, if more than half of a marble was covered with bedding. A greater number of buried marbles was considered as an indication for increased repetitive behavior.

Statistical analysis

For analysis of direct reciprocal social interaction and ultrasonic vocalizations in juvenile mice, two-way ANOVAs with the between-subject factors genotypes (PV+/+, PV+/−, PV−/−) and treatment (vehicle vs. E2) plus the covariate age of subject mice (PND) were calculated. In order to test whether differences in direct reciprocal social interaction behavior and the emission of ultra-sonic vocalizations emerged over time during testing, ANOVAs for repeated measurements with the same between-subject factors plus the covariate age of subject mice and the within-subject factor test duration were performed. Paired t tests were used to compare the likelihood of the occurrence of a social behavior in response to a social behavior, and one-sample t tests for comparisons with chance levels. Three-way ANOVAs for repeated measurements with the within-subject factor preference (mouse vs. object) and the between-subject factors genotype and treatment (vehicle vs. E2) were used to analyze social approach behavior in the three-chamber assay. Marble-burying behavior was analyzed using a two-way ANOVA with the between-subject factors genotype and treatment (vehicle vs. E2). ANOVAs were followed by LSD post hoc analysis or paired/unpaired Student's t tests when appropriate. Western blot analysis was performed, and protein levels were compared between genotypes and treatments using planned Student's t tests. For all the experiments, a p value < 0.05 was considered statistically significant. Data were analyzed using IBM SPSS Statistics 22 (Armonk, USA) and GraphPad Prism software (San Diego, USA).

Results

Here, we demonstrate that E2 upregulates PV expression in PV+/− mice leading to an amelioration of the ASD-related phenotypes previously described for PV-deficient (PV+/−, PV−/−) mice [7]. Conversely, in most assays, E2 treatment of PV+/+ mice unexpectedly provoked ASD-like behaviors, whereas in PV−/− mice, E2 had no significant effect in all behavioral tests carried out.

PV upregulation via 17-β estradiol administration

Based on direct and indirect evidence linking PV expression levels with estradiol [12, 22], we investigated whether E2 upregulates PV expression in PV+/− mice. PV levels in PV+/− forebrain samples were significantly lower, i.e., in the order of 50% compared to PV+/+ samples ($p = 0.003$; Fig. 1), in line with previous findings [5, 31, 32] and PV was completely absent in PV−/− mouse extracts (not shown). Both E2 treatments (10 or 50 μg/day) did not significantly affect PV expression levels in PV+/+ animals at PND25. Importantly, E2 treatment of PV+/− mice in the period from PND5 to PND15 resulted in a persistent increase in PV determined at PND25 (10 μg E2: $p = 0.011$; 50 μg E2: $p = 0.041$; Fig. 1). Since no significant differences in the degree of recovery of PV expression were observed

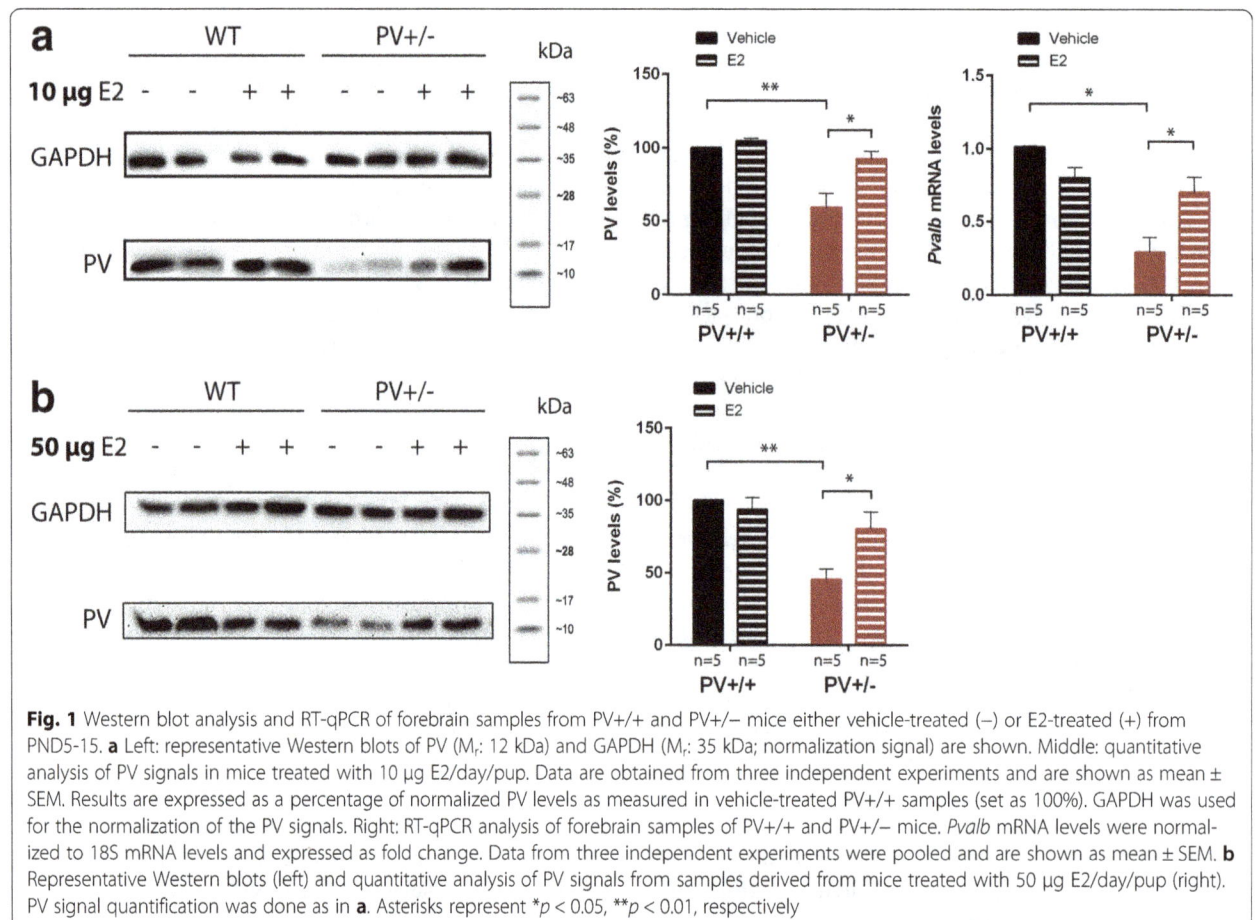

Fig. 1 Western blot analysis and RT-qPCR of forebrain samples from PV+/+ and PV+/− mice either vehicle-treated (−) or E2-treated (+) from PND5-15. **a** Left: representative Western blots of PV (M$_r$: 12 kDa) and GAPDH (M$_r$: 35 kDa; normalization signal) are shown. Middle: quantitative analysis of PV signals in mice treated with 10 μg E2/day/pup. Data are obtained from three independent experiments and are shown as mean ± SEM. Results are expressed as a percentage of normalized PV levels as measured in vehicle-treated PV+/+ samples (set as 100%). GAPDH was used for the normalization of the PV signals. Right: RT-qPCR analysis of forebrain samples of PV+/+ and PV+/− mice. *Pvalb* mRNA levels were normalized to 18S mRNA levels and expressed as fold change. Data from three independent experiments were pooled and are shown as mean ± SEM. **b** Representative Western blots (left) and quantitative analysis of PV signals from samples derived from mice treated with 50 μg E2/day/pup (right). PV signal quantification was done as in **a**. Asterisks represent *p < 0.05, **p < 0.01, respectively

in PV+/− animals treated with 10 or 50 μg E2, the lower dose was chosen for all behavioral experiments.

To evaluate how well *Pvalb* mRNA and protein expression levels correlate after E2 administration, we performed RT-qPCR analysis. *Pvalb* mRNA levels of E2-treated (10 μg) PV+/− mice were significantly increased, to a similar extent as PV protein levels (Fig. 1a), in comparison with PV+/− vehicle-treated mice ($p = 0.041$). This is suggestive of a modulation of PV via E2 at the transcriptional level, in line with previous studies [14]. No changes were seen in PV+/+ animals after E2 administration (Fig. 1a).

Direct reciprocal social interaction and ultrasonic vocalizations

Direct reciprocal social interaction was tested in PND25 ± 1 juvenile mice. The time spent in reciprocal social interactions was visibly affected by E2 treatment in a genotype-dependent manner (genotype: $p = 0.805$; treatment: $p = 0.848$; genotype x treatment: $p = 0.044$; Fig. 2a). In vehicle-treated PV−/− mice, we observed a tendency to engage less in reciprocal social interactions (− 28% interaction time) compared to PV+/+ littermate controls ($p = 0.077$), while the decrease was found insignificant in PV+/− mice ($p = 0.269$). In a previous study, a similar decrease in social interaction time had been observed; however, the overall effect was slightly larger (− 36%) and also significant in the PV+/− mouse group [7]. While in the group of E2-treated PV+/+ mice, the time spent in reciprocal social interactions was significantly decreased compared to the vehicle-treated PV+/+ mice ($p = 0.037$); no differences in interactions were observed in E2-treated PV+/− and PV−/− mice in comparison to corresponding vehicle-treated mice ($p = 0.475$ and $p = 0.147$, respectively). However, there was a notable tendency of increase in comparison to the E2-treated PV+/+ littermate controls ($p = 0.056$ and $p = 0.073$, respectively), an effect that was mostly attributable to a "worsening" of the E2-treated PV+/+ mice. Along the 5-min examination period, the time spent in social interactions was rather constant in all groups, with a trend for a decrease towards the end (Fig. 2b). When analyzing the social behavior repertoire in detail, its richness and reciprocal character were found to be strongly dependent on genotype (Fig. 2c). While vehicle-treated PV+/+ mice displayed a significant preference for engaging in another social behavior following a previous one in ~ 65% of the cases (~ 35% for non-social behavior; $p = 0.011$ vs. chance level), no such preference was seen in vehicle-treated PV+/− and PV−/− mice, with social behaviors following in ~ 57 and ~ 53% of cases, respectively ($p = 0.165$ and $p = 0.665$ vs. chance level, respectively). The genotype-dependent effect size was approximately of the same magnitude as observed in our previous study (compared to Fig. 1d in [7]). In E2-treated mice, however, a different pattern emerged (Fig. 2c'). Most remarkably, in E2-treated PV+/− mice, a social behavior was followed by another one in ~ 62% of cases ($p = 0.024$ vs. chance level), almost reaching the situation prevailing in "normal," i.e., vehicle-treated PV+/+ mice. While E2 treatment had no prominent effect in PV−/− mice, with social behaviors following in ~ 57% of cases ($p = 0.359$ vs. chance level), E2 treatment had detrimental effects in PV+/+ mice, with social behaviors following in only ~ 55% of cases ($p = 0.614$ vs. chance level). Representative ethograms of mouse pairs are depicted in Fig. 2d, d'. There was no evidence for genotype × treatment interaction effects on non-social behaviors, including rearing, grooming, and digging behavior (Fig. 2d, d', all p values > 0.100). The different social behavior components (e.g., facial sniffing, following, etc.) as shown in the ethograms (Fig. 2d, d') were statistically analyzed in more detail, i.e., for each behavior component independently and results are presented in Additional file 1. Only in one of the social behaviors (social grooming), we observed a weak genotype × treatment interaction ($p = 0.03$) indicating that behaviors grouped as "social behavior" represent general effects that cannot be fragmented into meaningful individual social behavior components.

Ultrasonic vocalization emission rates during reciprocal social interactions tended to be weakly affected by E2 treatment in a genotype-dependent manner (genotype: $p = 0.355$; treatment: $p = 0.298$; genotype × treatment: $p = 0.090$; Fig. 3a). Numbers of vocalizations were significantly decreased in vehicle-treated PV−/− mice compared to the corresponding PV+/+ group ($p = 0.047$; Fig. 3a). An intermediate phenotype was observed in vehicle-treated PV+/− mice, although the decrease in vocalization numbers compared to PV+/+ was not significant ($p = 0.303$), likely due to the large variations between individual mice of all genotype and treatment groups (Fig. 3a). Of note, genotype differences in vehicle-treated mice were less prominent than observed previously [7], possibly as the result of extensive/prolonged mouse handling during daily E2 or vehicle treatments (see discussion). Call numbers were significantly decreased in E2-treated PV+/+ compared to vehicle-treated PV+/+ mice ($p = 0.025$), but call numbers were essentially unchanged in E2- or vehicle-treated PV+/− and also PV−/− groups ($p = 0.723$ and $p = 0.582$, respectively) (Fig. 3a). The time course of vocalizations, i.e., the highest numbers of calls occurring within the first 2 min after the addition of the second mouse, followed by a gradual decline (Fig. 3b) was similar as reported before [7].

There was no evidence for genotype × treatment interaction effects on acoustic call features, including call duration (Fig. 3c), peak frequency (Fig. 3d; all p values > 0.100) and frequency modulation ($p = 0.083$; Fig. 3e). Irrespective of genotype and treatment, the emission of ultrasonic vocalizations was highly positively correlated

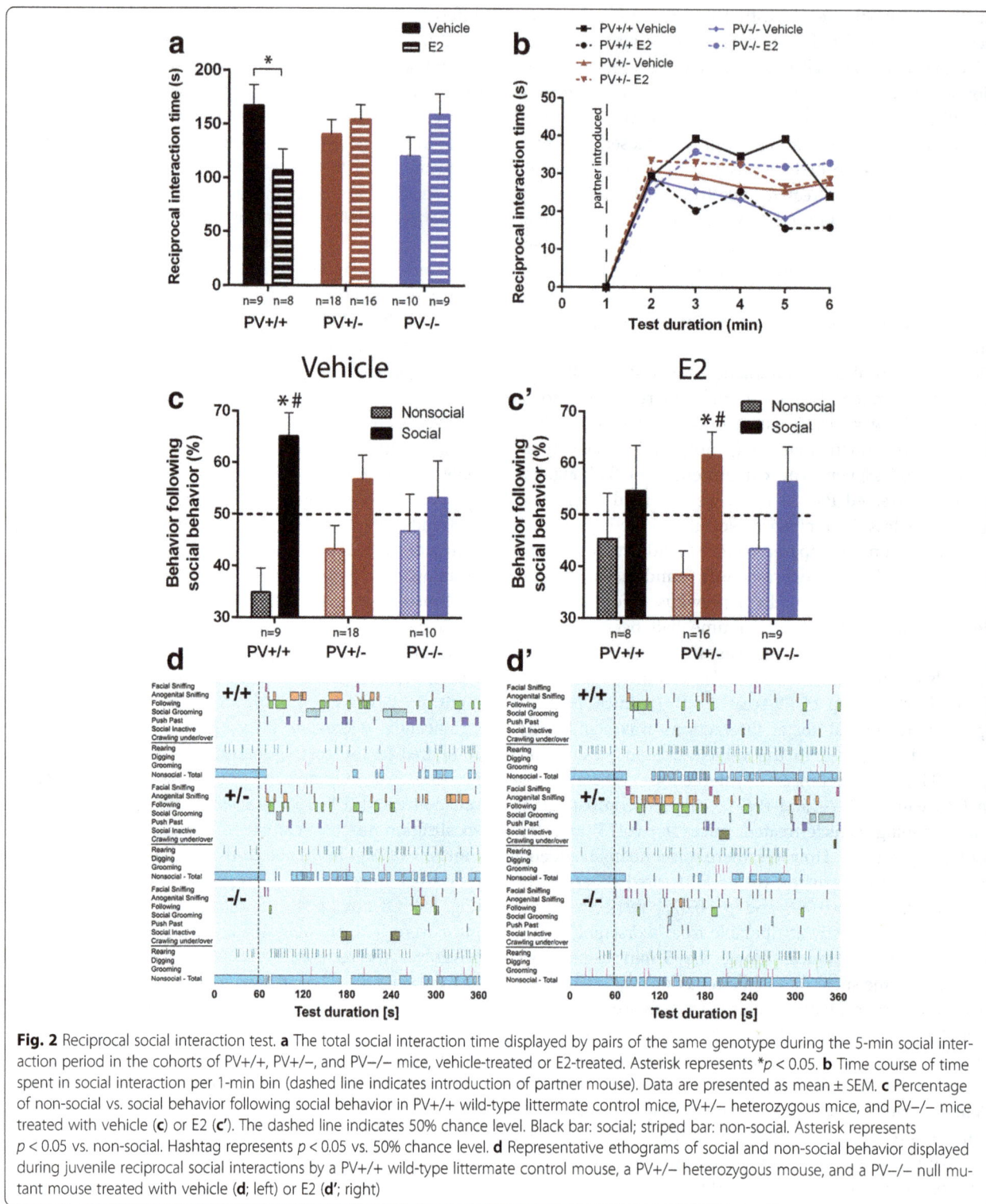

Fig. 2 Reciprocal social interaction test. **a** The total social interaction time displayed by pairs of the same genotype during the 5-min social interaction period in the cohorts of PV+/+, PV+/−, and PV−/− mice, vehicle-treated or E2-treated. Asterisk represents *$p < 0.05$. **b** Time course of time spent in social interaction per 1-min bin (dashed line indicates introduction of partner mouse). Data are presented as mean ± SEM. **c** Percentage of non-social vs. social behavior following social behavior in PV+/+ wild-type littermate control mice, PV+/− heterozygous mice, and PV−/− mice treated with vehicle (**c**) or E2 (**c'**). The dashed line indicates 50% chance level. Black bar: social; striped bar: non-social. Asterisk represents $p < 0.05$ vs. non-social. Hashtag represents $p < 0.05$ vs. 50% chance level. **d** Representative ethograms of social and non-social behavior displayed during juvenile reciprocal social interactions by a PV+/+ wild-type littermate control mouse, a PV+/− heterozygous mouse, and a PV−/− null mutant mouse treated with vehicle (**d**; left) or E2 (**d'**; right)

with the time spent in reciprocal social interaction ($r = 0.791$, $p < 0.001$; Fig. 3f). Representative spectrograms are depicted in Fig. 3g for a pair of vehicle-treated or E2-treated PV+/− mice; the other four groups of mice revealed very similar patterns of calls (not shown).

Social approach behavior in the three-chamber assay

In the often applied three-chamber test [29], sociability is defined as preference for a novel mouse (subject; S) over a novel object (empty wire cup; O). Preference is typically assessed by means of time spent in chambers containing

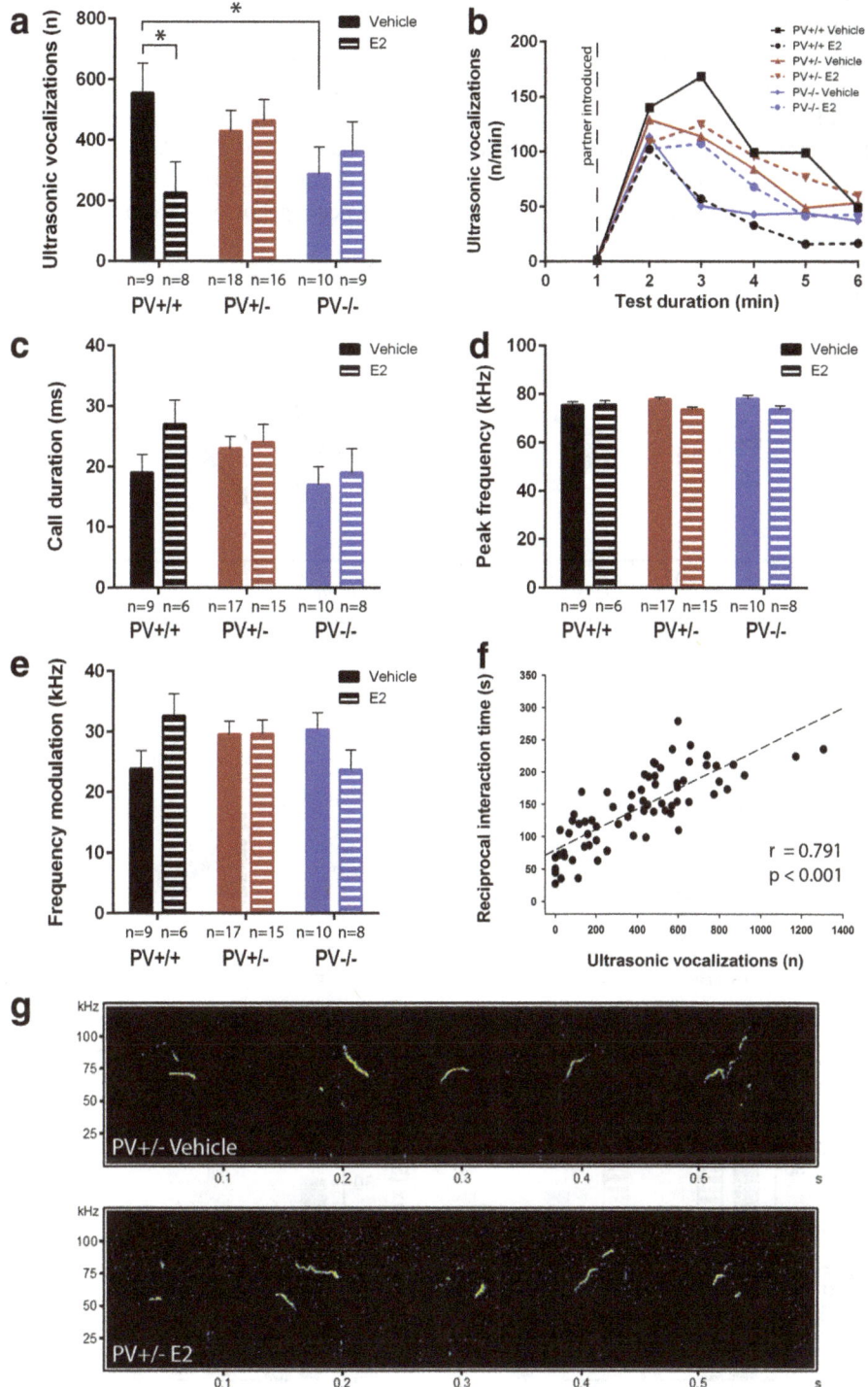

Fig. 3 Analysis of ultrasonic vocalizations between PV+/+, PV+/−, and PV−/− mouse pairs. Irrespective of treatment, all genotypes displayed similar call emission patterns. **a** Total number of calls emitted during the 5-min social interaction period; asterisks represent *$p < 0.05$. **b** Time course for the number of ultrasonic vocalizations emitted for each 1-min time bin across the 5-min social interaction period, plus 1 min habituation (dashed line indicates introduction of partner mouse). Data are presented as mean ± SEM. **c** Average call duration, **d** peak frequency and **e** frequency modulation of emitted calls during the 5-min social interaction period. **f** Correlation between ultrasonic vocalizations and time spent in social interaction for each animal. **g** Representative spectrograms of ultrasonic vocalizations emitted during juvenile reciprocal social interactions of a vehicle-treated (upper traces) and an E2-treated (lower traces) PV+/− mouse are shown

the novel mouse versus the novel object. This preference was clearly genotype-dependent (preference: $p = 0.002$; preference × genotype: $p = 0.014$; Fig. 4a; data are additionally presented as bar graphs in Additional file 1: Figure S3A). Vehicle-treated PV+/+ mice showed a strong preference for the chamber containing the novel mouse compared to the one with the novel object ($p = 0.001$), while no such preference was observed in vehicle-treated PV+/− and PV−/− mice (all p values > 0.100). Mice from the latter two groups (PV+/−, PV−/−) showed an almost equal interest in the two chambers. E2 treatment slightly decreased the S/O ratio in PV+/+ mice; however, mice still spent significantly more time in the S chamber ($p = 0.046$). E2 treatment of PV+/− and PV−/− mice did not affect the time spent in the S and O compartments (preference × treatment: $p = 0.165$; preference × genotype × treatment: $p = 0.335$).

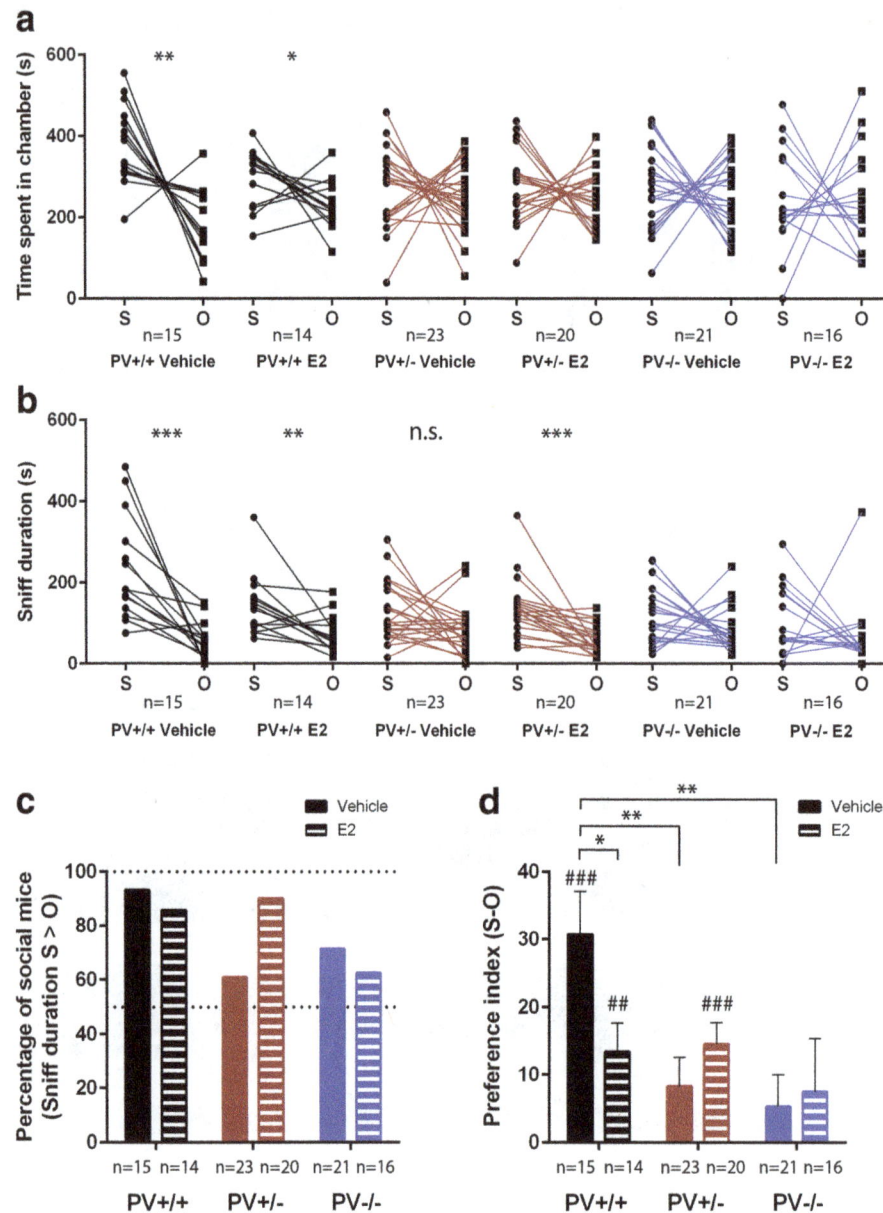

Fig. 4 E2 administration differently affected sociability of PV+/+, PV+/−, and PV−/− mice tested in the three-chamber assay. **a** Paired graphs of time spent in the chamber with the novel mouse (S) or the object (O) during the 10-min social interaction period plotted for each mouse; a negative slope (S > O) is characteristic of a "social" mouse. **b** Sniffing/exploration time spent close to the subject mouse, i.e., within 2 cm from the stranger/empty wired cup. **c** Percentage of "social" mice defined as animals with sniff duration time (S) > (O) during the 10-min test phase. **d** Preference index (stranger vs. object sniffing time divided by the total exploration time in the compartments containing S and O) fold change. Values close to "0" indicate no preference for the stranger mouse. Asterisks represent *$p < 0.05$; **$p < 0.01$; ***$p < 0.001$; n.s.: not significant. Hashtags represent significant preference for the stranger mouse over the object ##$p < 0.01$; ###$p < 0.001$

More relevant than a mouse's simple presence in the S- and O-containing chamber of the cage and thus representing a more sensitive measure of sociability is the measurement of sniff duration, i.e., the time spent within a 2-cm distance from the wire cup [16, 33]. With this measurement, genotype differences were even more prominent (preference: $p < 0.001$; preference × genotype: $p = 0.009$; Fig. 4b; data presented as bar graphs in Additional file 1: Figure S3B). In congruence with the results shown in Fig. 4a, vehicle-treated PV+/+ mice spent significantly more time in sniffing the novel mouse than the novel object ($p < 0.001$), while vehicle-treated PV+/− mice showed a much weaker (if any; $p = 0.057$) and PV−/− mice no such preference for the novel mouse ($p = 0.126$). The more sensitive sociability-related measure "sniff duration" further revealed that the preference for the novel mouse over the novel object was clearly modulated by E2 treatment in a genotype-dependent manner (preference × treatment: $p = 0.265$; preference × genotype × treatment: $p = 0.042$; Fig. 4b and Additional file 1: Figure S3B). E2 treatment of PV+/− mice considerably increased the duration of sniffing the novel mouse, resulting in a substantial preference towards it ($p < 0.001$), to levels observed in E2-treated or vehicle-treated PV+/+ mice. In the E2-treated PV+/− group, the percentage of mice with S > O sniff time rose to 90%, similar to values in the vehicle- (14 out of 15; 93.3%) and E2-treated (12 out of 14; 85.7%) PV+/+ group (Fig. 4c), indicative of an almost complete E2-mediated rescue in otherwise less social PV+/− mice. Such a change was not observed in E2-treated PV−/− mice ($p = 0.342$). E2-treated PV+/+ mice still displayed a preference for the novel mouse (S) over the novel object (O) ($p = 0.008$); however, such a preference was notably decreased. Of note, the results obtained in the three-chamber social approach assay were robust insofar, as the result pattern did not change depending on whether climbing on the cup was included in the sniffing analysis or not. In fact, the time that mice spent on top of either the stimulus (S) or object (O) cup closely resembled the picture observed for sniff time, simply on a much smaller time scale (compare Additional file 1: Figures S3B and S4A).

In an additional exploratory approach, this genotype effect was also evident when comparing the often used preference index, defined as the numerical difference between time spent exploring the targets (subject vs. object, S-O) divided by the total time spent in the two compartments containing either target, as described previously [34, 35]. A clear preference for the novel mouse was observed in vehicle-treated PV+/+ mice ($p < 0.001$), while such a preference was very weak for vehicle-treated PV+/− mice ($p = 0.070$) and not observed in PV −/− mice ($p = 0.277$), resulting in significant group differences ($p = 0.005$ and $p = 0.002$ vs. PV+/+, respectively;

Fig. 4d). E2 treatment significantly increased the preference index in PV+/− mice ($p < 0.001$), while this was not the case for E2-treated PV−/− mice ($p = 0.356$). There was still a significant, however, smaller (compared to vehicle-treated PV+/+) preference for the novel mouse in E2-treated PV+/+ mice ($p = 0.008$). In line with the results on reciprocal social interactions (Fig. 2a), sociability tested in the social approach assay was again decreased in E2-treated PV+/+ mice compared to vehicle-treated PV+/+ mice (Fig. 4d; $p = 0.034$), supporting the adverse effect of E2 treatment in "healthy" PV+/+ mice.

To exclude the possibility that the observed differences in preference might be the result of impaired or reduced locomotor activity in the six groups, the number of entries into the two chambers was determined and found to be unchanged (preference: $p = 0.843$; preference × genotype: $p = 0.201$; preference × treatment $p = 0.818$; preference × genotype × treatment: $p = 0.693$). However, general locomotor activity was affected (genotype: $p = 0.003$; treatment: $p = 0.896$; genotype × treatment: $p = 0.009$). In fact, under vehicle conditions genotypes did not differ ($p = 0.765$), yet under E2 treatment conditions, genotypes differed ($p = 0.001$) and PV+/− mice displayed more entries than PV+/+ and PV−/− mice ($p = 0.001$ and $p = 0.006$, respectively), possibly reflecting their more vigorous attempts to establish social contact (Additional file 1: Figure S3C).

Marble-burying test

To test repetitive behavior, we performed the marble-burying test [28]. Marble burying was visibly affected by E2 treatment in a genotype-dependent manner (genotype: $p = 0.471$; treatment: $p = 0.982$; genotype x treatment: $p = 0.009$; Fig. 5a). Vehicle-treated PV+/− and PV−/− mice buried more marbles compared to the corresponding PV+/+ mice ($p = 0.046$ and $p = 0.053$, respectively), in support of increased repetitive behavior in mice with reduced or absent PV levels [7]. While E2 treatment of PV+/+ mice increased their marble burying behavior ($p = 0.051$), E2-treated PV+/− mice buried less marbles than their corresponding vehicle-treated PV+/− group ($p = 0.011$). No E2 effects were observed in PV−/− mice ($p = 0.832$). Also the marble-burying test hints towards a common effect of E2 administration: an increase (worsening) in ASD-associated behaviors in PV+/+ and an attenuation (improvement) of ASD-associated behaviors in PV+/− mice (Fig. 5b), closely approaching the behavior of vehicle-treated PV+/+ mice.

Discussion

PV-deficient mice (PV+/−, PV−/−) represent a new genetic mouse model of ASD, displaying a behavioral phenotype characterized by impairments in social interaction, communication, and perseveration [7]. In these mice, PV expression levels are downregulated/absent, while the

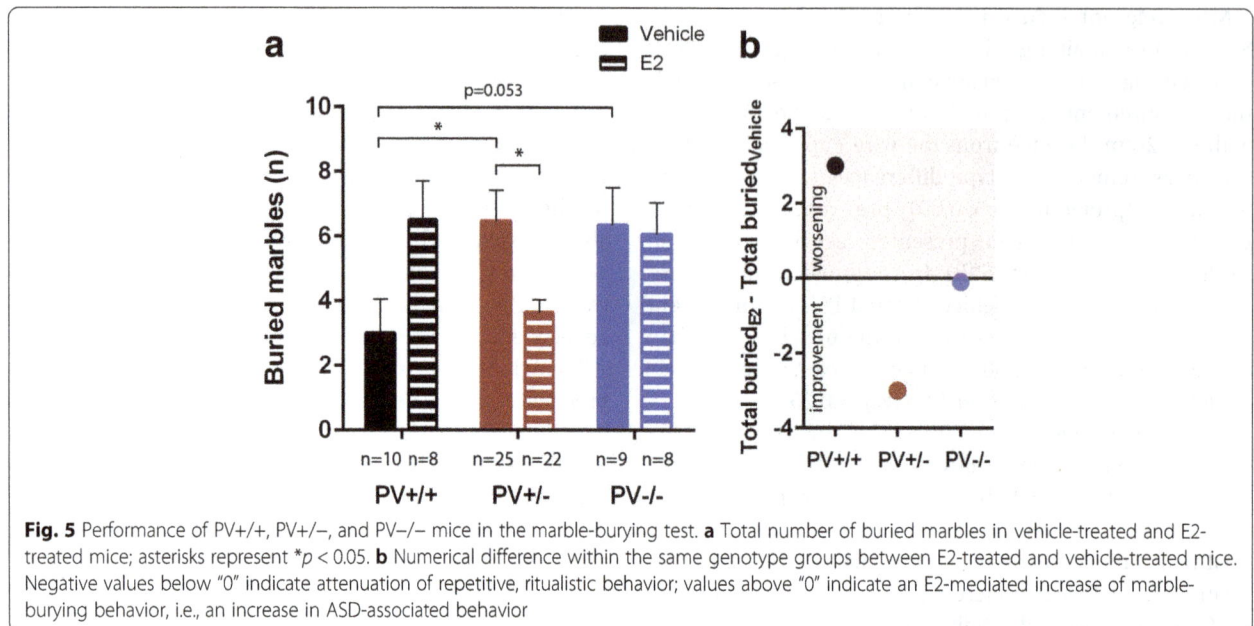

Fig. 5 Performance of PV+/+, PV+/−, and PV−/− mice in the marble-burying test. **a** Total number of buried marbles in vehicle-treated and E2-treated mice; asterisks represent *p < 0.05. **b** Numerical difference within the same genotype groups between E2-treated and vehicle-treated mice. Negative values below "0" indicate attenuation of repetitive, ritualistic behavior; values above "0" indicate an E2-mediated increase of marble-burying behavior, i.e., an increase in ASD-associated behavior

number of Pvalb neurons is unaltered compared to PV+/+ mice [5]. The same holds true for *Shank1−/−*, *Shank3−/−*, and VPA mice [6, 36], three well-established mouse models for ASD [28, 37–41]. Thus, we addressed the question whether the direct upregulation of PV via neonatal administration of E2 might ameliorate or even abrogate the ASD phenotype displayed by male juvenile PV+/− mice. E2 administration in PV+/− mice increased PV expression to levels closely approaching vehicle-treated PV+/+ mice; at the behavioral level, this coincided with an attenuation of the ASD-related phenotypes. Most evidently, the richness and reciprocal character of E2-treated PV+/− mice was substantially increased, as quantified by a preference for engaging in another social behavior following a previous one. Such a preference was repeatedly reported in mice displaying intact sociability, including, but not limited to [42], i.e., control (PV+/+) mice [7]. Consistently, a preference for engaging in another social behavior following a previous one was also seen in vehicle-treated PV+/+ mice in the present study, but not in PV+/− and PV−/− mice. Importantly, such a preference was also evident in E2-treated PV+/− mice, almost reaching the situation of vehicle-treated PV+/+ mice, while E2 treatment had no positive effect in PV−/− mice. This suggests that our recently established approach to quantify the preference for engaging in another social behavior following a previous one offers a new and unique possibility to assess treatment effects on the richness and the heterogeneity of the direct reciprocal social behavior repertoire displayed by juvenile mice. However, while this appears a promising strategy, our approach to quantify the preference for engaging in another social behavior is new and its validity and potential in revealing treatment effects thus would

merit an independent dedicated validation study. There, comparing several ASD mouse models with known social deficits would reveal whether this parameter might be helpful for the identification/validation of an ASD-like phenotype in mice.

Supporting the results from the direct reciprocal social interaction test, the "sniff duration" time, being the most sensitive parameter in the three-chamber social approach assay, revealed a pro-social effect of E2 treatment exclusively in PV+/− mice. The lack of social preference seen in vehicle-treated PV+/− and PV−/− mice is consistent with their altered reciprocal social interaction behavior when compared to PV+/+ mice. Only in PV+/− mice, E2 treatment considerably increased the sniffing S/O ratio of individual mice; 90% showed a preference for the novel mouse vs. 61% in vehicle-treated animals, indicative of an E2-mediated increase in sociability in otherwise "non-social" PV+/− mice.

Communication deficits in PV+/− and PV−/− mice observed before [7], were also seen in vehicle-treated PV+/− and PV−/− mice, but were only significant in PV−/− mice. E2 treatment had no effect in PV+/− and PV−/− mice but caused a reduction of call number in PV+/+ mice. The absence of a treatment effect on ultrasonic vocalizations might be attributable to the prolonged postnatal handling during E2/vehicle administration. In agreement, the average number of calls in vehicle-treated PV+/+ mice (556) was much higher than in the previous study where mice were subjected to substantially less handling (average 355 in PV+/+ mice; [7]). It is known that neonatal handling increases call emission in pups, which in turn, serves to increase maternal care [43, 44]. The stressful context associated with extensive handling [45] is the most likely explanation for the increased production of ultrasonic vocalizations in all genotypes compared to our previous study [7], possibly masking genotype-dependent effects of E2. As assessment of repetitive behaviors, we performed the marble-burying test; E2-treated PV+/− animals performed better (i.e., buried less marbles) than vehicle-treated PV+/− mice, consistent with previous findings showing that female sex hormone levels modulate marble-burying behavior [46, 47]. Moreover, the overall rather low numbers of marbles buried is likely the result of the juvenile age (PND31), when mice were tested; a significant age-dependent increase in marble-burying behavior from PND24 ($\approx 10\%$) to PND40 ($\approx 30\%$ marbles buried) has been observed before [46].

Taken together, our results confirm that E2 can ameliorate the investigated ASD-like symptoms, in line with previous findings supporting a role for E2 as a promising candidate in amelioration of ASD-related phenotypes [22, 23]. In particular, we observed a $\approx$ "rescue effect" in sociability tests and amelioration of repetitive behaviors selectively in E2-treated PV+/− mice, but not in the PV +/+ and PV−/− groups. It is important to remark that E2 had no significant effect on PV protein levels in juvenile PV+/+ and PV−/− mice; thus, any effect observed in these mice after E2 treatment excludes PV being the effector of the putative changes. Nevertheless, E2 might have effects per se, previously evidenced by its role in modulation of social behavior [48] and modulation of neural circuits via direct or indirect activation of multiple downstream signaling pathways [49]. In contrast to primates, where brain circuits are primarily masculinized by the action of androgens, it is presumed that in the brain of rodents, such masculinizing effects are mainly mediated by estrogens [50]. Repetitive exposure to estrogens in neonatal PV+/+ males from PND5 to PND15 might thus induce an "extreme male brain," according to the theory proposed by Baron-Cohen [51]. This might explain the "anti-social" effect of E2 treatment in PV+/+ mice (reduced ultrasonic vocalizations, decreased sociability) as well as the increase of repetitive behaviors (higher number of buried marbles compared to controls).

Our results indicate that E2 is sufficient to partially reverse ASD-relevant behaviors, if it is associated with a reinstatement of PV levels similar to the ones seen in PV+/+ mice. The E2-mediated re-establishment of PV levels is assumed to also restore the electrophysiological phenotypes associated with the absence of PV, i.e., stronger short-term facilitation, increased excitability, increased regularity of fast-spiking interneuron firing in PV−/− mice [52]. The presumed functional restoration of the Pvalb-neuron containing networks is then likely to also restore the excitation/inhibition (E/I) ratio in E2-treated PV+/− mice, the E/I balance assumed to be a key factor in ASD [53, 54]. Our results in male PV+/+ mice, however, indicate that E2 treatment in a situation

defined by a balanced E/I ratio actually leads to a "worsening" in communication and sociability tasks and an increase in repetitive behaviors.

An optimal range of PV circuit function in the insular cortex has been proposed before, where either an imbalance towards more excitation or more inhibition was shown to impair multisensory integration in several ASD mouse models including *Shank3* and *Mecp2* knockout mice [55]. In the latter, the trajectory of functional maturation of Pvalb neurons in the primary visual cortex is accelerated upon vision onset (advanced onset and closure of the critical period), based on higher expression levels of PV and GAD67, vGAT, perineuronal nets, and enhanced GABA transmission among Pvalb neurons at PND15 [56]. In the ASD knockout mouse model for BMP/RA-inducible neural-specific protein 1 (Brinp1 −/−), the higher density of PV+ neurons in the somatosensory cortex and medial hippocampus in adult mice, without indication of altered neuronal proliferation and apoptosis during embryonic development, is indicative of increased PV levels associated with the ASD phenotype [57]. Thus, putative E2-mediated alterations in the trajectory of PV expression and/or associated Pvalb network maturation in E2-exposed PV+/+ mice might be responsible for the appearance of an ASD phenotype possibly linked to accelerated maturation.

The identification of targets for the E2-mediated negative effects on the behavior of PV+/+ mice requires further investigations. It remains to be investigated whether E2-mediated increases in PV in other ASD mouse models, including *Shank1*, *Shank2*, and *Shank3* knockouts [58, 59] or VPA mice consequently ameliorates ASD-associated behaviors. If successful, E2 treatment and/or other means of selective PV upregulation might represent a new avenue towards improvement, i.e., "normalization" of behavior in human ASD.

Conclusions

Our study confirms that PV-deficient mice (PV+/− and PV−/−) show a discernable ASD-like phenotype. ASD-associated behaviors (decreased social interaction, augmented repetitive behaviors) displayed by PV+/− mice are strongly ameliorated, if PV expression is restored close to PV+/+ levels via early postnatal E2 administration. In PV−/− mice, where E2 treatment has obviously no effect on PV levels, the ASD-like phenotype persists. Unexpectedly, in E2-treated PV+/+ mice, ASD-associated behaviors arise. Our results point towards a key role of PV upregulation in PV+/− mice with regard to the amelioration of ASD-like behaviors. An increase in PV expression mediated by E2 in other ASD mouse models with reduced PV levels might also improve ASD-like behavior and possibly represent a point of convergence facilitating the search for new therapeutic approaches in ASD.

Additional file

Additional file 1: Supplemental information on experimental details. Figure S1 A) Details on mouse husbandry and **B**) selection of the tested mice. **Figure S2** Methodological details on mouse handling, E2 administration and mouse weights. **Figure S3** Results from 3-chamber social approach assay presented as bar graphs (**A** and **B**) and number of entries in S and O chamber (**C**). **Figure S4** Analysis of cup climbing time during the 3-chamber social approach assay. **Table S1** Component analysis of behaviors scored in social reciprocal interaction. (DOCX 3208 kb)

Abbreviations
ASD: Autism spectrum disorders; E2: 17-β estradiol; ERβ: Estrogen receptor β; FSI: Fast-spiking interneurons; GABA: Gamma aminobutyric acid; GAD67: Glutamic acid decarboxylase 67; O: Object; PND: Postnatal day; PV: Parvalbumin; rl: Reeler; S: Subject; SYT2: Synaptotagmin 2; vGAT: Vesicular GABA transporter; VPA: Valproic acid

Acknowledgements
The authors wish to thank Simone Eichenberger and Martine Steinauer, University of Fribourg, for the maintenance of the animal facility and technical support, respectively. The help of Gabriella Fernandes and Alessio Lavio, University of Fribourg, in the behavioral experiments is highly appreciated.

Funding
This study was supported by grants from the Swiss National Science Foundation (310030_155952/1 to B.S.), the Novartis Foundation (grant nr. 16C172), and the Deutsche Forschungsgemeinschaft (DFG WO 1732/1-1 to M.W.).

Authors' contributions
BS conceived the study and participated in data analyses and in the writing of the manuscript. FF carried out the experiments, performed statistical analysis, and participated in writing of the manuscript. EL carried out the experiments, performed statistical analysis, and participated in writing of the manuscript. KJV participated in analysis of behavioral data. MW participated in the design of the study, carried out experiments, and participated in the statistical analysis and writing of the manuscript. All authors read and approved the final manuscript.

Competing interests
The authors declare that they have no competing interests.

Author details
[1]Anatomy Unit, Section of Medicine, University of Fribourg, Route Albert-Gockel 1, CH-1700 Fribourg, Switzerland. [2]Behavioral Neuroscience, Faculty of Psychology, Philipps-University of Marburg, Gutenbergstraße 18, 35032 Marburg, Germany. [3]Marburg Center for Mind, Brain, and Behavior (MCMBB), Hans-Meerwein-Straße 6, 35032 Marburg, Germany.

References
1. de la Torre-Ubieta L, Won H, Stein JL, Geschwind DH. Advancing the understanding of autism disease mechanisms through genetics. Nat Med. 2016;22(4):345–61.
2. Ergaz Z, Weinstein-Fudim L, Ornoy A. Genetic and non-genetic animal models for autism spectrum disorders (ASD). Reprod Toxicol. 2016;64:116–40.
3. Politte LC, McDougle CJ. Atypical antipsychotics in the treatment of children and adolescents with pervasive developmental disorders. Psychopharmacology. 2014;231(6):1023–36.
4. Sahin M, Sur M. Genes, circuits, and precision therapies for autism and related neurodevelopmental disorders. Science. 2015;350(6263).
5. Filice F, Vörckel KJ, Sungur AO, Wöhr M, Schwaller B. Reduction in parvalbumin expression not loss of the parvalbumin-expressing GABA interneuron subpopulation in genetic parvalbumin and shank mouse models of autism. Mol Brain. 2016;9:10.
6. Lauber E, Filice F, Schwaller B. Prenatal valproate exposure differentially affects parvalbumin-expressing neurons and related circuits in the cortex and striatum of mice. Front Mol Neurosci. 2016;9:150.
7. Wöhr M, Orduz D, Gregory P, Moreno H, Khan U, Vorckel KJ, Wolfer DP, Welzl H, Gall D, Schiffmann SN, et al. Lack of parvalbumin in mice leads to behavioral deficits relevant to all human autism core symptoms and related neural morphofunctional abnormalities. Transl Psychiatry. 2015;5:e525.
8. Hashemi E, Ariza J, Rogers H, Noctor SC, Martinez-Cerdeno V. The number of parvalbumin-expressing interneurons is decreased in the medial prefrontal cortex in autism. Cereb Cortex. 2017;27(3):1931-43.
9. Zikopoulos B, Barbas H. Altered neural connectivity in excitatory and inhibitory cortical circuits in autism. Front Hum Neurosci. 2013;7:609.
10. Parikshak NN, Swarup V, Belgard TG, Irimia M, Ramaswami G, Gandal MJ, Hartl C, Leppa V, Ubieta LT, Huang J, et al. Genome-wide changes in lncRNA, splicing, and regional gene expression patterns in autism. Nature. 2016;540(7633):423–7.
11. Blurton-Jones M, Tuszynski MH. Estrogen receptor-beta colocalizes extensively with parvalbumin-labeled inhibitory neurons in the cortex, amygdala, basal forebrain, and hippocampal formation of intact and ovariectomized adult rats. J Comp Neurol. 2002;452(3):276–87.
12. Ross NR, Porter LL. Effects of dopamine and estrogen upon cortical neurons that express parvalbumin in vitro. Brain Res Dev Brain Res. 2002;137(1):23–34.
13. Sotonyi P, Gao Q, Bechmann I, Horvath TL. Estrogen promotes parvalbumin expression in arcuate nucleus POMC neurons. Reprod Sci. 2010;17(12):1077–80.
14. Fujimoto N, Igarashi K, Kanno J, Honda H, Inoue T. Identification of estrogen-responsive genes in the GH3 cell line by cDNA microarray analysis. J Steroid Biochem Mol Biol. 2004;91(3):121–9.
15. Corvino V, Di Maria V, Marchese E, Lattanzi W, Biamonte F, Michetti F, Geloso MC. Estrogen administration modulates hippocampal GABAergic subpopulations in the hippocampus of trimethyltin-treated rats. Front Cell Neurosci. 2015;9:433.
16. Silverman JL, Yang M, Lord C, Crawley JN. Behavioural phenotyping assays for mouse models of autism. Nat Rev Neurosci. 2010;11(7):490–502.
17. Wöhr M, Scattoni ML. Behavioural methods used in rodent models of autism spectrum disorders: current standards and new developments. Behav Brain Res. 2013;251:5–17.
18. Gorski RA. Perinatal effects of sex steroids on brain development and function. Prog Brain Res. 1973;39:149–63.
19. Alcantara S, Ferrer I, Soriano E. Postnatal development of parvalbumin and calbindin D28K immunoreactivities in the cerebral cortex of the rat. Anat Embryol. 1993;188:63–73.
20. del Rio JA, de Lecea L, Ferrer I, Soriano E. The development of parvalbumin-immunoreactivity in the neocortex of the mouse. Brain Res Dev Brain Res. 1994;81(2):247–59.
21. Gandal MJ, Nesbitt AM, McCurdy RM, Alter MD. Measuring the maturity of the fast-spiking interneuron transcriptional program in autism, schizophrenia, and bipolar disorder. PLoS One. 2012;7(8):e41215.
22. Macrì S, Biamonte F, Romano E, Marino R, Keller F, Laviola G. Perseverative responding and neuroanatomical alterations in adult heterozygous reeler mice are mitigated by neonatal estrogen administration. Psychoneuroendocrinology. 2010;35(9):1374–87.

23. Hoffman EJ, Turner KJ, Fernandez JM, Cifuentes D, Ghosh M, Ijaz S, Jain RA, Kubo F, Bill BR, Baier H, et al. Estrogens suppress a behavioral phenotype in zebrafish mutants of the autism risk gene, CNTNAP2. Neuron. 2016;89(4):725–33.

24. Schwaller B, Dick J, Dhoot G, Carroll S, Vrbova G, Nicotera P, Pette D, Wyss A, Bluethmann H, Hunziker W, et al. Prolonged contraction-relaxation cycle of fast-twitch muscles in parvalbumin knockout mice. Am J Physiol (Cell Physiol). 1999;276(2 Pt 1):C395–403.

25. Moreno H, Burghardt NS, Vela-Duarte D, Masciotti J, Hua F, Fenton AA, Schwaller B, Small SA. The absence of the calcium-buffering protein calbindin is associated with faster age-related decline in hippocampal metabolism. Hippocampus. 2012;22(5):1107–20.

26. Aiello TP, Whitaker-Azmitia PM. Sexual differentiation and the neuroendocrine hypothesis of autism. Anat Rec (Hoboken). 2011;294(10):1663–70.

27. Patisaul HB, Fortino AE, Polston EK. Neonatal genistein or bisphenol-A exposure alters sexual differentiation of the AVPV. Neurotoxicol Teratol. 2006;28(1):111–8.

28. Sungur AO, Vorckel KJ, Schwarting RK, Wöhr M. Repetitive behaviors in the Shank1 knockout mouse model for autism spectrum disorder: developmental aspects and effects of social context. J Neurosci Methods. 2014;234:92–100.

29. Yang M, Silverman JL, Crawley JN. Automated three-chambered social approach task for mice. Curr Protoc Neurosci. 2011;56:8.26.1–8.26.16.

30. Thomas A, Burant A, Bui N, Graham D, Yuva-Paylor LA, Paylor R. Marble burying reflects a repetitive and perseverative behavior more than novelty-induced anxiety. Psychopharmacology. 2009;204(2):361–73.

31. Caillard O, Moreno H, Schwaller B, Llano I, Celio MR, Marty A. Role of the calcium-binding protein parvalbumin in short-term synaptic plasticity. Proc Natl Acad Sci U S A. 2000;97(24):13372–7.

32. Schwaller B, Tetko IV, Tandon P, Silveira DC, Vreugdenhil M, Henzi T, Potier MC, Celio MR, Villa AE. Parvalbumin deficiency affects network properties resulting in increased susceptibility to epileptic seizures. Mol Cell Neurosci. 2004;25(4):650–63.

33. Silverman JL, Turner SM, Barkan CL, Tolu SS, Saxena R, Hung AY, Sheng M, Crawley JN. Sociability and motor functions in Shank1 mutant mice. Brain Res. 2011;1380:120–37.

34. Wang X, McCoy PA, Rodriguiz RM, Pan Y, Je HS, Roberts AC, Kim CJ, Berrios J, Colvin JS, Bousquet-Moore D, et al. Synaptic dysfunction and abnormal behaviors in mice lacking major isoforms of Shank3. Hum Mol Genet. 2011;20(15):3093–108.

35. Won H, Lee HR, Gee HY, Mah W, Kim JI, Lee J, Ha S, Chung C, Jung ES, Cho YS, et al. Autistic-like social behaviour in Shank2-mutant mice improved by restoring NMDA receptor function. Nature. 2012;486(7402):261–5.

36. Filice F, Schwaller B. Parvalbumin and autism: different causes, same effect? Oncotarget. 2017;8(5):7222–3.

37. Sungur AO, Schwarting RK, Wöhr M. Early communication deficits in the Shank1 knockout mouse model for autism spectrum disorder: developmental aspects and effects of social context. Autism Res. 2016;9(6):696–709.

38. Wöhr M, Roullet FI, Hung AY, Sheng M, Crawley JN. Communication impairments in mice lacking Shank1: reduced levels of ultrasonic vocalizations and scent marking behavior. PLoS One. 2011;6(6):e20631.

39. Peca J, Feliciano C, Ting JT, Wang W, Wells MF, Venkatraman TN, Lascola CD, Fu Z, Feng G. Shank3 mutant mice display autistic-like behaviours and striatal dysfunction. Nature. 2011;472(7344):437–42.

40. Mabunga DF, Gonzales EL, Kim JW, Kim KC, Shin CY. Exploring the validity of valproic acid animal model of autism. Exp Neurobiol. 2015;24(4):285–300.

41. Peixoto RT, Wang W, Croney DM, Kozorovitskiy Y, Sabatini BL. Early hyperactivity and precocious maturation of corticostriatal circuits in Shank3B(−/−) mice. Nat Neurosci. 2016;19(5):716–24.

42. Sungur AÖ, Stemmler L, Wöhr M, Rust MB. Impaired object recognition but normal social behavior and ultrasonic communication in Cofilin1 mutant mice. Front Behav Neurosci 2018:doi: https://doi.org/10.3389/fnbeh.2018.00025.

43. Bell RW, Nitschke W, Gorry TH, Zachman TA. Infantile stimulation and ultrasonic signaling: a possible mediator of early handling phenomena. Dev Psychobiol. 1971;4(2):181–91.

44. Raineki C, Lucion AB, Weinberg J. Neonatal handling: an overview of the positive and negative effects. Dev Psychobiol. 2014;56(8):1613–25.

45. Pare WP, Glavin GB. Restraint stress in biomedical research: a review. Neurosci Biobehav Rev. 1986;10(3):339–70.

46. Boivin JR, Piekarski DJ, Wahlberg JK, Wilbrecht L. Age, sex, and gonadal hormones differently influence anxiety- and depression-related behavior during puberty in mice. Psychoneuroendocrinology. 2017;85:78–87.

47. Piekarski DJ, Boivin JR, Wilbrecht L. Ovarian hormones organize the maturation of inhibitory neurotransmission in the frontal cortex at puberty onset in female mice. Curr Biol. 2017;27(12):1735–45. e1733

48. Reilly MP, Weeks CD, Topper VY, Thompson LM, Crews D, Gore AC. The effects of prenatal PCBs on adult social behavior in rats. Horm Behav. 2015;73:47–55.

49. Marino M, Galluzzo P, Ascenzi P. Estrogen signaling multiple pathways to impact gene transcription. Curr Genomics. 2006;7(8):497–508.

50. Wu MV, Manoli DS, Fraser EJ, Coats JK, Tollkuhn J, Honda S, Harada N, Shah NM. Estrogen masculinizes neural pathways and sex-specific behaviors. Cell. 2009;139(1):61–72.

51. Baron-Cohen S. The extreme male brain theory of autism. Trends Cogn Sci. 2002;6(6):248–54.

52. Schwaller B. The use of transgenic mouse models to reveal the functions of Ca^{2+} buffer proteins in excitable cells. Biochim Biophys Acta. 2012;1820(8):1294–303.

53. Rubenstein JL, Merzenich MM. Model of autism: increased ratio of excitation/inhibition in key neural systems. Genes Brain Behav. 2003;2(5):255–67.

54. Xiong Y, Liu X, Han L, Yan J. The ongoing balance of cortical excitation and inhibition during early development. Neurosci Biobehav Rev. 2011;35(10):2114–6.

55. Gogolla N, Takesian AE, Feng G, Fagiolini M, Hensch TK. Sensory integration in mouse insular cortex reflects GABA circuit maturation. Neuron. 2014;83(4):894–905.

56. Krishnan K, Wang BS, Lu J, Wang L, Maffei A, Cang J, Huang ZJ. MeCP2 regulates the. MD: modeling autism by SHANK gene mutations in mice. Neuron. 2013;78(1):8–27.

57. Berkowicz SR, Featherby TJ, Qu Z, Giousoh A, Borg NA, Heng JI, Whisstock JC, Bird PI. Brinp1(−/−) mice exhibit autism-like behaviour, altered memory, hyperactivity and increased parvalbumin-positive cortical interneuron density. Molecular Autism. 2016;7:22.

58. Jiang YH, Ehlers MD. Modeling autism by SHANK gene mutations in mice. Neuron. 2013;78(1):8–27.

59. Yoo J, Bakes J, Bradley C, Collingridge GL, Kaang BK. Shank mutant mice as an animal model of autism. Philos Trans R Soc Lond Ser B Biol Sci. 2014;369(1633):20130143.

Self-reported sex differences in high-functioning adults with autism

R. L. Moseley[*] ⓘ, R. Hitchiner and J. A. Kirkby

Abstract

Background: Sex differences in autistic symptomatology are believed to contribute to the mis- and missed diagnosis of many girls and women with an autism spectrum condition (ASC). Whilst recent years have seen the emergence of clinical and empirical reports delineating the profile of young autistic girls, recognition of sex differences in symptomatology in adulthood is far more limited.

Methods: We chose here to focus on symptomatology as reported using a screening instrument, the Ritvo Autism Asperger Diagnostic Scale-Revised (RAADS-R). In a meta-analysis, we pooled and analysed RAADS-R data from a number of experimental groups. Analysis of variance (ANOVA) searched for the presence of main effects of Sex and Diagnosis and for interactions between these factors in our sample of autistic and non-autistic adults.

Results: In social relatedness and circumscribed interests, main effects of Diagnosis revealed that as expected, autistic adults reported significantly greater lifetime prevalence of symptoms in these domains; an effect of Sex, in circumscribed interests, also suggested that males generally reported more prevalent symptoms than females. An interaction of Sex and Diagnosis in language symptomatology revealed that a normative sex difference in language difficulties was attenuated in autism. An interaction of Sex and Diagnosis in the sensorimotor domain revealed the opposite picture: a lack of sex differences between typically developing men and women and a greater prevalence of sensorimotor symptoms in autistic women than autistic men.

Conclusions: We discuss the literature on childhood sex differences in relation to those which emerged in our adult sample. Where childhood sex differences fail to persist in adulthood, several interpretations exist, and we discuss, for example, an inherent sampling bias that may mean that only autistic women most similar to the male presentation are diagnosed. The finding that sensorimotor symptomatology is more highly reported by autistic women is a finding requiring objective confirmation, given its potential importance in diagnosis.

Keywords: Sex, Gender, Self-report, RAADS-R

Background

Females with autism are historically underdiagnosed. In cognitively impaired children, autism diagnosis is currently estimated at two boys to every girl in cognitively impaired children, whereas in those who are higher-functioning, estimates range from 5.7, 11 or 15.7 boys to every girl (see [1, 2]). Most recently within the UK (Scotland, specifically), diagnostic ratios were put at 3.5 males to every female in autistic children and adolescents,

and two males to every female in adults [3]. A recent review of diagnosis internationally came to a similar diagnostic ratio, in children, of three boys diagnosed to every girl [4]. Convincing arguments from genetic research, beyond the scope of the present article, suggest that the prevalence of autism could be genuinely lower in females [2, 5–8], but in so far as those who are diagnosed, diagnostic rates appear to reflect a kind of 'bimodal distribution', with the more severely impaired autistic females likely to be detected in childhood and those without intellectual disability and with subtler presentations likely to be either missed or diagnosed later in life [1, 9]. The fact

* Correspondence: rmoseley@bournemouth.ac.uk
Department of Psychology, Bournemouth University, Fern Barrow, Poole, Dorset BH12 5BB, UK

that age of diagnosis is on average later in autistic females than males corroborates the known difficulty identifying girls and women and corroborates the calls from the autistic and the scientific community for research into the female autistic phenotype [5, 10].

Clinical reports and empirical studies continue to crystallise the female phenotype as it appears in young girls, though it must be noted that differences in sampling techniques and methodologies make comparison of findings somewhat opaque. Several studies of early childhood suggest that differences may become more apparent with age, finding no significant differences between male and female infants and toddlers in autistic symptomatology within broad domains [11–13]. A more detailed look at each symptom category, as children age, reveals the emergence of considerable differences. With consideration of the core diagnostic impairments in social communication and interaction [14], girls with autism are believed to be equivalent to their male peers in core difficulties with social *understanding* [5, 15]; reports that autistic girls exhibit greater social impairment [16–18] may be subject to the fact that less severe presentations of autism (i.e. high-functioning autism) are less likely to be recognised and thus diagnosed in girls [19–22]). The *expressive* behaviours of girls with autism, such as in making reciprocal conversation and displaying appropriate non-verbal behaviour and gestures, do however tend to outpass male peers [5, 23]; this is starkly illustrated by Hiller et al. [24], who found that whilst girls are more likely to use social gestures, their usage does not reflect underlying understanding. The fact that gestures may be unusually 'vivid', characterised by increased energy [23], could potentially say something of their learned nature. Young girls with autism are also known to be far more likely than boys to engage in complex imitation [24], which is problematic given the central featuring of imitative abilities in gold-standard diagnostic tests.

Autistic girls are more likely to correspond to Wing and Gould's [25] 'active but odd' category and tend away from 'autistic aloneness' [26, 27]. Indeed, where males with autism may withdraw from the more active games of their peers [24, 28], autistic girls are believed to be more socially motivated [29, 30] and, like non-autistic girls, to spend time chatting with friends as opposed to engaging in activities like sports or gaming [30–32]. Whilst these studies highlight similarities between autistic and non-autistic girls in female friendships, they do note that autistic girls struggle with managing conflict in relationships, and that social time is exhausting to them. This may be because, unlike autistic boys, autistic girls appear especially adept at skilfully managing social interaction through mimicking and rote-learnt strategies [24, 33, 34]. Qualitative investigation of these strategies suggest masterful adaptation where girls describe empathetic approaches as piggybacking on excellent memory and adherence to a learnt "social code" via observation

and subsequent imitation [35]. Quantitative attempts to capture these abilities show a discrepancy between the scores of women on mentalising tests and core autistic traits (measuring internal disposition and core ability) and their outwards sociocommunicative performance in the Autism Diagnostic Observation Schedule (ADOS-G) [36]. The masking skills of girls and women can unfortunately confound diagnosis, as does a lack of awareness of the female autistic phenotype in professionals and the gender stereotypes which cast socially impaired girls as 'shy' and socially impaired boys as 'unresponsive' [37]. Less disruptive, with fewer externalising and more internalising problems at school age [38–41], autistic girls are more likely to be mothered or accepted by non-autistic girls as fringe members of female social groups at least until adolescence, when female friendships require considerable social adroitness [35].

Autistic girls are also less likely than boys to stand out in the diagnostic domain of restricted and repetitive interests and behaviour, where they tend to exhibit fewer classically autistic symptoms like lining objects up and fascination with small parts [15, 17, 42–46]. Indeed, fascination with small parts and mechanical objects, in early-diagnosed children, is predictive of their being male [24]. Special interests, in girls, tend to be less eccentric and more age- and gender-appropriate (for example ponies or boybands), collecting things like stickers or shells, or obsessional behaviour with toys [24] but equal to those of autistic boys (and different from non-autistic girls) in their intensity [5, 33]. Autistic girls are more likely to engage in pretend play than autistic boys and may appear to have rich inner lives which under closer scrutiny may be seen to be extraordinarily scripted and repetitive [33, 39, 40, 47]. Sensory processing differences, which also fall within this diagnostic domain, are apparently equally apparent [33, 48], but research in this domain is limited; others report greater abnormalities in touch, taste and smell in autistic girls [49].

With the literature focused on childhood presentation, autistic adults are a neglected population in research and less is known about whether these sex differences in autistic symptomatology persist. Both autistic men and women differ from *non-autistic adults* in the attention they pay to faces [50], though interestingly this study did not replicate the trend seen in autistic males to fixate more on the mouth area [51, 52]. These three studies found abnormalities in social attention (as reflected by eye-gaze) to correlate with social competence, emotion recognition and autistic symptomatology respectively [50–52], so it is therefore perhaps unsurprising that difficulties with emotion recognition remain equally prevalent and equivalent in autistic men and women [1, 53], and likewise no differences were seen in empathy and systemizing, the drive to fit the world into rule-based systems [53, 54]. This last finding is particularly note-worthy given that normative sex differences in these domains appear to be attenuated in men and women with autism, a finding corroborated by a large-scale survey that revealed that men and women with autism are more similar to each other than are typically developing men and women [55].

Notwithstanding these similarities, other reports suggest that autism continues to present differently in males and females once they reach adulthood. Lai et al. [53] observed lower scores for women on the sociocommunicative aspects of the ADOS-G [56], seemingly consistent with the expressive skills of autistic females mentioned above, and reports of more sensory issues. There have been some reports of advantages for autistic women over autistic men in executive function and processing speed [1, 54, 57], which may partially explain their success in camouflage [34, 35, 58, 59]. Not all studies, however, have found differences between autistic men and women in executive function (for example, a lack of difference in response inhibition [54]): it is important to note that 'executive function', as a construct, in fact consists of multiple processes, each with distinct developmental trajectories, which are difficult to tease apart and to test in an ecologically valid way, hence the inconsistencies across autism research [60]. Indeed, some reports of sex differences in executive function in autistic children have reported patterns in the reverse, with poorer response inhibition and greater perseveration in autistic girls than boys [61, 62].

Outside of comparative tests in the laboratory, few studies have compared the real life outcomes in autistic men and women. A qualitative analysis by Baldwin and Costley [63] suggested that women might also have greater success than men in being able to study in higher education, though they also self-reported higher rates of mental illness. The same study suggested some interesting reversals of childhood trends: women were more likely than men to highlight difficulties with social interaction as the worst aspects of their employment history, were less likely to aspire to marriage or romantic relationships and more likely to prefer their own company, in contrast to the apparently higher social motivation seen in childhood. Whilst this study featured an impressive sample size, quantitative validation of these tantalising hints would be important.

A common theme throughout the limited literature in adults concerns the struggles that autistic women face in obtaining a diagnosis [1, 58, 59, 63]. The implications of this difficulty are potentially immense, such that many individuals lack support and treatment for their symptomatology [22, 64]. For this reason, the present study aimed to further the limited literature on the symptomatic differences between autistic men and women. We chose to do so utilising an established screening test which is employed in local diagnostic services in South-West England: the Ritvo Autism Asperger Diagnostic Scale-Revised (RAADS-R [65]). Sample size is always immensely problematic in comparing males and females

with autism, given the diagnostic bottleneck which results in many more males than females being identified [22]. For this reason, we sought to supplement our own data by pooling it with that from participating researchers who had also used the RAADS-R. We thus examined self-report ratings made by autistic and nonautistic adults of symptomatology in four domains: social relatedness, circumscribed interests, language and sensorimotor abnormalities.

Methods

We adopted the two-factorial design recommended by Lai et al. [5]: by comparing autistic men and women to each other as well as to typically developing men and women, it is possible to tease out normative sex differences in cognition which may or may not be present in autism. The focus for comparison was scores in the RAADS-R domains of social relatedness, circumscribed interests, sensory motor (henceforth sensorimotor) and language symptoms.

To supplement data gathered by our research group, we conducted a meta-analysis of studies which had used the RAADS-R. Below we describe our final selection of participants and the process of our meta-analysis, but details of the participant cohorts involved are given fully in Additional file 1. Ethical approval for the study was given by Bournemouth University Ethics Committee.

Participants

We obtained a total 961 datasets: 179 typically developing (TD) men, 528 typically developing women, 118 autistic men, and 136 autistic women (see Additional file 1) (Table 1). To ensure data quality, some control participants who scored particularly highly on the RAADS-R (and so might potentially be undiagnosed autistics) were removed (see Additional file 1, for details), leaving 137 TD men, 464 TD women, 118 autistic men, and 136 autistic women. In attempts to objectively create more evenly sized and age-matched groups, we used freely available software [66] to reduce the number of TD females by selecting those best matched in age to the other groups. Therefore, the final participants included in our analysis were 137 TD men, 136 TD women, 118 autistic men, and 136 autistic women. Whilst significant age differences remained between all four groups (F [3, 523] = 3.230, p = .022), no significant age differences remained in three of the four contrasts of interest for this analysis: namely, between TD men and men with autism spectrum conditions (ASC) (p = .192), TD females and females with ASC (p = .944), and between autistic men and women (p = .194). TD women included in the study were significantly older than TD men (t [271] = 2.635, p = .009).

As we were unable to obtain details of IQ, we were unable to match participants in this variable; however, all individuals are assumed to be of average or above-average IQ

Table 1 Average age in years (standard deviation in brackets) for each experimental group. The number of participants included from each source is displayed to the right

	Age (years)	Source
Typically developing men ($n = 137$)	33.1 (13.5)	Bournemouth University ($n = 30$) Kirkovski/Fitzgerald group ($n = 12$) Libero/Kana group ($n = 13$) Schwartzman/Kapp group ($n = 82$)
Typically developing women ($n = 136$)	37.4 (13.8)	Bournemouth University ($n = 16$) Kirkovski/Fitzgerald group ($n = 4$) Schwartzman/Kapp group ($n = 116$)
Autistic men ($n = 118$)	35.3 (13.4)	Bournemouth University ($n = 34$) Kirkovski/Fitzgerald group ($n = 13$) Libero/Kana group ($n = 5$) Schwartzman/Kapp group ($n = 84$)
Autistic women ($n = 136$)	37.5 (14)	Bournemouth University ($n = 35$) Kirkovski/Fitzgerald group ($n = 12$) Libero/Kana group ($n = 14$) Schwartzman/Kapp group ($n = 57$)

due to the nature of the recruitment process and the studies they participated in (see Additional file 1). We do not possess details of comorbid psychiatric disorders or use of psychotropic medication for all datasets, and so cannot confirm that all participants were medication-free or without additional psychiatric conditions.

Materials

The Ritvo Autism Asperger Diagnostic Scale-Revised (RAADS-R [65]) is an 80-item self-report questionnaire recommended by the National Institute of Health and Care Excellence [67] in Great Britain to screen adults of average to above-average intelligence for an autism spectrum condition. Although it has been used in research as a self-report measure, the RAADS-R was designed to be completed in clinical settings with the assistance of a clinician. 'Diagnostic Scale' is somewhat misleading [68]: this test functions rather as a screening instrument or, as the authors intended, as just one part of a comprehensive assessment rather than a standalone diagnostic instrument. The revised version of the original scale was standardised on 201 autistic individuals (145 males) and 578 non-autistic TD (248 males), collected in nine centres on three continents, and like the original is based on diagnostic criteria for autism and Asperger syndrome in DSM-IV-TR and ICD-10 (criteria that were retained in DSM-V). In this large study, the test showed high specificity in its ability to distinguish between TD and autistic individuals whose diagnoses had been independently confirmed (no false positives). Only six of 201 autistic participants scored below 65 and were consequently unidentified (97% sensitivity). The test also showed good test-retest reliability and high concurrent validity (95.59%) with other popular tests for ASC such as the Social Responsiveness Scale Adult Research version [69]. It has been validated for use in other languages [70] and shortened to a 14-item

version with demonstrated capacity to discriminate between ASC and some commonly comorbid psychiatric conditions [71].

The RAADS-R yields four subscales based on symptom areas from DSM-IV-TR [72] and ICD-10 [73], which themselves have high internal consistency. These domains are social relatedness (e.g. 'I often don't know how to act in social situations'), circumscribed interests (e.g. 'I only like to talk to people who share my special interests'), sensorimotor (e.g. 'I always notice how food feels in my mouth. This is more important to me than how it tastes') and language (e.g. 'I have a hard time figuring out what some phrases mean, like "you are the apple of my eye"'). Each item is scored in order of its emergence and current occurrence, with 'True now and when I was young' scored at 3; 'True only now' scored at 2; 'True only when I was younger than 16' scored at 1; and 'Never true' scored at 0. (This scoring is reversed for negative items, such as 'I can put myself in other people's shoes').

Procedure

In order to obtain a sizeable sample, we supplemented our data with that collected by other authors in a meta-analysis [74]. Inclusion criteria were that (1) studies must include clinically diagnosed autistic and non-autistic participants, on whom the RAADS-R had been conducted; (2) participants must be adults (that is, aged 18 or above); and (3) only studies using the RAADS-R, not the original Ritvo Autism Asperger Diagnostic Scale or the newer 14-item version [71] would be included. This therefore stipulated criteria 4), that only studies occurring between 2011 (the publication of the RAADS-R) and the present year of 2017 would be included. Exclusion criteria included (1) studies involving other clinical but non-autistic populations which were being screened for autistic traits (e.g. [65, 75]); (2) studies which used the RAADS-R to assume the presence of autism but did not confirm the diagnosis with participants (e.g. [76]); (3) studies written in languages other than English; and 4) or reviews citing the RAADS-R which did not include actual data.

We searched three online databases (Web of Science, PubMed, Science Direct) with the search command: 'Ritvo Autism Asperger Diagnostic Scale-Revised'. We also used Google Scholar to identify all publications which had cited Ritvo et al.'s publication of their scale. With some overlap and much redundancy, we obtained 6 search results from Web of Science, 4 from PubMed, 87 from Science Direct, and 85 from Google Scholar (see Additional file 1). Sorting through these citations with our criteria in mind, we identified 16 relevant studies and contacted 8 research groups (see Additional file 1). We received useable datasets from three of these (see Additional file 1). We ensured the data was numerically coded in the same way as our own (one for female, two

for male, for example) before collating it in SPSS (Statistical Programme for the Social Sciences).

Statistical analysis examined scores on the social relatedness, circumscribed interests, language and sensorimotor subscales of the RAADS-R. For each domain, separate two-way ANOVAs included between-subjects factors of Diagnosis (autistic vs. TD) and Sex (female vs. male). Interactions between Diagnosis and Sex, in this context, indicate that sex differences are attenuated or increased by the presence or lack of an autism diagnosis. The presence of an interaction thus motivated post hoc comparisons between males and females within the TD and within the autistic group.

Results

Effects of sex and diagnosis were examined for each RAADS-R domain independently and averages for each group can be seen in Fig. 1. In the social relatedness

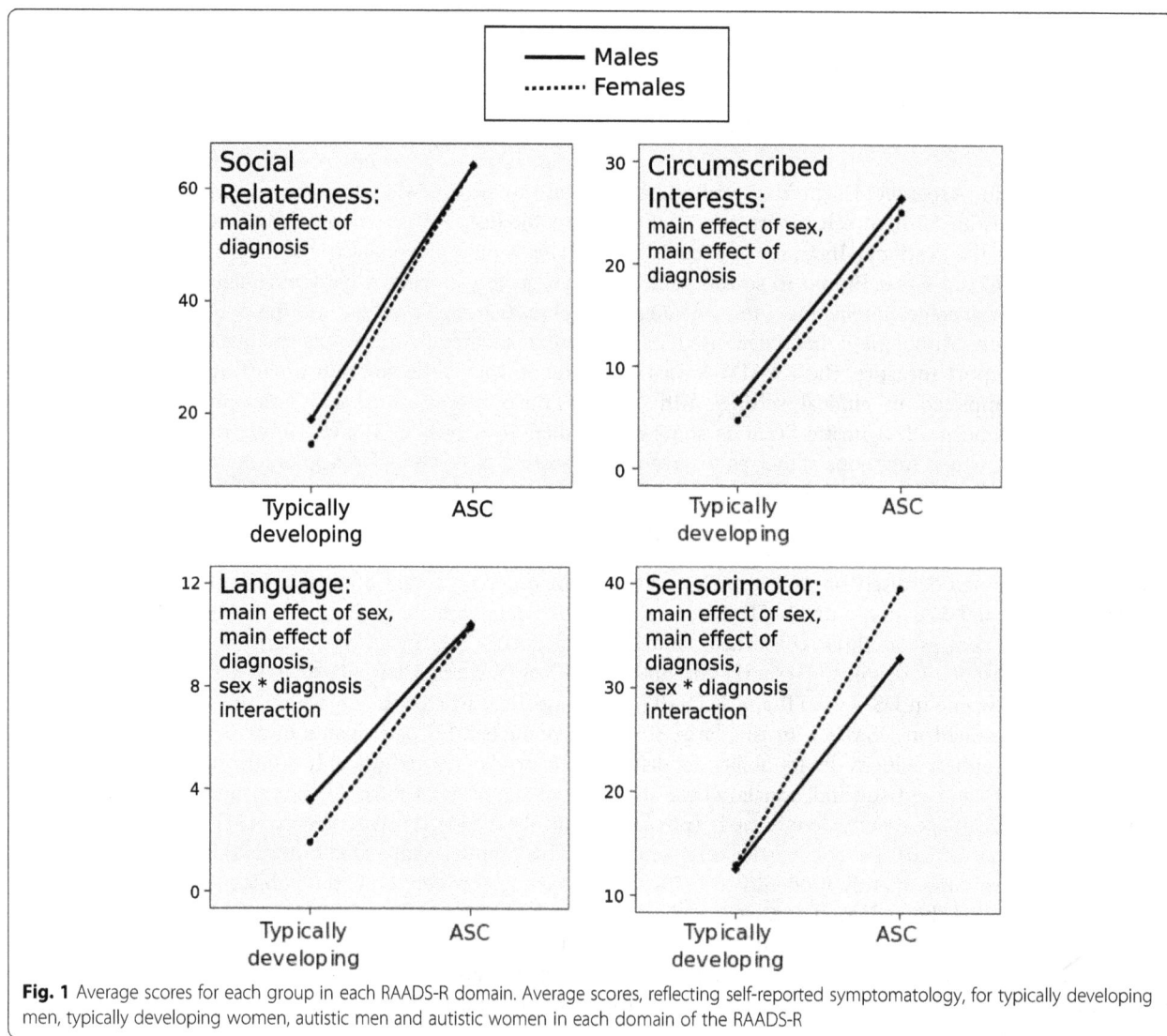

Fig. 1 Average scores for each group in each RAADS-R domain. Average scores, reflecting self-reported symptomatology, for typically developing men, typically developing women, autistic men and autistic women in each domain of the RAADS-R

domain, typically developed men scored an average of 18.9 (SD 10.8), typically developing women an average of 14.5 (SD 10.9), autistic men an average of 64.2 (SD 23) and autistic women an average of 64.2 (SD 19.7). A main effect of Diagnosis (F [1, 523] = 1068.299, p = .000) reflected that autistic participants reported significantly higher prevalence of social problems than typically developed individuals—a finding corroborating the original paper [65] and subsequent validations of the test [70, 71]. In the same vein, examination of the circumscribed interests domain revealed a main effect of Diagnosis (F [1, 523] = 904.268, p < .001), with typically developing men and women reporting lower symptoms on average (men 6.7 [SD 4.9], women 4.7 [SD 4.1]) than autistic men and women (men 26.4 [SD 10.1], women 25 [SD 9.8]). There was also a main effect of Sex (F [1, 523 = .6.080, p = .014) reflecting that males generally report more behaviours than women in the circumscribed interests domain.

In the language domain, typically developing men scored on average 3.6 (SD 2.5); women an average 1.9 [SD 1.8]); autistic men an average 10.4 [SD 4.6]; and autistic women an average 10.3 [SD 5.2]. A main effect of Sex (F [1, 523] = 7.333, p = .007) and a main effect of Diagnosis (F [1, 523] = 542.630, p < .001) reflected that women generally reported lower scores in autistic language symptomatology than men and that, as expected, individuals with autism reported significantly more symptoms than TD controls. A significant interaction between Sex and Diagnosis (F [1, 523, p = 5.707, p = .017) motivated post hoc tests, which revealed that scores differed significantly between typically developing men and women (t [271] = 6.311, p < .001) but not between autistic men and women (p = .866).

Highest scores in the sensorimotor domain were seen in autistic women (average 39.6 [SD 12.6]), followed by autistic men (average 32.9 [SD 11.6]), typically developing women (average 12.9 [SD 7.6]) and typically developing men (average 12.5 [SD 7.2]). A significant main effect of Sex (F [1, 523] = 16.235, p < .001) reflected lower self-reported sensorimotor abnormalities in women, and a main effect of Diagnosis (F [1, 523] = 726.807, p < .001) reflected greater symptomatology in the autistic group. An interaction between Sex and Diagnosis (F [1, 523, p = .12.983, p < .001), in this domain, reflected a surprising lack of difference between TD men and women (p = .252) and a significant difference between autistic men and women (t [252] = 4.346, p < .001).

Discussion

For the purpose of early identification, prior investigations of sex differences in autism have predominantly focused on child samples. Given the known difficulty identifying females with autism and the aptitude of many female and *male* individuals to camouflage their symptoms [32, 34, 35, 58, 59, 63], a substantial unidentified population reach

adulthood before being diagnosed [1, 64]. We consequently aimed to extend the small literature on how autistic symptomatology presents in autistic men and women through investigating a commonly used self-report measure, the Ritvo Autism Asperger Diagnostic Scale Revised (RAADS-R [65]). Studying sex differences as and if they emerge in screening instruments may be particularly important if these are considered frontline measures used in triage, as the RAADS-R happens to be in our area. To increase the power of our analysis, we conducted a meta-analysis, gathering data from several research groups. We discuss first the areas in which autistic men and women presented similarly and then the domain in which they differed.

Whilst the now extensive literature on sex differences in autistic children emphasises the divergence between girls and boys, previous investigations in autistic adults have reported similar competence in emotion recognition [1, 53] and even the *attenuation* of normative sex differences in empathising and systemising [53–55]. These findings align with a theoretical perspective that links ASC with the masculinization of brain and behaviour [77–80]. In the domain of social relatedness, we did not find that normative sex differences were attenuated in autism but that autistic men and women were alike in their quantification of symptomology. This is consistent with childhood impairments in the social domain, which appear to be of equal severity in boys and girls [15]. Previous studies have, however, noted a stark divergence between core social understanding and outward expressive social interaction in females [24], which indeed appears to be somewhat more typical due to skilled social mimicry [5, 23, 24, 33]. Our data appears to reflect the shared core disability in social understanding, as the social difficulties of autistic women were reported as no less prominent than those of autistic men. A qualitative difference previously reported relating to autistic women's heightened concern over social interaction [63] was not here quantified in reports of greater prevalence of social problems. Of note, however, is the self-report nature of our data: this greater concern over social competence could possibly have served to hide the better *expressive* social skills evinced in previous studies, if autistic women are inaccurate reporters. As in other studies of sex differences in autistic adults [53], the validity of our self-report measures depends on the self-reflective capacity of participants, differences, or in this case *lack* of sex differences, thus require independent, objective ratification.

This point holds true when we consider a lack of sex differences between autistic men and women in the circumscribed interests domain, despite a main effect of sex reflecting a general tendency for men to report more symptomatology in this domain. The 'circumscribed interests' domain of the RAADS-R aligns itself with the repetitive and restricted behaviours and interest (RRBI) diagnostic criterion [14], including items describing fixated and unusual interests which dominate conversation, detail-level focusing, adherence to fixed routines and difficulties with change, and enjoyment of lists and categorisation. It differs, however, from RRBI as conceptualised in diagnostic instruments such as the ADOS-G [56] and the Autism Diagnostic Interview (ADI-R [81], placing motor stereotypies and stimming (behaviours such as spinning, flicking or twiddling) into the sensorimotor domain. RRBI is the domain where sex differences are most likely to occur in children and young people [2, 5, 15], with boys showing significantly greater symptomatology. A sex difference in self-reported symptoms in adulthood seems to contradict this finding, but the non-equivalence of 'circumscribed interests' to the RRBI domain makes interpretation somewhat challenging, as RRBI includes sensory and motor abnormalities which we discuss separately below.

In the language domain, an interaction of sex and diagnosis revealed that where normative sex differences appeared between typically developing men and women (perhaps reflecting the commonly held belief of female superiority in communication [82]); there were no statistical differences in the language symptomatology reported by autistic adults. This finding corroborates previous reports of attenuated sex differences in autistic individuals [53–55]. In self-report form, our autistic participants did not corroborate previous suggestions that language skills may be superior in autistic females [5, 21, 24]. We note, however, the rather narrow coverage of the language domain: of these seven items, four relate to literal interpretation of language (e.g. 'The phrase "I've got you under my skin" makes me very uncomfortable'), and only one relates to the ability to engage in reciprocal conversation, which is the area where the camouflage of autistic women serves them well. As such, it is possible that the language measure of the RAADS-R lacks the refinement to pick up a genuine sex difference.

Indeed, at this point, let us further discuss and attempt to interpret the lack of statistical difference between autistic men and women in the social relatedness, circumscribed interests and language domains. The data informs us that autistic women do not rate themselves as significantly more or less symptomatic than men in any one of these domains, but whether these findings reflect a genuine equalisation of childhood differences is equivocal. We have noted, above, the differences that may emerge between studies using self-report data vs. objective observations. A further interpretation of the lack of differentiation seen here and in some other studies of male and female autistics at different ages [11–13] is that it reflects unsuccessful attempts to quantify these differences at domain level [5]. Particularly rich, clinically useful data has come from studies conducting

detailed analysis of diagnostic criteria within domains (see Hiller et al. [20] for example). Unfortunately, such scrutiny of individual items was impossible in this meta-analysis where we received only domain scores.

Another interpretation for the lack of differentiation in these domains concerns the diagnostic bottleneck or 'ascertainment bias' [5, 15, 22, 35, 57]. This and previous studies of the female autistic phenotype are limited by an inherent selection bias in participants. The current conceptualisation of autism, and the diagnostic tools and screening instruments used to detect it, are undeniably androcentric, being developed and standardised according to male cases. The same can be said of the original and revised Ritvo scale, given the heavy male bias in the original and the standardisation sample. As such, when studies examine diagnosed women who could conceivably more closely match the androcentric symptom presentation defined by the tests, similarities to autistic men may be artificially inflated. Studies have attempted to mitigate this problem in several ways: some have included women who do not reach cut-offs in gold-standard tests but whose diagnoses have been confirmed by experience clinicians [53], whereas others have recruited late-diagnosed women whose growing up undiagnosed suggests they did not fit the archetypal presentation of autism [58]. Nevertheless, the potential exclusion of swathes of less stereotypical autistic women casts a modicum of uncertainty on many findings. Future targets for research may be precisely those women referred for diagnosis whom fail to reach cut off on the androcentric instruments of diagnosis but who fulfil criteria for a developmental social and communication disorder on more dimensional scales, such as the Diagnostic Interview for Social and Communication Disorders (DISCO [83]). Here, differences in cognition, emotion and behaviour not only between autistic men and women but between classically diagnosed and subthreshold women might be highly illuminative and reveal a broader female spectrum.

An interesting finding of potential import for diagnosis and conceptualization of autism was the divergence between autistic men and women in the sensorimotor domain. This documents hypersensitivity and extraordinarily negative reactions to the textures of foods and clothes, sounds, noises, lights and being touched by others; hyposensitivity to pain and sensation-seeking behaviours like hand-fiddling, rocking or spinning; experiencing the same sensations as variably too intense or not registering them; and movement coordination problems.[1] Here, a main effect of sex revealed that females generally reported more sensorimotor differences than males, and a main effect of diagnosis corroborated the established sensorimotor abnormalities associated with autism [84, 85]. An interaction of sex and diagnosis revealed, however, that autistic women reported disproportionately more sensorimotor symptoms than their male counterparts. There are extensive reports of sensorimotor abnormalities in autism (see [86, 87] for review), but as usual these are strongly androcentric with few or no female cases. Comparisons with neurotypical peers suggest that motor symptoms are certainly present in autistic girls [88], as are sensory abnormalities [33]; comparisons between males and females on the spectrum, however, are much more scarce. Whilst some imply that sensorimotor abnormalities are equivalent [27, 48], one small study using the Japanese version of the CARS [89] found autistic girls between 5 and 9 years of age to show significantly greater abnormality than autistic boys in their responses to taste, smell and touch, and lesser abnormality in their activity level and bodily movements [49]. Interestingly, women generally obtain higher scores than men on this RAADS-R domain, with autistic women reporting the greatest number of symptoms [70]; the same pattern is seen in the 14-item version of the test [71]. Lai et al. [53] created a composite sensory abnormality score from three items of the ADI-R [81] tapping unusual sensory interests, noise hypersensitivity and extraordinarily negative responses to sensory stimuli. According to caregivers who completed the interview, these items were significantly more prevalent in autistic women.

If sensorimotor abnormalities are indeed a more prevalent feature of female autism than, say, the stereotypical manifestation of repetitive and restricted interests [15, 17, 24, 42–45], this finding would have important diagnostic implications. Sensorimotor abnormalities are downplayed in gold-standard diagnostic tests such as the ADOS-G and the ADI-R, which could, in this context, bias the tests away from detecting females. The suggestion must, however, be treated with caution, based as it is on one study with a small sample [49] and one with a measure lacking sensitivity to sensorimotor abnormalities [53]. It has been proposed that autistic women may have greater capacity for self-reflective awareness in symptom reporting [1, 53], although in our study they did not rate themselves more symptomatic than men in other domains. In line with the general sex difference in the RAADS-R sensorimotor domain [70], some studies suggest that women are generally more likely to report symptoms they perceive as abnormal and indeed to utilise medical services [90, 91], and this may be a normative sex difference that exists in both autistic and non-autistic people. As such, the particular focus that autistic women place on sensorimotor symptoms should be validated by independent, objective measures to investigate whether it has a basis in fact. 'Sensory subtypes' have recently been proposed in childhood autism, although gender did not appear to modulate a child's sensory profile

[92]. With a sample of 203 boys and 25 girls in this study, however, this might be worth investigating in a more balanced child and adult sample.

Alongside the avenues for future research suggested by our findings, the nature of the present study leaves several limitations on which further work could build. Primarily, although we were able to obtain a large dataset from other researchers to compliment the data we obtained from local clinics, we received only scores for each domain (social relatedness, circumscribed interests, language and sensorimotor) as a whole. This lack of scores for individual items *within* domains precluded other types of analysis, such as those exploring the factor structure of the RAADS-R and potential differences in the same between males and females. The original authors did not focus on sex differences and so reported a factor structure from a heavily male-dominated sample. Notably, however, they did report the emergence of a different factor than the sensorimotor one that remains in popular usage of the test: a factor identified as social anxiety. Lacking access to the scores to individual items, we were unable to calculate scores in this alternative domain for our male and female participants—however, it seems highly possible that social anxiety is an area where autistic males and females might diverge, given the suggested greater social motivation of autistic females [29, 30].

It is furthermore important to consider the potential influence of several variables which we were unable to control for in the present analysis. Firstly, we unfortunately lacked information regarding psychiatric comorbidities and even additional neurodevelopmental conditions (such as ADHD) in our participants. Whilst neurological conditions were controlled to an extent in some of the data we obtained, we were not privy to information regarding psychiatric comorbidities in any of the participants, thus precluding a more refined analysis. We thus cannot speculate on the effects of psychiatric comorbidities on responses to the RAADS-R (furthermore, we note with interest that the original authors did not appear to screen out additional psychiatric comorbidities in their standardisation sample). This may be highly important, given the greatly elevated prevalence of mental illness in ASC [93], and indeed the high likelihood of autistic females to be misdiagnosed with psychiatric conditions or to come to the attention of clinicians due to other conditions [33].

Race and ethnicity, socioeconomic status and education are other important variables which we were unable to control for in our multi-dataset analysis and which may affect responses to the RAADS-R. The RAADS-R was developed and standardised in Western populations. Although we cannot ascertain the precise ethnicity of each of our participants, it can be surmised with high probability that they were predominantly Caucasian, based on the ethnic diversity of the areas where they were recruited. Alongside sex, these are variables which can notably affect symptom presentation and the likelihood of obtaining an ASC diagnosis. In the UK, age of diagnosis is on average earlier in children with highly educated parents from higher socioeconomic backgrounds [94]; in America, autism diagnoses are substantially higher in the higher socioeconomic groups [95–97]. These statistics are explained largely (although not entirely) by another kind of bottleneck or bias in the diagnostic services: that highly educated parents with greater incomes are more likely and more *able* to approach clinicians with concerns, since many low-income families will lack access to these specialised services. There is, of course, a strong relationship between ethnicity and socioeconomic status. Autistic people from ethnic minority groups are also later to be diagnosed [97–99] and less likely to be diagnosed [97, 100], despite one report of more severe language symptoms in autistic toddlers from minority groups. Culture influences both the manifestation of autistic symptoms [101, 102] and their interpretation by parents and other observers [103]. As is typical of autism research in general, the majority of work in this area focuses on children: much less is known about how these variables affect symptom presentation and the likelihood of obtaining a diagnosis in adulthood, and whether they interact with sex, reflecting a clear need for future study.

As concerns sex, genetic evidence suggests a very real possibility that autism may not be *equally* prevalent in males and females [2–6, 104, 105]. Nevertheless, given their indubitable existence, it is imperative that investigation of the female autistic phenotype remains a high priority, given the suffering reported by late-diagnosed individuals [58, 63]. Maintaining the visibility of this topic is necessary to disseminate this kind of research to professionals within and outside the healthcare fields. A recent, startling finding from Hiller et al. [24] was that the majority of school-age autistic boys had been flagged up by their teachers in the pre-school years, whereas children who had never been a cause for concern were 13 times more likely to be female. The current study furthers investigation of how sex differences present in adulthood, through one screening instrument, the Ritvo Autism Asperger Diagnostic Scale [65]). Our inclusion of a large sample is a strength of the study, but it leaves many openings for future research which should control for psychiatric comorbidities and intellectual function. We may assume from the recruitment techniques and the samples collected (see Additional file 1) that our participants were of average to above-average intelligence. However, the findings cannot speak to the more nuanced issue of how intellectual disability might affect sex differences in autistic symptomatology in adults, and our discussion speaks only to symptom presentation in high-functioning individuals who had completed a self-report measure.

Conclusions

In these high-functioning individuals, the data from our meta-analysis reveals that autistic women did not statistically differ from autistic men in self-reported symptomatology in domains related to social-relatedness, language and circumscribed interest, but should be ratified by objective measures. It also highlights again the need for research to take into account the so-called ascertainment bias in studying those women who have reached diagnostic cut-offs on androcentric measures, and so whom may plausibly display a more male-like profile. Given the frequent use of child, adolescent and adult screening instruments by diagnostic services, whether these tools can adequately detect more unusual female presentations and subtle camouflaging, as implied in the qualitative literature [34, 35, 58], is of serious concern. An emergent emphasis by autistic women on their sensorimotor symptoms, however, is of potential clinical relevance, given the traditional downplaying of these items in diagnostic instruments and criteria, and requires further investigation.

Endnotes

[1]Unusually, four of the twenty items within this domain describe difficulties modulating vocal tone, pitch and volume which in other diagnostic instruments are related rather to differences in language and social communication [56, 81]. The apparent incongruence of these items within this domain is corroborated by the fact that the factor analysis conducted by the original authors [65] found these items loaded instead on factors related to social relatedness and social blindness. The sensorimotor domain, inadequately specific for autism, was subsequently removed from the RAADS-14 [71]

Abbreviations

ADI-R: Autism Diagnostic Interview Revised; ADOS-G: Autism Diagnostic Observation Schedule; ASC: Autism spectrum conditions; RAADS-R: Ritvo Autism Asperger Diagnostic Scale Revised; RRBI: Repetitive and restricted behaviours and interest; TD: Typically developing

Acknowledgements

We would like to acknowledge and thank our colleagues at Bournemouth University for their support, most especially Dr. Bernhard Angele, who provided statistical advice. We would like to thank the students who assisted in TD data collection, Ms. Asia Rose, Ms. Holly Stevens, Ms. Rebecca-Ann Jakeman, and Ms. Lana Gilbert, and all the participants who took part. This study would not have been possible without the assistance of the Community Adult Autism Service in Dorset, for providing us with the Bournemouth autism dataset, and the researchers we communicated with, who so generously shared their data with us—we extend our sincerest gratitude to all involved.

Authors' contributions

Data was collected by all three researchers. Dr. RLM wrote the manuscript, which was edited and contributed to by Dr. JAK and Ms. RH. All authors read and approved the final manuscript.

Competing interests

The authors declare that they have no competing interests.

References

1. Lehnhardt FG, Falter CM, Gawronski A, Pfeiffer K, Tepest R, Franklin J, et al. Sex-related cognitive profile in autism spectrum disorders diagnosed late in life: implications for the female autistic phenotype. J Autism Dev Disord. 2016;46:139–54.
2. Werling DMDM, Geschwind DHDH. Sex differences in autism spectrum disorders. Curr Opin Neurol [Internet] 2013;26:146–153. Available from: http://journals.lww.com/co-neurology/Abstract/2013/04000/Sex_differences_in_autism_spectrum_disorders.6.aspx%5Cn, http://www.pubmedcentral.nih.gov/articlerender.fcgi?artid=4164392&tool=pmcentrez&rendertype=abstract
3. Rutherford M, McKenzie K, Johnson T, Catchpole C, O'Hare A, McClure I, et al. Gender ratio in a clinical population sample, age of diagnosis and duration of assessment in children and adults with autism spectrum disorder. Autism [Internet]. 2016;20(5):628–34. Available from: http://www.ncbi.nlm.nih.gov/pubmed/26825959.
4. Loomes R, Hull L, Mandy WPL. What is the male-to-female ratio in autism spectrum disorder? A systematic review and meta-analysis. J Am Acad Child Adolesc Psychiatry 2017;56:466–474. Available from: http://www.ncbi.nlm.nih.gov/pubmed/28545751%0A, http://linkinghub.elsevier.com/retrieve/pii/S0890856717301521
5. Lai M-C, Lombardo M V., Auyeung B, Chakrabarti B, Baron-Cohen S. Sex/gender differences and autism: setting the scene for future research. J. Am. Acad. Child Adolesc. Psychiatry [Internet]. Elsevier; 2015 [cited 2014 Dec 18];54:11–24. Available from: https://www.jaacap.org/article/S0890-8567(14)00725-4/abstract
6. Sato D, Lionel AC, Leblond CS, Prasad A, Pinto D, Walker S, et al. SHANK1 Deletions in Males with Autism Spectrum Disorder. Am. J. Hum. Genet. [Internet]. 2017;90:879–87. Available from: https://doi.org/10.1016/j.ajhg.2012.03.017
7. Hallmayer J, Cleveland S, Torres A, Phillips J, Cohen B, Torigoe T, et al. Genetic heritability and shared environmental factors among twin pairs with autism. Arch. Gen. Psychiatry [Internet]. 2011 [cited 2014 Jul 26];68:1095–102. Available from: http://www.ncbi.nlm.nih.gov/pubmed/21727249
8. Robinson EB, Lichtenstein P, Anckarsater H, Happe F, Ronald A. Examining and interpreting the female protective effect against autistic behavior. Proc Natl Acad Sci [Internet]. 2013;110:5258–62. Available from: http://www.pnas.org/cgi/doi/10.1073/pnas.1211070110
9. Ratto AB, Kenworthy L, Yerys BE, Bascom J, Wieckowski AT, White SW, Scarpa A. What about the girls? Sex-based differences in autistic traits and adaptive skills. J Autism Dev Disord. 2018;48(5):1698-1711.
10. Halladay AK, Bishop S, Constantino JN, Daniels AM, Koenig K, Palmer K, et al. Sex and gender differences in autism spectrum disorder: summarizing evidence gaps and identifying emerging areas of priority. Mol Autism. 2015;6:1–5.
11. Andersson GW, Gillberg C, Miniscalco C. Pre-school children with suspected autism spectrum disorders: do girls and boys have the same profiles? Res Dev Disabil. 2013;34:413–22.
12. Fulton AM, Paynter JM, Trembath D. Gender comparisons in children with ASD entering early intervention. Res Dev Disabil. 2017;68:27–34.
13. Postorino V, Fatta LM, De Peppo L, Giovagnoli G, Armando M, Vicari S, et al. Longitudinal comparison between male and female preschool children with autism spectrum disorder. J Autism Dev Disord. 2015;45:2046–55.
14. American Psychiatric Association. Diagnostic and statistical manual of mental disorders (DSM-5®). Arlington: American Psychiatric Pub; 2013.
15. Van Wijngaarden-Cremers PJM, Van Eeten E, Groen WB, Van Deurzen PA, Oosterling IJ, Van Der Gaag RJ. Gender and age differences in the core triad of impairments in autism spectrum disorders: a systematic review and meta-analysis. J Autism Dev Disord. 2014:627–35.
16. Holtmann M, Bölte S, Poustka F. Autism spectrum disorders: sex differences in autistic behaviour domains and coexisting psychopathology. Dev Med Child Neurol. 2007;49:361–6.
17. Frazier TW, Georgiades S, Bishop SL, Hardan AY. Behavioral and cognitive characteristics of females and males with autism in the Simons Simplex Collection. J Am Acad Child Adolesc Psychiatry. 2014;53(3):329–340.e3.
18. McLennan JD, Lord C, Schopler E. Sex differences in higher functioning people with autism. J Autism Dev Disord [Internet]. 1993;23(2):217–27. Available from: http://link.springer.com/10.1007/BF01046216
19. Begeer S, Mandell D, Wijnker-Holmes B, Venderbosch S, Rem D, Stekelenburg F, et al. Sex differences in the timing of identification among children and adults with autism spectrum disorders. J. Autism Dev. Disord. [Internet]. 2013 [cited 2015 Apr 1];43:1151–6. Available from: http://www.ncbi.nlm.nih.gov/pubmed/23001766
20. Giarelli E, Wiggins LD, Rice CE, Levy SE, Kirby RS, Pinto-Martin J, et al. Sex differences in the evaluation and diagnosis of autism spectrum disorders among children. Disabil. Health J. [Internet]. Elsevier Inc; 2010 [cited 2015 Apr 1];3:107–16. Available from: http://www.ncbi.nlm.nih.gov/pubmed/21122776
21. Dworzynski K, Ronald A, Bolton P, Happé F. How different are girls and boys above and below the diagnostic threshold for autism spectrum disorders? J. Am. Acad. Child Adolesc. Psychiatry [Internet]. Elsevier Inc.; 2012 [cited 2015 Feb 4];51:788–97. Available from: http://www.ncbi.nlm.nih.gov/pubmed/22840550
22. Kirkovski M, Enticott PG, Fitzgerald PB. A review of the role of female gender in autism spectrum disorders. J. Autism Dev. Disord. [Internet]. 2013 [cited 2015 Mar 3];43:2584–603. Available from: http://www.ncbi.nlm.nih.gov/pubmed/23525974
23. Rynkiewicz A, Schuller B, Marchi E, Piana S, Camurri A, Lassalle A, et al. An investigation of the "female camouflage effect" in autism using a computerized ADOS-2 and a test of sex/gender differences. Mol. Autism. 2016;7:1–8.
24. Hiller R, Young RL, Weber N. Sex differences in pre-diagnosis concerns for children later diagnosed with autism spectrum disorder. Autism. 2016;20:75–84.
25. Wing L, Gould J. Severe impairments of social interaction and associated abnormalities in children: epidemiology and classification. J Autism Dev Disord. 1979;9:11–29.
26. Kopp S, Gillberg C. Girls with social deficits and learning problems: autism, atypical Asperger syndrome or a variant of these conditions. Eur Child Adolesc Psychiatry. 1992;1:89–99.
27. Rivet TT, Matson JL. Review of gender differences in core symptomatology in autism spectrum disorders. Res. Autism Spectr. Disord. [Internet]. Elsevier Ltd; 2011 [cited 2015 Feb 21];5:957–76. Available from: http://linkinghub.elsevier.com/retrieve/pii/S1750946710001264
28. Wainscot JJ, Naylor P, Sutcliffe P, Tantam D, Williams JV. Relationships with peers and use of the school environment of mainstream secondary school pupils with Asperger syndrome (high-functioning autism): a case-control study. Int J Psychol Psychol Ther. 2008;8:25–38.

29. Head AM, McGillivray J A, Stokes M A. Gender differences in emotionality and sociability in children with autism spectrum disorders. Mol. Autism [Internet]. Molecular Autism; 2014 [cited 2015 Mar 19];5:19. Available from: http://www.pubmedcentral.nih.gov/articlerender.fcgi?artid=3945617&tool=pmcentrez&rendertype=abstract

30. Sedgewick F, Hill V, Yates R, Pickering L, Pellicano E. Gender differences in the social motivation and friendship experiences of autistic and non-autistic adolescents. J Autism Dev Disord. 2016;46:1297–306.

31. Kuo MH, Orsmond GI, Cohn ES, Coster WJ. Friendship characteristics and activity patterns of adolescents with an autism spectrum disorder. Autism [Internet]. 2013;17:481–500. Available from: http://www.ncbi.nlm.nih.gov/pubmed/22087043

32. Foggo RSV, Webster AA. Understanding the social experiences of adolescent females on the autism spectrum. Res. Autism Spectr. Disord. 2017;35:74–85.

33. Gould J, Ashton-Smith J. Missed diagnosis or misdiagnosis? Girls and women on the autism spectrum. Good Autism Pract. 2011;12:34–41.

34. Hull L, Petrides KV, Allison C, Smith P, Baron-Cohen S, Lai MC, et al. "Putting on my best normal": social camouflaging in adults with autism spectrum conditions. J Autism Dev Disord. 2017:1–16.

35. Tierney S, Burns J, Kilbey E. Looking behind the mask: social coping strategies of girls on the autistic spectrum. Res Autism Spectr Disord. 2016;23:73–83.

36. Lai M-C, Lombardo M V, Ruigrok AN, Chakrabarti B, Auyeung B, Szatmari P, et al. Quantifying and exploring camouflaging in men and women with autism. Autism [Internet]. 2016;1–13. Available from: http://www.ncbi.nlm.nih.gov/pubmed/27899710

37. Goldman S. Opinion: sex, gender and the diagnosis of autism—a biosocial view of the male preponderance. Res. Autism Spectr. Disord. 2013;7:675–9.

38. Bauminger N, Solomon M, Rogers SJ. Predicting friendship quality in autism spectrum disorders and typical development. J Autism Dev Disord. 2010;40:751–61.

39. Solomon M, Miller M, Taylor SL, Hinshaw SP, Carter CS. Autism symptoms and internalizing psychopathology in girls and boys with autism spectrum disorders. J. Autism Dev. Disord. [Internet]. 2012 [cited 2015 Feb 6];42:48–59. Available from: http://www.pubmedcentral.nih.gov/articlerender.fcgi?artid=3244604&tool=pmcentrez&rendertype=abstract

40. Hiller RM, Young RL, Weber N. Sex differences in autism spectrum disorder based on DSM-5 criteria: evidence from clinician and teacher reporting. J. Abnorm. Child Psychol. [Internet]. 2014 [cited 2015 Feb 4];42:1381–93. Available from: http://www.ncbi.nlm.nih.gov/pubmed/24882502

41. May T, Cornish K, Rinehart N. Does gender matter? A one year follow-up of autistic, attention and anxiety symptoms in high-functioning children with autism spectrum disorder. J Autism Dev Disord. 2014;44:1077–86.

42. Mandy W, Chilvers R, Chowdhury U, Salter G, Seigal A, Skuse D. Sex differences in autism spectrum disorder: evidence from a large sample of children and adolescents. J Autism Dev Disord. 2012;42:1304–13.

43. Park S, Cho SC, Cho IH, Kim BN, Kim JW, Shin MS, et al. Sex differences in children with autism spectrum disorders compared with their unaffected siblings and typically developing children. Res. Autism Spectr. Disord. [Internet]. 2012;6:861–70. Available from: https://www.sciencedirect.com/science/article/pii/S1750946711001978.

44. Zwaigenbaum L, Bryson SE, Szatmari P, Brian J, Smith IM, Roberts W, et al. Sex differences in children with autism spectrum disorder identified within a high-risk infant cohort. J. Autism Dev. Disord. [Internet]. 2012;42:2585–96. Available from: http://www.ncbi.nlm.nih.gov/pubmed/22453928

45. Szatmari P, Liu XQ, Goldberg J, Zwaigenbaum L, Paterson AD, Woodbury-Smith M, et al. Sex differences in repetitive stereotyped behaviors in autism: implications for genetic liability. Am J Med Genet Part B Neuropsychiatr Genet. 2012;159 B:5–12.

46. Tillmann J, Ashwood K, Absoud M, Bölte S, Bonnet-Brilhault F, Buitelaar JK, De Bildt A. Evaluating Sex and Age Differences in ADI-R and ADOS Scores in a Large European Multi-site Sample of Individuals with Autism Spectrum Disorder. J Autism Dev Disord. 2018;1-16.

47. Knickmeyer RC, Wheelwright S, Baron-Cohen S. Sex-typical play: masculinization/defeminization in girls with an autism spectrum condition. J Autism Dev Disord. 2008;38:1028–35.

48. Nguyen C, Sc M, Ronald A. How do girls with low functioning autism compare to boys with autism and typically developing girls with regard to behavior, cognition, and psychopathology? Scand J Child Adolesc Psychiatry Psychol [Internet] 2014;2:55–65.

49. Kumazaki H, Muramatsu T, Kosaka H, Fujisawa TX, Iwata K, Tomoda A, et al. Sex differences in cognitive and symptom profiles in children with high functioning autism spectrum disorders. Res Autism Spectr Disord. 2015;13:1–7.

50. Ketelaars MP, In't Velt A, Mol A, Swaab H, Bodrij F, van Rijn S. Social attention and autism symptoms in high functioning women with autism spectrum disorders. Res Dev Disabil. 2017;64:78–86.

51. Klin A, Jones W, Schultz R, Volkmar F, Cohen D. Visual Fixation Patterns During Viewing of Naturalistic Social Situations as Predictors of Social Competence in Individuals With Autism. Arch. Gen. Psychiatry [Internet]. 2002;59:809. Available from: http://archpsyc.jamanetwork.com/article.aspx?doi=10.1001/archpsyc.59.9.809

52. Kliemann D, Dziobek I, Hatri A, Steimke R, Heekeren HR. Atypical reflexive gaze patterns on emotional faces in autism spectrum disorders. J Neurosci [Internet]. 2010;30:12281–7. Available from: http://www.jneurosci.org/cgi/doi/10.1523/JNEUROSCI.0688-10.2010

53. Lai MC, Lombardo MV, Pasco G, Ruigrok ANV, Wheelwright SJ, Sadek SA, et al. A behavioral comparison of male and female adults with high functioning autism spectrum conditions. PLoS One. 2011;6

54. Lai MC, Lombardo MV, Ruigrok ANV, Chakrabarti B, Wheelwright SJ, Auyeung B, et al. Cognition in males and females with autism: similarities and differences. PLoS One. 2012;7(10):e47198

55. Baron-Cohen S, Cassidy S, Auyeung B, Allison C, Achoukhi M, Robertson S, et al. Attenuation of typical sex differences in 800 adults with autism vs. 3,900 controls. PLoS One. 2014;9(7):e102251.

56. Lord C, Risi S, Lambrecht L, Cook EH, Leventhal BL, Dilavore PC, et al. The autism diagnostic observation schedule-generic: a standard measure of social and communication deficits associated with the spectrum of autism. J Autism Dev Disord. 2000;30:205–23.

57. Bolte S, Duketis E, Poustka F, Holtmann M. Sex differences in cognitive domains and their clinical correlates in higher-functioning autism spectrum disorders. Autism. 2011;15:497–511.

58. Bargiela S, Steward R, Mandy W. The experiences of late-diagnosed women with autism spectrum conditions: an investigation of the female autism phenotype. J Autism Dev Dsorders. 2016;46:3281–94.

59. Hendrickx S. Women and girls with autism spectrum disorder: understanding life experiences from early childhood to old age. London: Jessica Kingsley Publishers; 2015.

60. Kenworthy L, Yerys BE, Anthony LG, Wallace GL. Understanding executive control in autism spectrum disorders in the lab and in the real world. Neuropsychol Rev. 2008;18(4):320–38.

61. Lemon JM, Gargaro B, Enticott PG, Rinehart NJ. Executive functioning in autism spectrum disorders: a gender comparison of response inhibition. J Autism Dev Disord. 2011;41:352–6.

62. Memari AH, Ziaee V, Shayestehfar M, Ghanouni P, Mansournia MA, Moshayedi P. Cognitive flexibility impairments in children with autism spectrum disorders: links to age, gender and child outcomes. Res Dev Disabil. 2013;34:3218–25.

63. Baldwin S, Costley D. The experiences and needs of female adults with high-functioning autism spectrum disorder. Autism. 2016;20:483–95.

64. Lai MC, Baron-Cohen S. Identifying the lost generation of adults with autism spectrum conditions. The Lancet Psychiatry. 2015;2(11):1013–27.

65. Ritvo RA, Ritvo ER, Guthrie D, Ritvo MJ, Hufnagel DH, McMahon W, et al. The Ritvo Autism Asperger Diagnostic Scale-Revised (RAADS-R): a scale to assist the diagnosis of autism spectrum disorder in adults: an international validation study. J Autism Dev Disord. 2011;41:1076–89.

66. Van Casteren M, Davis MH. Match: a program to assist in matching the conditions of factorial experiments. Behav Res Methods. 2007;39:973–8.

67. National Institute of Health and Care Excellence. Autism spectrum disorder in adults: diagnosis and management [Internet]. NICE Guidel. 2012 [cited 2017 Dec 30]. Available from: https://www.nice.org.uk/guidance/cg142/chapter/1-guidance

68. Stoesz BM, Montgomery JM, Smart SL, Hellsten L-AM. Review of five instruments for the assessment of Asperger's disorder in adults. Clin Neuropsychol [Internet] 2011;25:376–401. Available from: http://www.informaworld.com/smpp/title~content=t713721659%5Cnhttp://dx.doi.org/10.1080/13854046.2011.559482%5Cn, http://www.informaworld.com/%5Cn, http://www.psypress.com/tcn

69. Frazier TW, Ratliff KR, Gruber C, Zhang Y, Law P A, Constantino JN. Confirmatory factor analytic structure and measurement invariance of quantitative autistic traits measured by the Social Responsiveness Scale-2.

Autism [Internet]. 2014;18:31–44. Available from: http://www.ncbi.nlm.nih.gov/pubmed/24019124

70. Andersen LMJ, Näswall K, Manouilenko I, Nylander L, Edgar J, Ritvo RA, et al. The Swedish version of the Ritvo Autism and Asperger Diagnostic Scale: Revised (RAADS-R). A validation study of a rating scale for adults. J Autism Dev Disord. 2011;41:1635–45.

71. Eriksson JM, Andersen LM, Bejerot S. RAADS-14 Screen: validity of a screening tool for autism spectrum disorder in an adult psychiatric population. Mol. Autism [Internet]. 2013;4:49. Available from: http://www.pubmedcentral.nih.gov/articlerender.fcgi?artid=3907126&tool=pmcentrez&rendertype=abstract

72. American Psychiatric Association. Diagnostic and statistical manual of mental disorders (4th Edition, Revision). Fourth. Washington, DC: American Psychiatric Association; 2000.

73. Organization WH. The ICD-10 classification of mental and behavioural disorders: clinical descriptions and diagnostic guidelines. World Health Organization [Internet]. 1992;1–267. Available from: http://apps.who.int/iris/handle/10665/37958%5Cn, http://scholar.google.com/scholar?hl=en&btnG=Search&q=intitle:The+ICD-10+Classification+of+Mental+and+Behavioural+Disorders#1

74. Field AP, Gillett R. How to do a meta-analysis. Br J Math Stat Psychol. 2016; 63:665–94.

75. Vagni D, Moscone D, Travaglione S, Cotugno A. Using the Ritvo Autism Asperger Diagnostic Scale-Revised (RAADS-R) disentangle the heterogeneity of autistic traits in an Italian eating disorder population. Res. Autism Spectr. Disord. 2016;32:143–55.

76. Satterfield D, Lepage C, Ladjahasan N. Preferences for online course delivery methods in higher education for students with autism spectrum disorders. Procedia Manuf. 2015;3

77. Baron-Cohen. The extreme male brain theory of autism. Trends Cogn. Sci. [Internet]. 2002;6:248–54. Available from: https://www.ncbi.nlm.nih.gov/pubmed/12039606

78. Baron-Cohen S, Baron-Cohen S. The hyper-systemizing, assortative mating theory of autism. Prog Neuro-Psychopharmacol Biol Psychiatry. 2006;30(5): 865–72. Prog. Neuro-Psychopharmacology Biol. Psychiatry. 2006;30:865–72

79. Baron-Cohen S, Auyeung B, Nørgaard-Pedersen B, Hougaard DM, Abdallah MW, Melgaard L, et al. Elevated fetal steroidogenic activity in autism. Mol. Psychiatry [Internet]. 2015;20:369–76. Available from: http://www.ncbi.nlm.nih.gov/pubmed/24888361

80. Auyeung B, Taylor K, Hackett G, Baron-Cohen S. Foetal testosterone and autistic traits in 18 to 24-month-old children. Mol Autism. 2010;1:11.

81. Le Couteur A, Lord C, Rutter M. The autism diagnostic interview-revised (ADI-R). Los Angeles: Western Psychological Services; 2003.

82. Wallentin M. Putative sex differences in verbal abilities and language cortex: a critical review. Brain Lang. 2009;108:175–83.

83. Wing L, Leekam SR, Libby SJ, Gould J, Larcombe M. The diagnostic interview for social and communication disorders: background, inter-rater reliability and clinical use. J Child Psychol Psychiatry Allied Discip. 2002;43: 307–25.

84. Klintwall L, Holm A, Eriksson M, Carlsson LH, Olsson MB, Hedvall Å, et al. Sensory abnormalities in autism. A brief report. Res Dev Disabil. 2011;32: 795–800.

85. Marco EJ, Hinkley LBN, Hill SS, Nagarajan SS. Sensory processing in autism: a review of neurophysiologic findings. Pediatr Res. 2011;69

86. Fournier KA, Hass CJ, Naik SK, Lodha N, Cauraugh JH. Motor coordination in autism spectrum disorders: a synthesis and meta-analysis. J Autism Dev Disord. 2010;40:1227–40.

87. Moseley RL, Pulvermüller F. What can autism teach us about the role of sensorimotor systems in higher cognition? New clues from studies on language, action semantics, and abstract emotional concept processing. Cortex. 2018;100:149-190

88. Kopp S, Beckung E, Gillberg C. Developmental coordination disorder and other motor control problems in girls with autism spectrum disorder and/or attention-deficit/hyperactivity disorder. Res Dev Disabil. 2010;31:350–61.

89. Schopler E, Van Bourgondien ME, Wellman GJ, Love SR. The childhood autism rating scale. Los Angeles: WPS; 1980.

90. Ladwig KH, Marten-Mittag B, Formanek B, Dammann G. Gender differences of symptom reporting and medical health care utilization in the German population. Eur J Epidemiol. 2000;16:511–8.

91. Green CA, Pope CR. Gender, psychosocial factors and the use of medical services: a longitudinal analysis. Soc Sci Med. 1999;48:1363–72.

92. Lane AE, Molloy CA, Bishop SL. Classification of children with autism spectrum disorder by sensory subtype: a case for sensory-based phenotypes. Autism Res. 2014;7:322–33.

93. Croen LA, Zerbo O, Qian Y, Massolo ML, Rich S, Sidney S, et al. The health status of adults on the autism spectrum. Autism [Internet]. 2015;19:814–23. Available from: http://www.ncbi.nlm.nih.gov/pubmed/25911091

94. Fountain C, King MD, Bearman PS. Age of diagnosis for autism: individual and community factors across 10 birth cohorts. J Epidemiol Community Health. 2011;65:503–10.

95. Croen LA, Grether JK, Selvin S. Descriptive epidemiology of autism in a California population: who is at risk? J Autism Dev Disord. 2002;32:217–24.

96. Durkin MS, Maenner MJ, Meaney FJ, Levy SE, di Guiseppi C, Nicholas JS, et al. Socioeconomic inequality in the prevalence of autism spectrum disorder: evidence from a U.S. cross-sectional study. PLoS One. 2010;5

97. Thomas P, Zahorodny W, Peng B, Kim S, Jani N, Halperin W, et al. The association of autism diagnosis with socioeconomic status. Autism [Internet]. 2012;16:201–13. Available from: http://journals.sagepub.com/doi/10.1177/1362361311413397

98. Mandell DS, Novak MM, Zubritsky CD. Factors associated with age of diagnosis among children with autism spectrum disorders. Pediatrics [Internet]. 2005;116:1480–6. Available from: http://www.ncbi.nlm.nih.gov/pubmed/16322174%5Cn, http://www.pubmedcentral.nih.gov/articlerender.fcgi?artid=PMC2861294

99. Mandell DS, Listerud J, Levy SE, Pinto-Martin JA. Race differences in the age at diagnosis among Medicaid-eligible children with autism. J. Am. Acad. Child Adolesc. Psychiatry [Internet]. 2002;41:1447–53. Available from: http://www.sciencedirect.com/science/article/pii/S0890856709607395

100. Begeer S, Bouk S El, Boussaid W, Terwogt MM, Koot HM. Underdiagnosis and referral bias of autism in ethnic minorities. J Autism Dev Disord 2009;39:142–148.

101. Matson JL, Worley JA, Fodstad JC, Chung K-M, Suh D, Jhin HK, et al. A multinational study examining the cross cultural differences in reported symptoms of autism spectrum disorders: Israel, South Korea, the United Kingdom, and the United States of America. Res. Autism Spectr. Disord. [Internet]. 2011;5:1598–604. Available from: http://linkinghub.elsevier.com/retrieve/pii/S1750946711000705

102. Matson JL, Matheis M, Burns CO, Esposito G, Venuti P, Pisula E, et al. Examining cross-cultural differences in autism spectrum disorder: a multinational comparison from Greece, Italy, Japan, Poland, and the United States. Eur Psychiatry. 2017;42:70–6.

103. Ennis-Cole D, Durodoye BA, Harris HL. The impact of culture on autism diagnosis and treatment: considerations for counselors and other professionals. Fam J Couns Ther Couples Fam. 2013;21:279–87.

104. Hallmayer J, Cleveland S, Torres A, Phillips B, Torigoe T, Miller J, et al. Genetic heritability and shared environmental factors among twin pairs with autism. Arch. Gen. Psychiatry [Internet]. 2011;68:1095. Available from: http://archpsyc.jamanetwork.com/article.aspx?doi=10.1001/archgenpsychiatry.2011.76

105. Robinson EB, Lichtenstein P, Anckarsäter H, Happé F, Ronald A. Examining and interpreting the female protective effect against autistic behavior. Proc. Natl. Acad. Sci. U. S. A. [Internet]. 2013;110:5258–62. Available from: http://www.pubmedcentral.nih.gov/articlerender.fcgi?artid=3612665&tool=pmcentrez&rendertype=abstract

16

Practice patterns and determinants of wait time for autism spectrum disorder diagnosis in Canada

Melanie Penner[1,2], Evdokia Anagnostou[1,2] and Wendy J. Ungar[3,4*]

Abstract

Background: Inefficient diagnostic practices for autism spectrum disorder (ASD) may contribute to longer wait times, delaying access to intervention. The objectives were to describe the diagnostic practices of Canadian pediatricians and to identify determinants of longer wait time for ASD diagnosis.

Methods: An online survey was conducted through the Canadian Paediatric Society's developmental pediatrics, community pediatrics, and mental health sections. Participants were asked for demographic information, whether they diagnosed ASD, and elements of their diagnostic assessment. A multiple linear regression of total wait time (time from referral to communication of the diagnosis to the family) as a function of practice characteristics was conducted.

Results: A total of 90 participants completed the survey, of whom 57 diagnosed ASD in their practices (63.3%). Respondents reported varied use of multi-disciplinary teams, with 53% reporting participation in a team. No two identically composed teams were reported. Respondents also had varied use of diagnostic tools, with 21% reporting no use of tools. The median reported total wait for ASD diagnosis time was 7 months (interquartile range 4–12 months). Longer time spent on assessment was the only variable that remained significantly associated with longer wait time in multiple regression ($p = 0.002$). Use of diagnostic tools did not significantly affect wait time.

Conclusion: Canadian ASD diagnostic practices vary widely and wait times for these assessments are substantial—7 months from referral to receipt of diagnosis. Time spent on the assessment is a significant determinant of wait time, highlighting the need for efficient assessment practices.

Keywords: Autism spectrum disorder, Diagnosis, Early detection, Pediatrics, Health services research

Background

Autism spectrum disorder (ASD), a neurodevelopmental disorder defined by impairment in social communication and the presence of restricted repetitive behaviors [1], has steadily increased in reported prevalence over the past decade [2]. Pediatricians are frequently involved in ASD diagnosis in pre-school age children in Canada [3]. Numerous guidelines have been published for diagnostic assessment for ASD, with varied recommendations for personnel and tools in the assessment [4–9]. A concern about models for diagnostic assessment is how they may extend the waiting period to receive intervention. Waiting for an ASD diagnostic assessment occurs during a critical period of brain development [10] and an extended wait time may delay receipt of intervention and reduce effectiveness [11]. To date, little work has been done looking specifically at wait times for ASD diagnosis, and how diagnostic practices influence wait times.

Age at diagnosis has often been used as a proxy to understand wait times; however, other factors beyond diagnostic demand and supply influence this metric. Milder ASD subtypes have been associated with a later age at diagnosis [12]. These children may not show significant impairment associated with ASD until their

* Correspondence: wendy.ungar@sickkids.ca
[3]Technology Assessment at Sick Kids (TASK), Child Health Evaluative Sciences, The Hospital for Sick Children Research Institute, Toronto, Canada
[4]Institute of Health Policy, Management and Evaluation, University of Toronto, Toronto, Canada
Full list of author information is available at the end of the article

skills are exceeded by social demands, which will occur later for more mildly affected children. Additional studies have shown that severe language impairment/regression, unusual mannerisms, and toe walking were features of the clinical presentation associated with younger age at diagnosis [13, 14]. Co-occurring or alternative diagnoses such as attention deficit hyperactivity disorder may delay diagnostic evaluation for ASD [15]. Factors external to the child also decrease the age at diagnosis, including older maternal age [15] and having relatives with ASD [14], both of which may be indicative of caregivers who are more aware of the possibility of ASD. Lower socioeconomic status, being a visible minority, and living in a rural setting are all associated with an older age at diagnosis [13, 14, 16]. The number of potential confounders makes it difficult to isolate the impact of wait times for assessment on the diagnosis age.

Few studies have reported current ASD diagnostic practices and their association with wait times. One USA study evaluated factors related to wait times for diagnosis, which was 13 months on average in their sample [17]. Reported associations in this study were mostly between wait times and patient demographic factors, but there was no association between the use of a standardized diagnostic tool and mean age of first ASD diagnosis. One chart review of 70 children's cases from Scotland found that receiving more information prior to the assessment, such as contextual information and results of other assessments, reduced the number of assessment visits needed and decreased the total wait for diagnosis [18]. This sample was taken from only eight children's services, and therefore provides little insight on between-provider variability in practice and its impact on wait times.

Further information on diagnostic assessment and wait times from diverse clinical practices is needed to inform ASD service planning in constrained health care systems. The study objectives were to (1) document the diversity of practices of Canadian pediatricians with regard to their diagnostic assessment for ASD; and (2) to identify the elements of clinical diagnostic practice that are associated within a longer wait times for ASD diagnosis.

Methods
Study design
This was a cross-sectional survey of pediatricians across Canada to investigate ASD diagnostic practices. The study was approved by the Research Ethics Board of The Hospital for Sick Children and participants were informed that survey completion indicated their consent.

Target population
The Canadian Paediatric Society (CPS) is the national association of Canadian pediatricians, representing over

3000 pediatricians and pediatric trainees [19]. In Canada, most primary care is provided by family physicians, who consult pediatricians if the child's care needs exceed their scope of practice. Developmental pediatricians are subspecialists, some of whom only accept referrals from pediatricians, necessitating multiple referrals before reaching this level of expertise. There are no uniform ASD diagnostic requirements across Canada, making it an ideal setting to explore varying diagnostic practices and their impact on wait times. Three sections were chosen for survey distribution based on their likelihood of participating in ASD diagnosis: developmental pediatrics, community pediatrics, and mental health. Current members of these sections who were practicing pediatrics in Canada and who were able to complete the survey in English were eligible to participate.

Survey administration
The survey instrument was designed based on a review of the literature and clinical experiences of the researchers (Additional file 1). The survey collected information on provider demographics, (age, sex, province, catchment area, years in pediatric practice, type of health professional, training in child development). For those that diagnosed ASD in their practice, the survey asked about the participants' current wait time in months for the first visit of the diagnostic assessment and the current wait time in weeks from the first assessment visit to communication of the ASD diagnosis to the family. The survey was piloted in November 2014 with two Ontario developmental pediatricians and two general pediatricians. Minor changes were made to improve clarity. The main survey was administered in March 2015. Using an electronic mail list serve, the CPS sent all potential participants an email containing an online link to complete an electronic version of the survey created using REDCap (Research Electronic Data Capture) [20]. Participants had 3 weeks to complete the survey, during which they were sent two reminder emails.

Statistical analysis
All data were exported from the online database to R for statistical analysis (Vienna, Austria, 2014). Descriptive statistics were calculated for all question responses. Demographic characteristics for participants who diagnose ASD were compared to those who do not diagnose ASD using non-parametric statistics. The median amount billed per clinic visit was calculated. Time-based billing codes were excluded from the analysis as the total amount billed per visit could not be calculated without knowledge of the amount of time spent on each visit. Wait times for ASD diagnosis are defined in Fig. 1. The wait time between receiving the referral and the first

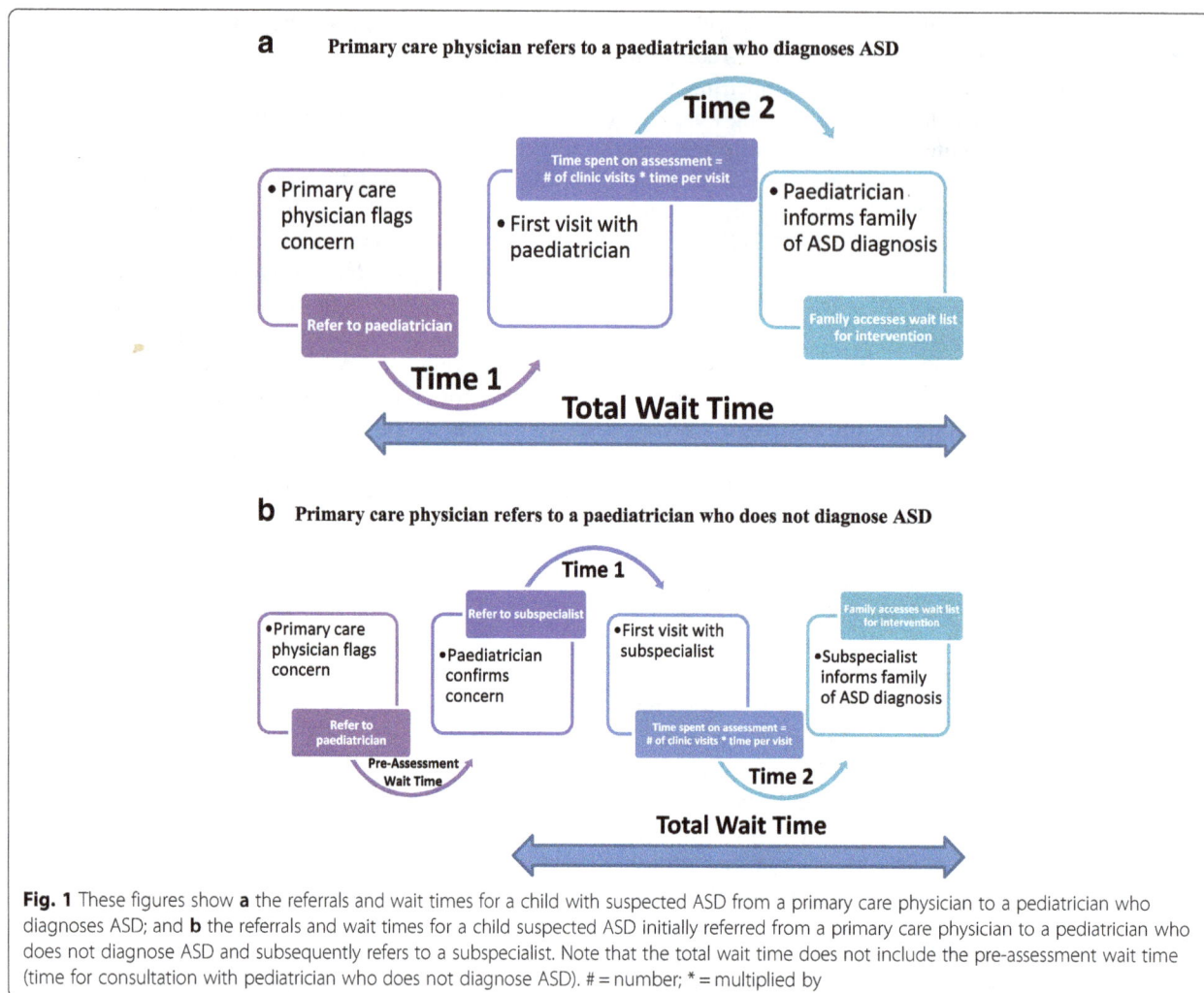

Fig. 1 These figures show **a** the referrals and wait times for a child with suspected ASD from a primary care physician to a pediatrician who diagnoses ASD; and **b** the referrals and wait times for a child suspected ASD initially referred from a primary care physician to a pediatrician who does not diagnose ASD and subsequently refers to a subspecialist. Note that the total wait time does not include the pre-assessment wait time (time for consultation with pediatrician who does not diagnose ASD). # = number; * = multiplied by

scheduled visit of the diagnostic assessment (time 1) was reported in months and converted to days in the analysis. The wait time from the first visit of the diagnostic assessment to the communication of the diagnosis to the family (time 2) was reported in weeks and converted to days for the analysis. The total wait time (in days) was calculated for each participant by adding time 1 and time 2. Times are reported in months for ease of interpretation.

A multiple linear regression of total wait time as a function of diagnostic assessment characteristics was conducted. A subspecialized assessor (a developmental pediatrician) and practicing in a multi-disciplinary team (MDT) were each hypothesized to be independently positively correlated with a longer wait time due to constraints on availability. Province of practice was included as a covariate, as provincial policies may dictate necessary elements of the assessment [4]. The clinician's catchment area was included because a larger service population may increase wait times [14]. Accepting referrals from family physicians was hypothesized to be

associated with longer wait times due to a higher volume of referrals for assessment. More junior clinicians have been reported to work fewer hours [21, 22], which may increase their wait times.

Time spent on assessment was calculated for each participant by multiplying the number of diagnostic visits by the average reported length of each visit selected from a list of options for visit length (Additional file 1); the mid-range value was taken as the average length of each visit. Longer time spent on assessment was hypothesized to be positively correlated with wait time due to fewer clinic slots available for new assessments.

A series of bivariate analyses to test the association between hypothesized covariates and total wait time were initially performed to determine which explanatory variables to include in the regression model. The significance level for inclusion in the model was set at 0.2. Because none of the variables were normally distributed, non-parametric tests including Spearman correlation for continuous variables and Kruskal-Wallis and Wilcoxon tests for categorical variables were used to determine the significance of the observed associations. Non-parametric tests were used to determine the relationship between all potential covariates. Two variables were considered to be collinear when they were significantly associated ($p < 0.05$); these variables were not tested together in the model. The dependent variable and each of the variables that were significant in the bivariate analyses were entered one by one to build a forward multivariate linear regression model. If a variable was significantly correlated with the dependent variable ($p < 0.05$), it remained in the model. As the dependent variable total wait time was skewed, it was transformed to a natural logarithm (ln), with normal distributions of the residuals confirmed for the ln-transformed analyses. Goodness of fit was tested with R^2. Back transformation of the ln-transformed dependent variable was performed by calculating the Duan smearing estimate [23]. The predicted values of wait time were multiplied by the smearing estimate to determine the mean adjusted wait times (with 95% confidence intervals) based on the included covariate(s).

An additional analysis was conducted to assess the association between wait time and diagnostic tool use. The total wait time was compared between respondents who did and did not report use of various diagnostic tools using Wilcoxon tests.

Results

Of 639 individuals solicited, 91 responses were received (response rate of 14%). One participant who was a speech language pathologist (not a pediatrician) was removed from the sample, leaving 90 respondents. Eighty-five respondents completed all mandatory questions (5 incomplete). The demographic information for the total sample is displayed in Table 1. A majority of participants (66%) were female. The sample included representation from all Canadian provinces with the exception of PEI, and from two territories (no responses from the Northwest Territories), with a proportionally larger representation from Ontario.

Practice characteristics

Practice characteristics were summarized separately for those who did not diagnose ASD ($n = 33$) and those who did ($n = 57$) and are compared in Table 1. There were no statistically significant differences between these two groups in their ages, years in practice, sex, province of practice, or catchment areas. Significant differences were seen between the two groups in the types of professionals, with all but one developmental pediatrician indicating they diagnose ASD, and in additional training in child development, where all participants who had undertaken a developmental pediatrics fellowship were in the diagnosing group.

Participants who did not diagnose ASD were pediatricians who would either confirm or refute a developmental concern raised by a primary care physician (Fig. 1). The median wait time for consultation with this group (pre-assessment wait time, Fig. 1b) was 70 days (range 14 to 560), with 60.1% of participants reporting a visit length of 46–75 min. The median amount billed for a developmental consultation was $171.82 (full list of reported billing codes for this group is presented in Appendix 1).

General information about ASD diagnosticians is reported in Table 2. Fifteen (26.3%) respondents provided a definitive assessment in more than half of their cases, although responses were missing for 44% of participants for this optional question. The majority of respondents (87.7%) reported that they referred to regional developmental intervention services for some or all of their assessments thereby obtaining input from other disciplines. Commonly ordered tests included hearing (80.7% of respondents ordered this in the majority of assessments), chromosomal microarray (68.4%), and Fragile X (64.9%).

A wide range of billing codes and amounts for ASD assessment was observed (Appendix 2). The first visit was associated with a median billing of $229.15 (range $47 to $411.87). The second visit had a median billing of $187 (range $76.71 to $300.70), and the third visit also had a median billing of $187 (range $92.40 to $300.70).

Participants indicated using a variety of tools in the assessment for ASD, including the Autism Diagnostic Observation Schedule (ADOS), the Autism Diagnostic Interview–Revised (ADI-R), and the Childhood Autism Rating Scale (CARS). Forty percent of participants (23 participants) used more than one tool as part of their assessment, though the most commonly reported tool employed was the ADOS alone (11 participants) followed by the ADOS and ADI-R combined (6 participants). Twelve participants (21.1%) reported using no tools in the assessment. The number of participants using each tool, along with the time spent on administration and scoring, is included in Appendix 3.

Although 52.6% of diagnosticians reported practicing as part of a MDT, no two MDTs across the country had the same composition, even when limiting to team members involved in the majority of assessments. While 57% of respondents indicated that psychologists participated in the majority of diagnostic assessments, 5 of the 30 respondents belonging to MDTs did not have access to a psychologist. Speech language pathologists and occupational therapists were also frequently identified team members. The frequencies of clinicians available to MDTs, as well as those included in the majority of diagnostic assessments, are shown in Fig. 2.

Table 1 Demographics and practice patterns

Characteristic	Total sample (n = 90)		Diagnose ASD (n = 57)		Do not diagnose ASD (n = 33)		p
	n	%	n	%	n	%	
Age (years), median; range; IQR	54; 29–77; 42–63		52; 29–77; 41–60		57; 31–76; 45–64		0.17[a]
Years in practice, median; range; IQR	21; 0.5–46; 8–30.5		18; 0.5–46; 7–28		26; 1–44; 13–35		0.08[b]
Sex							
Male	30	33.3%	19	33.3%	11	33.3%	
Female	60	66.7%	38	66.7%	22	66.7%	1
Province of practice							
Ontario	39	43.3%	27	47.4%	12	36.3%	
Alberta	15	16.7%	11	19.3%	4	12.1%	
Quebec	12	13.3%	4	7%	8	24.2%	
British Columbia	6	6.7%	3	5.3%	3	9.1%	
New Brunswick	4	4.4%	4	7%	–	–	
Newfoundland and Labrador	4	4.4%	2	3.5%	2	6.1%	
Nova Scotia	4	4.4%	1	1.8%	3	9.1%	
Manitoba	2	2.2%	1	1.8%	1	3%	
Saskatchewan	2	2.2%	2	3.5%	–	–	
Nunavut	1	1.1%	1	1.8%	–	–	
Yukon	1	1.1%	1	1.8%	–	–	0.14[c]
Catchment							
Within regional health authority	28	31.1%	20	35.1%	8	24.2%	
Within city only	23	25.6%	15	26.3%	8	24.2%	
Within province/territory	20	22.2%	15	26.3%	5	15.1%	
No defined catchment	17	18.9%	7	12.3%	10	30.3%	
Missing	2	2.2%	–	–	2	6.1%	0.07[c]
Type of professional							
General pediatrician	64	70%	33	57.9%	31	93.9%	
Developmental pediatrician	23	25.6%	22	38.6%	1	3%	
Neonatologist	2	2.2%	1	1.8%	1	3%	
Pediatrician + allergist	1	1.1%	1	1.8%	–	–	< 0.01[c]
Extra training in child development							
None	57	63.3%	28	49.1%	29	87.9%	
Fellowship in developmental pediatrics	22	24.4%	22	38.6%	–	–	
General pediatrics training with additional child development	5	5.6%	3	5.3%	2	6.1%	
Continuing medical education	2	2.2%	1	1.8%	1	3%	
Fellowship in pediatric neurology	2	2.2%	2	3.5%	–	–	
Participation in a MDT	1	1.1%	1	1.8%	–	–	
Missing	1	1.1%	–	–	1	3%	< 0.01[c]

IQR interquartile range, MDT multi-disciplinary team; percentages may not sum to 100% due to rounding
[a]Wilcoxon rank sum test W = 803
[b]Wilcoxon rank sum test W = 758
[c]Using Fisher's exact test

Wait times

Wait times for a first visit (time 1) varied from 1 to 24 months (interquartile range 3–9 months). Wait times for a diagnosis (time 2) also had a wide range, with half of the respondents reporting an interval of between 0.5 and 1.5 months, with some respondents indicating a much longer wait. The total wait time varied from 2 to 24 months, with a median of 7 months (Table 3).

Table 2 Practice patterns for participants who diagnose ASD (n = 57)

Practice characteristic	n	%
Accepts referrals from family doctor		
Yes	44	77.2%
No	12	21.1%
Missing	1	1.8%
Number of visits to make a diagnosis of ASD		
1 visit	8	14.0%
2 visits	33	57.9%
3 visits	11	19.3%
4 visits	4	7.0%
5 visits	1	1.8%
Reported typical visit length		
< 30 min	3	5.3%
31–60 min	20	35.1%
61–90 min	19	33.3%
91–120 min	8	14.0%
121–180 min	5	8.8%
> 180 min	2	3.5%
For what percentage of cases of ASD do you provide a definitive assessment?		
0–25%	6	10.5%
26–50%	11	19.3%
51–75%	4	7.0%
76–100%	11	19.3%
Missing	25	43.9%
Practice in MDT		
Yes	30	52.6%
No	27	47.4%
Percentage of cases assessed with MDT		
1–25%	4	7.0%
26–50%	3	5.3%
51–75%	5	8.8%
76–100%	18	31.6%
(Did not practice in team) 0%	27	47.4%
Percentage of assessments with consultation with regional speech-language pathology		
0%	1	1.8%
1–25%	17	29.8%
26–50%	12	21.1%
51–75%	9	15.8%
76–100%	17	29.8%
Missing	1	1.8%
Percentage of assessments with consultation with regional developmental early intervention staff		
0%	7	12.3%

Table 2 Practice patterns for participants who diagnose ASD (n = 57) (Continued)

Practice characteristic	n	%
1–25%	20	35.1%
26–50%	13	22.8%
51–75%	6	10.5%
76–100%	10	17.5%
Missing	1	1.8%
Percentage of assessments with consultation with regional occupational therapist		
0%	5	8.8%
1–25%	27	47.4%
26–50%	11	19.3%
51–75%	6	10.5%
76–100%	7	12.3%
Missing	1	1.8%
Tests ordered for the majority of assessments		
Hearing	46	80.7%
Chromosomal microarray	39	68.4%
Fragile X	37	64.9%
Vision	22	38.6%
Metabolic screening	9	15.8%
MRI brain	4	7.0%
MECP2	3	5.3%
EEG	0	–
Other[a]	2	3.5%
None	1	1.8%

[a]Text response: "Depends on presentation"; *ASD* autism spectrum disorders, *EEG* electroencephalogram, *MDT* multidisciplinary team, *MECP2* methyl cytosine phosphate guanine binding protein 2 (genetic testing for Rett syndrome), *MRI* magnetic resonance imaging; percentages may not sum to 100% due to rounding; respondents could select more than one test and these percentages will not sum to 100% as a result

The results of bivariate analyses exploring potentially significant demographic and practice factors explaining total wait time are presented in Table 4. Time spent on assessment was significantly positively correlated with total wait time ($r = 0.31$, $p = 0.02$). The type of assessor was significant with general pediatricians having a longer median total wait time compared with developmental pediatricians, which was contrary to expectations. Further analysis showed that general pediatricians had a shorter median time 1 (4 versus 6 months for developmental pediatricians), and an identical median time 2 (1 month), though their combined time 1 and 2 was longer. The differences in total wait times between provinces were sufficiently significant to merit inclusion in the model, with total wait time varying from 5 months in Alberta to 14.5 months in Quebec. As type of assessor was significantly associated with time spent on assessment (Kruskal-Wallis chi-squared = 5.59; degrees of

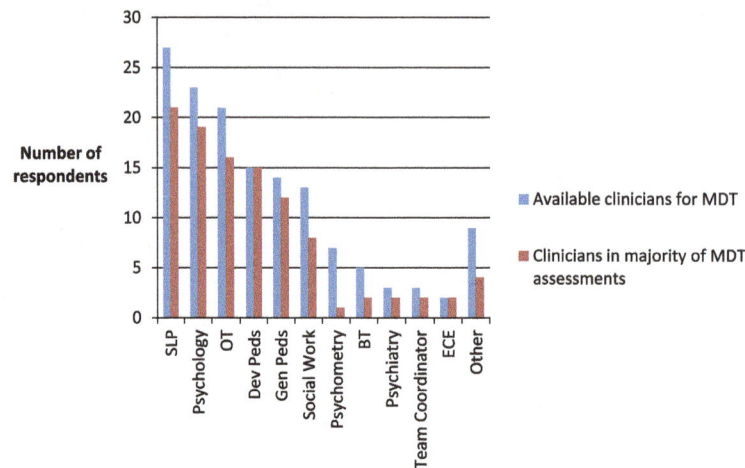

Fig. 2 This figure shows the number of respondents indicating participation of each type of clinician available to the MDT for involvement in diagnostic assessments (blue bars) and those that participate in the majority of assessments (red bars). SLP = speech language pathology; OT = occupational therapy; Dev Peds = developmental pediatrics; Gen Peds = general pediatrics; BT = behavior therapy; ECE = early childhood educator; other is comprised of clinicians reported only once: ASD service provider, audiology, clinical genetics, dietician, family liaison, gastroenterology, neurology, neuropsychology, and nursing

freedom [d.f.] = 2; $p = 0.003$), these two variables were not tested together in the multiple regression model. In the multi-variate model, time spent on assessment remained significantly associated with total wait time ($\beta = 0.004$, $p = 0.002$). It remained marginally significant when controlling for province ($\beta = 0.003$, $p = 0.05$), but province itself was not significantly associated with total wait time (partial F test = 0.88, $p = 0.56$). Type of assessor was not significantly associated with total wait time in the multi-variate model. The R^2 for the full data set model was 0.17. The mean adjusted total wait time after back transformation was 8.5 months (95% confidence interval 7, 10). Adjusted values for the full data set are plotted in Fig. 3.

The total wait time was also analyzed based on use of the various diagnostic tools (Table 5). There were no significant differences in total wait time between respondents who did or did not use a particular tool. There was also no significant difference in total wait time between those who used diagnostic tools (median 7 months) and those who did not (median 6.3 months; Wilcoxon $W = 295.5$, $p = 0.54$).

Discussion

This study is the first to examine detailed self-reported practice patterns and wait times for ASD diagnosis among pediatricians across Canada. There was wide variation in reported practices for the diagnosis of ASD, including personnel and tools used in the assessment. There were no two identically composed MDTs across the country, which may reflect the lack of uniformity in guidance documents regarding the necessary personnel for ASD diagnostic assessment [4, 5, 9, 24].

A longer time spent on the assessment was significantly associated with longer total wait from referral to diagnosis, indicating that clinical decisions regarding necessary assessment elements have an important impact on wait times for families. Physicians with longer assessment times will likely have fewer available clinic slots and as a result will see fewer patients, lengthening their queue for ASD assessment. Use of a diagnostic tool was not significantly associated with total wait time, though statistical power may have limited our ability to detect a significant association, making this question worthy of further study. A wide range of reported wait times between the first clinic visit and the completion of the assessment was also observed. This period may represent a particularly stressful time for families as they likely know their child is being assessed for ASD but do not have the diagnosis required (in most jurisdictions) to access intervention. Each component of diagnostic delay may put the child at risk for suboptimal developmental outcomes [11].

Given the increase in prevalence of ASD diagnoses [2], demand for diagnostic assessments may exceed available resources, leading to wait times. As such, our results are relevant to all jurisdictions that provide publicly funded ASD diagnostic assessments. A study from the UK using data from 2001 to 2002 found that only 19% of assessments occurred within the recommended time frame of 30 weeks [25]. The time period between referral and receipt of ASD diagnosis has been repeatedly described as a highly stressful time for families, increasing the impetus to provide timely access to diagnosis [26, 27]. Parental stress and dissatisfaction are significantly associated with a higher number of professionals seen during

Table 3 Wait times for ASD diagnostic assessment (n = 57)

	n	%	Median	Range	Interquartile range
Wait time for first visit (time 1)			6	1–24	3–9
1 month	3	5.3%			
2 months	7	12.3%			
3 months	10	17.5%			
4 months	4	7.0%			
5 months	1	1.8%			
6 months	10	17.5%			
7 months	2	3.5%			
8–9 months	5	8.8%			
10–12 months	7	12.3%			
13–18 months	5	8.8%			
19–24 months	3	5.3%			
Wait time from first visit to diagnosis (time 2)			1	0–6.5	0.5–2
0 months	7	12.3%			
0.25 months	3	5.3%			
0.5 months	5	8.8%			
0.75 months	5	8.8%			
1 month	18	31.6%			
1.5 months	2	3.5%			
2 months	7	12.3%			
3 months	4	7.0%			
4.5 months	2	3.5%			
≥ 6 months	4	7.0%			
Total wait from referral to diagnosis			7	2–26	4–12
< 2 months	3	5.3%			
2–3 months	6	10.5%			
4 months	6	10.5%			
5–6 months	7	12.3%			
7–8 months	9	15.8%			
9–10 months	8	14.0%			
11–12 months	2	3.5%			
13–14 months	6	10.5%			
15–18 months	3	5.3%			
19–22 months	4	7.0%			
23–26 months	3	5.3%			

Percentages may not sum to 100 due to rounding

the diagnostic process [26, 28]. To meet diagnostic demand, clinical guidelines for ASD diagnosis have focused on the need to train more providers to perform ASD assessments [4] and to fund more MDTs [5]. Our results suggest that further work is needed to determine the optimal balance between accuracy, quality, and efficiency in ASD assessments, allowing a higher volume of assessments to be completed and reducing wait times.

Our analysis revealed intriguing findings regarding the types of clinicians involved in the diagnostic assessment. Many pediatricians conducted developmental consultations (with wait times and billing costs) but did not provide ASD diagnoses in their practices. Though general pediatricians had a trend toward a shorter time to first visit of the diagnostic assessment, they trended toward a longer overall time to completion of the assessment. General pediatricians

Table 4 Bivariate analyses of associations between continuous putative variables and total wait time

Continuous variables		Test (r_s)	p
Time spent on assessment (minutes)		0.31	0.02[a]
Years in practice		−0.13	0.34
Categorical variables	Median wait time (months)	Test	p
Type of assessor		Kruskal-Wallis chi-squared = 3.66	0.16[a]
Developmental pediatrician	6.5		
General pediatrician	7.5		
Other	3		
Accepts referral from family doctor		Wilcoxon rank sum test W = 200	0.24
Yes	7		
No	6		
Practices in team		Wilcoxon rank sum test W = 308.5	0.25
Yes	9		
No	6.5		
Catchment		Kruskal-Wallis chi-squared = 2.85	0.42
Within city only	6.5		
Within regional health authority	9		
Within province/territory	6.5		
No defined catchment	6.5		
Province of practice		Kruskal-Wallis chi-squared = 13.67	0.19[a]
British Columbia	9.5		
Alberta	5		
Ontario	6.5		
Quebec	14.5		
New Brunswick	8.5		
Other[b]	7.5		

[a]Variable meets cutoff of p < 0.2 to be included in regression analysis
[b]"Other" is the median wait time for provinces with one respondent (Manitoba, Saskatchewan, Nova Scotia, Newfoundland and Labrador, Yukon, and Nunavut) that have been collapsed in the displayed results to prevent identification of individual respondents' wait times

who diagnose ASD may avert the need for an additional referral to a developmental pediatrician or MDT in the diagnostic journey for families. Further work is needed to ensure that a general pediatrician diagnosis of ASD is accurate, acceptable to families, and that it is completed in an expedient manner. A qualitative study of general pediatricians in Ontario, Canada has shown varying willingness to diagnose ASD in their practices [29]. While many of those interviewed felt they were able to provide quality assessments that helped families access services faster than they would have if they waited for a subspecialist, there were identified barriers to conducting ASD diagnostic assessments, including uncertainty about the role of the general pediatrician in ASD diagnosis, inadequate training, and inadequate remuneration. In order to deal with diagnostic uncertainty, solo general pediatricians talked to other clinical staff in their office or reached out to subspecialist colleagues for "hallway consultations." Similar to the results of this survey, participants reported differing use of diagnostic tools, including the ADOS, an abbreviated form of the ADOS, and using a screening tool such as the Modified Checklist for Autism in Toddlers [30] to structure their diagnostic interview. Participants identified barriers beyond identifying ASD, including disclosure of the diagnosis to families and knowledge of available resources in a fragmented system; as such, efforts to increase diagnostic capacity in general pediatricians must consider aspects of diagnostic assessment beyond accuracy, including communication skills and availability of service navigation.

A number of study limitations were present. The low response rate and the voluntary nature of the survey increase the potential for volunteer bias with respondents more likely to have an interest in ASD. As such, caution should be taken in extrapolating the results to all Canadian pediatricians. The study

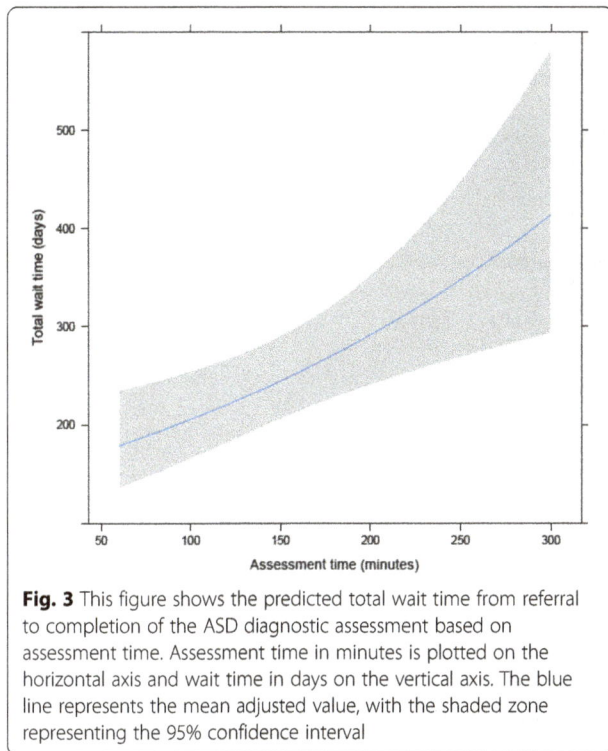

Fig. 3 This figure shows the predicted total wait time from referral to completion of the ASD diagnostic assessment based on assessment time. Assessment time in minutes is plotted on the horizontal axis and wait time in days on the vertical axis. The blue line represents the mean adjusted value, with the shaded zone representing the 95% confidence interval

assessment pathway. The use of the single wait time for ASD diagnosis was chosen so that the influence of diagnostic practices on wait time would not be diluted by adding the wait times for other physician referrals. The total number of respondents limited the statistical power, though the response rate is similar to other Canadian physician surveys [31]. With a larger sample size, additional significant determinants of wait times may have been identified. The findings are nevertheless highly informative as they represent the first study looking at this critical question of capacity in the face of growing ASD prevalence.

Results of this study have identified an important association between the length of the ASD diagnostic assessment and wait times, although far more research is needed to determine the optimal balance between efficiency and comprehensiveness for a complex condition such as ASD. Further analysis is needed at the individual patient level, such as through health administrative or insurance databases, to determine the proportion of children/adults receiving their diagnoses from various providers/teams. This could be compared across jurisdictions with differing requirements for ASD diagnosis, including analysis of resource use and wait times. The variability in diagnostic assessment models reported in this study demands further evaluation of the accuracy of assessment types, such as MDT versus solo assessment and subspecialist versus general pediatrician assessment. Any system-wide strategy for improving efficiency of ASD diagnostic assessments should have accompanying qualitative examination related to uptake of new recommendations and requirements in all relevant stakeholders.

sample did not include psychologists and psychiatrists, who may also be involved in the diagnosis of ASD. Wait times in the survey were self-reported by clinicians, leading to the potential for reporting bias. To minimize the possibility of recall bias, participants were asked to report their current wait time, as opposed to estimating an average over a previous interval. Participants were carefully instructed in the consent form that they would be asked for their current wait time for ASD diagnostic assessment and to have this information prepared. This information could not be verified and is an acknowledged limitation of the work. The total wait time in this analysis only considered the wait time for one referral; this will underestimate wait times for diagnostic journeys that include non-productive referrals to non-diagnosing practitioners at early stages of the

Conclusion

In conclusion, Canadian pediatric practices for ASD diagnosis vary substantially. Assessment time is a significant determinant of total wait time for ASD diagnosis. Further work is needed to identify efficient assessment strategies that preserve reasonable accuracy and quality while allowing families to access timely diagnosis.

Table 5 Wait times by diagnostic tool use

Test	n using tool	Median total wait among those endorsing use	Median total wait among those not endorsing use	p
ADOS	29	7.4	6.1	0.12
ADI-R	15	7	6.9	0.99
CARS	9	8	6.9	0.62
SRS	8	8.2	6.9	0.12
VABS	7	9.8	6.9	0.2
No test	12	6.3	7	0.54

Wait time reported in months; p value based on Wilcoxon estimate. *ADI-R* Autism Diagnostic Interview–Revised, *ADOS* Autism Diagnostic Observation Schedule, *CARS* Childhood Autism Rating Scale, *SRS* Social Responsiveness Scale, *VABS* Vineland Adaptive Behavior Scale

Appendix 1

Table 6 Billing codes reported by participants who do not diagnose ASD

Billing codes used:	n	%
BC–00511 ($411.87)	2	5.9%
BC–00554 ($166.51)	1	2.9%
Alberta 03.08A CMXV30 ($229.15)	4	11.8%
Ontario–A265 ($167)	5	23.5%
Ontario–K122 ($80.30/30 min)	1	2.9%
Ontario–K123 ($91.10/30 min)	1	2.9%
Quebec–09165 ($187.25)	4	11.8%
Quebec–09127 ($56.65)	1	2.9%
Nova Scotia–03.08 ($171.82)	3	5.9%
Newfoundland–101 ($174.04	1	2.9%
Other[a]	2	5.9%
Do not know	2	5.9%

[a]Written responses: "Alternate payment" and "Psychosocial visit under remuneration mixte"

Appendix 2

Table 7 Billing codes used in the ASD diagnostic assessment

Billing code	Amount	First visit (n)	Second visit (n)	Third visit (n)	Fourth visit (n)
Alberta-3.08A	$198.04	3	–	–	–
Alberta-03.08A CMXC30	$229.15	3	5	1	–
Alberta-03.08A + 03.08J	$198.04 + $59.41 per 15 min unit after 30 min	2	–	–	–
Alberta-03.08A CMXC30 + 03.08J	$229.15 + $59.41 per 15 min unit after 30 min	1	1	–	–
Alberta-03.03F	$99.02	–	2	–	–
Alberta-03.03F + 03.03FA	$99.02 + $59.41 per 15 min unit after 30 min	–	1	–	–
Alberta-03.03F CMXV30 + 03.03FA	$130.13 + $59.41 per 15 min unit after 30 min	–	1	–	–
BC-00511	$411.87	2	–	–	–
BC-00512	$99.19	–	–	1	–
BC-00554	$76.71	–	1	–	–
Manitoba-8552	$48.65 per 15 min unit (includes report writing)	1	–	–	–

Table 7 Billing codes used in the ASD diagnostic assessment (Continued)

Billing code	Amount	First visit (n)	Second visit (n)	Third visit (n)	Fourth visit (n)
New Brunswick-14.1-93	$217	3	–	–	–
New Brunswick-14.1-94	$133	–	1	–	–
New Brunswick-14.2-85	$92.40	–	–	1	–
New Brunswick-14.8C-91	$263.20	–	1	–	–
Newfoundland-101	$174.04	1	–	–	–
Newfoundland-113	$93.37	–	1	–	–
Nova Scotia-03.08	$171.82	1	–	–	–
Ontario-A265	$167	10	–	–	–
Ontario-A667	$395.65	10	–	–	–
Ontario-A260	$300.70	3	1	1	–
Ontario-A2662	$395.65	2	–	–	–
Ontario-A2661	$68.80	0	1	–	–
Ontario-K119	$100.00	1	–	–	–
Ontario-K122	$80.30 per 30 min unit	–	4	1	–
Ontario-K123	$91.10 per 30 min unit	–	12	5	2
Quebec-09127	$57	–	–	–	–
Quebec-09165	$187	2	1	1	–
Quebec-09129	$47	1	–	–	–
Quebec-15164	$55.05 per 15 min unit	–	2	1	–
Saskatchewan-9C	$125	1	–	–	–
Saskatchewan-3C	$89.40	–	1	–	–
Nunavut K1/K2	(unable to determine)	1	1	1	–
NB-90 + 2172	(unable to determine)	–	1	–	–
Do not know		5	8	1	–
Alternate funding plan		3	2	1	1
No response		1	1	1	1
Total		57	49	16	3

The number of participants indicating use of each billing code or billing code combination is displayed. The fifth clinic visit and any additional visits are not displayed and are described in the text. Where the respondent selected more than one billing code per visit but only one of those selected could be used for a patient visit according to the province's fee schedule, the billing code with the higher amount was included in the analysis

Appendix 3

Table 8 Time spent administering and scoring diagnostic tools

Tools	Number using tool	Median (min)	Range (min)	Interquartile range (min)
Autism Diagnostic Observation Schedule (ADOS)	29	60	30–120	60–79
Autism Diagnostic Interview–Revised (ADI-R)	15	90	20–120	53–105
Childhood Autism Rating Scale	9	20	15–60	15–30
Social Responsiveness Scale	8	10	5–45	10–15
Vineland Adaptive Behavior Scales	7	45	18–90	38–60
Social Communication Questionnaire	4	23	10–45	18–30
M-CHAT	4	NS	–	–
Adaptive Behavior Assessment System	2	10	–	–
"DSM-5 criteria"	2	NS	–	–
"Cognitive assessment"	2	90	–	–
Mullen Scales of Early Learning	1	60	–	–
"Neurodevelopmental assessment"	1	45	–	–
"Academic screen"	1	40	–	–
Peabody Picture Vocabulary Test	1	30	–	–
Beery-Butenica Test of Visual-Motor Integration	1	20	–	–
Bayley Scales of Infant Development	1	NS	–	–
Diagnostic Interview for Social and Communication Disorders	–	–	–	–
None	12			

NS not specified, responses appearing in quotations are written-in responses not corresponding with an identified tool

Abbreviations
ADI-R: Autism Diagnostic Interview–Revised; ADOS: Autism Diagnostic Observation Schedule; ASD: Autism spectrum disorder; CARS: Childhood Autism Rating Scale; CPS: Canadian Pediatric Society; d.f.: Degrees of freedom; ln: Natural logarithm; MDT: Multidisciplinary team; PEI: Prince Edward Island; REDCap: Research Electronic Data Capture; USA: United States of America

Acknowledgements
Not applicable.

Funding
MP received salary funding from the Clinician Investigator Program at the University of Toronto, a Canada Graduate Scholarship, and a salary award from the Department of Paediatrics at the University of Toronto to complete this work.

Authors' contributions
MP co-developed the research question, drafted the survey, conducted data analysis, and drafted the manuscript. EA provided input on the survey and co-interpreted the results. WU supervised MP, co-developed the research question, provided input on the survey, and co-interpreted the results. All authors read and approved the final manuscript.

Competing interests
MP and WU have no competing interests to declare. EA has served as a consultant to Roche, has received grant funding from SanofiCanada and SynapDx, has received royalties from APPI and Springer, and has received in kind support from AMO Pharmaceuticals.

Author details
[1]Autism Research Centre, Bloorview Research Institute, Holland Bloorview Kids Rehabilitation Hospital, Toronto, Canada. [2]Department of Paediatrics, University of Toronto, Toronto, Canada. [3]Technology Assessment at Sick Kids (TASK), Child Health Evaluative Sciences, The Hospital for Sick Children Research Institute, Toronto, Canada. [4]Institute of Health Policy, Management and Evaluation, University of Toronto, Toronto, Canada.

References
1. American Psychiatric Association. Diagnostic and statistical manual of mental disorders (DSM-5). Arlington: American Psychiatric Association; 2013.
2. Centre for Disease Control National Center on Birth Defects and Developmental Disabilities. Prevalence of autism spectrum disorder among children aged 8 years—autism and developmental disabilities monitoring network, 11 sites, United States, 2010. MMWR Surveill Summ. 2014;63:1–21.

3. Siklos S, Kerns KA. Assessing the diagnostic experiences of a small sample of parents of children with autism spectrum disorders. Res Dev Disabil. 2007;28(1):9–22.

4. Dua V. Standards and guidelines for the assessment and diagnosis of young children with autism spectrum disorder in British Columbia. An evidence-based report prepared for the British Columbia Ministry of Health Planning. 2003.

5. The Miriam Foundation. Canadian Best Practice Guidelines. Screening, assessment and diagnosis of autism spectrum disorders in young children; 2008.

6. National Collaborating Centre for Women's and Children's Health. Autism: recognition, referral and diagnosis of children and young people on the autism spectrum. London: RCOG Press; 2011.

7. Filipek PA, Accardo PJ, Ashwal S, Baranek GT, Cook EH Jr, Dawson G, et al. Practice parameter: screening and diagnosis of autism: report of the quality standards subcommittee of the American Academy of Neurology and the Child Neurology Society. Neurology. 2000;55(4):468–79.

8. Johnson CP, Myers SM. American Academy of Pediatrics Council on children with disabilities. Identification and evaluation of children with autism spectrum disorders. Pediatrics. 2007;120(5):1183–215.

9. Volkmar F, Siegel M, Woodbury-Smith M, King B, McCracken J, State M, et al. Practice parameter for the assessment and treatment of children and adolescents with autism spectrum disorder. J Am Acad Child Adolesc Psychiatry. 2014;53(2):237–57.

10. Dawson G. Early behavioral intervention, brain plasticity, and the prevention of autism spectrum disorder. Dev Psychopathol. 2008;20(3):775–803.

11 Perry A, Cummings A, Dunn Geier J, Freeman N, Hughes S, Managhan T, et al. Predictors of outcome for children receiving intensive behavioral intervention in a large, community-based program. Res Autism Spectr Disord. 2011;5:592–603.

12 Ouellette-Kuntz HM, Coo H, Lam M, Yu CT, Breitenbach MM, Hennessey PE, et al. Age at diagnosis of autism spectrum disorders in four regions of Canada. Can J Public Health. 2009;100(4):268–73.

13 Mandell DS, Novak MM, Zubritsky CD. Factors associated with age of diagnosis among children with autism spectrum disorders. Pediatrics. 2005; 116(6):1480–6.

14 Valicenti-McDermott M, Hottinger K, Seijo R, Shulman L. Age at diagnosis of autism spectrum disorders. J Pediatr. 2012;161(3):554–6.

15 Frenette P, Dodds L, MacPherson K, Flowerdew G, Hennen B, Bryson S. Factors affecting the age at diagnosis of autism spectrum disorders in Nova Scotia, Canada. Autism. 2013;17(2):184–95.

16 Fountain C, King MD, Bearman PS. Age of diagnosis for autism: individual and community factors across 10 birth cohorts. J Epidemiol Community Health. 2011;65(6):503–10.

17 Wiggins LD, Baio J, Rice C. Examination of the time between first evaluation and first autism spectrum diagnosis in a population-based sample. J Dev Behav Pediatr. 2006;27(2 Suppl):S79–87.

18 McKenzie K, Forsyth K, O'Hare A, McClure I, Rutherford M, Murray A, et al. Factors influencing waiting times for diagnosis of autism Spectrum disorder in children and adults. Res Dev Disabil. 2015;45(46):300–6.

19 Canadian Paediatric Society. About the Canadian Paediatric Society 2015. Available from: http://www.cps.ca/en/about-apropos. [cited 25 Apr 2015].

20 Harris PA, Taylor R, Thielke R, Payne J, Gonzalez N, Conde JG. Research electronic data capture (REDCap)—a metadata-driven methodology and workflow process for providing translational research informatics support. J Biomed Inform. 2009;42(2):377–81.

21 Royal College of Physicians and Surgeons of Canada. NPS Primer, June, 2013: Work Hours 2013. Available from: http://nationalphysiciansurvey.ca/wp-content/uploads/2013/10/OFFICIAL-RELEASE_NPS-2013-Backgrounder_EN.pdf. [cited 20 May 2013].

22 Staiger DO, Auerbach DI, Buerhaus PI. Trends in the work hours of physicians in the United States. JAMA. 2010;303(8):747–53.

23 Duan N. Smearing estimate: a nonparametric retransformation method. J Am Stat Assoc. 1983;78(3838):605–10.

24 Anagnostou E, Zwaigenbaum L, Szatmari P, Fombonne E, Fernandez BA, Woodbury-Smith M, et al. Autism spectrum disorder: advances in evidence-based practice. Can Med Assoc J. 2014;186(7):509–19.

25 Preece P, Mott J. Multidisciplinary assessment at a child development centre: do we conform to recommended standards? child: care. Health Dev. 2006;32(5):559–63.

26 Moh TA, Magiati I. Factors associated with parental stress and satisfaction during the process of diagnosis of children with autism spectrum disorders. Res Autism Spectr Disord. 2012;6(1):293–303.

27 Howlin P, Moore A. Diagnosis in autism: a survey of over 1200 patients in the UK. Autism. 1997;1(2):135–62.

28 Goin-Kochel RP, Mackintosh VH, Myers BJ. How many doctors does it take to make an autism spectrum diagnosis? Autism. 2006;10(5):439–51.

29 Penner M, King GK, Hartman L, Anagnostou E, Shouldice M, Moore Hepburn C. Community general pediatricians' perspectives on providing autism diagnoses in Ontario, Canada: a qualitative study. J Dev Behav Pediatr. 2017;38:593–602.

30 Robins D, Fein D, Barton M. Modified Checklist for Autism in Toddlers. 2009.

31 The College of Family Physicians of Canada, Canadian Medical Assocation, The Royal College of Physicians and Surgeons of Canada. National Physician Survey. 2010.

17

Does stereopsis account for the link between motor and social skills in adults?

Danielle Smith[1], Danielle Ropar[2] and Harriet A Allen[2*] (ORCID)

Abstract

Background: Experimental and longitudinal evidence suggests that motor proficiency plays an important role in the development of social skills. However, stereopsis, or depth perception, may also play a fundamental role in social skill development either indirectly through its impact on motor skills or through a more direct route. To date, no systematic study has investigated the relationship between social skills and motor ability in the general adult population, and whether poor stereopsis may contribute to this association. This has implications for clinical populations since research has shown associations between motor abnormalities and social skills, as well as reduced depth perception in autism spectrum disorder and developmental coordination disorder.

Methods: Six hundred fifty adults completed three validated questionnaires, the stereopsis screening inventory, the Adult Developmental Coordination Disorder Checklist, and the Autism Spectrum Quotient.

Results: An exploratory factor analysis on pooled items across all measures revealed 10 factors that were largely composed of items from a single scale, indicating that any co-occurrence of poor stereopsis, reduced motor proficiency, and difficulties with social interaction cannot be attributed to a single underlying mechanism. Correlations between extracted factor scores found associations between motor skill and social skill.

Conclusions: Mediation analyses suggested that whilst fine motor skill and coordination explained the relationship between stereopsis and social skill to some extent, stereopsis nonetheless exerted a substantial direct effect upon social skill. This is the first study to demonstrate that the functional significance of stereopsis is not limited to motor ability and may directly impact upon social functioning.

Keywords: Stereopsis, Stereoability, Depth perception, Motor skills, Social skills, Factor analysis, Path analysis

Background

Motor ability exhibits rich and complex relationships with regards to other cognitive domains [1]. A basic movement repertoire of functional actions involving both fine (such as pointing a finger, eye movements) and gross (such as arm gestures, walking together) motor domains aids in the initiation and sustainment of successful social interactions [2]. For instance, motor control plays an important role in joint attention (e.g. head-turning, reaching, pointing) and imitation [3], both crucial components of social relations [4]. A relationship between social and motor abilities has been identified in typically developing children as young as 8 months [5], with development from crawling to walking encouraging the use of more advanced social behaviours, such as initiation of bids for joint attention and directed gestures [6, 7]. Other research, using longitudinal designs, reported relationships between motor function at 5–6 years and a range of social behaviours at 6–7 years [8], and between motor abilities at 6–7 years and social status with peers at 9–10 years [9]. Additionally, a reduction in social play and increased social reticence has been noted in children with poor motor skills [10].

Although there appears to be sufficient evidence to support a link between motor and social skills, our understanding of this relationship still has important gaps that need to be addressed. Firstly, although evidence for a relationship between motor and social skills has been demonstrated in several studies with typically developing children, it remains unclear whether this relationship would extend into early adulthood. Secondly, previous literature exploring the link between motor and social

* Correspondence: h.a.allen@nottingham.ac.uk
[2]School of Psychology, University of Nottingham, Nottingham NG7 2RD, UK
Full list of author information is available at the end of the article

functioning has neglected important visual skills, such as depth perception, which may help contribute to the relationship between these two domains. For example, there are clear links between depth perception in terms of stereoacuity (the estimation of depth from combining information from two eyes) and the physical manipulation of objects, which may help explain poor coordination or clumsiness. More specifically, the shape of the hand is wider and less accurate when reaching and grasping, and the time taken for the reach is much slower in individuals where stereopsis is reduced or absent in adults [11–14], with even larger errors in these tasks for children with reduced stereoacuity [15–17]. Poor depth perception can also impact upon gross motor skills such as walking; adults with reduced stereoacuity also demonstrate differences in gait with a more cautious approach, higher toe clearance, and increased hesitation [18, 19]. All of these skills may have implications for the likelihood of taking part in team, motor, and social activities; however, this relationship has rarely been studied.

Depth perception and stereopsis may also impact on social skills more directly by influencing social behaviour, perhaps via social norms. When interacting with another individual, we need to determine and maintain an appropriate amount of personal space. Stereo depth cues are most useful in this peri-personal space [20] suggesting those with reduced ability to judge this might inadvertently violate these norms. Good stereo ability requires good alignment and vergence of the eyes, but there is also evidence that those with strabismus (i.e. poor alignment of the eyes) experience social exclusion [21]. There are also preliminary links between poorly regulated eye contact and social abilities [22]. Finally, Kuang et al. [23] found a relationship between stereopsis and quality of life in older people, but the mechanisms for this are, as yet, unclear. There are, therefore several ways in which depth perception might impact upon social skills either indirectly through motor skills, or through a more direct route. To date, however, research has only investigated the links between motor and social ability and the links between motor and visual abilities separately.

The potential relationship between motor, social, and visual abilities has important implications for understanding developmental disorders [24–26]. Poor social skills are central to the diagnostic criteria of ASD [27]. Gross and fine motor impairment as well as difficulties in motor planning have been reported in up to 90% of those with ASD [28–33]. Significant correlations between motor skills and socialisation [34] and degree of social impairment [35–37] have been found in children with ASD. Motor dysfunction is also central to the diagnosis of DCD (also referred to as 'dyspraxia' and affects around 5% of the population [31]), and there has been an increasing interest in the social functioning of individuals with DCD

in recent years. Both clinical and screening studies have reported significant relationships between motor abilities and parent-reported peer or social problems [38–41], showing children with impaired motor skills engaging in more solitary-type activities and generally being more isolated from their peers. There is also evidence from parental report and empirical work that individuals with autism show violations of personal space with others which might impact upon social acceptance [42]. Finding a relationship between stereopsis, motor ability, and social ability might provide a useful avenue for understanding, and perhaps treating these developmental disorders.

From the few studies that have made a direct comparison between ASD and DCD, it would appear that both disorders exhibit a similar range of social and motor difficulties [43, 44]. Importantly, however, it may be that the co-occurrence of these impairments is attributable to another underlying factor. The majority of studies reporting stereoacuity in ASD indicate that those with ASD are less sensitive to binocular disparity than their TD counterparts or normative data [45–51]. There is one contradictory finding. Milne, Griffiths, Buckley, and Scope [52] used the Frisby stereotest and found no significant group difference in stereoacuity between the TD and ASD groups. However, Anketell et al. [46, 47] found differences using this stereotest. A general stereopsis deficit has also been observed in those with DCD; Creavin, Lingam, Northstone, and Williams [53] reported that those with DCD were on average 8 percentage points more likely to have impaired stereopsis (i.e. stereoacuity of higher than 60 arc s) than their TD peers (a 44.5% relative increase), and those with severe DCD were more likely to show evidence of poor depth perception than those with moderate DCD.

The current study

Despite the suggestion from within clinical groups that poor depth perception, or stereopsis, may be linked to both motor skills and social abilities, there has been little research to investigate the relationship between these three abilities. Furthermore, previous work that has investigated the relationship between motor and social skills has focused on children, with a remarkable paucity of research involving adults. It is essential to initially establish the links between stereopsis, motor, and social skills in a larger general population where these skills vary before exploring these relationships in clinical populations, such as ASD, which are often complicated with other co-occurring conditions. Through measuring autistic traits in a large sample within the general population, this study will be able to identify any potential links, either direct or indirect, between depth perception and social skills. This work will help define more specific questions to explore this area further in ASD populations. This study has two primary aims. The first is to extend the previous research linking motor and social skill impairment in children to a typical adult sample, identifying the possible later consequences of early deficit in these domains. Secondly, to examine which particular aspects of motor and social skill impairment were contributed to by reduced stereopsis; that is, if the effects of poor stereoacuity are strong enough to be able to affect social skill either directly or through mediation by motor ability.

Methods
Participants and recruitment
Ethical permission from the University of Nottingham's School of Psychology Ethics Committee was granted prior to recruitment. Participants were sampled opportunistically from Reddit (www.reddit.com; $n = 311$, 47.8%), social media and email ($n = 193$, 29.7%), and an internal recruitment system for undergraduate students at the University of Nottingham for partial completion of course credit ($n = 146$, 22.5%).

Potential participants were provided with a paragraph explaining the study and a hyper-link taking them to the survey website. Although all materials used were originally developed as 'pen-and-paper' questionnaires, it appears there is little variation in responses when questionnaires are presented on-line [54, 55]. Individuals were advised the completion of the study would take approximately 20 min. All participants were offered the chance to enter into a prize draw for one of two £15 vouchers.

The sample included 650 participants aged between 16 and 70 (mean 26.46 ± 10) years. Demographic data in the form of gender, age, and occupation were collected, though these were optional. There were 227 males (age 27.01 ± 10.31; range = 16–67 years), 369 females (age 26.24 ± 9.79; range = 16–70 years), and 6 who identified as "other" (age 25.33 ± 4.23; range = 21–33 years). The age values were not of a normal univariate distribution for any gender group; all groups had positively skewed age distributions, and the ages of the "male" and "other" genders were platykurtic. However, age distributions for each group were roughly equivalent according to a two-sample Kolmogorov-Smirnov test (male vs female $D = 0.1$, $p = 0.08$; male vs other $D = 0.3$, $p = 0.6$; female vs other $D = 0.4$, $p = 0.2$).

Of the participants who reported an occupation (89.5%, $n = 582$), 54.1% ($n = 315$) reported that they were enrolled in secondary or tertiary education, 38% ($n = 221$) were in employment, and 6.19% ($n = 36$) were not in work or education. More details regarding occupation, including a breakdown by industry, can be seen in Additional file 1: Table S1. Diagnoses were not collected as part of the demographical data. However, a number of participants (3.69%, $n = 24$) disclosed various psychiatric or organic illness via the feedback section of the questionnaire. 0.92% ($n = 6$) reported they had been

diagnosed with an ASD (all self-described as Asperger's syndrome), and 1.85% ($n = 12$) reported amblyopia, strabismus or general "poor vision". All diagnostic disclosures are summarised in Additional file 2: Table S2.

Materials
The questionnaires were presented in a fixed order, beginning with the Stereopsis Screening Inventory [56], then the autostereogram self-asssessment, followed by the Adult Developmental Disorder Checklist [57] and the Autism Spectrum Quotient [58]. Finally, demographics including age and gender were requested, but these were optional.

Stereoacuity
The Stereopsis Screening Inventory (SSI) is a self-report screening inventory for stereopsis [56]. It is composed of 10 statements with 5 response options (never, seldom, occasionally, frequently, and always). Coren and Hakstian [56] demonstrated that the scores obtained using the SSI correlate highly ($r = .8$) with laboratory measures of stereopsis such as the TNO test, with others demonstrating a moderate relationship [59] between these measures ($r = .34$). Recommended cut-offs are 17 for moderate stereopsis deficit and 30 for major stereopsis deficit.

The Autostereogram Self-Assessment (ASA) is a short four-item survey created for the present study where the participant self-assesses their autostereogram skill. Based upon short reports by Wilmer and Backus [59] and Cisarik, Davis, Kindy, and Butterfield [60], the questions asked the subject to identify two autostereograms (Fig. 1). The respondent was offered four possible choices plus an 'I don't know' option. Correct answers were designated a score of 1, all other answers were given a 0. Respondents were also asked how difficult they found viewing the autostereograms (on a scale from 1 to 5, where 1 was extremely difficult and 5 very easy), and whether they had successfully perceived stereopsis in an autostereogram previously ('yes' answers were given a score of 1, all others a 0). Self-reported skill to perceive depth in autostereograms has been found to be predictive of stereoacuity, as measured by the TNO test ($r = .45$; [59, 60]).

Motor skills
The Adult Developmental Coordination Disorder Checklist (ADC) is a validated screening tool for identifying the difficulties experienced by adults with DCD [57]. The ADC consists of three sub-scales; the first relates to difficulties that the individual experienced as a child (10 items). The second (10 items) and third sub-scales (20 items) relate to current difficulties. The second sub-scale focuses on the individual's perception of their performance, whereas the third sub-scale relates to current feelings about their performance as reflected upon by others. All items are rated on a four-point scale

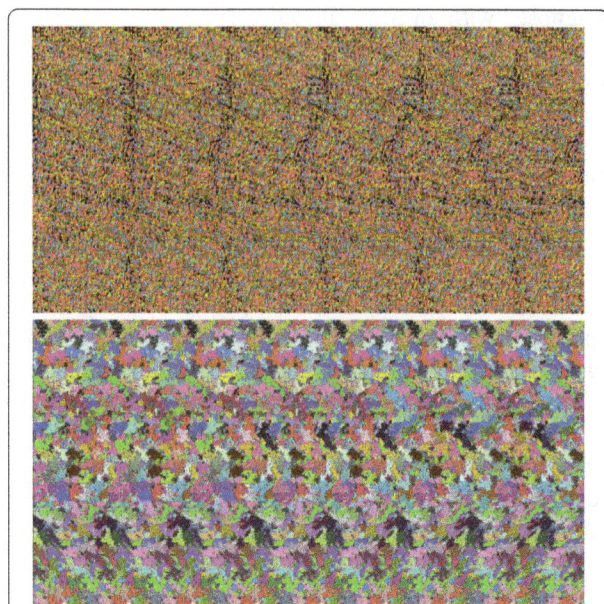

Fig. 1 The two autostereograms used in the current study. The top autostereogram contains a shark [115], and the bottom a teapot [116]. The instructions for viewing are as follows: "Above is an autostereogram or Magic Eye© picture - to reveal the hidden 3D illusion, you must diverge your eyes (i.e. focus beyond the image). First, bring your face close to the page (so that you are almost touching it with your nose). The image should appear blurry. Focus as though you are looking through the image into the distance. Very slowly move away from the page until you begin to perceive depth in the image. At this point, hold very still and the hidden image will slowly appear"

(never, sometimes, frequently or always), resulting in possible scores ranging from 0 to 120. Recommended cut-off scores include 56 for "at risk of DCD" and 65 for "probable DCD" [57]. The latent structure of the ADC has not yet been confirmed using factor analysis.

Social or autism-related traits

The Autism Spectrum Quotient (AQ) is a self-report questionnaire comprising of 50 statements [58]. It was designed as a measure of autistic characteristics in the general population. Although a 4-point response format is used, it is typically scored in a binary manner, where a response is scored as a one if it indicates an autistic trait and zero if this is not the case; this yields a score that can range from 0 to 50. Using this scoring approach, Baron-Cohen et al. [58] determined the optimal cut-off for identifying people with clinically significant levels of autistic traits to be 32 or above. The AQ can also be scored according to the 4-point response option [61, 62], which potentially yields a more sensitive index of ASD severity. In the current study, binary scoring was used to determine the proportion of participants that scored above the 32-point threshold mentioned previously. For all other analyses, including the exploratory factor analysis, the 4-point response was used. Past factor analyses

of AQ items have been inconsistent, with studies finding two, three or four factors rather than five [63].

Missing data

If a participant left more than 10% of responses across all items blank, the data were excluded from the analysis ($n = 0$; highest proportion of missing data for a single participant was 8.308%). The proportion of missing data for any individual questionnaire item ranged from 0 to 30%. Closer inspection of the pattern of missingness revealed that two items relating to driving ability in the Adult Developmental Coordination Disorder Checklist ("Did it take you longer than others to learn to drive?" and "If you are a driver, do you have difficulty parking a car?") accounted for the highest amount of missing data (28.154% and 30% respectively). When the data from these questions were removed from the analysis, the highest proportion of missing data for a single item was reduced to 10.154%.

Although the number of subjects in the study was 650, 290 cases were missing a response for at least one item. Homoscedasticy of the data was tested using the TestMCARNormality function [64], which is part of the MissMech package in R. The test of homoscedasticy was rejected, indicating that the data was not missing completely at random (MCAR). The R package missForest [65] was used to impute the missing data. This has been demonstrated to introduce the least imputation error and has the smallest prediction difference from actual non-imputed values [66].

Data analysis

Statistical analyses were performed using R 3.0.1. The relationship between scores on the ADC, AQ, ASA, and SSI were first examined using Pearson correlation analysis. The data were then randomly split into two equally sized groups ($n = 325$) to act as training and test data in a cross validation procedure. All items from all measures (minus the two ADC items mentioned above) within the training data set were subjected to exploratory factor analysis (EFA). Oblique rotation was specified for the EFA, given that the factors were expected to correlate with one another based on theoretical and empirical grounds [67]. Parallel analysis and Velicier's Minimum Average Partial Test (available as part of the psych package) were used to determine the number of factors to retain. Factors were further interpreted if the grouping of the loading variables made conceptual sense. Given the fairly large sample size, items were considered to load onto a factor if their loading was ≥ .32 [68].

Cross-validation was then performed using the test data set, with the factors extracted using EFA being used to specify the factor structure for confirmatory factor analysis (CFA). In CFA, there is no single definitive indicator of model fit. The overall model fit was therefore assessed in terms of five measures from two perspectives: absolute fit and comparative fit to a base model, with index cut-offs (seen in brackets) informed by recommendations in the literature [69–72]. Absolute fit measures included the model chi-square/degrees of freedom ($\chi2$/df; 3.0), standardised root mean square residual (SRMR; .08), and root mean square error of approximation (RMSEA; .06). The comparative measures were comparative fit index (CFI; .9) and Tucker-Lewis index (TLI; .9). Post hoc modification indices were applied to improve model fit. These indices were only used when modifications could be supported with theory as suggested by the literature; here, modifications consisted of allowing correlated residuals between items that loaded on to the same factor [73].

In the case where CFA fit indices indicated an adequate fit to the test data, bivariate correlations and subsequent moderation and mediation analyses in the form of structural equation modelling were conducted upon the extracted factor scores from the CFA to determine how they related to one another.

Results

Descriptive statistics
Tests of multi- and uni-variate normality indicated that the scores across all items did not meet the assumption of normality (Royston's H test [74]; $H = 11,580.473$, $p = < 0.001$). For large sample sizes, significant results can be derived even in the case of a small deviation from normality [75].

All scales demonstrated acceptable internal consistency—see Table 1 for these and other descriptive data including the percentage of the total sample who met cut-off scores indicating clinically significant impairment for each measure. Of note is a higher incidence than would be expected of participants meeting cut-offs for clinically significant impairment for each standardised measure. These are higher incidences than would be expected from participants drawn from the general population (where DCD has a prevalence of approximately 5% [31]), ASD 1.1–2.4%

[76, 77] and stereopsis deficit 40% [78]); however, one must be cautious when comparing rates of diagnosis in the clinic to questionnaire based estimates, see the "Discussion" section. It was not uncommon for participants who had a score above threshold for one measure to also score above threshold for at least one of the other measures (see Additional files 1, 2, and 3).

Correlation of measure totals
Bivariate correlations of measure scores revealed a number of significant associations. A strong positive relationship was observed between AQ and ADC total scores ($r(648) = 0.628$, $p = < 0.001$), meaning that those with higher levels of autistic traits were also likely to exhibit higher levels of dyspraxic traits. Small-to-moderate positive correlations were observed between SSI, and both AQ ($r(648) = 0.277$, $p = < 0.001$) and ADC ($r(648) = 0.268$, $p = < 0.001$) scores, indicating that higher levels of autistic and dyspraxic traits were associated with an increased degree of stereoscopic deficit. A small negative relationship was also observed between ASA and ADC scores ($r(648) = - 0.106$, $p = 0.007$), denoting that those with increased dyspraxic traits tended to be worse at perceiving autostereograms. No significant relationship was found between ASA and either AQ ($p = 0.056$) or (surprisingly) SSI scores ($p = 0.502$).

Exploratory factor analysis
The aim of this study was to assess the existence of latent variables, thus EFA was used to determine the dimensional structure of pooled items across the four measures previously described.

For the training dataset ($n = 325$) the Kaiser-Meyer-Olkin coefficient of sampling adequacy was good (.857; .6 is recommended by Cerny and Kaiser [79]) and Bartlett's test of sphericity [80] was significant (χ^2 (5151) = 17,439.845, $p = < 0.001$), indicating that the data were suitable for factor analysis. Parallel analysis [81] and Velicer's minimum average partial test [82] recommended that 10 factors be extracted from the data [83, 84]. Factor loadings

Table 1 Descriptive statistics for the Adult Developmental Coordination Disorder Checklist (ADC), Autism Spectrum Quotient (AQ), autostereogram self-assessment (ASA), and Stereopsis Screening Inventory (SSI) ($n = 650$). Clinically significant impairment is based on Coren and Hakstian [56], Kirby et al. [57], and Baron-Cohen e al. [58]

	M (SD)	Range	Cut-off scores indicating clinically significant impairment	% of participants meeting cut-off	Skewness	Kurtosis	Cronbach's α
ADC	41.7 (21.97)	0–116	"DCD at risk" = 56–64	2.31%	0.75	3.09	0.94
			"Probable DCD" = ≥ 65	13.08%			
AQ	121.52 (22.5)	78–179	≥ 32	24.92%; note, 6 participants disclosed ASD diagnosis	0.29	2.16	0.91
ASA	3.6 (2.53)	1–8	Data not available	N/A	0.61	1.82	0.72
SSI	24.14 (9.28)	9–45	Moderate deficit = 17–29	34.62%	− 0.07	1.78	0.87
			Major deficit = ≥ 30	35.08%			

were calculated using principal axis factoring with oblmin (oblique) rotation on 102 of 104 Likert scale questions across all four measures (omitting the two items of the ADC which had a high proportion of missing data, see the "Methods" section) and are shown in Table 2. Labels have been provided for the 10 extracted factors, based on an interpretation of the items that constitute them; 'social skill', 'stereopsis', 'attention to detail', 'fine motor skill', 'organisation', 'Magic Eye proficiency', 'isolation due to motor proficiency', 'coordination', 'imagination', and 'multitasking'. All items loading on to these factors are shown in Table 2.

Confirmatory factor analysis

The factor structure suggested by EFA was cross-validated by means of CFA, using the lavaan package. The 'test' data ($n = 325$) were analysed using the MLR estimator, which is robust to the non-normality of the observed variables [85]. In the first model, items (indicators in CFA terminology) which had a sufficiently high factor loading in the initial EFA ($\geq .32$) were estimated as free parameters; all other items were fixed to zero. The factors (or latent variables) were allowed to covary freely. Though the initial model showed a reasonable fit on some of the indicators, it did not meet criteria for acceptable fit for the comparative fit indices ($\chi^2/df = 2.013$, CFI = 0.782, TLI = 0.771, SRMR = 0.08, RMSEA = 0.056). This is to be expected, as the initial model to be tested through CFA had more stringent restrictions than the factor model obtained through EFA, where no factor loadings were fixed to zero. In studies using cross-validation procedures such as those performed here, it is recommended that a less constrained model is tested where some parameters are freed [86]. Modification indices were allowed in the creation of an adjusted model, though with restrictions upon which changes could be reasonably made to the initial model.

After modification indices were applied, where the residuals between indicators loading on to the same latent variable were allowed to correlate with one another if this significantly improved the fit of the model, all indices indicated an acceptable fit ($\chi^2/df = 1.485$, CFI = 0.899, TLI = 0.89, SRMR = 0.069, RMSEA = 0.039). A scaled chi-square difference test [87] showed that this modification-index-adjusted model exhibited a significantly better fit compared to the initial model ($\Delta\chi^2(88) = 1261.05$, $p = < 0.001$). Factor scores were calculated from the adjusted CFA model using simple regression [88] for each participant. These scores were then used to perform mediation analyses in order to better understand the relationships between the factors or latent variables.

Mediation

Factors were only included in this aspect of the analysis where strong a-priori hypotheses could be made: stereopsis, Magic Eye proficiency, fine motor skill, coordination,

isolation due to motor proficiency, and social skill factor scores were retained. As can be seen in Table 3, the majority of these factors showed medium-to-large correlations with one another. All mediation analyses reported here were performed using lavaan's structural equation modelling (SEM) framework.

Motor skills may mediate the link between stereopsis and social skills

Fine motor skill, coordination, and isolation due to motor proficiency were entered into a multiple mediation analysis to investigate the relationship between stereopsis impairment and reduced social ability. A significant total effect of stereopsis on social skills emerged, $\beta = - 0.312$, $z = - 6.143$, $p = < 0.001$. When dividing this total effect into the direct effect of stereopsis, and the total indirect effects of all three mediators, the direct effect of stereopsis remained significant after adjusting for all three mediators, $\beta = - 0.216$, $z = - 4.615$, $p = < 0.001$. The total indirect effect was also significant, $\beta = - 0.096$, $z = - 3.441$, $p = < 0.001$. Of the three mediator variables, only fine motor skill contributed significantly to the indirect effect of stereopsis upon social skills (12.436% of the total effect; $\beta = - 0.039$, $z = - 2.276$, $p = 0.02$). Neither coordination nor isolation exhibited a significant amount of mediation ($p = 0.061$ and 0.178, respectively).

Motor skills mediate the link between stereopsis and isolation

To investigate why individuals with worse stereopsis reported increased isolation due to motor proficiency, a multiple mediation analysis was performed with the mediator variables being fine motor skill and coordination. A significant total effect of stereopsis on isolation emerged, $\beta = 0.179$, $z = 3.47$, $p = < 0.001$. When dividing this total effect into the direct effect of stereopsis, and the total indirect effects of both mediators, the direct effect of stereopsis was no longer significant, $\beta = 0.02$, $z = 0.772$, $p = 0.44$, but the total indirect effect was significant, $\beta = 0.158$, $z = 3.545$, $p = < 0.001$. Both mediator variables contributed significantly to the indirect effect of stereopsis upon isolation due to motor proficiency, though coordination exhibited a greater proportion of mediation (75.3% of the total effect; $\beta = 0.134$, $z = 3.471$, $p = < 0.001$) than fine motor skills (13.273% of the total effect; $\beta = 0.024$, $z = 2.294$, $p = 0.02$).

Isolation may mediate the link between coordination/fine motor skills and social skills

Two final mediation models indicated that isolation due to motor proficiency was a significant mediator both in the relationship between coordination and social skills (39.772% of the total effect; $\beta = - 0.211$, $z = - 2.533$, $p = 0.01$) and fine motor skill and social skills (40.941% of the total

Table 2 Factor loadings of a 10-factor EFA solution for items pooled across all measures. Principal axis factoring, oblmin rotation. Loadings below .32 (which explain less than 10% of the variance in that item) are not highlighted and are considered to be negligible loadings for the purposes of analysis

Measure	Item	Social	Stereo	Detail	Fine motor	Org	Magic Eye	Isolation	Coord	Imagine	Multi
AQ	Enjoy social chitchat	**0.70**	0.01	−0.06	−0.09	−0.06	−0.03	−0.04	0.07	0.01	0.08
AQ	Good at social chitchat	**0.70**	0.04	0.02	−0.05	0.03	0.12	0.03	0.01	−0.05	−0.03
AQ	Find social situations easy	**0.67**	−0.05	0.07	−0.01	0.01	0.03	0.01	0.00	0.02	−0.08
AQ	Prefer people over things	**0.59**	−0.01	−0.12	−0.04	0.02	0.04	−0.01	−0.04	0.04	0.09
AQ	Enjoy social occasions	**0.56**	−0.07	−0.10	−0.14	0.02	−0.02	−0.10	−0.09	0.08	0.01
AQ	Enjoy meeting new people	**0.53**	−0.07	−0.12	0.02	0.00	0.02	−0.04	−0.20	0.05	0.04
ADC	Choose to spend leisure time on own	**−0.48**	0.05	0.09	0.20	−0.02	0.02	0.25	−0.01	0.01	0.06
AQ	Easily keep track of several conversations	**0.44**	−0.03	0.15	0.00	−0.08	−0.01	0.01	0.07	0.19	−0.19
AQ	Can work out what someone is feeling from their face	**0.43**	−0.02	0.00	−0.06	−0.08	−0.01	−0.02	0.06	**0.34**	−0.10
AQ	Prefer to do things with others	**0.43**	0.05	0.02	0.13	−0.11	−0.02	−0.11	0.02	−0.22	−0.05
AQ	Find it hard to make new friends	**−0.41**	−0.06	0.30	−0.05	−0.04	−0.06	0.20	0.15	−0.16	−0.06
AQ	New situations bring on anxiety	**−0.35**	0.08	0.11	−0.11	0.01	0.06	0.17	0.09	−0.08	0.24
AQ	Don't know how to keep conversation going	**−0.33**	−0.04	0.22	0.04	0.02	−0.09	0.11	−0.00	−0.25	0.11
AQ	Can easily 'read between the lines'	**0.32**	−0.03	0.02	−0.10	−0.03	0.10	0.06	0.03	0.31	−0.14
SSI	Do you think you need glasses	0.03	**0.94**	0.02	0.05	0.01	−0.01	−0.03	−0.03	0.03	0.01
SSI	Glasses/contact lens wearer	−0.05	**0.90**	−0.00	−0.00	0.01	0.02	−0.02	−0.02	0.02	−0.00
SSI	W/out correction, clearness of vision in LEFT eye	0.08	**0.89**	0.02	0.03	−0.04	−0.01	0.07	−0.05	−0.04	0.05
SSI	W/out correction, clearness of vision in RIGHT eye	−0.08	**0.88**	−0.06	−0.03	0.00	0.02	−0.02	0.03	0.06	−0.03
SSI	Vision as good as other people's	0.06	**0.87**	0.02	−0.03	0.03	−0.04	−0.00	−0.00	−0.06	−0.01
SSI	Correction needed for reading	−0.02	**0.53**	0.01	−0.04	−0.02	0.05	−0.09	0.21	−0.05	−0.08
AQ	Notice patterns in things all the time	−0.13	0.05	**0.67**	−0.08	0.10	0.02	−0.03	−0.08	0.05	−0.05
AQ	Notice car number plates or similar	−0.01	0.02	**0.56**	−0.03	0.04	0.06	0.03	−0.01	−0.02	−0.07
AQ	Tend to notice details that others do not	−0.14	−0.02	**0.55**	0.12	0.06	−0.00	−0.10	0.01	0.30	−0.09
AQ	Strong interests, get upset if can't pursue	0.01	0.04	**0.55**	0.14	−0.02	−0.04	0.05	−0.03	0.03	0.16
AQ	Notice small sounds	−0.13	0.07	**0.47**	0.07	0.07	0.06	0.01	0.05	0.18	0.07
AQ	Get strongly absorbed in one thing	−0.24	0.12	**0.46**	−0.06	0.18	−0.02	−0.02	−0.01	−0.03	−0.02
AQ	Enjoy collecting information about categories	−0.01	−0.07	**0.45**	0.13	−0.08	0.02	0.04	0.09	−0.07	0.05
AQ	Repetitive topic of conversation	0.06	0.03	**0.45**	0.11	0.03	−0.01	0.13	−0.01	−0.18	0.01
AQ	Tend to dominate conversation	0.18	0.03	**0.43**	0.05	−0.06	0.06	0.09	−0.02	−0.04	0.12
AQ	Fascinated by numbers	−0.07	−0.05	**0.41**	0.07	0.03	0.03	−0.07	0.04	−0.08	−0.06
AQ	Difficult to work out people's intentions	−0.06	0.06	**0.39**	−0.00	0.04	−0.03	0.06	−0.00	−0.29	0.16
AQ	Difficulty imagining being someone else	0.08	−0.09	**0.37**	0.14	−0.01	−0.12	0.09	−0.06	−0.16	0.19
AQ	Say impolite things without realising	0.09	−0.02	**0.36**	0.14	−0.12	−0.03	0.12	0.02	−0.04	0.25
AQ	Difficulty speaking in turns on phone	−0.01	0.03	**0.35**	0.13	0.07	−0.05	0.10	0.09	−0.05	0.10
AQ	Difficultly working out characters' intentions in story	0.12	0.01	**0.34**	0.06	−0.04	0.14	0.13	0.13	−0.24	0.02
ADC	Others find it difficult to read your writing	0.01	0.04	0.00	**0.79**	−0.07	0.01	0.05	−0.07	0.01	−0.06
ADC	Difficulty with writing neatly AND quickly	−0.06	0.02	−0.03	**0.73**	0.03	−0.04	0.02	−0.02	0.03	0.09
ADC	Difficulty with neat writing when child	−0.07	−0.01	0.07	**0.70**	0.13	−0.04	0.07	−0.11	0.00	0.00
ADC	Difficulties reading own writing	−0.04	0.07	−0.05	**0.66**	−0.04	0.03	−0.08	0.18	−0.01	−0.15
ADC	Difficulties with writing as fast as peers	0.00	−0.04	0.07	**0.65**	0.06	0.03	−0.04	0.09	−0.12	0.05
ADC	Difficulty with fast writing as child	0.04	−0.06	0.06	**0.62**	0.15	0.03	0.01	0.06	−0.07	0.06

Table 2 Factor loadings of a 10-factor EFA solution for items pooled across all measures. Principal axis factoring, oblmin rotation. Loadings below .32 (which explain less than 10% of the variance in that item) are not highlighted and are considered to be negligible loadings for the purposes of analysis *(Continued)*

Measure	Item	Social	Stereo	Detail	Fine motor	Org	Magic Eye	Isolation	Coord	Imagine	Multi
ADC	Difficulty copying without mistakes	−0.09	−0.06	−0.09	**0.43**	0.10	−0.02	−0.15	0.27	0.04	0.08
ADC	Difficulty with organisation	−0.04	0.07	−0.06	0.14	**0.71**	0.07	−0.09	0.02	−0.00	−0.03
ADC	Difficulties with organisation as child	−0.01	0.09	−0.05	0.06	**0.68**	−0.02	0.10	−0.06	−0.01	−0.09
ADC	Others call you disorganised	0.06	0.00	0.11	0.08	**0.66**	0.09	0.01	0.02	−0.04	0.00
ADC	Tend to lose possessions	0.01	−0.09	−0.03	0.04	**0.58**	−0.04	0.15	0.03	0.05	0.03
ADC	Difficulty sitting still	−0.08	−0.07	0.23	0.05	**0.52**	−0.04	−0.02	−0.05	0.07	0.18
ADC	Difficulty planning ahead	−0.08	0.03	0.09	−0.02	**0.48**	0.04	−0.14	0.02	−0.18	0.29
ADC	Bump into, spill, or break things	−0.00	−0.07	−0.02	−0.04	**0.43**	−0.10	**0.41**	0.19	0.04	0.02
ADC	Difficulty managing money	−0.02	−0.04	0.05	0.01	**0.43**	0.04	−0.17	0.23	−0.03	0.15
ADC	Can lose attention in certain situations	−0.02	0.05	0.12	0.02	**0.42**	−0.02	−0.05	0.04	−0.07	0.31
ADC	Bumped into objects more than other children	0.03	−0.07	0.09	0.05	**0.38**	−0.13	**0.36**	0.20	−0.02	−0.03
MEA	Identify shape in autostereogram [shark]	−0.05	0.00	−0.03	0.01	−0.00	**0.91**	0.04	0.01	0.01	0.02
MEA	Identify shape in autostereogram [teapot]	0.05	−0.00	0.01	−0.03	0.04	**0.91**	0.00	0.06	−0.06	−0.03
MEA	Ease of perceiving shapes in autostereograms above	0.03	−0.02	0.03	0.04	0.01	**0.85**	0.01	−0.03	0.06	0.04
MEA	Previous successful completion of autostereogram	−0.09	0.10	0.09	−0.01	−0.01	**0.35**	0.22	−0.15	0.04	−0.04
ADC	If do sport, likely to be on your own	−0.16	−0.01	0.04	0.05	−0.04	0.06	**0.63**	−0.08	−0.04	−0.03
ADC	Avoid team games/sports	−0.18	0.11	0.05	0.02	0.00	0.09	**0.60**	0.03	0.02	0.08
ADC	Difficulties playing team games as child	−0.04	0.13	−0.01	0.14	0.02	0.01	**0.47**	0.17	−0.05	0.12
ADC	Others commented on clumsiness as child	0.13	0.02	0.06	0.01	**0.35**	−0.16	**0.44**	0.23	−0.04	−0.06
ADC	Difficulties with hobbies requiring good coordination	−0.03	0.10	−0.10	0.02	0.09	−0.03	0.25	**0.57**	0.03	0.05
ADC	Difficulties eating with utensils	−0.03	−0.08	0.06	0.08	0.01	0.05	−0.09	**0.57**	−0.09	0.06
ADC	Self-care difficulties	−0.08	0.02	0.05	0.19	0.07	−0.08	−0.01	**0.48**	−0.08	0.08
ADC	Avoid hobbies that require good coordination	−0.02	0.13	−0.08	0.02	−0.02	−0.02	**0.36**	**0.45**	−0.03	0.15
AQ	Can easily imagine what characters in story look like	0.00	−0.01	0.08	−0.16	−0.08	0.08	−0.00	0.05	**0.52**	−0.00
AQ	Easily play games with children involving pretending	0.28	−0.07	−0.05	−0.10	0.05	0.05	0.08	−0.15	**0.43**	0.14
AQ	Easy to create a picture using imagination	0.01	−0.01	0.25	−0.03	−0.08	0.08	−0.09	−0.01	**0.42**	0.02
AQ	Is a good diplomat	0.28	0.02	−0.00	0.05	−0.08	−0.00	−0.11	−0.01	**0.37**	−0.05
AQ	Making up stories is easy	0.06	0.00	0.23	−0.08	0.08	0.05	0.12	−0.08	**0.37**	−0.02
ADC	Difficulty performing concurrent tasks	−0.11	0.04	0.02	0.20	0.10	−0.02	−0.05	0.24	0.08	**0.41**
ADC	Difficulty with distance estimation	0.06	0.12	0.02	−0.06	0.14	−0.07	0.23	0.13	−0.04	**0.39**
AQ	Easy to do more than one thing at once	0.28	0.04	0.04	−0.05	−0.02	0.02	0.03	−0.09	0.13	**−0.34**
ADC	Difficulty with navigation	0.00	0.09	−0.09	0.09	0.03	−0.07	0.18	0.16	−0.06	0.32
ADC	Difficulty packing suitcase to go away	0.03	−0.05	0.13	0.09	0.21	0.00	−0.05	0.26	−0.02	0.29
ADC	Difficulty learning to ride bike as child	0.06	0.05	0.04	0.12	0.04	−0.03	0.25	0.13	0.02	0.28
ADC	Difficulty preparing meal from scratch	−0.03	−0.02	0.14	−0.01	0.04	−0.05	−0.09	0.27	−0.16	0.25
AQ	Prefer to do things the same way over and over	−0.05	0.00	0.30	0.16	−0.10	−0.06	0.11	0.02	0.04	0.25
AQ	Know if someone listening to me is getting bored	0.27	−0.05	−0.10	0.03	−0.05	−0.04	−0.07	−0.07	0.29	−0.23
ADC	Difficulties with self-care when child	0.10	−0.03	0.01	0.18	0.15	−0.12	0.18	0.26	0.07	0.22
ADC	Difficulty folding and putting away clothes	0.11	0.07	0.13	0.28	0.24	0.00	−0.01	0.20	−0.03	0.22
AQ	Not upset if daily routine is disturbed	0.27	−0.12	−0.06	0.05	0.06	0.04	−0.05	−0.04	0.04	−0.21
AQ	Enjoy doing things spontaneously	0.29	−0.16	−0.09	0.08	0.15	0.10	−0.13	−0.18	0.06	−0.21

Table 2 Factor loadings of a 10-factor EFA solution for items pooled across all measures. Principal axis factoring, oblimin rotation. Loadings below .32 (which explain less than 10% of the variance in that item) are not highlighted and are considered to be negligible loadings for the purposes of analysis *(Continued)*

Measure	Item	Social	Stereo	Detail	Fine motor	Org	Magic Eye	Isolation	Coord	Imagine	Multi
AQ	Quickly go back to previous activity after interruption	0.19	−0.04	−0.01	0.04	−0.10	0.09	0.08	−0.01	0.23	−0.21
ADC	Slower at getting ready	−0.00	0.07	0.08	0.17	0.28	0.07	−0.03	0.12	−0.13	0.20
AQ	When younger, enjoyed pretend games with others	0.10	0.04	−0.25	−0.08	0.08	0.10	0.03	−0.20	0.29	0.19
AQ	Carefully plan any activities participated in	−0.13	0.06	0.31	0.07	−0.27	−0.07	0.09	0.14	0.16	0.19
SSI	Book too close to eyes when reading	−0.09	0.29	0.03	−0.09	0.09	−0.05	0.18	0.09	−0.09	−0.18
AQ	Not very good at remembering phone numbers	−0.01	0.04	−0.24	0.19	−0.08	−0.03	0.14	0.01	0.11	0.18
SSI	Experience temporary loss of vision	−0.05	0.16	0.03	0.04	0.13	−0.15	0.00	0.30	0.10	−0.17
AQ	Not good at remembering people's date of birth	−0.09	−0.02	−0.15	0.20	0.11	0.04	0.12	−0.17	0.09	0.17
AQ	Don't enjoy reading fiction	0.10	−0.02	0.07	0.03	0.02	0.04	0.06	−0.01	−0.06	0.15
AQ	Rather go to library than a party	−0.24	0.12	0.22	0.08	−0.05	0.04	0.25	0.09	0.08	−0.13
AQ	Concentrate on whole rather than parts	0.13	−0.04	−0.23	−0.05	0.09	0.02	0.00	0.07	0.11	−0.11
ADC	Do you avoid going to clubs/dancing	−0.30	0.09	0.15	0.08	0.06	0.01	0.25	−0.06	−0.04	−0.06
AQ	Last to understand the point of a joke	0.14	0.00	0.32	0.01	0.05	−0.14	0.09	0.16	−0.12	0.05
AQ	Fascinated by dates	0.07	0.03	0.26	−0.02	−0.06	0.10	−0.03	0.14	−0.03	−0.05
AQ	Don't notice small changes	0.01	0.12	0.02	0.20	−0.02	−0.00	0.11	−0.13	−0.20	0.03
AQ	Rather go to the theater than to a museum	0.29	0.01	−0.09	−0.10	−0.05	−0.05	−0.18	0.18	0.04	0.03
ADC	Difficulties playing music instrument when child	0.04	−0.03	−0.03	0.21	0.18	−0.17	0.18	0.15	−0.01	0.01
SSI	Difference between items 8 and 9	0.01	0.05	0.08	−0.01	−0.04	−0.10	0.04	0.03	0.02	−0.01
SSI	Eyes feel 'tired'	0.09	0.30	−0.02	0.10	0.06	−0.07	−0.03	0.25	0.04	−0.00

effect; $\beta = -0.214$, $z = -4.477$, $p = < 0.001$). Partial mediation occurred in both cases, as coordination and fine motor skill were still significant predictors of social skills after adjusting for the indirect effect of isolation (coordination: $\beta = -0.32$, $z = -3.647$, $p = < 0.001$, fine motor skills: $\beta = -0.309$, $z = -4.605$, $p = < 0.001$).

Path analysis

The above mediation models were aggregated into a larger path model. This final model included relationships with Magic Eye proficiency as detailed in Table 3. This model had a good fit, with $\chi^2/\mathrm{df} = 0.418$, CFI = 1, TLI = 1.011, SRMR = 0.017, and RMSEA = < 0.001. The results of the path analysis with standardised regression coefficients are presented in Fig. 2. The relationship between stereopsis and social skills, as well as stereopsis and isolation (both mediated by fine motor skill and coordination) held in this larger model. The effect of isolation due to motor proficiency acting as a mediator between fine motor skill/coordination and social skills did not hold in this larger model. Whilst fine motor skill and coordination were responsible for full mediation of the relationship between stereopsis and isolation due to motor proficiency, there was no serial mediation from the fine motor/coordination variables to social skills via the isolation variable. Finally, Magic Eye proficiency was not a significant independent variable within the context of the path model.

Discussion

The aim of the present study was to explore the relationship between stereopsis, motor ability, and social skills in a sample of adults. The current research builds upon prior work by investigating whether the impact of motor impairment upon social functioning persists in adulthood, as well as incorporating a variable, stereopsis, which may underlie deficits in motor ability and thus have an impact upon social skill. The results indicated that impaired stereopsis both directly and indirectly affected social skills, in the latter case through mediation

Table 3 Spearman correlation coefficients for factor scores extracted using confirmatory factor analysis (CFA)

	Stereo	Magic Eye	Social	Isolation	Coord
Magic Eye	0.14*	–			
Social	−0.34***	0.05	–		
Isolation	0.21**	−0.12	−0.53***	–	
Coord	0.20**	−0.18**	−0.55***	0.86***	–
Fine motor	0.19**	−0.08	−0.54***	0.64***	0.67***

Significant relationships are indicated by asterisks. *$p < 0.05$, **$p < 0.01$, ***$p < .001$. Significance values Bonferroni corrected in order to adjust for multiple comparisons

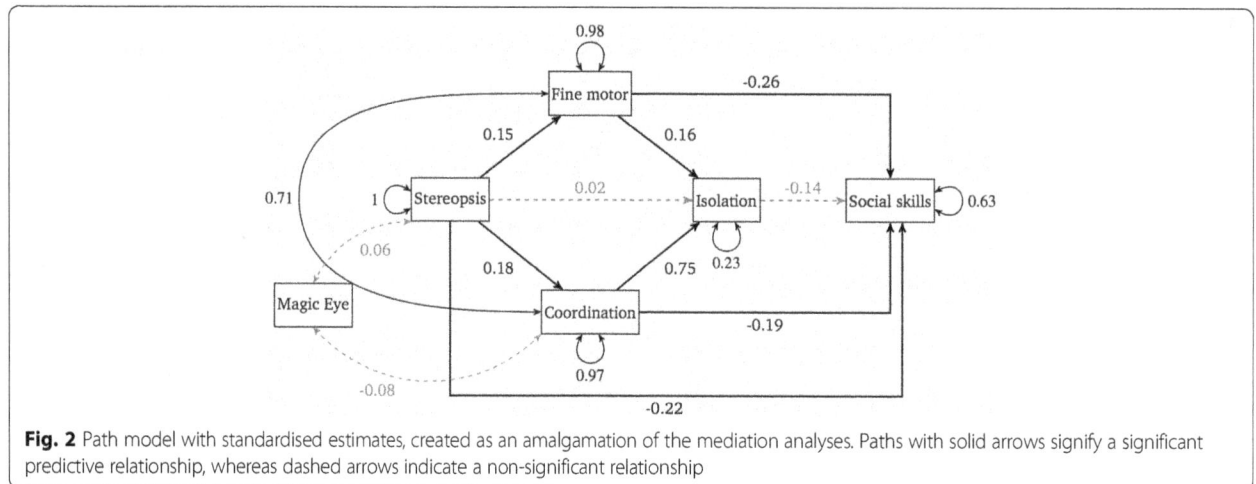

Fig. 2 Path model with standardised estimates, created as an amalgamation of the mediation analyses. Paths with solid arrows signify a significant predictive relationship, whereas dashed arrows indicate a non-significant relationship

by coordination and fine motor skill. Additionally, both fine motor skill and coordination fully mediated the relationship between stereopsis and isolation due to motor proficiency, with coordination explaining much larger proportion of variance. However, in the full model, isolation due to motor proficiency did not have a significant relationship with social skills.

Overall, the results of this study suggest that stereopsis impairment can affect both motor skill proficiency and social skills. Additionally, as the final aggregate path model was a good fit for the data, preliminary support is provided for the validity of the causal pathways in the model.

Associations between stereopsis, motor skills, and isolation
The findings reported here support the hypothesis of links between impaired stereopsis and both fine and gross motor skills. In the current study, there was also a relationship between stereopsis impairment and coordination/daily living skills. Little previous research has looked at this more functional consequence of impaired stereopsis. It has been observed that the sensation of depth afforded by binocular viewing is important for certain gross motor skills, such as obstacle avoidance whilst walking [18] and intercepting thrown objects [89], but only two studies have specifically looked at the contribution of reduced stereopsis to daily living skills.

In a group of older individuals (aged 65 years), Kuang, Hsu, Chou, Tsai, and Chou [23] found no effect of stereopsis on daily living tasks such as cooking and writing, but they did observe that those with poor stereopsis exhibited a reduction in reported energy/vitality, suggesting that more effort may be required to accomplish daily living tasks. Cao and Markowitz [90] noted that in a group of older subjects (aged 50 years) with age-related macular degeneration, those with reduced stereopsis experienced difficulty with visual motor skills required for daily living. The observers in the current study were

younger than the groups surveyed by Kuang et al. [23] and Cao and Markowitz [90], with 92.6% of the participants who disclosed their age being under 60 years old, thus, here we extend the finding of a relationship between stereopsis and daily living skills to younger and middle-aged adult populations.

Whilst there was a relationship between stereopsis and both types of motor proficiency, the size of this effect was small within the context of the path model. A much stronger association was present between fine motor skill/coordination and isolation. Of these two facets of motor skill that showed links with isolation, it was coordination/daily living skills (which require gross motor ability) that exhibited the largest amount of mediation between stereopsis and isolation. Whilst there is already evidence that motor ability correlates with feelings of isolation and social standing with peers [8–10, 40, 91], these studies do not tend to differentiate between fine and gross motor skill. Future work might look at whether social isolation is due to simple impairment in gross motor skills or if it might be more specifically attributed to a reduction in daily living skills; such knowledge would allow more targeted treatment (such as physical therapy for gross motor skills versus occupational therapy for daily living skills).

The impact of impaired stereopsis on social skills
Impaired stereopsis may affect social skill by causing a reduction in general motor ability. The current results are consistent with those who have previously found an association between motor proficiency and social competence [8, 34–37, 92, 93]. Whilst fine motor skill and coordination did mediate the relationship between stereopsis and social skill, this effect was only partial (the mediation model accounted for around a third of the variance in the relationship between stereopsis and social skill). Fine motor skill, coordination, and stereopsis all exhibited a

similar strength of effect in their relationship with social skill. That the mediators between stereopsis and social skill accounted for only a small amount of variance suggests that there are other unmeasured factors that play a part in the relationship between impaired stereopsis and reduced social skill. The findings here suggest that stereopsis may prove useful in other, as yet unexplored, domains related to social interaction—for instance, the estimation of interpersonal distance.

It is interesting to speculate on the underlying mechanisms between impaired stereopsis and social skills. Theories from autism research have attempted to link visual and social abilities, via a common, generalised, cause [94]. Pellicano and Burr [95] use a Bayesian framework to argue that flattened priors may account for the changes in autism. They argue that many of the traits underlying autism are related to a failure to update perception from prior experience. It is not clear whether this general deficit extends to depth and stereo-disparity processing, however, since people with and without autism integrate depth cues similarly [51]. An alternative theory proposes that autistic individuals have enhanced perceptual function (EPF) [96] in early associative areas of sensory processing (e.g. visual discrimination), resulting in greater locally oriented processing. This account suggests that higher-order processing is not always engaged or mandatory in autism, when a task can be carried out using lower-level perceptual processing. Therefore, when presented with complex and fast moving social stimuli (e.g. a person speaking), a strong focus on low-level perceptual features may result in information overload and an inability to attend to the relevant visual cues. This account appears to conflict with the current results in that we find a link between impaired, rather than enhanced, perceptual function and social isolation. It is worth noting, however, that the perceptual losses described here are likely to predominantly come from issues at the earliest stages of perceptual processing such as lack of eye alignment (strabismus or squint) as well as, possibly, more neurological deficits. The links proposed between EPF and social abilities are usually described as more complex cognitive biases which are not necessarily linked to depth perception [51]. It is important, therefore, to consider the impact of both peripheral perceptual and cognitive differences to understand social behaviour.

An alternative explanation for the link between stereopsis and social abilities and behaviours is that the link is environmentally mediated and is due to selective reinforcement of behaviours. As discussed in the introduction, stereopsis cues to depth are most useful in peri-personal space [20] and thus would be useful for judging social distance and interpersonal space. Furthermore, optical conditions that impair depth perception, such as amblyopia or strabismus, have also been linked to social exclusion and reduced quality of life measures [21, 97]. Under this explanation, poor stereopsis reduces the opportunity to develop social skills, especially in childhood, and this extends into adulthood. This explanation must also be viewed with caution, not least because it is not clear whether the deficits in those with strabismus are due to the condition itself or the treatment [98]. Further work to test the whether the predictions of clinical models extend to the general population is necessary.

Isolation due to motor proficiency does not predict general social ability

In contrast to previous research which has established that perceived and/or actual social isolation causes individuals to change their behaviour and have lower-quality social interactions [99–101], we did not find that isolation due to motor proficiency significantly predicted social skill in the full path model. It is likely that motor ability (represented by the fine motor skill and coordination variables) is responsible for this relationship, especially considering the items that constitute the isolation factor all relate to motor proficiency, specifically in the context of sport and team games. When isolation is characterised more fully, including indicators such as social network size, participation in a range of social activities (not just those that require motor proficiency), and perceived lack of social support, the relationship between isolation and social ability is likely to hold true.

Limitations

It is assumed that the greater correlations between the AQ and ADC scores compared to the SSI score, and the motor (fine motor and coordination) and social skills factor scores compared to the stereopsis factor score reflect a greater interdependence of social and motor skills in development. However, it is possible that the stronger correlation may be an artefact of the questionnaires used, with the two questionnaires with the largest number of questions and covering a range of domains (the AQ and ADC) correlating most strongly. Coren and Hakstian [56] have established that whilst the SSI has a relatively high specificity, the sensitivity is relatively poor (59.7%). A lab- or clinic-derived measure of stereoacuity might highlight relatively larger (or smaller, dependent on whether the stereopsis factor extracted in the current study actually measures this function) correlations with social and motor skills. Related to this point, whilst self-report questionnaires are easy to administer to a large number of individuals, their subjective nature may result in biased responses [102]. However, the questionnaires used in this study are well standardised and have demonstrable construct validity. The ADC and AQ in particular are commonly employed as research and screening tools.

It is interesting to note that our correlations between stereoacuity and Magic Eye proficiency factor scores were relatively low, although significant (see Table 3); there was no significant correlation between the ASA and SSI total scores. For the factor scores, our correlation value is slightly lower than the value of 0.34 previously found by Wilmer and Backus [59] in a similar comparison. Our comparison was slightly different to that previous study in that we asked people to report their difficulty resolving the autostereogram image, which could account for some of the difference. Furthermore, to be successful with the auto-stereogram, participants require good near convergence which is not covered by the SSI stereoacuity measure [103]. As above, conclusions regarding stereoacuity based on questionnaires must be cautious until they are followed up with controlled clinic or laboratory measurement.

Our sample was non-stratified and was biased towards university students; however, we note that the number of participants sampled was markedly higher than the majority of studies, which administer the AQ in a non-clinical sample (which is by far the most commonly reported questionnaire of the ones used in the current study [104]). The recruitment strategies used for the current study are similar to the trends noted for other research involving the AQ, including part of the participant sample being drawn from participant databases maintained by universities, and the use of online survey tools to reach a broader audience [104].

There was a relatively high proportion of participants who surpassed the threshold for clinically significant levels of impairment across all of the standardised questionnaires we used. This may be due to self-selection bias as the study was advertised as a "survey on correlations between visual ability, coordination, and autistic traits". Individuals who perceived themselves as clumsy, having poor social skills, or problems with visual perception may have been more likely to take part, creating an opportunistic selection bias. The particularly high proportion of participants meeting or exceeding the AQ cut-off may reflect the large proportion of individuals either pursuing a STEM degree or in a STEM career, who are more likely to score higher on the AQ than those in non-STEM education or career paths [105]. Furthermore, whilst only six participants disclosed a diagnosis of autism or Asperger's syndrome, more specified that they were first-degree relatives of someone with the condition. It is thought that autistic traits may be expressed to a greater degree in close relatives of people with an ASD, even though they might not meet the criteria for clinical diagnosis [106], a concept termed the broader autism phenotype [107–109]. However, our final sample showed a broad range of individual differences in the scores of the SSI, AQ, and ADC, indicating that whilst self-selection bias may have occurred, there was still sufficient variability in the data to allow us to conduct our analyses.

Clinical implications

The first and most important clinical implication of this study is that visual deficits such as reduced stereopsis can have far reaching implications on behaviour. Interventions to improve stereopsis itself have had limited success but are probably not sufficiently developed to be recommended to ameliorate the issues described here [110–112]. Nevertheless, it would be important to address the sensory and motor issues in the clinic. Stereopsis is not the only cue to depth; many other cues to depth such as texture gradient, size, occlusion are available. Those with reduced stereopsis are likely to use cues differently to those with good or normal stereopsis [51]. For many tasks, simply adding a pattern to a surface can improve the ability to judge and use depth cues, by providing more size and texture gradient cues. This can improve activities such as walking and stepping [113, 114] so may have implications for problems of dexterity and clumsiness. For social skills, it is possible that therapies which guide those with reduced stereopsis to use alternative cues to judge critical distances such as interpersonal distance might be particularly effective. For instance, training people to use rules such as keeping an arm's length away rather than relying on implicit cues might be helpful. Finally, it is possible that the link between stereopsis and social skill is because the perceptual deficits reduce the likelihood that people engage in social activities. Thus, in this case, it would be the clinician's role to support the child (or adult) to find social activities which are not affected by a loss of stereopsis.

Conclusions

This study has demonstrated the presence of a relationship between stereopsis, motor ability, and social skill. Using a large group of adults, this work complements research previously conducted with children, in addition to providing evidence for an underlying contributor to impairment in both motor and social skill. Preliminary support for causal pathways between stereopsis, motor ability, and social skill has been provided, but further evidence is needed to clarify the mechanisms responsible, especially in clinical populations. The repercussions of poor stereopsis have been demonstrated to be far-reaching, limiting not only motor skill, but also social competence.

Additional files

Additional file 1: Table S1. A detailed breakdown of self-reported occupation, including faculty for those in education (where available) and sector for those in employment. (DOCX 25 kb)

Additional file 2: Table S2. The psychiatric or organic illnesses self-disclosed in the feedback section of the questionnaire. Note that diagnoses were not collected routinely as part of the demographical data. The data below represent a number of co-morbidities: 32 diagnoses were disclosed by 24 participants (3.7% of the sample). (DOCX 24 kb)

Additional file 3: Figure S1. Depicted is a 3-set Venn diagram where the size of the ovals indicates relative magnitude and the numbers within portray the number of participants who scored above threshold on th(at|ose) measure(s). Note that for the SSI, the higher threshold boundary indicating major stereopsis deficit was used. Descriptive statistics for questionnaire responses: It was not uncommon for participants who had a score above threshold for one measure to also score above threshold for at least one of the other measures. The most substantial amount of overlap between measures was for the AQ and the SSI, with 10.615% of the total participant sample scoring above threshold on both of these measures (note that the higher SSI threshold indicating major stereopsis deficit was used in this case). However, the largest degree of overlap was between the ADC and AQ, with 71.765% of participants who met the threshold for 'probable developmental coordination disorder' also scoring above threshold on the AQ. (PNG 54 kb)

Abbreviations
3D: Three-dimensional; ADC: Adult Developmental Coordination Disorder Checklist; AQ: Autism Spectrum Quotient; ASA: Autostereogram Self-Assessment; ASD: Autism spectrum disorder; CFA: Confirmatory factor analysis; CFI: Comparative Fit Index; DCD: Developmental coordination disorder; EFA: Exploratory factor analysis; MCAR: Missing completely at random; RMSEA: Root mean square error of approximation; SEM: Structural equation modelling; SRMR: Standardised root mean square residual; SSI: Stereopsis Screening Inventory; TLI: Tucker-Lewis Index

Funding
This work was supported by the Economic and Social Research Council [grant number ES/J500100/1], by a PhD studentship to DS. The funders had no role in the study design, data collection, analysis, decision to publish, or preparation of the manuscript.

Authors' contributions
All authors developed the study concept and design. DS created the survey website, recruited participants, analysed the data, and wrote the first draft of the article, under supervision of HA and DR. All authors contributed to the final paper and approved the final version for submission.

Competing interests
The authors declare that they have no competing interests.

Author details
[1]Research and Development Department, Cumbria Partnership NHS Foundation Trust, Carleton Clinic, Carlisle CA1 3SX, UK. [2]School of Psychology, University of Nottingham, Nottingham NG7 2RD, UK.

References
1. Leonard HC, Hill EL. Review: the impact of motor development on typical and atypical social cognition and language: a systematic review. Child Adolesc Ment Health. 2014;19:163–70.
2. Lippold T, Burns J. Social support and intellectual disabilities: a comparison between social networks of adults with intellectual disability and those with physical disability. J Intellect Disabil Res. 2009;53:463–73.
3. Kenny L, Hill E, Hamilton AFD. The Relationship between Social and Motor Cognition in Primary School Age-Children. Front in Psychol. 2016;7. https://doi.org/10.3389/fpsyg.2016.00228.
4. Bhat AN, Landa RJ, Galloway JC. Current perspectives on motor functioning in infants, children, and adults with autism spectrum disorders. Phys Ther. 2011;91:1116–29.
5. Lamb ME, Garn SM, Keating MT. Correlations between sociability and motor performance scores in 8-month-olds. Infant Behav Dev. 1982;5:97–101.
6. Clearfield MW, Osborne CN, Mullen M. Learning by looking: infants' social looking behavior across the transition from crawling to walking. J Exp Child Psychol. 2008;100:297–307.
7. Karasik LB, Tamis-LeMonda CS, Adolph KE. Transition from crawling to walking and infants' actions with objects and people. Child Dev. 2011;82:1199–209.
8. Bart O, Hajami D, Bar Haim Y. Predicting school adjustment from motor abilities in kindergarten. Infant Child Dev. 2007;16:597–615.
9. Ommundsen Y, Gundersen KA, Mjaavatn PE. Fourth graders' social standing with peers: a prospective study on the role of first grade physical activity, weight status, and motor proficiency. Scand J Educ Res. 2010;54:377–94.
10. Bar Haim Y, Bart O. Motor function and social participation in kindergarten children. Soc Dev. 2006;15:296–310.
11. Grant S, Melmoth DR, Morgan MJ, Finlay AL. Prehension deficits in amblyopia. Investig Opthalmology Vis Sci. 2007;48:1139–48.
12. Melmoth DR, Finlay AL, Morgan MJ, Grant S. Grasping deficits and adaptations in adults with stereo vision losses. Invest Ophthalmol Vis Sci. 2009;50:3711–20. https://doi.org/10.1167/iovs.08-3229.
13. Niechwiej-Szwedo E, Goltz HC, Chandrakumar M, Wong AMF. The effect of sensory uncertainty due to amblyopia (lazy eye) on the planning and execution of visually-guided 3D reaching movements. PLoS One. 2012;7:e31075.
14. Schiller PH, Kendall GL, Kwak MC, Slocum WM. Depth perception, binocular integration and hand-eye coordination in intact and stereo impaired human subjects. J Clin Exp Ophthalmol. 2012;3:1–12.
15. Grant S, Suttle C, Melmoth DR, Conway ML, Sloper JJ. Age- and stereovision-dependent eye-hand coordination deficits in children with amblyopia and abnormal binocularity. Invest Ophthalmol Vis Sci. 2014;55:5687–57015.
16. Hrisos S, Clarke MP, Kelly T, Henderson J, Wright CM. Unilateral visual impairment and neurodevelopmental performance in preschool children. Br J Ophthalmol. 2006;90:836–8.
17. Suttle CM, Melmoth DR, Finlay AL, Sloper JJ, Grant S. Eye-hand coordination skills in children with and without amblyopia. Invest Ophthalmol Vis Sci. 2011;52:1851–64.
18. Buckley JGJ, Panesar GKG, MacLellan MMJ, Pacey IE, Barrett BT. Changes to control of adaptive gait in individuals with long-standing reduced stereoacuity. Invest Ophthalmol Vis Sci. 2010;51:2487–95. http://www.iovs.org/content/51/5/2487.short. Accessed 4 Apr 2013.
19. Ooi TL, He ZJ. Space perception of Strabismic observers in the real world environment. Invest Ophthalmol Vis Sci. 2015;56:1761–8.
20. Cutting JE, Vishton PM. Perceiving layout and knowing distances: the integration, relative potency, and contextual use of different information about depth. Perception. 1995;5:1–37.
21. Satterfield D, Keltner JL, Morrison TL. Psychosocial-Aspects of Strabismus Study. Arch Ophthalmol. 1993;111:1100–5. https://doi.org/10.1001/archopht.1993.01090080096024.
22. Jones CR, Swettenham J, Charman T, Marsden AJ, Tregay J, Baird G, et al. No evidence for a fundamental visual motion processing deficit in adolescents with autism spectrum disorders. Autism Res. 2011;4:347–57.
23. Kuang TM, et al. "Impact of stereopsis on quality of life." Eye. 2005;19(5):540–5.

24. Diamond A. Close interrelation of motor development and cognitive development and of the cerebellum and prefrontal cortex. Child Dev. 2000; 71:44–56.

25. Hartman E, Houwen S, Scherder E, Visscher C. On the relationship between motor performance and executive functioning in children with intellectual disabilities. J Intellect Disabil Res. 2010;54:468–77.

26. Kim H, Carlson AG, Curby TW, Winsler A. Relations among motor, social, and cognitive skills in pre-kindergarten children with developmental disabilities. Res Dev Disabil. 2016;53–54:43–60.

27. American Psychiatric Association. DSM 5: diagnostic and statistical manual of mental disorders: American Psychiatric Press Inc.; 2013.

28. Gillberg C. Asperger syndrome in 23 Swedish children. Dev Med Child Neurol. 1989;31:520–31.

29. Green D, Charman T, Pickles A, Chandler S, Loucas T, Simonoff E, et al. Impairment in movement skills of children with autistic spectrum disorders. Dev Med Child Neurol. 2009;51:311–6.

30. Klin A, Volkmar FR, Sparrow SS, Cicchetti DV, Rourke BP. Validity and neuropsychological characterization of Asperger syndrome: convergence with nonverbal learning disabilities syndrome. J Child Psychol Psychiatry. 1995;36:1127–40.

31. Lingam R, Hunt L, Golding J, Jongmans M, Emond A. Prevalence of developmental coordination disorder using the DSM-IV at 7 years of age: a UK population{\textendash}based study. Pediatrics. 2009;123:e693–700.

32. Manjiviona J, Prior M. Comparison of Asperger syndrome and high-functioning autistic children on a test of motor impairment. J Autism Dev Disord. 1995;25:23–39.

33. Ming X, Brimacombe M, Wagner GC. Prevalence of motor impairment in autism spectrum disorders. Brain and Development. 2007;29:565–70.

34. Sipes M, Matson JL, Horovitz M. Autism spectrum disorders and motor skills: the effect on socialization as measured by the baby and infant screen for children with aUtIsm traits (BISCUIT). Dev Neurorehabil. 2011;14:290–6.

35. Dyck MJ, Piek JP, Hay DA, Hallmayer JF. The relationship between symptoms and abilities in autism. J Dev Phys Disabil. 2007;19:251–61.

36. Hilton CL, Wente L, LaVesser P, Ito M, Reed C, Herzberg G. Relationship between motor skill impairment and severity in children with Asperger syndrome. Res Autism Spectr Disord. 2007;1:339–49.

37. Hilton CL, Zhang Y, White MR, Klohr CL, Constantino JN. Motor impairment in sibling pairs concordant and discordant for autism spectrum disorders. Autism. 2011;16:1362361311423018–441.

38. Cummins A, Piek JP, Dyck MJ. Motor coordination , empathy, and social behaviour in school-aged children. Clin Psychol. 2005;47:437–42.

39. Green D, Baird G, Sugden D. A pilot study of psychopathology in developmental coordination disorder. Child Care Health Dev. 2006;32:741–50.

40. Jarus T, Lourie-Gelberg Y, Engel-Yeger B, Bart O. Participation patterns of school-aged children with and without DCD. Res Dev Disabil. 2011;32:1323–31.

41. Wagner MO, Bös K, Jascenoka J, Jekauc D, Petermann F. Peer problems mediate the relationship between developmental coordination disorder and behavioral problems in school-aged children. Res Dev Disabil. 2012;33:2072–9.

42. Kennedy DP, Adolphs R. Violations of personal space by individuals with autism spectrum disorder. PLoS One. 2014.

43. Dewey D, Cantell M, Crawford SG. Motor and gestural performance in children with autism spectrum disorders, developmental coordination disorder, and/or attention deficit hyperactivity disorder. J Int Neuropsychol Soc. 2007;13:246–56.

44. Green D, Baird G, Barnett AL, Henderson L, Huber J, Henderson SE. The severity and nature of motor impairment in Asperger's syndrome: a comparison with specific developmental disorder of motor function. J Child Psychol Psychiatry. 2002;43:655–68.

45. Adams RJ, Dove CN, Drover JR, Norman BR, Birch EE, Wang Y-Z, et al. Assessing Eye and Visual Functioning in Children and Young Adults with Autism Spectrum Disorder; 2010. p. 93057.

46. Anketell PM, Saunders KJ, Gallagher SM, Bailey C, Little J-A. Visual findings in children with autistic Spectrum disorder. In: Association for Research in Vision & Ophthalmology; 2013.

47. Anketell PM, Saunders KJ, Gallagher SM, Bailey C, Little JA. Accommodative function in individuals with autism Spectrum disorder. Optom Vis Sci. 2018; 95:193–201.

48. Black K, McCarus C, Collins MLZ, Jensen A. Ocular manifestations of autism in ophthalmology. Strabismus. 2013;21:98–102.

49. Coulter RA, Tea Y, Bade A, Fecho G, Amster D, Jenewein E, et al. Vision testing of children and adolescents with ASD: what are we missing? In: International meeting for autism research; 2013.

50. Scharre JE, Creedon MP. Assessment of visual function in autistic children. Optom Vis Sci. 1992;69:433–9.

51. Smith D, Ropar D, Allen HA. The integration of occlusion and disparity information for judging depth in autism spectrum disorder. J Autism Dev Disord. 2017;47:3112–24.

52. Milne E, Griffiths H, Buckley D, Scope A. Vision in children and adolescents with autistic Spectrum disorder: evidence for reduced convergence. J Autism Dev Disord. 2009;39:965–75. https://doi.org/10.1007/s10803-009-0705-8.

53. Creavin AL, Lingam R, Northstone K, Williams C. Ophthalmic abnormalities in children with developmental coordination disorder. Dev Med Child Neurol. 2014;56:164–70.

54. Van De Looij-Jansen PM, De Wilde EJ. Comparison of web-based versus paper-and-pencil self-administered questionnaire: effects on health indicators in Dutch adolescents. Health Serv Res. 2008;43(5p1):1708–21.

55. Wu RC, Thorpe K, Ross H, Micevski V, Marquez C, Straus SE. Comparing administration of questionnaires via the internet to pen-and-paper in patients with heart failure: randomized controlled trial. J Med Internet Res. 2009;11:e3.

56. Coren S, Hakstian R. Screening for stereopsis without the use of technical equipment: scale development and cross-validation. Int J Epidemiol. 1996;25: 146–51.

57. Kirby A, Edwards L, Sugden D, Rosenblum S. The development and standardization of the adult developmental co-ordination disorders/dyspraxia checklist (ADC). Res Dev Disabil. 2010;31:131–9.

58. Baron-Cohen S, Wheelwright S, Skinner R, Martin J, Clubley E. The autism-spectrum quotient (AQ): evidence from asperger syndrome/high-functioning autism, males and females, scientists and mathematicians. J Autism Dev Disord. 2001;31:5–17.

59. Wilmer JB, Backus BT. Self-reported Magic Eye stereogram skill predicts stereoacuity. Perception. 2008;37:1297–300.

60. Cisarik P, Davis N, Kindy E, Butterfield B. A comparison of self-reported and measured autostereogram skills with clinical indicators of vergence and accommodative function. Perception. 2012;41:747–54.

61. Austin EJ. Personality correlates of the broader autism phenotype as assessed by the autism spectrum quotient (AQ). Pers Individ Dif. 2005;38:451–60.

62. Hoekstra RA, Vinkhuyzen AAE, Wheelwright S, Bartels M, Boomsma DI, Baron-Cohen S, et al. The construction and validation of an abridged version of the autism-spectrum quotient (AQ-short). J Autism Dev Disord. 2011;41:589–96.

63. Hoekstra RA, Bartels M, Cath DC, Boomsma DI. Factor structure, reliability and criterion validity of the autism-Spectrum quotient (AQ): a study in Dutch population and patient groups. J Autism Dev Disord. 2008;38:1555–66.

64. Jamshidian M, Jalal S. Tests of homoscedasticity, normality, and missing completely at~random for incomplete multivariate data. Psychometrika. 2010;75:649–74.

65. Stekhoven DJ, Buhlmann P. MissForest--non-parametric missing value imputation for mixed-type data. Bioinformatics. 2011;28:112–8.

66. Waljee AK, Mukherjee A, Singal AG, Zhang Y, Warren J, Balis U, et al. Comparison of imputation methods for missing laboratory data in medicine. BMJ Open. 2013;3:e002847.

67. Fabrigar LR, Wegener DT, MacCallum RC, Strahan EJ. Evaluating the use of exploratory factor analysis in psychological research. Psychol Methods. 1999;4:272.

68. Tabachnick BG, Fidell LS. Using Multivariate Statistics. Boston: Pearson; 2013.

69. Hooper D, Coughlan J, Mullen M. Structural equation modelling: guidelines for determining model fit. Electron J Bus Res Methods. 2008;6:53–60.

70. Hu L, Bentler PM. Cutoff criteria for fit indexes in covariance structure analysis: conventional criteria versus new alternatives. Struct Equ Model A Multidiscip J. 1999;6:1–55.

71. Marsh HW, Hau K-T, Wen Z. In search of Golden rules: comment on hypothesis-testing approaches to setting cutoff values for fit indexes and dangers in overgeneralizing Hu and Bentler's (1999) findings. Struct Equ Model A Multidiscip J. 2004;11:320–41.

72. Schermelleh-Engel K, Moosbrugger H. Evaluating the fit of structural equation models: tests of significance and descriptive goodness-of-fit measures. Methods Psychol Res online. 2003;8:23–74.

73. Jackson DL, Gillaspy JA, Purc-Stephenson R. Reporting practices in confirmatory factor analysis: an overview and some recommendations. Psychol Methods. 2009;14:6–23.

74. Royston JP. Some techniques for assessing multivarate normality based on the shapiro-wilk w. Appl Stat. 1983.

75. Öztuna D, Elhan AH, Tüccar E. Investigation of four different normality tests in terms of type 1 error rate and power under different distributions. Turkish J Med Sci. 2006;36:171–6.

76. Brugha T, Cooper SA, McManus S, Purdon S, Smith J. Estimating the prevalence of autism spectrum conditions in adults: extending the 2007 adult psychiatric morbidity survey. London: NHS; 2012. https://digital.nhs.uk/data-and-information/publications/statistical/estimating-the-prevalence-of-autism-spectrum-conditions-in-adults/estimating-the-prevalence-of-autism-spectrum-conditions-in-adults-extending-the-2007-adult-psychiatric-morbidity-survey.

77. Zablotsky B, Black LI, Maenner MJ, Schieve LA, Blumberg SJ. Estimated Prevalence of Autism and Other Developmental Disabilities Following Questionnaire Changes in the 2014 National Health Interview Survey. Natl Health Stat Report. 2015;(87):1–20.

78. Bosten JM, Goodbourn PT, Lawrance-Owen AJ, Bargary G, Hogg RE, Mollon JD. A population study of binocular function. Vis Res. 2015;110(Pt A):34–50.

79. Cerny BA, Kaiser HF. A study of a measure of sampling adequacy for factor-analytic correlation matrices. Multivariate Behav Res. 1977;12:43–7.

80. Bartlett MS. Tests of significance in factor analysis. Br J Stat Psychol. 1950;3:77–85.

81. Horn JL. A rationale and test for the number of factors in factor analysis. Psychometrika. 1965;30:179–85.

82. Velicer WF. Determining the number of components from the matrix of partial correlations. Psychometrika. 1976;41:321–7.

83. Costello AB, Osborne JW. Best practices in exploratory factor analysis: four recommendations for getting the most from your analysis. Pr Assess Res Eval. 2005;10:1–9.

84. Ledesma RD, Valero-Mora P. Determining the number of factors to retain in EFA: an easy-to-use computer program for carrying out parallel analysis. Pract Assessment, Res Eval. 2007;12:1–11.

85. Li C-H. Confirmatory factor analysis with ordinal data: comparing robust maximum likelihood and diagonally weighted least squares. Behav Res Methods. 2015.

86. van Prooijen J-W, van der Kloot WA. Confirmatory analysis of Exploratively obtained factor structures. Educ Psychol Meas. 2001;61:777–92.

87. Satorra A, Bentler PM. A scaled difference chi-square test statistic for moment structure analysis. Psychometrika. 2001;66:507–14.

88. Thurstone LL. The vectors of mind. Chicago: University of Chicago Press; 1935.

89. Mazyn LIN, Lenoir M, Montagne G, Savelsbergh GJP. The contribution of stereo vision to one-handed catching. Exp Brain. 2004;157:383–90.

90. Cao KY, Markowitz SN. Residual stereopsis in age-related macular degeneration patients and its impact on vision-related abilities: a pilot study. J Optom. 2014;7:100–5.

91. Smyth MM, Anderson HI. Coping with clumsiness in the school playground: social and physical play in children with coordination impairments. Br J Dev Psychol. 2000;18:389–413.

92. Wang MV, Lekhal R, Aarø LE, Schjølberg S. Co-occurring development of early childhood communication and motor skills: results from a population-based longitudinal study. Child Care Health Dev. 2012;40:77–84.

93. Perry A, Flanagan HE, Dunn Geier J, Freeman NL. Brief report: the Vineland adaptive behavior scales in young children with autism spectrum disorders at different cognitive levels. J Autism Dev Disord. 2009;39:1066–78.

94. Simmons DR, Robertson AE, McKay LS, Toal E, McAleer P, Pollick FE. Vision in autism spectrum disorders. Vis Res. 2009;49:2705–39. https://doi.org/10.1016/j.visres.2009.08.005.

95. Pellicano E, Burr D. When the world becomes "too real": a Bayesian explanation of autistic perception. Trends Cogn Neurosci. 2012;16:504–10. https://doi.org/10.1016/j.tics.2012.08.009.

96. Mottron L, Dawson M, Soulières I, Hubert B, Burack J. Enhanced perceptual functioning in autism: an update, and eight principles of autistic perception. J Autism Dev Disord. 2006;36:27–43. https://doi.org/10.1007/s10803-005-0040-7.

97. Paysse EA, Steele EA, McCreey KMB, Wilhelmus KR, Coats DK. Age of the emergence of negative attitudes toward strabismus. Journal of Aapos. 20015. p. 361–6. https://doi.org/10.1067/mpa.2001.119243.

98. Collins MLZ. Strabismus in cerebral palsy: When and why to operate. Am Orthopt J. 2014;64:17–20. https://doi.org/10.3368/aoj.64.1.17.

99. Cacioppo JT, Hawkley LC. People thinking about people: The vicious cycle of being a social outcast in one's own mind. In: Williams KD, Forgas JP, von Hippel W, editors. The Social Outcast Ostracism, Social Exclusion, Rejection, and Bullying. New York: The social outcast: Ostracism; 2005. p. 91–108.

100. Cacioppo JT, Hawkley LC. Perceived social isolation and cognition. Trends Cogn Sci. 2009;13:447–54.

101. Hawkley LC, Hughes ME, Waite LJ, Masi CM, Thisted RA, Cacioppo JT. From social structural factors to perceptions of relationship quality and loneliness: the Chicago health, aging, and social relations study. J Gerontol B Psychol Sci Soc Sci. 2008;63:S375–84.

102. Van Vaerenbergh Y, Thomas TD. Response Styles in Survey Research: A Literature Review of Antecedents, Consequences, and Remedies. International Journal of Public Opinion Research. 2013;25:195–217. https://doi.org/10.1093/ijpor/eds021.

103. Gómez AT, Lupón N, Cardona G, Aznar-Casanova JA. Visual mechanisms governing the perception of auto-stereograms. Clin Exp Optom. 2011;95:146–52.

104. Ruzich E, Allison C, Smith P, Watson P, Auyeung B, Ring H, et al. Measuring autistic traits in the general population: a systematic review of the Autism-Spectrum Quotient (AQ) in a nonclinical population sample of 6,900 typical adult males and females. Mol Autism. 2015;6:1–12.

105. Ruzich E, Allison C, Chakrabarti B, Smith P, Musto H, Ring H, et al. Sex and STEM occupation predict autism-Spectrum quotient (AQ) scores in half a million people. PLoS One. 2015;10:1–15.

106. Hoekstra RA, Bartels M, Verweij CJH, Boomsma DI. Heritability of autistic traits in the general population. Archives of Pediatrics & Adolescent Medicine. 2007;161:372–7. https://doi.org/10.1001/archpedi.161.4.372.

107. Bolton P, Macdonald H, Pickles A, Rios P, Goode S, Crowson M, et al. A case-control family history study of autism. J Child Psychol Psychiatry Allied Discip. 1994.

108. Piven J, Palmer P, Jacobi D, Childress D, The AS. Broader autism phenotype evidence from a family study of multiple incidence autism families. Am J Psychiatry. 1997.

109. Sucksmith E, Roth I, Hoekstra RA. Autistic Traits Below the Clinical Threshold: Re-examining the Broader Autism Phenotype in the 21st Century. Neuropsychology Review. 2011;21:360–89. https://doi.org/10.1007/s11065-011-9183-9.

110. Ding J, Levi DM. Recovery of stereopsis through perceptual learning in human adults with abnormal binocular vision. Proceedings of the National Academy of Sciences of the United States of America. 2011;108:E733–E741.

111. Barrett BT. A critical evaluation of the evidence supporting the practice of behavioural vision therapy. Ophthalmic and Physiological Optics. 2009;29:4–25. https://doi.org/10.1111/j.1475-1313.2008.00607.x.

112. Whitecross S. Vision therapy: Are you kidding me? Problems with current studies. Am Orthopt J. 2013;63:36–40. https://doi.org/10.3368/aoj.63.1.36.

113. Schofield AJ, et al. "Reduced sensitivity for visual textures affects judgments of shape-from-shading and step-climbing behaviour in older adults." Experimental Brain Research. 2017;235(2):573–83.

114. Lord SR, Menz HB. "Visual contributions to postural stability in older adults." Gerontology. 2000;46(6):306–10.

115. Hsu F. Autostereogram Tutorial Random Dot Shark. 2005.

116. Winfree E, Fleischer A, Barr A. https://apod.nasa.gov/apod/ap050130.html.

18

Intranasal administration of exosomes derived from mesenchymal stem cells ameliorates autistic-like behaviors of BTBR mice

Nisim Perets[1], Stav Hertz[2], Michael London[2] and Daniel Offen[1,3]*

Abstract

Autism spectrum disorders (ASD) are neurodevelopmental disorders characterized by three core symptoms that include social interaction deficits, cognitive inflexibility, and communication disorders. They have been steadily increasing in children over the past several years, with no effective treatment. BTBR T+tf/J (BTBR) mice are an accepted model of evaluating autistic-like behaviors as they present all core symptoms of ASD. We have previously shown that transplantation of human bone marrow mesenchymal stem cells (MSC) to the lateral ventricles of BTBR mice results in long lasting improvement in their autistic behavioral phenotypes. Recent studies point exosomes as the main mediators of the therapeutic effect of MSC. Here, we tested whether treatment with the exosomes secreted from MSC (MSC-exo) will show similar beneficial effects. We found that intranasal administration of MSC-exo increased male to male social interaction and reduced repetitive behaviors. Moreover, the treatment led to increases of male to female ultrasonic vocalizations and significant improvement in maternal behaviors of pup retrieval. No negative symptoms were detected following MSC-exo intranasal treatments in BTBR or healthy C57BL mice. The marked beneficial effects of the exosomes in BTBR mice may translate to a novel, non-invasive, and therapeutic strategy to reduce the symptoms of ASD.

Introduction

Autism spectrum disorders (ASD) are neurodevelopmental disabilities characterized by three core symptoms: severe impairment of social interactions and communication skills, increased repetitive behaviors, and cognitive inflexibility [1]. In this study, we used the inbred mouse strain BTBR T+tf/J (BTBR) that incorporates multiple behavioral phenotypes relevant to all three diagnostic symptoms of autism. BTBR present significantly reduced social approach, low reciprocal social interactions, and impaired juvenile play in comparison to the C57BL controls [2, 3]. Using this model, we have recently shown that MSC transplantation to the lateral ventricles of the brain of BTBR mice has the ability to ameliorate their core autistic-like behaviors [4].

Moreover, the behavioral effect of MSC on BTBR mice had lasted for 6 months despite the fact that the MSC themselves do not survive in the transplanted tissue for such an extended period [5]. Such phenomenon has been reported in the literature under the title "hit and run" meaning MSC have the ability to leave a lasting "memory" on the tissue, even after the MSC cells have been degraded [6]. It has been suggested that the MSC therapeutic effect is mainly mediated by their secretome to the tissue [7]. The secretome is referred to as the complete repertoire of molecules and extracellular vesicles secreted from MSC. Yet, it has been found that the nano-vesicles, exosomes, are the major mediators between the MSC and the tissue [8, 9].

Exosomes were initially thought to be a mechanism for removing unneeded membrane proteins from reticulocytes. However, recent studies have shown that they are also used for cell to cell communication through the carrying of genetic information from between cells [10].

* Correspondence: danioffen@gmail.com
[1]Sagol School of Neuroscience, Tel Aviv University, Tel Aviv, Israel
[3]Sacklar School of Medicine, Department of Human Genetics and Biochemistry, Tel Aviv University, Tel Aviv, Israel
Full list of author information is available at the end of the article

Several studies have reported that MSC-exo have functions similar to those of MSC, such as repairing damaged tissue, suppressing inflammatory responses, and modulating the immune system [11, 12]. Exosomes contain mainly proteins, as well as RNA and a large number of micro RNAs. Approximately, 25% of these proteins and RNA play a role in cell growth and maintenance [13, 14]. A key advantage of MSC-exo over MSC is their ability to enter the brain with ease following intranasal administration [15, 16]. We have previously demonstrated that exosomes loaded with gold nanoparticles can cross the blood-brain barrier via intranasal administration and can be visualize in vivo inside the brain [17].

Here, we show that BTBR mice that were treated with MSC-exo via intranasal administration present significant improvement in the social interaction domain, ultrasonic communication, and repetitive behavior. Moreover, we show for the first time that BTBR mothers that were treated with MSC-exo presented significant improvement in maternal pup retrieval behavior.

Results

MSC-exo characterization

MSC-exo were characterized by NanoSight. The average size was 114 ± 2.9 nm, and the average concentration was 3.81×10^8 particles/μL (Fig. 1a, b). Western blot analysis indicates that the MSC-exo express CD9 and CD63, while we could not detect it in the MSC lysate (not shown). In contrast, Calnexin was undetectable in the MSC-exo and found in the MSC lysate, indicating for the purity of the exosomes [18] (Fig. 1c).

MSC-exo improves male to male social interaction and reduces repetitive behaviors during social interaction

Mice were tested for male to male interaction before and after MSC-exo or saline administration. Intra-subject analysis showed that the BTBR MSC-exo mice group had spent significantly more time in social interactions after the treatment whereas the BTBR saline and C57BL saline groups did not show any change (paired t test, $t_5 < 0.0001$). Comparison analysis between the groups showed that the BTBR mice of both groups had spent significantly less time engaging in social interaction in comparison to C57BL basal behavior (ANOVA1, $F_{2,18} = 14.4$, $p < 0.01$, Bonferroni). Exosome treatment dramatically increased social interactions in the BTBR MSC-exo group in comparison to BTBR mice treated with saline and is comparable to the C57BL mice group (ANOVA1, $F_{2,16} = 9.44$, $p < 0.01$, Bonferroni) (Fig. 2a, Additional files 1 and 2).

During the social interaction test, the repetitive behavior was also measured. Intra-subject analysis showed that the BTBR MSC-exo-treated group spent significantly less time in repetitive behaviors while both the BTBR saline and C57BL saline mice groups did not show any changes in comparison to their basal behaviors (paired t test, $t_5 < 0.001$). A comparison analysis between groups showed that before treatment, there was no difference between BTBR MSC-exo and BTBR saline basal behaviors, and that both groups significantly differed from the basal behavior of the C57BL saline group (ANOVA1, $F_{2,18} = 13.71$, $p < 0.001$, Bonferroni). After treatment, The BTBR MSC-exo group was not significantly different from the BTBR saline group and the

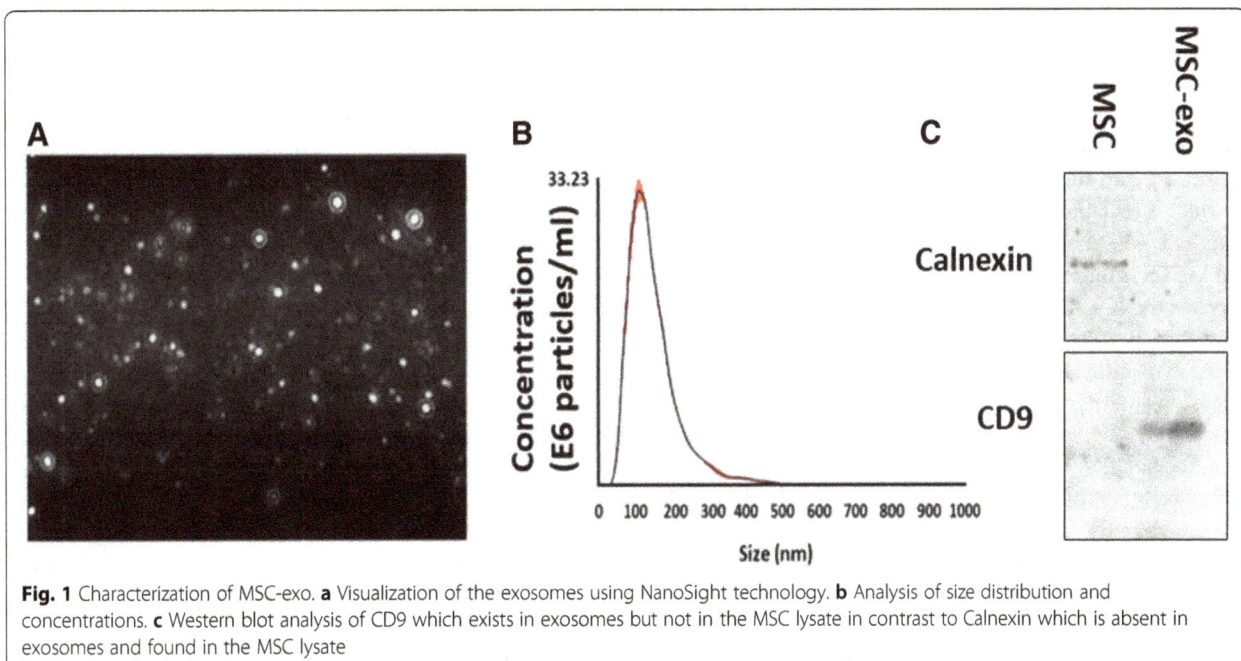

Fig. 1 Characterization of MSC-exo. a Visualization of the exosomes using NanoSight technology. b Analysis of size distribution and concentrations. c Western blot analysis of CD9 which exists in exosomes but not in the MSC lysate in contrast to Calnexin which is absent in exosomes and found in the MSC lysate

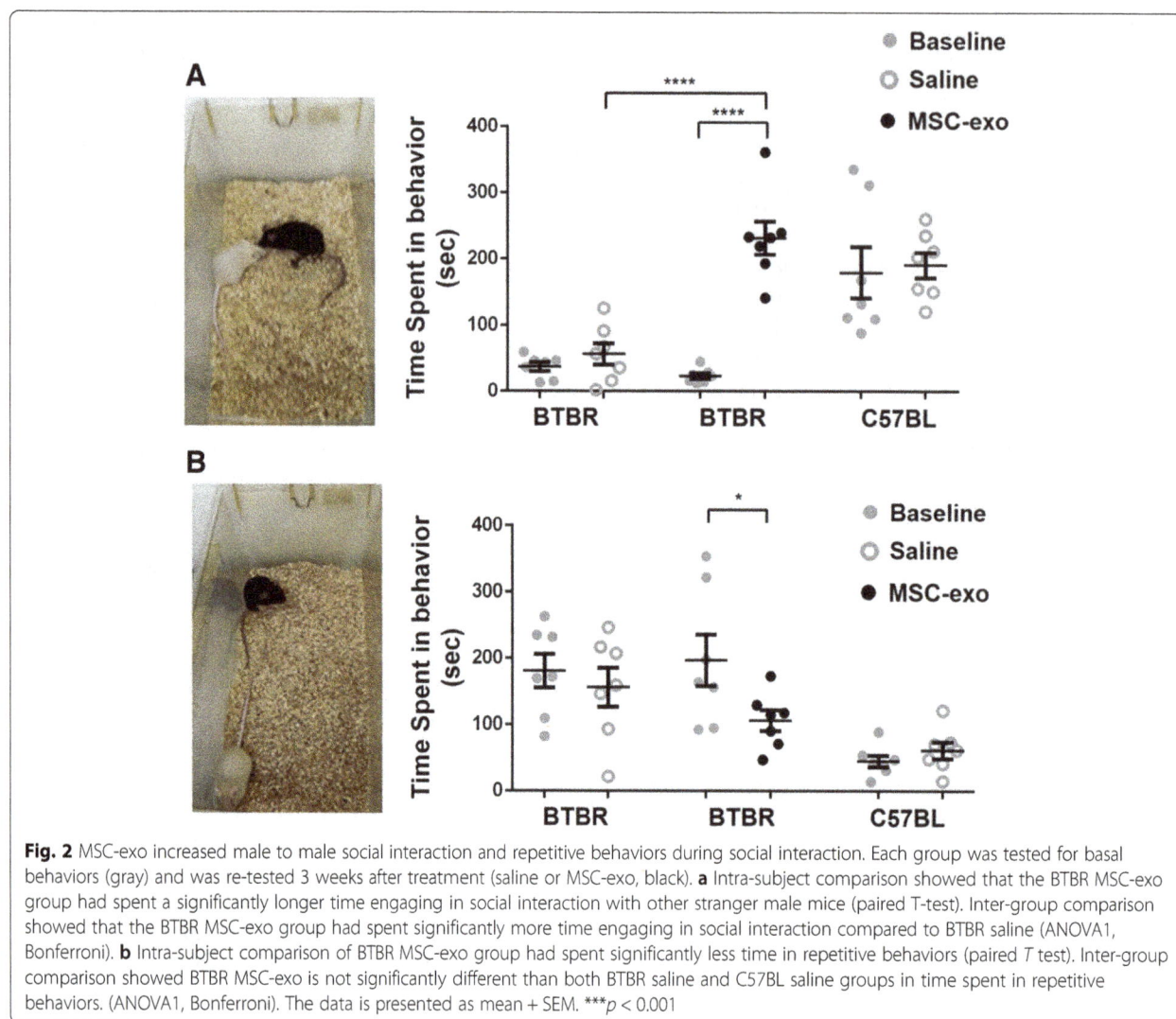

Fig. 2 MSC-exo increased male to male social interaction and repetitive behaviors during social interaction. Each group was tested for basal behaviors (gray) and was re-tested 3 weeks after treatment (saline or MSC-exo, black). **a** Intra-subject comparison showed that the BTBR MSC-exo group had spent a significantly longer time engaging in social interaction with other stranger male mice (paired T-test). Inter-group comparison showed that the BTBR MSC-exo group had spent significantly more time engaging in social interaction compared to BTBR saline (ANOVA1, Bonferroni). **b** Intra-subject comparison of BTBR MSC-exo group had spent significantly less time in repetitive behaviors (paired T test). Inter-group comparison showed BTBR MSC-exo is not significantly different than both BTBR saline and C57BL saline groups in time spent in repetitive behaviors. (ANOVA1, Bonferroni). The data is presented as mean + SEM. ***$p < 0.001$

C57BL group (Fig. 2b). In repetitive behavior tests that were outside of the context of social interaction, BTBR MSC-exo spent significantly less time in repetitive grooming and digging in intra-subject analysis compared to their basal behaviors ($t_5 < 0.05$). In groups, comparisons showed that they were significantly different from the BTBR saline group but not from the C57BL saline group (ANOVA1, $F_{2,18} = 13.83$, $p < 0.01$, Bonferroni) (Additional file 5: Figure S1). Importantly, C57BL MSC-exo mice did not present any behavioral differences in neither social interactions, antisocial interactions, nor repetitive behaviors during social contact (Additional file 5: Figure S2A). In comparison between MSC-exo to exosomes isolated from neuronal stem cells (NSC-exo), we found that only the MSC-exo-treated group presented a significant increase in social interaction, a reduction in repetitive behaviors, and a significant increase in communication while NSC-exo-treated mice did not present the same behavioral differences

compared to saline-treated group (ANOVA1, $F_{2,14} = 4.28$, $p < 0.05$, Bonferroni). Importantly, MSC-exo and saline groups were also used as a biological replication of the social interaction with different seven mice per group (Additional file 5: Figure S3).

MSC-exo improved male to female ultrasonic vocalizations

In general, male mice emitted a large number of complex ultrasonic vocalizations (USVs) when interacting with adult females (Fig. 3a, experimental demonstration). As seen qualitatively from the spectrograms in our study, BTBR MSC-exo vocalizations became more complex and longer compared to the BTBR saline group, making them more similar to C57BL (Fig. 3b). During the first 5 min of interaction with females, BTBR saline mice emitted 317 ± 39.4 syllables, BTBR MSC-exo emitted 571 ± 74 (180% more), and C57BL emitted 854.5 ± 65.2 syllables (Fig. 3c, ANOVA1, $F_{2,18} = 19.2$, $p < 0.001$,

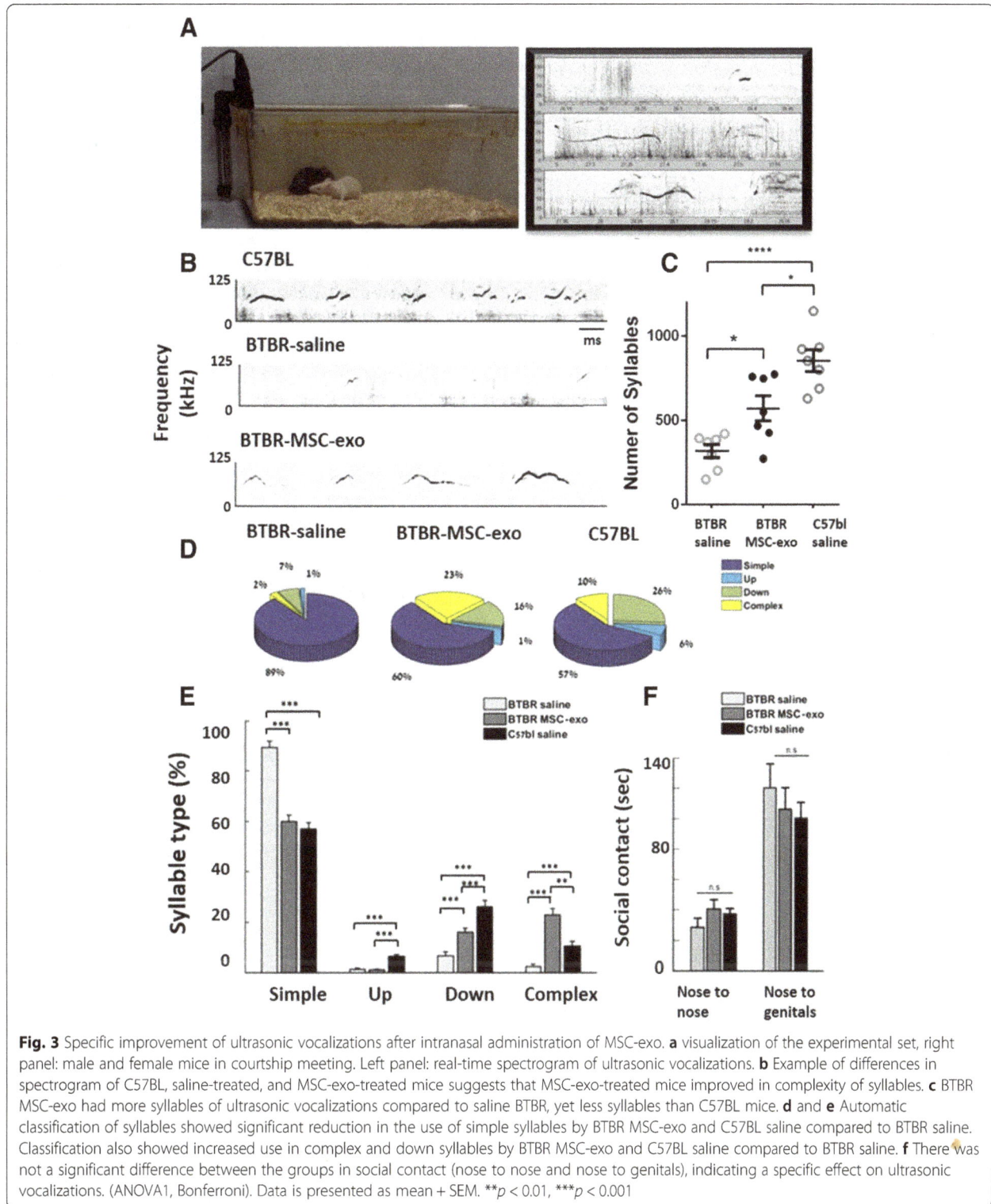

Fig. 3 Specific improvement of ultrasonic vocalizations after intranasal administration of MSC-exo. **a** visualization of the experimental set, right panel: male and female mice in courtship meeting. Left panel: real-time spectrogram of ultrasonic vocalizations. **b** Example of differences in spectrogram of C57BL, saline-treated, and MSC-exo-treated mice suggests that MSC-exo-treated mice improved in complexity of syllables. **c** BTBR MSC-exo had more syllables of ultrasonic vocalizations compared to saline BTBR, yet less syllables than C57BL mice. **d** and **e** Automatic classification of syllables showed significant reduction in the use of simple syllables by BTBR MSC-exo and C57BL saline compared to BTBR saline. Classification also showed increased use in complex and down syllables by BTBR MSC-exo and C57BL saline compared to BTBR saline. **f** There was not a significant difference between the groups in social contact (nose to nose and nose to genitals), indicating a specific effect on ultrasonic vocalizations. (ANOVA1, Bonferroni). Data is presented as mean + SEM. **$p < 0.01$, ***$p < 0.001$

Bonferroni). Classification of syllables revealed significant differences between the syllable types used by BTBR saline and BTBR MSC-exo (Fig. 3d, e). For simple syllables, BTBR saline used 89%, BTBR MSC-exo used 57%, and C57BL saline used 60% (ANOVA1, $F_{2,18}$ = 49.44, $p < 0.001$, Bonferroni). For complex syllables, BTBR saline used 2%, BTBR MSC-exo used 23%, and C57BL saline used 10% (ANOVA1, $F_{2,18} = 30.61$, $p <$

0.001, Bonferroni). For down syllables, BTBR saline used 7%, BTBR MSC-exo used 16%, and C57BL saline used 26% (ANOVA1, $F_{2,18} = 25.23$, $p < 0.001$, Bonferroni). For up syllables, BTBR saline used 1%, BTBR MSC-exo used 1%, and C57BL saline used 6% (ANOVA1, $F_{2,18} = 41.22$, $p < 0.001$, Bonferroni).

There was no significant difference between groups in time spent sniffing the female's genitals or faces, meaning that the effect seen in the ultrasonic vocalizations was not impacted by the pheromones of the females (Fig. 3f). C57BL mice that were treated with MSC-exo showed similar number of syllables compared to C57BL saline group (Additional file 5: Figure S2B). In comparison between MSC-exo and NSC-exo, only the BTBR MSC-exo group presented a significant increase in number of syllables compared to BTBR saline group (ANOVA1, $F_{2,14} = 9.44$, $p < 0.01$, Additional file 5: Figure S3B). This result also used as biological replication of the vocalizations test.

MSC-EXO improves pup retrieval behavior

We have performed pup-retrieval tests for MSC-exo- or saline-treated mothers, naïve virgins, and experienced virgins [19, 20]. The C57BL saline mothers retrieved all pups (15/15), and their total average time for retrieval

was 10.4 s ± 1.08 s. In contrast, only one of eight BTBR saline mothers retrieved two pups (in 156 s), without bringing them back to the nest. Altogether, only 2/24 pups were retrieved. After treatment, BTBR MSC-exo mothers retrieved all pups (18/18) at a mean time of 25.24 s ± 5.7 s (ANOVA1 on time of retrieval, $F_{2,48} = 332.5$, $p < 0.0001$). C57BL saline trained virgins retrieved all pups (15/15) with a total average time of 38.3 s ± 3.3 s. BTBR saline trained virgins mostly did not retrieve the pups besides for one female that had retrieved two pups with a mean time of 152 s. Altogether, 2/21 pups were retrieved by BTBR saline trained virgins. BTBR MSC-exo trained virgins retrieved 7/9 pups at a total average time of 83.3 ± 16.02 s (ANOVA1 on time of retrieval, $F_{2,42} = 29.47$, $p < 0.0001$). Neither the C57BL naïve virgins (0/21) nor the BTBR naïve virgins had retrieved the pups (0/21) (Fig. 4c, Additional files 3 and 4). We had assumed that the MSC-exo naïve virgins would also not retrieve the pups.

Visualization of MSC and exosomes after intranasal delivery

MAESTRO whole brain imaging was used to visualize PKH26-labeled MSC and MSC-exo. After intranasal and intravenous administration, MSC-exo can be visualized

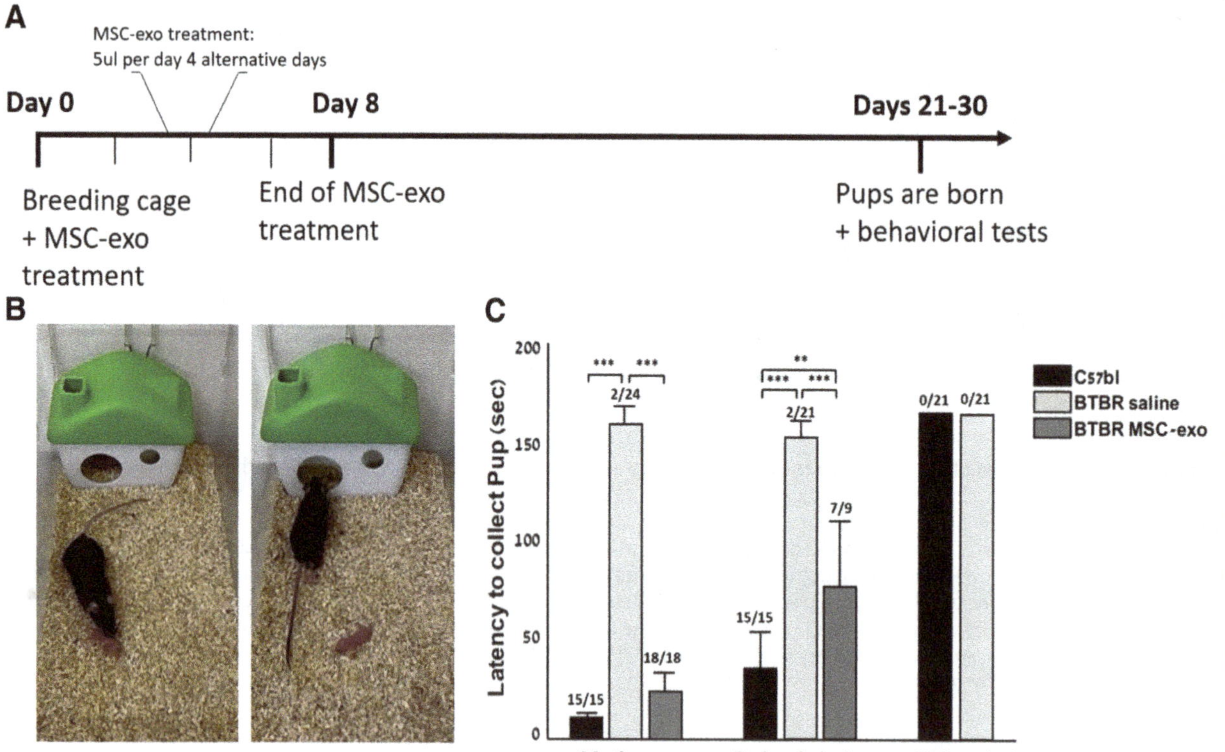

Fig. 4 MSC-exo improves maternal pup retrieval and learning of maternal pup retrieval behaviors. **a** Experiment's timeline. **b** Visualization of normal pup retrieval behavior vs. autistic-like behavior. **c** C57BL and BTBR mice groups were treated with saline or MSC-exo were tested for pup retrieval. Data is presented as mean + SEM. **$p < 0.01$, ***$p < 0.001$

fluorescently while MSC cannot be detected (Fig. 5a). Immunostaining indicated that MSC-exo penetrate the brain parenchyma and are found in the cells of the tissue (Fig. 5b, c).

MSC-exo migration and efficacy are dependent on their membrane proteins

The ability of MSC-exo to cross the blood-brain barrier and to be uptake by cells in the brain is critical for the therapeutic effect. To block the MSC-exo from being uptake by the cells in the brain and to use them as control, MSC-exo were treated with protease-k (ProtK) in order to remove the membrane proteins. Immunostainings of the tissue indicated that the MSC-exo-protk delivered intranasally have not been uptake into the cells at the same efficiency as MSC-exo (Fig. 6a as compared to Fig. 5b). To demonstrate the effectiveness of ProtK in degrading the proteins on the exosomes' membrane, we used Western blot analysis to CD9 and CD63 since they are known to be overexpressing on the membrane of the exosomes and are commonly used for exosomes detection and characterizations [42]. The Western blot showed deletion of the membrane proteins CD9 and a reduction of CD63 (Fig. 6b). NanoSight analysis showed no significant change in the number and size of MSC-exo-protK compared to MSC-exo (Fig. 6c). BTBR mice that were treated with MSC-exo-protK did not demonstrate behavioral differences in social interaction and repetitive behaviors (Fig. 6d).

Discussion

We have previously found that surgical transplantation of MSC to the brain ameliorates the autistic-like behaviors of BTBR mice [4]. Furthermore, we have shown that this effect could last for 6 months post a single treatment, even though MSC does not survive for an extended period in the brain [5]. We have also demonstrated that MSC-exo efficiently cross the blood-brain barrier after intranasal administration compares to intravenous injection, and can be visualized in vivo when they are loaded with gold nanoparticles [17]. In the current experiment, BTBR mice were treated via intranasal administration of MSC-exo followed by behavioral tests in all the ASD-like phenotypes presented by this model. Remarkably, the BTBR MSC-exo group presented significant improvements in all the tested ASD-like phenotypes.

In social interaction, the BTBR MSC-exo group spent a significantly longer time engaging in interaction with the stranger male compared to the saline-treated mice and their own basal behaviors. BTBR MSC-exo had also presented a significant decrease in repetitive behaviors of self-grooming and digging compared to their own basal behavior and to the BTBR saline group. Their scores had become closer to the C57BL saline group.

Deficits in social communication are a core symptom of ASD in children [1]. It has been reported that BTBR mice present unusual repertoire of male to female ultrasonic vocalizations compared to normal C57BL mice

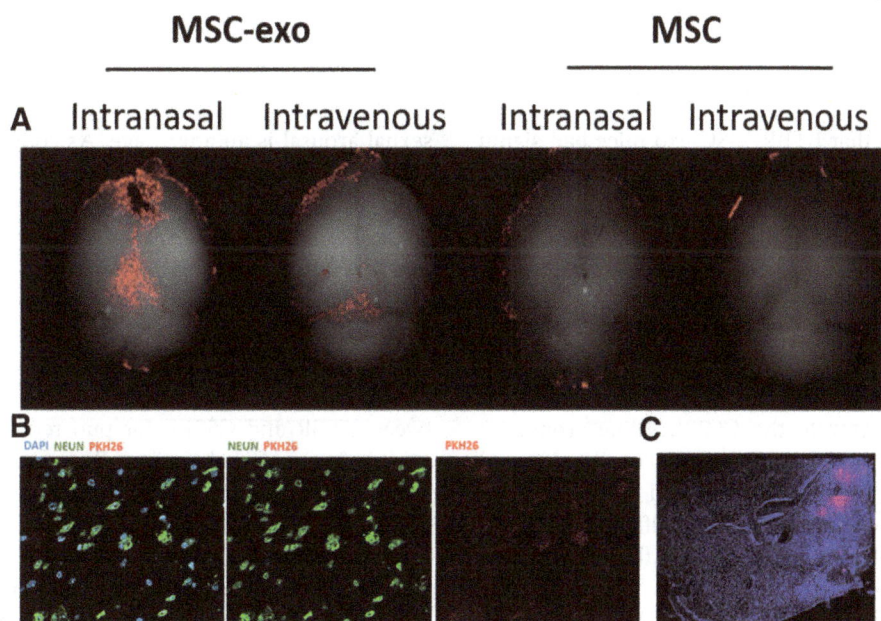

Fig. 5 Comparison between MSC-exo and MSC labeled with PKH26 visualization in the brain. **a** From left to right: MSC-exo intranasal, MSC-exo intravenous, MSC intranasal, and MSC intravenous. MSC-exo cross the blood brain barrier, both intranasally and intravenously, while MSC much less. **b** Immunostaining of neurons, DAPI and PKH26 labeled MSC-exo after intranasal administration. **c** Sagittal section of the BTBR MSC-exo brain after intranasal administration of PKH26 labeled MSC-exo (top) and Alan brain atlas (bottom)

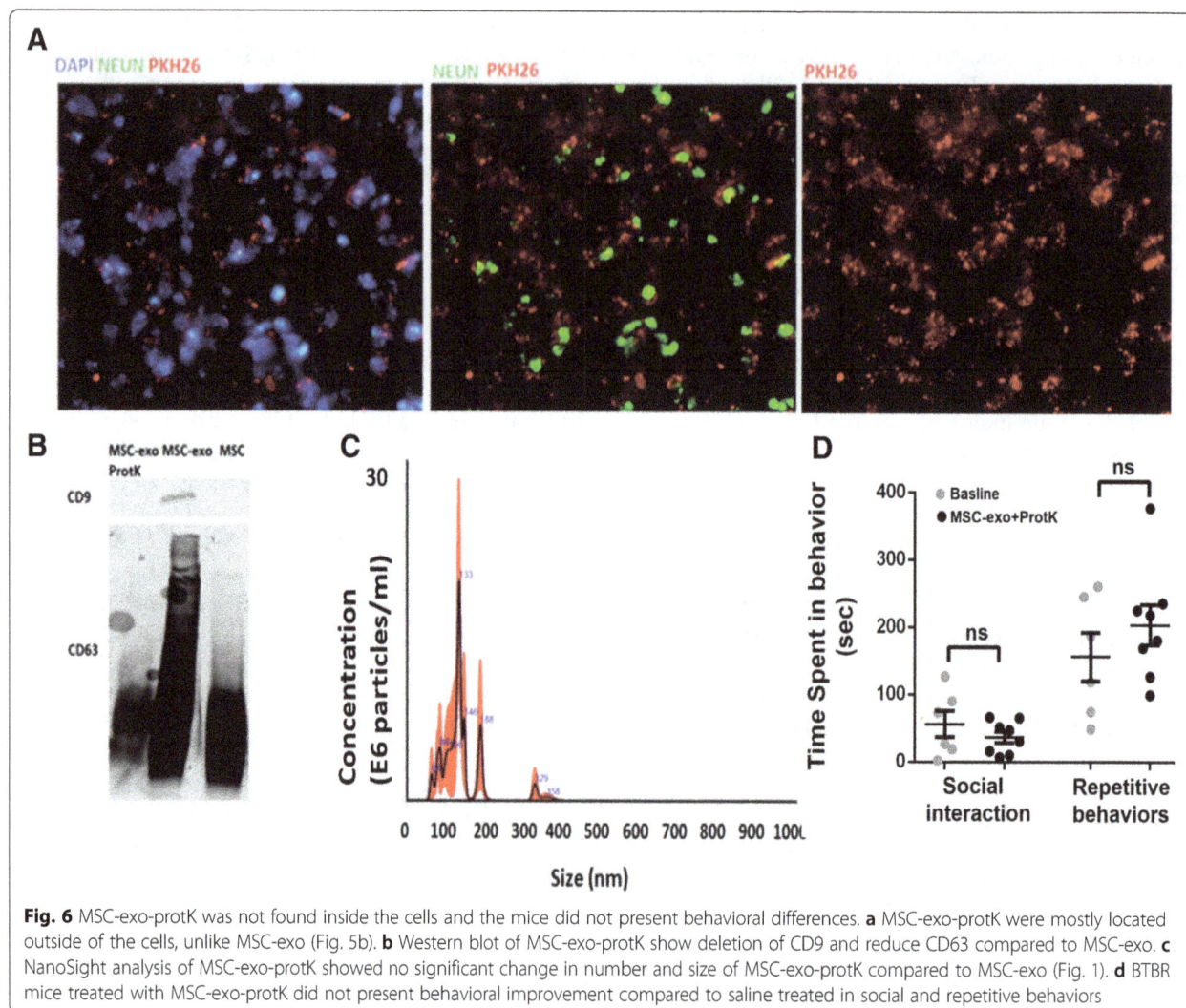

Fig. 6 MSC-exo-protK was not found inside the cells and the mice did not present behavioral differences. **a** MSC-exo-protK were mostly located outside of the cells, unlike MSC-exo (Fig. 5b). **b** Western blot of MSC-exo-protK show deletion of CD9 and reduce CD63 compared to MSC-exo. **c** NanoSight analysis of MSC-exo-protK showed no significant change in number and size of MSC-exo-protK compared to MSC-exo (Fig. 1). **d** BTBR mice treated with MSC-exo-protK did not present behavioral improvement compared to saline treated in social and repetitive behaviors

[21]. We reported that BTBR MSC-exo mice had significant improvement in the number of syllables compared to the control BTBR saline group. Their number of syllables was closer to the C57BL group. To examine other features of ultrasonic vocalizations, such as complexity and classification of syllables, we have used an advanced classification algorithm. This classification revealed significant improvement in the complexity of syllables of BTBR MSC-exo mice, making their ultrasonic vocalizations repertoire closer to the C57BL saline group. Importantly, the improvement in male-to-female ultrasonic vocalizations did not seem to be caused by higher sexual arousal as there was no significant difference between the duration of interaction initiated by the males toward the females in any of the groups. This finding was also observed in our previous studies after MSC transplantation to BTBR mice [5]. Considering the growing recognition that some adolescents and young adults with ASD may exhibit inappropriate sexual behaviors [22, 23], the fact that MSC-exo treatment also does not enhance

sexual arousal is an advantage. As compared, the C57BL MSC-exo group did not present behavioral changes in their ultrasonic vocalizations and social interactions toward both males and females. This finding may suggest that MSC-exo administration leads to beneficial effects and not to non-specific hyperactivity or behavioral side effects.

Maternal behavior of BTBR mice has yet to be studied extensively. Here, we observed significant differences between BTBR and C57BL for pup retrieval. C57BL mice exhibit "normal" behavior, and they created a nest for their pups. If the pup was separated, they had quickly retrieved it [18, 19]. In contrast, BTBR created a nest but reacted slowly to the pup separation and nearly always had not brought the pup within 3 min. Interestingly, BTBR MSC-exo mothers demonstrated high scores in the pup retrieval test, with results comparable to C57BL saline mothers. Furthermore, a naïve C57BL virgin who spent a few days with a mother can learn this "experienced" behavior. BTBR saline females did not manage to learn from other mothers (C57BL mothers) while BTBR MSC-exo had presented learning abilities. Maternal behavior, as well as social interaction, acquires high-level synchronization of sensory input and behavioral output. We suggest MSC-exo may play a role in the mechanisms of sensory integration, making its effect influential in the realms of the social domain symptoms. Sensory integration and coordination deficits have been suggested to be one of the underlying mechanism of the ASD patients [24–26].

Stem cell therapy has been previously used on ASD children with long-term beneficial effects [27]. Bone marrow MSC has been proven to be safe to use in several clinical trials [28–30]. Mechanistically, bone marrow MSC was found efficient in promoting tissue regeneration, immunomodulation, and inflammatory reduction [31–33]. We reported that the transplantation of MSC to the lateral ventricles of BTBR mice leads to increased neurogenesis and BDNF in the hippocampus [4]. Although it is clear that MSC have beneficial properties that can be used safely for clinical purposes, recent evidence shows that the therapeutic effect of MSC is largely mediated via the secretion of exosomes that contain important molecular information [34, 35]. Our findings support this concept, and our study demonstrates that a remarkable behavioral effect, on all ASD-like phenotypes of BTBR mice, can be achieved by simply using MSC-exo rather than MSC. We are aware that small number of mice per group is a limiting factor of our results, yet the behavioral difference post MSC-exo treatment is remarkable. Furthermore, in social interaction and repetitive behaviors, each mouse was compared to its own basal behavior and also to saline-treated group post the treatment, this experimental design was chosen to increase the confidence on the results. Mentionable, for the comparison between MSC-exo and NSC-exo, we used another MSC-exo-treated mice; therefore, the USV and social and repetitive behaviors post MSC-exo treatment were tested twice independently.

The contents of MSC-exo have been characterized using proteomics and RNA sequencing. Importantly, the capacity of the exosomes seems to be selectively packaged. Therefore, some of the proteins and miRNA that are over expressed in the cells are packaged in exosomes while others have over-representation [14, 36]. While exosomes contain numerous variations of RNA, their miRNA repertoire has been spotlighted as a major candidate for their effect in the host cell and the tissue. For example, miRNA-143 was found to be related to the immunomodulatory effect of MSC, and miRNA-10b was found related to their migration abilities [37, 38]. In addition, multiple miRNAs highly represented in MSC-exo (miR-191, miR-222, miR-21) regulate cell cycle progression and proliferation and modulate angiogenesis

(miR-222, miR-21) [39–41]. Yet, we are aware that MSC-exo are complex vesicles containing hundreds of proteins and RNA molecules; therefore, we cannot pinpoint on the specific factors that led to the behavioral difference and future study may be needed to uncover the mechanism of action that led MSC-exo-treated mice to behavioral amelioration. Moreover, since BTBR mice are multifactorial model of autism, it may be worth to test MSC-exo effect of other models, including genetically modified mice such as shank3 mutation as well.

Altogether, our findings suggest that MSC-exo may be tested as a safe noninvasive treatment to ameliorate behavioral symptoms of patients with ASD.

Materials and methods

Mesenchymal stem cells preparation

Human MSC were purchased from Lonza (cat:PT-2501, Basel, Switzerland). Cells were cultured and expanded as previously described [42]. Before exosome collection, the cells were cultured in exosome-free platelets for 3 days and this medium was then collected.

Exosomes purification protocol

The exosomes were purified by taking the culture fluid and centrifuging it for 10 min at 300g. The supernatant was recovered and centrifuged for 10 min at 2000g. Once again, the supernatant was recovered and centrifuged for 30 min at 10,000g. The supernatant was filtrated through a 0.22-μm filter and centrifuged for 70 min at 100,000g. The pellet containing the exosomes and proteins was washed in PBS and then centrifuged for 70 min at 100,000g. The pellet containing the purified exosomes was re-suspended in 200 μm of sterilized PBS. Each centrifugation occurred at 4 °C [43].

Neuronal stem cells preparation

Human neuronal stem cell lines (CTX0E03) were purchased from ReNeuron, UK. Cells were cultured and expanded according to the company's protocol. Cell lines were routinely cultured at 37 °C in tissue culture flasks freshly coated with mouse laminin (20 μg/ml in DMEM:F12). Growth medium supplemented with 4-OHT was changed three times per week. When 70–90% confluent, cells were passaged using trypsin (0.25%) for 5–10 min at 37 °C, followed by treatment with soybean trypsin inhibitor (0.25 mg/ml). Cells were spun down (800×g for 5 min at room temperature) and re-suspended at an appropriate density in full growth medium supplemented with 100 nM 4-OHT. The NSC-exo were purified at the same protocol as MSC-exo, and a number of particles were matched per mouse using NANOsight analysis (Merkel technologies LTD, Israel).

Exosomes characterization

NanoSight technology (Merkel technologies LTD, Israel) was used to characterize the size and concentration of the exosomes (3.81×10^8 particles/μL). Lysates of MSC-exo were subject for Western blot using SDS poly-acrylamide gel. Proteins were transferred to Immobilon®-P membranes (Millipore, Amsterdam, The Netherlands), incubated in 5% milk for 1 h, and probed overnight at 4 °C with CD9 antibody (ABCAM), CD63 (ABCAM), and Cal-nexin (ABCAM). After three washes in TBS-Tween 20, the membranes were incubated with the secondary antibody for 1 h and re-washed.

Exosomes labeling

Exosomes were labeled with PKH26 (Sigma-Aldrich) [44, 45]. PKH26 (2 μL) in 500 μL diluent was then added to 50 μL exosomes in PBS for 5 min of incubation. Exosomes were suspended in 70 ml PBS and were centrifuged for 90 min at 100,000g at 4 °C. The pellet was suspended in 200 μL of PBS.

Ex vivo imaging

Adult BTBR male mice (6–7 weeks) were given 5 μL of labeled exosomes or labeled MSC via intranasal administration ($N = 2$ per condition). Another adult BTBR male mice (6–7 weeks) were given 100 μL of intravenously with labeled exosomes or labeled MSC. (The tail vain was warmed using water and exosomes were directly injected to the vain, no anesthetics used, $N = 2$ per condition.) The number of exosomes per mouse was equal between the intranasal/intravenous administrations (19.05×10^8 particles) as well as the number of MSC. For 24-h post administration, mice were perfused and fixated with PBS and 4% paraformaldehyde (PFA). The brains were incubated in PFA for 24 h followed by 30% sucrose for 48 h and stored at 4 °C. Whole brain fluorescence imaging was taken with Maestro CRi, excitation filter 523, and emission filter 560. For immunostaining analysis, the brains were frozen in chilled 2-methylbutane (Sigma-Aldrich), stored at 4 °C, and subsequently sectioned into slices measuring 10 lm. Slides were incubated with blocking solution (5% goat/donkey serum, 1% BSA, 0.5% Triton X-100 in PBS) for 1 h. Thereafter, slides were incubated overnight at 4 °C with primary antibody in blocking solution (mouse anti-NueN, 1:500, Abcam) and secondary antibody in blocking solution (goat anti-mouse Alexa 488, 1:500, Molecular Probes, Invitrogen) for 1–2 h at room temperature. Next, nuclei were counterstained with DAPI (1:500; Sigma-Aldrich). Sections were ultimately mounted with fluorescent mounting solution (Fluoromount-G, Southern Biotech), covered with a cover slide, and sealed with nail polish.

Proteinase-k treatment to MSC-exo

Two hundred microliters of PKH26 labeled exosomes were incubated with 7 μL proteinase-K (Roche Diagnostica GmbH, Germany) and 750 μL BPS in 55 °C for 10 min [45]. Proteinase-K inhibitor (7 μL) (phenylmethanesulfonyl fluoride, Sigma) was added to the solution and was suspended for 2 h in 70 ml BPS for ultracentrifugation. Finally, the pellet (MSC-exo-protk) was re-suspended in 200ul PBS. For behavioral treatment, non-labeled MSC-exo-protk were used. Proteinase-k-treated MSC-exo were characterized with NANO-sight and Western blot.

Animals

Mice were placed under a 12-h light/12-h dark condition and grown in individual ventilated cages with access to food and water ad libitum. All experimental protocols were approved by the Tel Aviv University Committee of Animal Use for Research and Education. All methods were performed in accordance with relevant guidelines and regulations. BTBR mice were bred from adult pairs originally purchased from The Jackson Laboratory (Bar Harbor, ME). At 4 weeks of age, the first cohort of littermate male mice was randomly assigned for basal behavioral experiments followed by intranasal administration of saline (BTBR saline, $N = 7$) or MSC-exo (BTBR MSC-exo, $N = 7$). For the pup retrieval experiment, the first cohort of littermate female mice was randomly assigned at 5 weeks of age to saline or to MSC-exo. At the end of the treatment, random groups of females were placed at breeding colonies with BTBR male mice (1 male 2 females, BTBR mothers). At days 1–2 post whelping, random groups of virgin females were placed with the mothers for 4 days to gain experience (BTBR experienced virgins). The rest of the mice were left at their home cage (BTBR naïve virgins) (Additional file 5: Table S1 for number of females in each group).

C57BL mice were bred from adult pairs originally purchased from The Jackson Laboratory (Bar Harbor, ME). At 4 weeks of age, the first cohort of littermate male mice was randomly assigned for basal behavioral experiments followed by intranasal administration of saline (C57BL saline, $N = 7$) or MSC-exo (C57BL MSC-exo). For the pup retrieval experiment, the first cohort of littermate female mice was randomly assigned to saline at 5 weeks of age. At the end of the treatment, random groups of females were placed at breeding colonies with C57BL male mice (1 male 2 females, C57BL mothers). On days 1–2 post-whelping, random groups of virgin females were placed with the mothers for 4 days to gain experience (C57BL experienced virgins). The rest of the mice remained at their home cage (C57BL naïve virgins) (Additional file 5: Table S1 for number of females in each group).

For comparison between NSC-exo and MSC-exo, another group of mice was randomly assigned. They were raised as previously described and treated with intranasal administration of MSC-exo ($N = 7$), NSC-exo ($N = 5$), or saline ($N = 7$). For comparison between saline and MSC-exo+protK in behavioral experiments, another group of mice was randomly assigned. They were raised as previously described and treated with intranasal administration of MSC-exo+protK ($N = 8$) or saline ($N = 6$). Complete summary of all the mice in all the experiments is found in Table S2.

Mice were treated with intranasal MSC-exo or saline for 12 days, 5 µL a day, and every other day (total of 30 µL per mouse). Administration was done using a gentle pipette of 2.5 µL per nostril with no anesthetics.

Behavioral tests

Reciprocal dyadic social interaction test

The reciprocal dyadic social interaction test [46] was conducted using a 5-week-old male C57BL/6 stranger mouse as the social stimulus. The stranger mouse was placed in a $40 \times 40 \times 20$ cm cage with the test mouse. Prior to the test, both mice were isolated for 1 h. In addition, both mice were recorded for 20 min, with the last 10 min quantified by an observer blind to treatment. Cowlog V3 software was used to score the social contact initiated by the test mouse (Helsinki University, Helsinki, Finland). Scoring was determined by the duration that the mice had engaged the stranger mouse in social behaviors. The social behaviors that were quantified included nose to nose sniffing (i.e., approach to the front of the stranger), nose to genital sniffing (i.e., approach to the back of the stranger), and attacking (i.e., test mouse initiates a fight with the stranger mouse). Active avoidance (i.e., test mouse deliberately avoids interaction when the stranger mouse initiates it) was considered an antisocial behavior. During social interactions, the time spent in repetitive behaviors (i.e., self-grooming and digging) was also observed and quantified.

Repetitive behaviors not during social interaction

Mice were placed alone in an arena with dimensions $40 \times 40 \times 20$ cm for 20 min. The last 10 min was quantified for grooming and digging. While observing the grooming behavior, the mice were placed in a clean cage absent from wood-chips in order to prevent digging. Also, self-grooming was not measured while observing the digging behavior.

Ultrasonic vocalizations

Both BTBR and C57BL males met C57BL/6 females. Each male was placed in a separate cage for 1 h, and a female was then placed in the cage. Ultrasonic vocalizations were recorded for the first five minutes of encounter to prevent extremely high sexual arousal and mating behaviors. The encounters were filmed for male-female interaction analysis. In the study, all males and females were sexually naïve. Females were in the same cage in order to synchronize their estrus cycle and had met the males on the same day. Vocalizations were recorded with Avisoft-RECORDER v. 4.2.21 recording program. The settings included a sampling rate of 250 kHz and a format of 16 bit. For spectrogram generation, recordings were transferred to Avisoft-SASLab Pro Version 5.2.07 and a fast Fourier transformation (FFT) was conducted. Spectrograms were generated with an FFT length of 256 points and a time window overlap of 50% (100% Frame, FlatTop window). The number of syllables was quantified automatically by Avisoft-SASLab, and syllable classification was done by MATLAB using a classification algorithm [47] (Additional file 5: Supplementary Materials and Methods).

Pup retrieval

C57BL and BTBR females were tested for their latency to retrieve pups and bring them back to the nest. Each one was tested with three pups, and the duration of each trial was 180 s. In addition, the number of retrieved pups and time required for each pup retrieval was measured. During the test, all females were taken out of the home cage and were placed back one at a time for a 5-min acclimation with the pups prior to testing. Each of the pups was between 1 and 3 days old [18, 19]. The tests were filmed with a SAMSUNG 11mp camera.

Additional files

Additional file 1: BTBR male control male to male social interaction. (AVI 5543 kb)

Additional file 2: BTBR male MSC-exo male to male social interaction. (mov 6092 kb)

Additional file 3: BTBR mother control pup retrieval. (AVI 5543 kb)

Additional file 4: BTBR mother MSC-exo pup retrieval. (AVI 6092 kb)

Additional file 5: Figure S1. MSC-exo decreases repetitive behavior of self-grooming. Intra-subject comparison shows BTBR MSC-exo group spent significantly less time in repetitive behaviors, while BTBR saline and C57BL saline showed no difference between basal and post treatment behavior (paired T test). Inter-group comparison shows BTBR MSC-exo is significantly different than BTBR saline group in time spent in repetitive behaviors. (ANOVA1, Bonferroni). Data is presented as mean + SEM. **$p < 0.05$. **Figure S2.** MSC-exo had no significant effect on C57BL behavior. A. C57BL mice were tested for baseline behavior (baseline) and after MSC-exo intranasal administration (post-treatment) in the tests of social, antisocial interaction, and repetitive behaviors. No significant differences were found in any of the behaviors (paired T test, $p > 0.05$). B. C57BL MSC-exo mice presented no difference in their number of USV compared to saline-treated group (unpaired T test, $p > 0.05$). Data is presented as mean + SEM. **Figure S3.** MSC-exo but not NSC-exo significantly ameliorates male to male social interaction, repetitive behaviors, and male to female ultrasonic vocalizations of BTBR mice. A. male to male social interaction. B. repetitive behaviors. C. male to female ultrasonic vocalizations (ANOVA 1, Bonfferoni *$p < 0.05$, **$p < 0.01$, ***$p < 0.001$). Data is presented as mean +

SEM. **Figure S4.** Full Western blot gels: A. Calnexin as negative marker for MSC-exo B. CD9 as positive marker of MSC-exo. C. CD63 as positive marker of MSC-exo and for reduction after protK treatment. D. CD9 as positive marker of MSC-exo and for reduction after ProtK treatment. **Table S1.** Number of females tested in maternal behavioral experiment. **Table S2.** Number of mice at each group in the behavioral experiments. (DOCX 1010 kb)

Abbreviations

ASD: Autism spectrum disorders; BTBR: BTBR T+tf/J; MSC: Mesenchymal stem cells; MSC-exo: Exosomes secreted from MSC

Acknowledgements

The authors would like to thank the following for their contributions in the research: Shai Israel for his kind help in the MATLAB code and Michael Anbar for his kind help in consulting and helping with Western blots.

Funding

N.P. received funding scholarship from Sagol School of Neuroscience, Tel Aviv University.

Authors' contributions

NP was involved in the idea generation, all of the experiments, and writing the paper. SH developed the classification algorithm of the ultrasonic vocalizations in Fig. 3 and was involved in writing the paper. ML supervised SH with developing the algorithm and writing the paper. DO supervised NP and was involved in idea generation of the experiments and writing the paper. All authors read and approved the final manuscript.

Competing interests

DO and NP have submitted several patent applications related to exosomes. All were assigned to "Ramot at Tel Aviv University." Brainstorm Cell Therapeutics to "Stem Cell Medicine." The other authors have nothing to disclose.

Author details

[1]Sagol School of Neuroscience, Tel Aviv University, Tel Aviv, Israel. [2]Edmond and Lily Safra Center for Brain Sciences, Hebrew University, Jerusalem, Israel. [3]Sacklar School of Medicine, Department of Human Genetics and Biochemistry, Tel Aviv University, Tel Aviv, Israel.

References

1. Wilkins T, Pepitone C, Alex B, Schade RR. Diagnosis and management of IBS in adults. Am Fam Physician. 2012;86(5):419–26. https://doi.org/10.1136/bmj. d6238.
2. Meyza KZ, Defensor EB, Jensen AL, et al. The BTBR T+ tf/J mouse model for autism spectrum disorders in search of biomarkers. Behav Brain Res. 2013; 251:25–34. https://doi.org/10.1016/j.bbr.2012.07.021.
3. Yang M, Scattoni ML, Zhodzishsky V, et al. Social approach behaviors are similar on conventional versus reverse lighting cycles , and in replications across cohorts, in BTBR T + tf / J , C57BL / 6J , and vasopressin receptor 1B mutant mice. 2007;1(November):1–9. https://doi.org/10.3389/neuro.08/001. 2007.
4. Segal-Gavish H, Karvat G, Barak N, et al. Mesenchymal stem cell transplantation promotes neurogenesis and ameliorates autism related behaviors in BTBR mice. Autism Res. 2016;9(1):17–32. https://doi.org/10. 1002/aur.1530.
5. Perets N, Segal-Gavish H, Gothelf Y, Barzilay R, Barhum Y, Abramov N, Hertz S, Morozov D, London M, Offen D. Long term beneficial effect of neurotrophic factorssecreting mesenchymal stem cells transplantation in the BTBR mouse model of autism. Behav Brain Res. 2017. https://doi.org/10. 1016/j.bbr.2017.03.047.
6. Ankrum J a, Ong JF, Karp JM. Mesenchymal stem cells: immune evasive, not immune privileged. Nat Biotechnol. 2014;32(3):252–60. https://doi.org/10. 1038/nbt.2816.
7. Ng KS, Kuncewicz TM, Karp JM. Beyond hit-and-run: stem cells leave a lasting memory. Cell Metab. 2015;22(4):541–3. https://doi.org/10.1016/j.cmet. 2015.09.019.
8. Zhang Y, Chopp M, Liu XS, Katakowski M, Wang X. Exosomes derived from mesenchymal stromal cells promote axonal growth of cortical neurons. 2016. https://doi.org/10.1007/s12035-016-9851-0.
9. Braccioli L, Van Velthoven C, Heijnen CJ. Exosomes: a new weapon to treat the central nervous system. 2014:113–9. https://doi.org/10.1007/s12035-013-8504-9.
10. Valadi H, Ekström K, Bossios A, Sjöstrand M, Lee JJ, Lötvall JO. Exosome-mediated transfer of mRNAs and microRNAs is a novel mechanism of genetic exchange between cells. Nat Cell Biol. 2007;9(6):654–9. https://doi. org/10.1038/ncb1596.
11. Yu B, Zhang X, Li X. Exosomes derived from mesenchymal stem cells. Int J Mol Sci. 2014;15(3):4142–57. https://doi.org/10.3390/ijms15034142.
12. Xin H, Li Y, Buller B, et al. Exosome-mediated transfer of miR-133b from multipotent mesenchymal stromal cells to neural cells contributes to neurite outgrowth. Stem Cells. 2012;30(7):1556–64. https://doi.org/10.1002/ stem.1129.
13. Roubelakis MG, Pappa KI, Bitsika V, Antsaklis A, Anagnou NP. Molecular and proteomic characterization of human comparison to bone marrow mesenchymal stem cells. 2007;951:931–51. https://doi.org/10.1089/scd.2007. 0036.
14. Haraszti RA, Didiot MC, Sapp E, et al. High-resolution proteomic and lipidomic analysis of exosomes and microvesicles from different cell sources. J Extracell Vesicles. 2016;5(1):1–14. https://doi.org/10.3402/jev. v5.32570.
15. Haney MJ, Klyachko NL, Zhao Y, et al. Exosomes as drug delivery vehicles for Parkinson's disease therapy. J Control Release. 2015;207:18–30. https:// doi.org/10.1016/j.jconrel.2015.03.033.
16. Sun D, Zhuang X, Xiang X, et al. A novel nanoparticle drug delivery system: the anti-inflammatory activity of curcumin is enhanced when encapsulated in exosomes. Mol Ther. 2010;18(9):1606–14. https://doi.org/ 10.1038/mt.2010.105.
17. Betzer O, Perets N, Angel A, et al. In vivo neuroimaging of exosomes using gold. 2017. https://doi.org/10.1021/acsnano.7b04495.
18. Hansen S. Maternal behavior of female rats with 6-OHDA lesions in the ventral striatum: characterization of the pup retrieval deficit. Physiol Behav. 1994;55(4):615–20. https://doi.org/10.1016/0031-9384(94)90034-5.
19. Svirsky N, Levy S, Avitsur R. Prenatal exposure to selective serotonin reuptake inhibitors (SSRI) increases aggression and modulates maternal behavior in offspring mice. Dev Psychobiol. 2016;58(1):71–82. https://doi. org/10.1002/dev.21356.
20. Livshts MA, Khomyakova E, Evtushenko EG, et al. Isolation of exosomes by differential centrifugation: theoretical analysis of a commonly used protocol. Sci Rep. 2015;5(October):1–14. https://doi.org/10.1038/srep17319.
21. Scattoni ML, Ricceri L, Crawley JN. Unusual repertoire of vocalizations in adult BTBR T+tf/J mice during three types of social encounters. Genes Brain Behav. 2011;10(1):44–56. https://doi.org/10.1111/j.1601-183X.2010.00623.x.
22. Hayward B. Sexual behaviours of concern in young people with autism spectrum disorders; 2010. p. 17–8.
23. Sutton LR, Hughes TL, Huang A, et al. Identifying individuals with autism in a state facility for adolescents adjudicated as sexual offenders: a pilot study. Focus Autism Other Dev Disabl. 2013;28(3):175–83. https://doi.org/10.1177/ 1088357612462060.
24. Ayres a J, Tickle LS. Hyper-responsivity to touch and vestibular stimuli as a predictor of positive response to sensory integration procedures by autistic children. Am J Occup Ther Off Publ Am Occup Ther Assoc. 1980;34(6):375–81. https://doi.org/10.5014/ajot.34.6.375.

25. Iarocci G, McDonald J. Sensory integration and the perceptual experience of persons with autism. J Autism Dev Disord. 2006;36(1):77–90. https://doi.org/10.1007/s10803-005-0044-3.

26. Tomchek SD, Dunn W. Sensory processing in children with and without autism: a comparative study using the short sensory profile. Am J Occup Ther. 2007;61(2).

27. Dawson G, Sun JM, Davlantis KS, et al. Autologous cord blood infusions are safe and feasible in young children with autism Spectrum disorder: results of a single-center phase I open-label trial. Stem Cells Transl Med. 2017:1332–9. https://doi.org/10.1002/sctm.16-0474.

28. Petrou P, Gothelf Y, Argov Z, et al. Safety and clinical effects of mesenchymal stem cells secreting neurotrophic factor transplantation in patients with amyotrophic lateral sclerosis. JAMA Neurol. 2016;73(3):1. https://doi.org/10.1001/jamaneurol.2015.4321.

29. Duijvestein M, Vos ACW, Roelofs H, et al. Autologous bone marrow-derived mesenchymal stromal cell treatment for refractory luminal Crohn's disease: results of a phase I study. Gut. 2010;59:1662–9. https://doi.org/10.1136/gut.2010.215152.

30. Gothelf Y, Abramov N, Harel A, Offen D. Safety of repeated transplantations of neurotrophic factors-secreting human mesenchymal stromal stem cells. Clin Transl Med. 2014;3:21. https://doi.org/10.1186/2001-1326-3-21.

31. Shimizu S, Kitada M, Ishikawa H, Itokazu Y, Wakao S, Dezawa M. Peripheral nerve regeneration by the in vitro differentiated-human bone marrow stromal cells with Schwann cell property. Biochem Biophys Res Commun. 2007;359(4):915–20. https://doi.org/10.1016/j.bbrc.2007.05.212.

32. Wilkins A, Kemp K, Ginty M, Hares K, Mallam E, Scolding N. Human bone marrow-derived mesenchymal stem cells secrete brain-derived neurotrophic factor which promotes neuronal survival in vitro. Stem Cell Res. 2009;3(1):63–70. https://doi.org/10.1016/j.scr.2009.02.006.

33. Sotiropoulou P a, Papamichail M. Immune properties of mesenchymal stem cells. Methods Mol Biol. 2007;407(2):225–43. https://doi.org/10.1007/978-1-59745-536-7_16.

34. Baglio SR, Pegtel DM, Baldini N. Mesenchymal stem cell secreted vesicles provide novel opportunities in (stem) cell-free therapy. Front Physiol. 2012;3 SEP(September):1–11. https://doi.org/10.3389/fphys.2012.00359.

35. Lener T, Gioma M, Aigner L, et al. Applying extracellular vesicles based therapeutics in clinical trials - an ISEV position paper. J Extracell Vesicles. 2015;4:1–31. https://doi.org/10.3402/jev.v4.30087.

36. Baglio SR, Rooijers K, Koppers-Lalic D, et al. Human bone marrow- and adipose-mesenchymal stem cells secrete exosomes enriched in distinctive miRNA and tRNA species. Stem Cell Res Ther. 2015;6(1):127. https://doi.org/10.1186/s13287-015-0116-z.

37. Zhao X, Liu D, Gong W, et al. The toll-like receptor 3 ligand, Poly(I:C), improves immunosuppressive function and therapeutic effect of mesenchymal stem cells on sepsis via inhibiting MiR-143. Stem Cells. 2014;32(2):521–33. https://doi.org/10.1002/stem.1543.

38. Zhang F, Jing S, Ren T, Lin J. MicroRNA-10b promotes the migration of mouse bone marrow-derived mesenchymal stem cells and downregulates the expression of E-cadherin. Mol Med Rep. 2013;8(4):1084–8. https://doi.org/10.3892/mmr.2013.1615.

39. Nagpal N, Kulshreshtha R. miR-191: an emerging player in disease biology. Front Genet. 2014;5(APR):1–10. https://doi.org/10.3389/fgene.2014.00099.

40. Urbich C, Kuehbacher A, Dimmeler S. Role of microRNAs in vascular diseases, inflammation, and angiogenesis. Cardiovasc Res. 2008;79(4):581–8. https://doi.org/10.1093/cvr/cvn156.

41. Yoo JK, Kim J, Choi S-J, et al. Discovery and characterization of novel microRNAs during endothelial differentiation of human embryonic stem cells. Stem Cells Dev. 2012;21(11):2049–57. https://doi.org/10.1089/scd.2011.0500.

42. Sadan O, Melamed E, Offen D. Intrastriatal transplantation of neurotrophic factor-secreting human mesenchymal stem cells improves motor function and extends survival in R6/2 transgenic mouse model for Huntington's disease. PLoS Curr. 2012;4:e4f7f6dc013d4e. https://doi.org/10.1371/4f7f6dc013d4e.

43. Théry C, Clayton A, Amigorena S, Raposo G. Isolation and characterization of exosomes from cell culture supernatants. Curr Protoc Cell Biol. 2006:3.22.1-3.22.29.

44. Yu B, Kim HW, Gong M, et al. Exosomes secreted from GATA-4 overexpressing mesenchymal stem cells serve as a reservoir of anti-apoptotic microRNAs for cardioprotection. Int J Cardiol. 2015;182(C):349–60. https://doi.org/10.1016/j.ijcard.2014.12.043.

45. Fitzner D, Schnaars M, van Rossum D, et al. Selective transfer of exosomes from oligodendrocytes to microglia by macropinocytosis. J Cell Sci. 2011;124(Pt 3):447–58. https://doi.org/10.1242/jcs.074088.

46. Silverman JL, Pride MC, Hayes JE, et al. GABAB receptor agonist R-baclofen reverses social deficits and reduces repetitive behavior in two mouse models of autism. Neuropsychopharmacology. 2015;40(9):2228–39. https://doi.org/10.1038/npp.2015.66.

47. Wiaderkiewicz J, Głowacka M, Grabowska M, et al. Male mice song syntax depends on social contexts and influences female preferences. J Neurol Neurosurg Psychiatry. 2013;44(4):1–16. https://doi.org/10.1136/jnnp.44.7.600.

Savant syndrome has a distinct psychological profile in autism

James E A Hughes[1]* ⓘ, Jamie Ward[1], Elin Gruffydd[1], Simon Baron-Cohen[2], Paula Smith[2], Carrie Allison[2] and Julia Simner[1]

Abstract

Background: Savant syndrome is a condition where prodigious talent can co-occur with developmental conditions such as autism spectrum conditions (autism). It is not yet clear why some autistic people develop savant skills while others do not.

Methods: We tested three groups of adults: autistic individuals who have savant skills, autistic individuals without savant skills, and typical controls without autism or savant syndrome. In experiment 1, we investigated the cognitive and behavioural profiles of these three groups by asking participants to complete a battery of self-report measures of sensory sensitivity, obsessional behaviours, cognitive styles, and broader autism-related traits including social communication and systemising. In experiment 2, we investigated how our three groups learned a novel savant skill—calendar calculation.

Results: Heightened sensory sensitivity, obsessional behaviours, technical/spatial abilities, and systemising were all key aspects in defining the savant profile distinct from autism alone, along with a different approach to task learning.

Conclusions: These results reveal a unique cognitive and behavioural profile in autistic adults with savant syndrome that is distinct from autistic adults without a savant skill.

Keywords: Autism spectrum conditions, Savant syndrome, Sensory processing, Cognition, Perception, Talent, Skill learning

Background

People with savant syndrome are characterised by their remarkable talent in one or more domains (e.g. music, memory) but also by the presence of some form of developmental condition such as autism spectrum conditions (henceforth autism) [1]. Autism describes a set of symptoms involving difficulties in social communication, unusually repetitive/routine behaviours, unusually narrow interests, and atypical sensitivity to sensory stimuli [2]. Recent models of autism also focus on strengths associated with the condition (not just on their difficulties), in areas such as perceptual and cognitive processing [3], systemising [4], and attention to detail [5], as well as areas of interest, aptitude, and talents. In savant syndrome, talents and skills observed in such individuals far exceed their own overall level of intellectual or developmental functioning.

Exceptional cases of *prodigious* savant syndrome occur when an autistic individual's level of skill goes beyond that seen even in the general population. A well-known example of a prodigious savant is the artist Stephen Wiltshire who is capable of drawing hyper-detailed cityscapes from memory and who also has autism [6]. Savant skills can exist in a variety of areas, but most savants show skills in art (e.g. hyper-detailed drawings), music (proficiency in musical instrument playing), maths (fast mental arithmetic), calendar calculation (the ability to provide the day of the week for any given date), and memory recall of facts, events, numbers etc. [7].

Although savant syndrome can co-occur with a range of developmental conditions, most cases involve autism in some form [8, 9] and savant syndrome has been reported to occur in up to 37% of autistic individuals [10].

---

* Correspondence: james.hughes@sussex.ac.uk
[1]School of Psychology, Pevensey Building, University of Sussex, Brighton BN1 9QJ, UK
Full list of author information is available at the end of the article

The emergence of savant skills in autistic adults is not fully understood, and there is a lack of empirical evidence to support current theories. The motivation for the current research is to understand the condition of savant syndrome in more depth by contrasting a group of autistic savant individuals with a group of autistic individuals who do not have a savant skill. A third group of typical controls without autism or savant skills serve as a comparison. With this approach, we aim to separate features that are tied to savant syndrome from features that are tied to autism per se. We ask what individual differences lie within the autistic population that might allow some to develop savant skills while others do not. We first summarise current theoretical frameworks on the origins of savant skills. We then present two experiments that consider the development of savant skills at multiple levels of cognition, perception, and behaviour.

There is no consensus on exactly how savant skills are developed in autistic individuals. Bölte and Poustka [11] showed that savants do not show differences in standard intelligence compared to other autistic individuals. It could therefore be that their skills develop simply through many hours of extended practice. This would be similar to the abilities of neurotypical 'memory athletes' who can, for instance, memorise thousands of digits of pi using mnemonic techniques, with top performers relying on thousands of hours of practice—as in other sports [12–14]. Savants too appear to require practice, but here we ask exactly *why* they practice and whether they also have cognitive or perceptual differences beyond practice alone.

Two theoretical models have bridged the gap between need-for-practice and autistic symptoms in savants [15, 16]. Happé and Vital [15] proposed that one way in which savant skills might emerge could be through the autism-related trait of mind-blindness, which is the difficulty in attributing mental states to others [17, 18]. Happé and Vital [15] suggest that a lack of interest in the social world could serve to free up cognitive and time resources that are usually dedicated to monitoring social interactions. As a result, these extra resources could be re-allocated to the development of talent by permitting more time (i.e. practice) to the nurturing of restricted interests commonly observed in autistic individuals. Since these cognitive resources have been allocated away from monitoring social interactions, a further expected consequence might also be lower social and communication skills in savants and we explore this in experiment 1 below.

In contrast, Simner et al. [16] suggest that the hours spent achieving savant ability are the result not of mind-blindness, but of the autism-linked trait of obsessiveness—i.e. savants have an obsessive urge to over-rehearse their skills to prodigious levels. Tentative support for this comes from LePort et al. [19] who showed that a group of individuals with prodigious event-memory (some of whom are likely to be savants [16]) showed higher obsessional traits than controls. However, the controls they tested did not have autism, making it unclear whether obsession was tied to savant skills per se or simply to autism (or other co-occurring neurodevelopmental differences [20]). O'Connor and Hermelin [21] compared savants to controls with autism and drew similar conclusions about obsessiveness—but their questionnaire also contained items unrelated to obsessions (e.g. decision-making). In addition, they may not have corrected their question-by-question statistics for multiple comparisons, making it difficult to tie their findings to any particular trait. Similarly, Howlin et al. [10] used a questionnaire of just five questions, testing repetitive behaviours with a number of other traits (e.g. sensory sensitivity), again making it difficult to interpret their findings (of no difference between autistic-savants and autistic-nonsavants).

Finally, Bennet and Heaton [22] found higher scores for savant children on a five-question factor they named 'obsessions and special interests' compared to autistic-nonsavants, but traced this back to an individual question related to becoming absorbed in different topics. Given these differences across studies in their focus, questionnaire length, and testing groups, it remains unclear whether savants are particularly notable for their obsessional traits, above and beyond what we would expect from autism alone. Here we test both models described above, i.e. to see whether savants are particularly notable for their obsessional traits or for traits that are linked to mind-blindness (e.g. social and communication skills), compared to autistic individuals without savant skills.

Although both types of rehearsal (from mind-blindness or obsessiveness) could influence savant skills, this practice alone probably does not act as the only catalyst for talent to emerge. There may also be differences in certain cognitive abilities, linked to autism, which manifest themselves more strongly in individuals who acquire savant skills compared to those who do not. Specifically, we propose here and previously [16, 23] that talent could emerge from autism traits such as excellent attention-to-detail, hyper-systemising, and sensory differences. For example, the combination of attention-to-detail and hyper-systemising may predispose some autistic individuals to develop talent through the increased detection of 'if p, then q' rules [23]. These rules can be found in savant skills such as calendar calculation (i.e. stating the weekday for a given date) and can be learned from predictable patterns within the calendar itself.

A related proposal is Mottron et al.'s [24] 'veridical mapping' that links savant talent to the enhanced ability of autistic individuals to detect regularities within and between systems. Some savant skills do indeed depend on mapping regularities across systems (e.g. mapping from musical pitch to note-label in absolute pitch). In addition, savants appear to show a particular cognitive style of enhanced local processing, as outlined in the *enhanced perceptual functioning* model [3], and less global interference (e.g. in a target-detection task [25]) at least when activities demand active interaction [26]. Again, however, it is not clear whether these influences are tied to being a savant or simply having autism. Here we test groups of autistic individuals with and without savant syndrome to examine whether savants have a particular cognitive style (e.g. local bias), as well as elevated autism-related traits such as systemising.

Savant talent may also have important sensory components. Baron-Cohen et al. [23] argue that heightened sensory sensitivity may be the pre-requisite for excellent attention-to-detail, which they theorise as an autistic trait linked to savant syndrome. Subjective accounts of sensory irregularities in autism have been shown previously [27–30], and multiple studies have objectively demonstrated superior visual, auditory, and tactile sensory perception in autism [31–36]. These sensory differences may bring about the emergence of talent by affecting information processing at an early stage [23] although this suggestion is not universally supported [22].

One final sensory link between autism and savant syndrome is the presence of synaesthesia, where stimuli such as letters, numbers, and sounds invoke automatic and additional sensory experiences such as colours [37, 38]. Hughes et al. [39] found that synaesthesia occurs at higher levels among autistic individuals with savant skills (but not those without savant skills). Simner et al. [37] hypothesised that the obsessive over-rehearsal of savants may focus particularly on skills born out of synaesthesia, building on earlier work [25]. Elsewhere, we have already supported one branch of this model by showing that people with synaesthesia have elevated skills in savant domains (e.g. event recall [16]). Here we test the other branch of the model by examining whether their rehearsal is born out of obsessive traits [16] or mind-blindness which might predict lower social or communication skills [15]. Finally, we test the role of sensory sensitivities more generally, by comparing the sensitivities of autistic individuals with and without savant skills.

In our experiments, we look at two groups of autistic individuals, with and without a savant skill (specifically, *prodigious* talents which are above the skills of the general population). In experiment 1, we contrast our groups on cognitive and sensory self-report measures predicted by previous theoretical accounts. We test differences related to sensory sensitivity using the Glasgow Sensory Questionnaire (GSQ) [30], we test obsessive-behaviours using the Leyton Obsessional Inventory (LOI) [40], we test cognitive styles (e.g. local bias) using the Sussex Cognitive Styles Questionnaire (SCSQ) [41], and we test autistic traits such as systemising using the Systemising Quotient-Revised (SQ-Revised) [42] and the Autism Spectrum Quotient (AQ) [43]. In addition to our two groups of autistic individuals, with and without savant skills, we also test a typical control group with neither autism nor prodigious talents.

As stated above, there is very little empirical evidence to evaluate current theories of savant syndrome apart from tentative pointers towards increased obsessionality [16] and evidence for links to synaesthesia [16, 39]. Our goal is to test all theories directly; therefore, our predictions are based on the above theoretical frameworks. Following the theory by Baron-Cohen et al. [23], we predict that savants, relative to autistic individuals without a savant skill, will report more traits or behaviours related to sensory sensitivity, attention-to-detail, and systemising. We also predict they will report a more local (as opposed to global) cognitive style since this has previously been implicated in (e.g. visual search) advantages in autism and has been theorised to contribute to the development of savant skills [44]. Based on the model of autism-linked obsessive rehearsal [16], we predict that autistic-savants will report more obsessional behaviours compared to autism individuals without a savant skill. Alternatively, the rehearsal account based on mind-blindness [15] predicts that autistic savants would have lower social or communication skills (here measured using the AQ) compared to autistic individuals without a savant skill. Finally, we predict that both autism groups, regardless of the presence of a savant skill, will report heightened traits or behaviours in all of the above areas compared to the typical control group.

Experiment 2 investigates how a distinct psychological or behavioural profile in savants (explored in experiment 1) might influence performance on a behavioural task. We test the same three groups, to determine whether savants have a particular style of learning when presented with a novel savant skill: calendar calculation. As noted above, calendar calculation is the ability to give the correct day of the week for a given date in the past or future (e.g. 18th September 1990 was a Tuesday) and is considered one of the most characteristic savant abilities [7]. In experiment 2, three groups of participants (autistic-savants, autistic-nonsavants, controls) learned how to calendar calculate through a series of tutorials about different patterns and rules of the calendar. It is unclear whether calendar-calculating savants rely on rote memorisation of dates [45] or internalisation of the inherent rules of the calendar (e.g. 1st March 2013, 2014, 2015 = Friday, Saturday, Sunday respectively) or indeed whether they use some multi-faceted approach [44]. No studies to date have investigated the learning of calendar calculation skills in savants (who do not already possess this skill) compared to nonsavant autistic individuals and controls; therefore, our predictions below are again based on current theoretical models of savant syndrome.

If savant syndrome is linked to pre-existing abilities or dispositions (as opposed to practice alone), then we predict that savants may show a superior level of accuracy. In particular, the 'enhanced perceptual functioning' and 'veridical mapping' models predict more accurate performance by savants from their superiority in learning pattern/rule-based skills [3, 24, 44]. In contrast, accounts of savant skills that emphasise obsession or practice may not predict immediate advantages without extended training but might predict a different learning approach. Thus, if savants show increased repetitive/obsessive tendencies, we might expect them to engage in a slower, more careful approach to our calendar calculation task from, for example, increased answer checking.

In summary, our studies investigate savant syndrome by directly contrasting savants against a group of autistic individuals without a savant skill as well as a typical control group. Our investigation is the first to take an empirical approach to test a number of theoretical accounts of savant syndrome [15, 16, 23, 24, 44], some of which currently lack a clear empirical foundation.

Experiment 1: traits linked to savant syndrome
Methods
Participants

One hundred and eleven participants took part in the study. They comprised 44 autistic individuals with savant skills ('autistic-savants': 23 female; mean age 36.52, range 20–55, SD = 9.56), 36 autistic individuals without a savant skill ('autistic-nonsavants': 23 female; mean age 36.67, range 18–51, SD = 9.35), and 31 typical controls with neither autism nor a savant skill ('controls': 25 female; mean age 36.84, range 18–50, SD = 10.94). Participants were matched group-wise on age, with no significant differences across groups $F(2, 110) = .009$, $p = .991$.

Participants were recruited from two sources. Three of the 44 autistic-savants were recruited from The Savant Network, which is a group of individuals with a self-reported savant skill who have expressed an interest in taking part in research studies at the University of Sussex. The remaining autistic-savants were recruited from the Cambridge Autism Research Database (CARD). All autistic-nonsavant individuals and all controls also came from CARD, which holds status information of both autism and typical participants. To ensure that our autism participants had sufficient cognitive levels to independently provide consent, we sent our recruitment materials to high functioning autistic adults, as detailed in the CARD database of autistic participants. Participants volunteered to take part in our study in response to an

email advertisement that was sent to 4172 participants in these databases (553 autistic-savants, 930 autistic-nonsavants, and 2689 typical adults). The email did not describe the nature of our tests but invited participants to take part in studies that look into how people 'perceive and interact with the world around them'. Participants did not receive payment for taking part, and our study was approved through the Cross-Schools Science and Technology Research Ethics Committee at the University of Sussex. In addition to the 111 participants, we additionally recruited but subsequently excluded 12 further participants because they initially indicated autism but failed to meet our criteria when probed further (see the 'Procedure' section).

All individuals in the autism groups (autistic-savant; autistic-nonsavant) self-reported having a formal diagnosis of autism in our questionnaire (see the 'Materials' section): 9 autism, 64 Asperger syndrome, 1 pervasive developmental disorder not otherwise specified, and 6 other. These formal diagnoses had also been recorded for 77 of the 80 autistic individuals as part of their CARD recruitment procedure. There were no controls who reported autism. All autistic-savants, and no other group, self-reported having a savant skill (in our *Sussex Savant Questionnaire*; see below).

Materials

We administered the following questionnaires: the Sussex Savant Questionnaire (SSQ), the Glasgow Sensory Questionnaire (GSQ) [30], the Leyton Obsessional Inventory—short form (LOI) [40], the Sussex Cognitive Styles Questionnaire (SCSQ) [41], the Systemising Quotient-Revised (SQ-R) [42], and the Autism Spectrum Quotient (AQ) [43]. These are described below.

Sussex Savant Questionnaire

This questionnaire was created for the purposes of this study. An initial question asked 'Have you received a formal diagnosis of any of the following: Autism, Asperger Syndrome, Pervasive developmental disorder not otherwise specified; 'other'?'. Next, we provided a definition of *prodigious* savant syndrome and then asked: 'Do you think that you have any skills, abilities, or talents (e.g. art, maths, music etc.) that are beyond the abilities of the general population?' Participants who responded in the affirmative to this question were given a list of nine categories of savant skills to choose from and used check boxes to indicate the skills that were relevant to them (see Fig. 1). One option was 'other' with a text-box provided for elaboration.

Autism Spectrum Quotient

The AQ contains 50 items to measure autistic traits in adults of average or above average intelligence [43]. The AQ contains 10 statements for each of five different

What type of skills do you have?

Please select all that apply

☐ **Math** (fast mental arithmetic calculations, generation of prime numbers etc...)

☐ **Calendar calculation** (generation of the appropriate day of the week of a given date)

☐ **Musical instrument playing** (do you show a particular talent for playing an instrument?)

☐ **Music reproduction** (Can you reproduce a piece of music after hearing it for the first/only a few times?)

☐ **Absolute pitch** (can you identify the note of a pitch just by listening to it? For example a musical note on a piano or the buzzing of an electric fan)

☐ **Art** (drawing, painting, sculpting)

☐ **Memory** (Memorization of films, bus routes, maps, sports trivia etc...)

☐ **Mechanical** (building, creating, measuring distances)

☐ **Fluency for different languages**

☐ **Other** (please specify)

Fig. 1 Savant skill categories, as presented during the savant skills questionnaire

subscales: social skills, attention switching, attention-to-detail, imagination, and communication. Participants responded to each statement on a four-point scale (definitely agree, slightly agree, slightly disagree, definitely disagree). Example items included 'I find it hard to make new friends', 'It does not upset me if my daily routine is disturbed', and 'I find it difficult to imagine what it would be like to be someone else'. Approximately half of the questions are reverse coded. Responses were coded as 0 or 1, with total scores ranging from 0 to 50. Items were given a score of one point if the participant recorded an autistic trait (e.g. exceptional attention-to-detail or poor social skill) using the 'slightly' or 'definitely' response. A total score of 32 or above is used is a strong indicator of likely autism [43].

Systemising Quotient-Revised

The SQ-R contains 75 items with possible scores ranging from 0 to 150, where a higher score suggests a greater tendency to systemise. Systemising is defined as the drive to identify and analyse systematic relationships or patterns in rule-based information. Participants demonstrated their level of agreement with each statement using a four-point scale (definitely agree, slightly agree, slightly disagree, definitely disagree). An individual scores two points if he/she strongly displays a systemising response and one point if they slightly display a systemising response, and approximately half the items are reverse-coded. Example items included 'When I look at a building, I am curious about the precise way it was constructed' and 'If I were buying a stereo, I would want to know about its precise technical features'.

Glasgow Sensory Questionnaire

The GSQ contains 42 items (scored from 0 to 4, 'never' to 'always' respectively, with possible total scores ranging from 0 to 168) that explore unusual sensory behaviours, for example, 'Do you react very strongly when you hear an unexpected sound?' and 'Do bright lights ever hurt your eyes or cause a headache?'. The questionnaire measures sensory sensitivity across seven modalities that include visual, olfactory, auditory, gustatory, tactile, vestibular, and proprioception. Each of these modalities is represented by six items in the questionnaire, and this is further broken down into three items each in order to measure both hypo-sensitivity and hyper-sensitivity per modality.

Sussex Cognitive Styles Questionnaire

The SCSQ consists of 60 questions that assess the general cognitive profile of an individual and his/her style of thinking (e.g. visual/verbal cognitive styles). Each question has one of five answers (strongly disagree, disagree, neither agree nor disagree, agree, strongly agree). Each question is linked to one or more of six factors (imagery ability, technical/spatial abilities, language and word forms, need for organisation, global bias, and systemising). The factor of 'imagery ability' refers to the use of visual imagery in everyday life (e.g. 'I often use mental images or pictures to help me remember things'). The factor 'technical/spatial abilities' refers to technical interests (e.g. 'If I were buying a computer, I would want to know exact details about its hard drive capacity and processor speed'), mathematical abilities (e.g. 'I am fascinated by numbers'), and the use of spatial mental imagery (e.g. 'I can easily imagine and mentally rotate three-dimensional geometric figures'). The factor 'language and word forms' refers to an interest in the visual appearance of written language as opposed to spoken language abilities (e.g. 'When I hear a new word, I am curious to know how it is spelled'; 'When I read something, I always notice whether it is grammatically correct'). The factor 'need for organisation' refers to things relating to order and organisation (e.g. 'If I had a collection (e.g. CDs, coins, stamps), it would be highly organised'). The factor 'global bias' refers to the tendency to process stimuli holistically rather than by its local features (e.g. 'I usually concentrate on the whole picture, rather than the small details'). Reverse scored questions for this factor indicate more attention-to-detail or a local processing preference (e.g. 'I tend to focus on details in a scene rather than the whole picture'). Finally, the factor 'systemising tendency' refers to an interest in systems (e.g. 'I am fascinated by dates') and categorisation (e.g. 'When I look at an animal, I like to know the precise species it belongs to').

Leyton Obsessional Inventory—short form

The LOI consists of 30 questions that assess the presence or absence of obsessional symptoms using a 'true/false' format. Each question relates to one of four factors (contamination, doubts/repeating, checking/detail, and worries/just right) in the questionnaire. Factor 1—'contamination' is related to concerns about germs, dirty environments, obsessive cleanliness, and the excessive use of cleaning products (e.g. 'I avoid using the public telephone because of possible contamination'). Factor 2—'doubts/repeating' is related to uncomfortable thoughts, repeating behaviours, checking, and serious doubts about everyday things (e.g. 'I frequently get nasty thoughts and have difficulty getting rid of them'). Factor 3—'checking/detail' is specifically related to repeated checking, too much attention-to-detail, conscience/honesty concerns, and strict routine (e.g. 'I am more concerned than most people about honesty'). Factor 4—'worries/just right' is related to behaviours such as taking a long time to dress and to hang up and put away clothing, worrying about bumping into other people, and belief in unlucky numbers (e.g. 'some numbers are extremely unlucky').

Procedure

All participants were tested remotely via the online survey-hosting platform Qualtrics (www.qualtrics.com). Participants (autistic-savants, autistic-nonsavants, and controls) accessed the study by clicking on a URL provided to them electronically. After seeing the information sheet and consent page, participants saw the following questionnaires in order: SSQ, AQ, SQ-R, GSQ, SCSQ, and LOI. For those participants recruited from the CARD database, the AQ and SQ-R data were collected in a separate procedure as part of the standard protocol for participants when signing up to that database. In this, participants completed the AQ and SQ-R (among other tests) online during the sign-up stage of recruitment. Our procedure took approximately 20 min to complete, and participants were also asked a set of additional questions for publication elsewhere (concerning synaesthesia).

Results

Since some participants completed different elements of our tasks (e.g. because they left before the end of the study), we preface our results with the number of participants in each test. All data here and throughout approximated normal distributions and so parametric statistics were used. We conducted a series of ANOVA's to investigate group differences in each of our measures separately.

Autism Spectrum Quotient

AQ data was collected from 33 autistic-savants, 30 autistic-nonsavants, and 28 controls, and Fig. 2 shows every factor of the AQ. We conducted a 3×5 ANOVA contrasting group (autistic-savants, autistic-nonsavants, controls) and the individual AQ factors (social skills, attention switching, attention-to-detail, communication, imagination), and a main effect of group was found ($F(2, 88) = 96.96$, $p < .001$, $\eta p2 = .69$). There was also a main effect of factor ($F(4, 352) = 29.50$, $p < .001$, $\eta p2 = .25$) and an interaction between group and factor ($F(8, 352) = 7.44$, $p < .001$, $\eta p2 = .15$). Post hoc comparisons with Bonferroni correction revealed the same pattern of results for every factor, that is, a significant difference between autistic-savants and controls (all $p < .001$) and between autistic-nonsavants and controls (all $p < .001$), but not between autistic-savants and autistic-nonsavants (all $p > .05$).

Where we found null results between autistic-savants and autistic-nonsavants for the AQ, we calculated Bayes factors to determine whether null results indicated no difference or a lack of statistical power.[1] We selected an informed prior (i.e. the mean difference we might expect between our participant groups, and its standard error) from an earlier study [43] using the same dependent variable as the current study. This prior was generated by looking at the difference in AQ scores between UK Mathematics Olympiad winners ($N = 16$) and autistic individuals ($N = 58$), and we treat Mathematics Olympiad Winners as a comparable group to autistic-savants in our own study (i.e. both groups display some form of exceptional skill). This comparison was chosen because we are looking to see whether differences truly exist between our autistic-savants and autistic-nonsavants. Our Bayes factors suggested support for the null

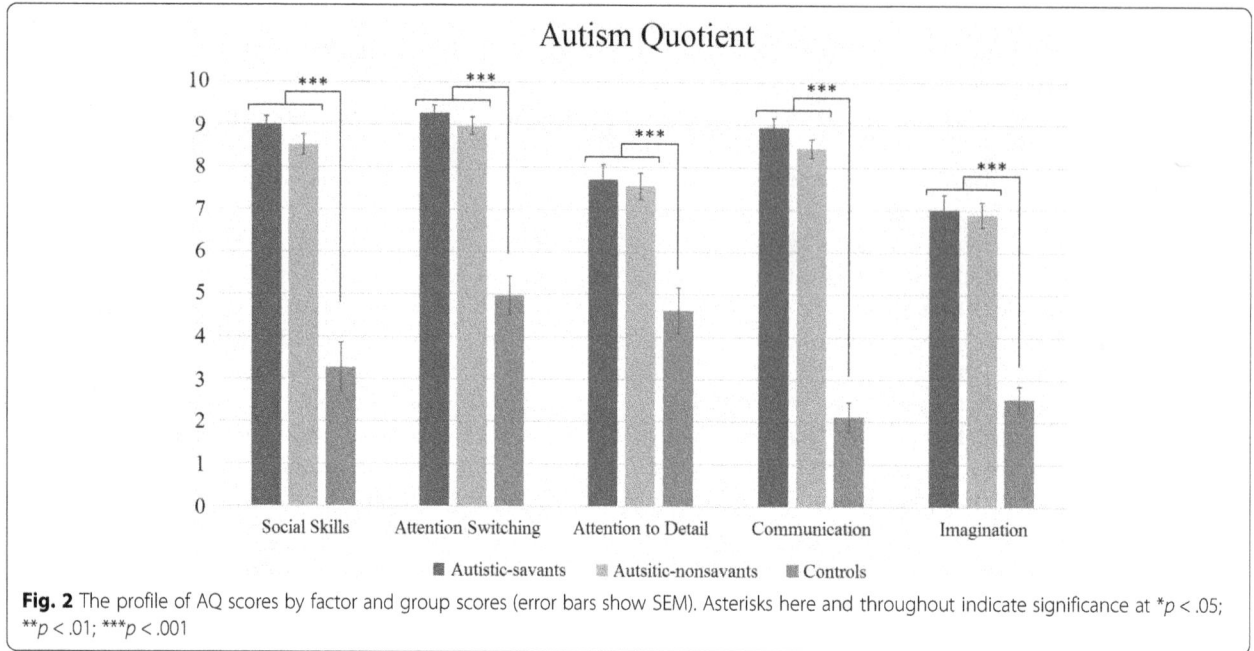

Fig. 2 The profile of AQ scores by factor and group scores (error bars show SEM). Asterisks here and throughout indicate significance at $*p < .05$; $**p < .01$; $***p < .001$

hypothesis (i.e. no differences between groups) for four of the five AQ factors (social skills BF < .33; communication BF < .33; attention switching BF < .33; imagination BF = .35) with the exception of attention-to-detail, for which no firm conclusions could be drawn (BF = 0.96). Refer to Additional file 1 for more information regarding our calculation of the above Bayes factors including our choice of parameters as well as a sensitivity analysis.

Systemising Quotient-Revised

SQ-R data was collected for 31 autistic-savants, 33 autistic-nonsavants, and 27 controls, and their data is shown in Fig. 3. A one-way ANOVA comparing these differences revealed a significant main effect, $F(2, 90) = 23.94$, $p < .001$, $\eta p2 = .35$. Post hoc comparisons with Bonferroni correction revealed significant differences between the autistic-savant and autistic-nonsavant group ($p = .022$), the autistic-savant and control group (p

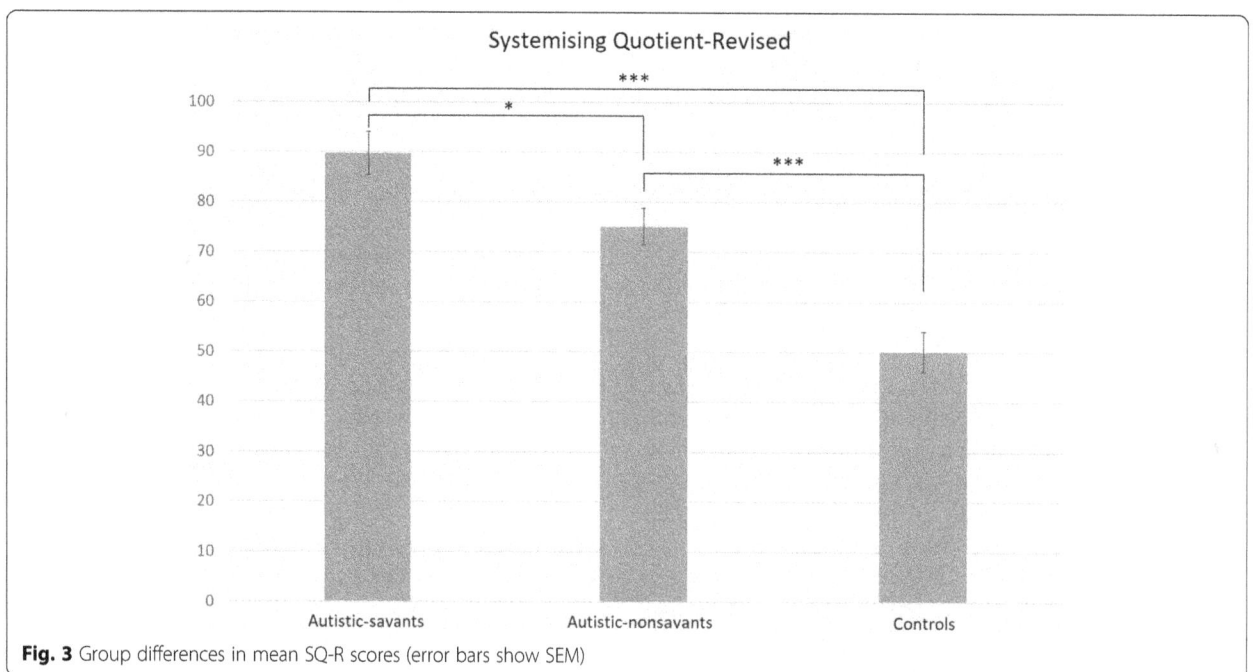

Fig. 3 Group differences in mean SQ-R scores (error bars show SEM)

< .001), and the autistic-nonsavant and control group (p < .001). In other words, the pattern was autistic-savants > autistic-nonsavants > controls.

Glasgow Sensory Questionnaire

All participants completed this test. Figure 4 displays participants' total GSQ scores for the autistic-savant, autistic-nonsavant, and control group. A one-way ANOVA comparing these differences revealed a significant main effect, $F(2, 110) = 29.35$, $p <$ .001, ηp2 = .35. Post hoc comparisons with Bonferroni correction revealed significant differences in total GSQ scores between the autistic-savant and autistic-nonsavant group (p = .030), the autistic-savant and control group ($p <$ .001), and the autistic-nonsavant and control group ($p <$ .001). In other words, the pattern again was autistic-savants > autistic-nonsavants > controls.

Sussex Cognitive Styles Questionnaire

All participants completed this test. Figure 5 shows all factors of the SCSQ. We conducted a 3 × 6 ANOVA contrasting group (autistic-savants, autistic-nonsavants, controls) and the individual SCSQ factors. We found a significant main effect of group ($F(2, 108) = 6.06$, p = .003, ηp2 = .10), a significant main effect of factor ($F(5, 540) = 31.84$, $p <$ .001, ηp2 = .23), and an interaction between group and factor ($F(10, 540) = 7.69$, $p <$ .001, ηp2 = .13).

Post hoc comparisons with Bonferroni correction revealed significant differences (all $p <$ .05) between autistic-savants and controls on technical/ spatial, need for organisation, global bias, and systemising. Significant differences (all $p <$ .05) were also found between autistic-nonsavants and controls on need for organisation, global bias, and systemising. A significant difference was also found between autistic-savants and

autistic-nonsavants on technical/spatial (p = .005). No significant differences were found between any group for 'imagery ability' or 'language and word forms'. As before, we calculated Bayes factors to determine whether these null results indicated no difference or a lack of statistical power. This time, however, no suitable previous studies exist from which to draw informed priors. We therefore used an uninformative prior with the H1 (prior distribution) modelled as a uniform distribution in which all effects within a specified interval are considered equally likely (given no previous evidence to inform our decision). Following the standard procedure, we entered the lowest and highest possible mean differences between groups (i.e. zero and [maximum score per factor minus minimum score] respectively). Our calculation of Bayes factors suggests evidence for the null hypothesis for both imagery (BF = .22) and language (BF = .30). In summary, we found that autistic individuals, irrespective of savant syndrome, scored higher than controls on need for organisation, systemising, and local bias (i.e. low global bias). In addition, autistic-savants out-performed controls and autistic-nonsavants in technical/spatial traits.

Leyton Obsessional Inventory—short form

All participants completed this test. Figure 6 shows all factors of the LOI across groups. We conducted a 3 × 4 ANOVA contrasting group (autistic-savants, autistic-nonsavants, controls) and the individual LOI factors (contamination, doubts/repeating, checking/detail, worries/just right). There was a significant main effect of group ($F(2, 108) = 16.28$, $p <$ .001, ηp2 = .23), a significant main effect of factor ($F(3, 324) = 90.78$, $p <$ .001, ηp2 = .46), and a significant interaction ($F(6, 324) = 2.85$, p = .01, ηp2 = .05).

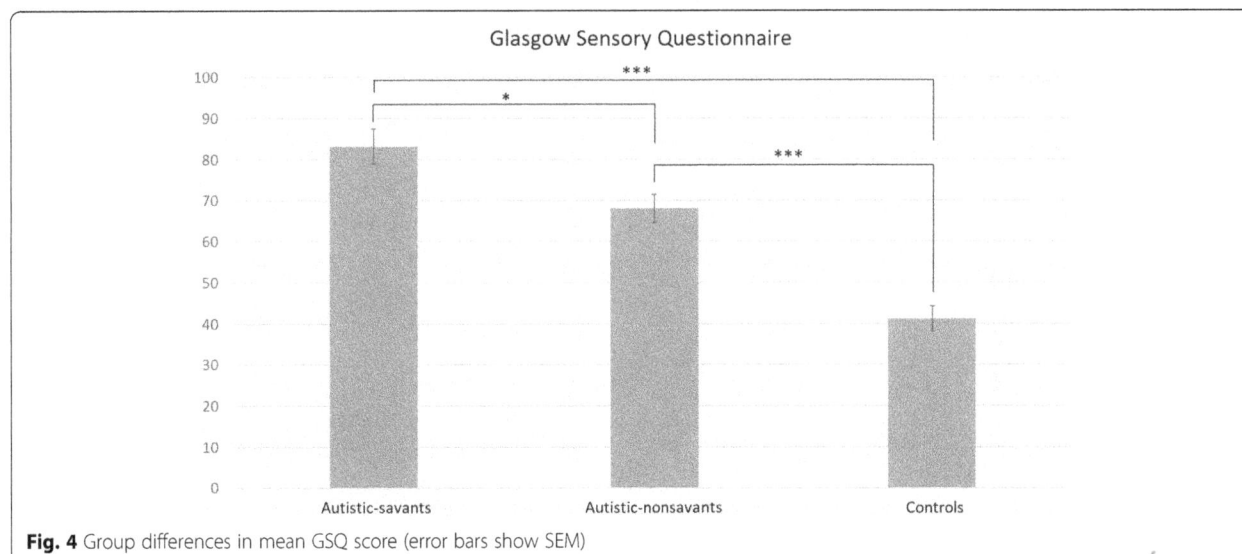

Fig. 4 Group differences in mean GSQ score (error bars show SEM)

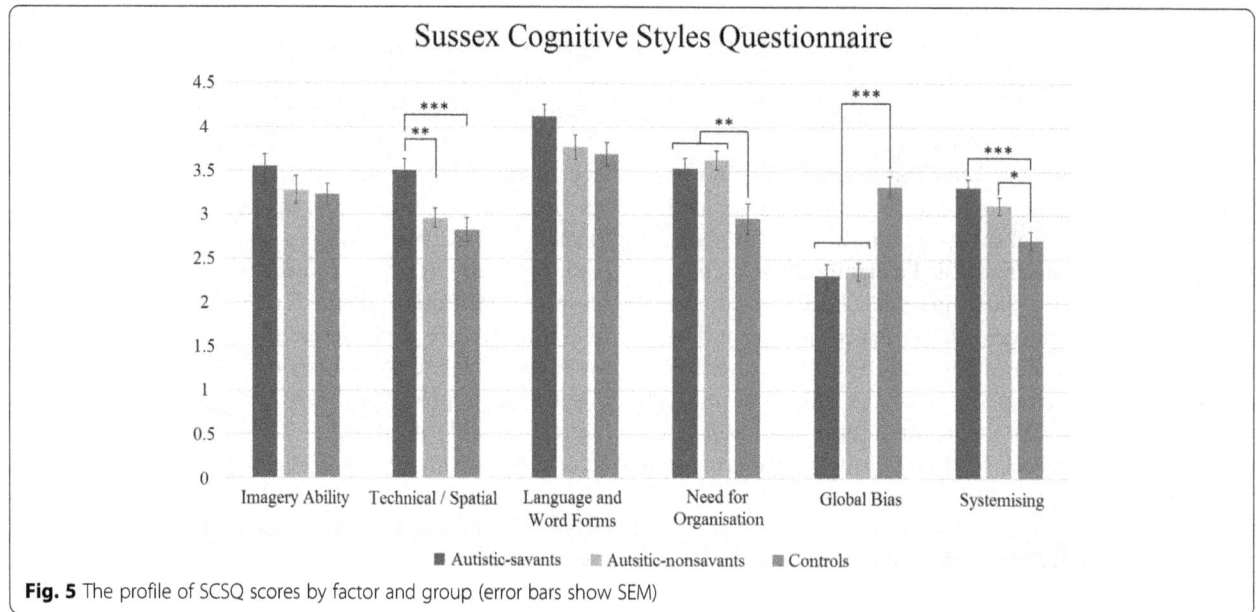

Fig. 5 The profile of SCSQ scores by factor and group (error bars show SEM)

Post hoc comparisons with Bonferroni correction revealed significant differences between autistic-savants and controls on every factor (all $p < .05$). Significant differences were also found between autistic-nonsavants and controls on every factor (all $p < .05$) apart from the worries/just right factor ($p = .58$). Finally, a significant difference between autistic groups emerged on the worries/just right factor with autistic-savants scoring higher than autistic-nonsavants ($p = .02$).

We also found that seven autistic-savants as well as two autistic-nonsavants and one control scored above the threshold of a score of 20 or more which suggests obsessive-compulsive disorder (OCD) symptoms. However,

a chi-square test of association between the rates of OCD symptoms in the three groups did not reach significance ($\chi^2(2) = 4.34$, $p = .11$).

Sussex Savant Questionnaire

All participants completed this test, whose aim had been to separate our autism sample into our two autism sub-groups (autistic-savants and autistic-nonsavants). Table 1 shows the categories of skills asked about during the study along with the number of cases of each skill reported by participants. For completeness, the Additional file 2 contain descriptive statistics for the various sub-scales of our above questionnaire measures broken

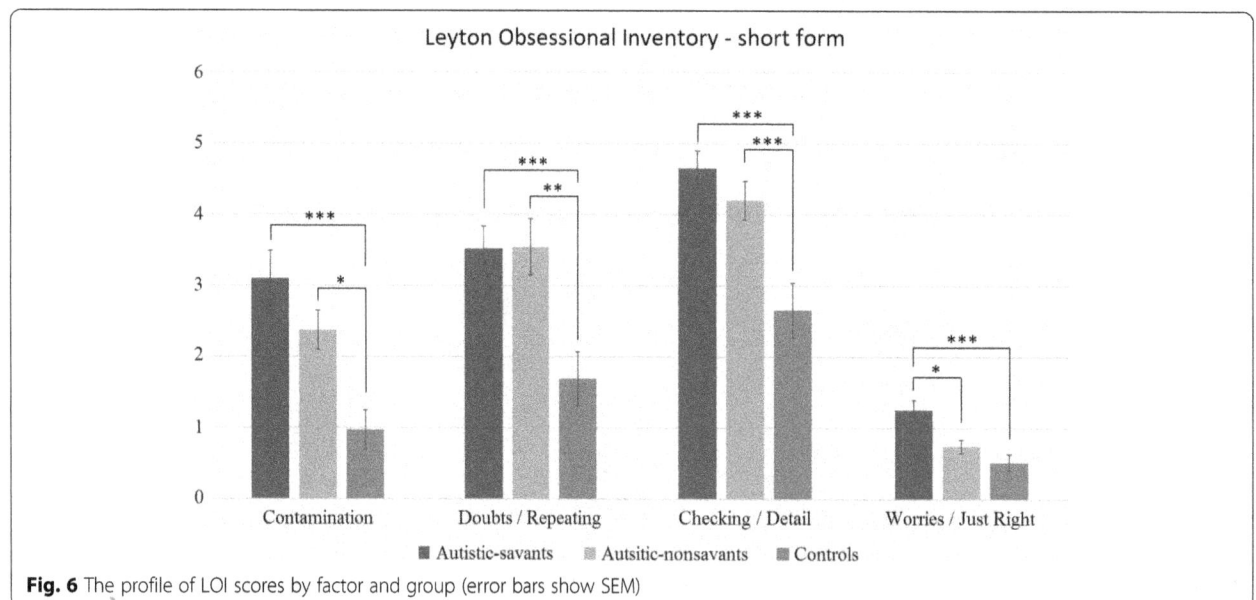

Fig. 6 The profile of LOI scores by factor and group (error bars show SEM)

Table 1 Types of savant skills reported by the autistic-savant group, some participants reported having multiple savant skills

Skill types	Number of cases
Math	16
Calendar calculation	3
Musical instrument playing	6
Music reproduction	9
Absolute pitch	12
Art	16
Memory	26
Mechanical (building)	8
Fluency for different languages	12
Other	25

down according to the presence or absence of particular savant skills, but we do not consider them in detail here due to the large number of measures and lack of power when smaller samples are divided in this way.

As an additional validation of our methodology, we looked again at the skills reported in Table 1, to see whether these self-reports could be directly tied to our measures. We found a 'dose-like' effect in the number of savant skills reported within our savant group. Here a significant correlation was found between the number of savant skills reported and the strength of the technical-spatial abilities found in our *Sussex Cognitive Styles Questionnaire* ($r = .43$, $p_{corrected} = .01$); none of our other above effects were significant (all $p's_{corrected} > .05$). Finally, we note that there were gender imbalances across our groups (see [46] for gender effects in autism). For an exploration of the effects of gender on all of our above measures, see footnote.[2]

Discussion
Our results reveal a distinct profile of group differences between autistic-savants and autistic-nonsavants. The autistic-savants differed from autistic-nonsavants in that the former had heightened sensory sensitivity, greater obsessional behaviours (relating to excessive worries and getting things 'just right'), more systemising traits, and increased technical/spatial traits (i.e. technical interests, mathematical abilities, and the use of spatial mental imagery). In all instances, these traits are features of autism more generally (i.e. they also discriminated between autistic-nonsavants and controls) but were particularly enhanced in savant syndrome specifically (i.e. discriminating autistic-savants from autistic-nonsavants). However, it is not the case that savants are simply shifted upwards along the autism spectrum. We did not find any differences between autistic-savants and autistic-nonsavants on the AQ or on subscales relating to attention-to-detail or social and communication skills,

which might otherwise have been expected based on previous theoretical accounts [15, 23]. The implications of these findings for other theoretical models are discussed in more depth in the 'General discussion' section.

Experiment 2: learning the novel savant skill of calendar calculation
The purpose of experiment 2 was to explore whether participants could be trained to perform a characteristic savant skill—calendar calculation—and to investigate whether autistic-savants would show differences in accuracy or learning-style compared to autistic-nonsavants. As before, controls without autism or savant skills were included to separate effects linked to autism from effects linked to savant syndrome. Participants learned a number of different calendar rules throughout a training session and were given a final test that tapped all the rules. For example, the 'matching month' rule states that within any non-leap year, certain months have matching structures (January = October; March = November = February; September = December; July = April; e.g. if 1 March is a Sunday, then it necessarily follows that 1 November and 1 February will also be Sundays in that year). Savants who have calendar calculating within their repertoire are already sensitive to these rules [47]. For instance, they are faster at saying that 1 November is Sunday if it has been 'primed' by a preceding question about 1 March (which has the same answer, as its 'matching month') than if preceded by 1 September (which has a different answer). As well as examining the overall ability to learn the task, we can use this pattern of response times (i.e. faster responses for primed answers) as a measure of the degree to which the rules have been internalised and are utilised by all subjects, and furthermore, whether savants perform differently in either accuracy or speed.

In summary, this study aimed to determine whether people with savant skills have a natural aptitude for learning this kind of information or whether they approach the task with different strategies. If so, we assess whether this is linked to autism per se or linked only to those autism subjects with pre-existing savant abilities (excluding calendar calculation). We predict that savants may show either a superior level of accuracy or a different style of approach to the question (this latter suggested by response time measures and/or a post hoc questionnaire).

Participants
Fifty-eight participants took part in experiment 2, 14 of whom also took part in experiment 1 above (6 autistic-savants, 6 autistic-nonsavants, and 2 controls). The participants comprised 13 autistic-savants (4 female; mean age 37.54, range 23–56, SD = 9.11), 10 autistic-nonsavants (5 female; mean age 39.20, range 27–51, SD = 9.02), and 35 controls (29 female; mean age 32.26, range 20–50, SD =

11.21). A one-way ANOVA showed no significant differences between groups on age, $F(2, 57) = 2.37$, $p = .10$, or highest qualification, $F(2, 57) = 2.23$, $p = .12$. All individuals in the autism groups (autistic-savant; autistic-nonsavant) self-reported having a formal diagnosis of autism in our questionnaire (see the 'Procedure' section): 3 autism, 18 Asperger syndrome, and 2 other. All autistic-savants, and no other group, self-reported having a savant skill.

Participants were recruited from two sources. Forty-two participants were recruited from CARD (13 autistic-savants, 10 autistic-nonsavants, 19 controls). The remaining 16 participants (all controls) were recruited from the University of Sussex community. Participants were entered into a £50 prize-draw for their participation, and our study was approved through the Cross-Schools Science and Technology Research Ethics Committee at the University of Sussex. In addition to the above participants, a further 22 were initially recruited but later excluded. These were 13 participants who used incorrect response buttons (i.e. the right-hand numeric keypad rather than the number keys) and 9 participants who were not engaging in the task. Three of these had response times that were not within a feasible range (i.e. < 700 ms; given the mean average RT for other subjects of 12.4 s; SD = 5.3) and 6 scored below chance, indicating they had not engaged with the calendar rules presented during our test.

Materials and procedure

All participants received an initial email invitation and accessed the study by clicking on a link embedded in the email that took them to the information and consent page. Participants then gave demographic information and next completed the Sussex Savant Questionnaire (SSQ) in the same way as in experiment 1 above. Participants then completed additional questionnaires to be published elsewhere (involving synaesthesia). All participants then completed a test of mental arithmetic (henceforth 'maths test') to ensure there were no a priori differences across groups in maths ability. In this, participants saw 20 questions requiring the addition of a pair of two-digit numbers (e.g. 76 + 43). Participants were required to calculate the answer as quickly as possible and type it into the box provided. Following the maths test, participants then began their calendar calculation training.

The calendar calculation training took place entirely online using Inquisit, an online experiment-hosting software and lasted around 35 min. Participants completed a training session (composed of three tutorials) followed by a final test at the end of the session. Each tutorial explained a set of patterns and calendar rules that can be used to calculate days of the week for certain dates. Tutorial 1 taught participants about the *matching-month rule* that explains that certain months cluster into

groups regarding their weekdays (see above for a further explanation). Tutorial 2 taught participants the *follow-on month rule* which states that months of the year can be arranged in a particular sequence to calculate days of the week faster (e.g. if 1 March 2015 is a Sunday, then it follows that 1 June is a Monday and 1 September is a Tuesday). Tutorial 3 focused on the *1-8-15-22-29 rule* which states that the 1st, 8th, 15th, 22nd, and 29th days of the month all fall on the same day of the week (e.g. in March 2015 all these dates fell on a Sunday). Each tutorial was accompanied by examples of calendar images to aid learning. At the end of each tutorial, participants were given 2 min to memorise the material just covered (without writing anything down) and then answered a set of tutorial questions based on those rules. At the end of all three tutorials, they completed the final calendar calculation test (see below).

For the purposes of this study, we focused only on teaching participants how to calculate days of the week for the year 2015 (due to the time limitations of a single study session). All questions (tutorial and final test) were forced choice with each answer being one of the seven days of the week. Participants answered using keys 1–7 on the keyboard and were given feedback ('correct'; or what the correct answer should have been e.g. 'Tuesday'). During the very first tutorial, participants with incorrect responses had to then select the correct answer to continue.

After all tutorials, participants completed the final calendar calculation test. The test contained 40 questions that spanned all the rules that had been taught previously and which again were dates that required participants to supply their weekday. Within these questions, there were 20 'primed' and 20 'unprimed' dates. Primed dates could be answered more easily than un-primed dates by reference to the question before, given the rule of 'matching months'. As noted above, this rule exploits the fact that 2015 has four groups of months, such that dates within each group fall on the same weekday (e.g. January and October are within the same group, so 8 January will fall on the same weekday at 8 October). Hence, 'primed' questions should be easier to answer because the response is the same as the question before (e.g. What weekday was 8 January? Answer: *Thursday*; PRIMED = What weekday was 8 October 2015? Answer: *Thursday*; UNPRIMED = What weekday was 8 November 2015? Answer: *Sunday*).

After the test, participants completed a questionnaire (see Additional file 2) with two sub-sections, asking how much they had enjoyed the study (Q7, Q8, Q9) and what strategies they used (Q1, Q2, Q3, Q4). These questions were presented on a 1–5 Likert scale (strongly disagree, disagree, neither agree nor disagree, agree, strongly agree). An additional question (Q5) was to ensure subjects were paying attention, and two final optional questions provided text boxes to enable participants to add further information if they wished (Q6 and Q10; not analysed). Once this enjoyment/strategy questionnaire was complete, participants saw a final screen thanking them for their time.

Results

Sussex Savant Questionnaire

Table 2 shows the categories of skills asked about during the study. Importantly, no autistic-savants reported calendar calculation as one of their savant skills, meaning they should not have an advantage to other groups based on prior abilities.

Maths pre-test

There were no significant differences in mental arithmetic accuracy between the autistic-savants ($M = 19.36$, SD = .51), autistic-nonsavants ($M = 19.1$, SD = 1.29), and controls ($M = 19.34$, SD = 1.06), $F(2, 55) = .76$, $p = .475$. There were also no significant differences in response times between the autistic-savants ($M = 6899$, SD = 1887), autistic-nonsavants ($M = 7675$, SD = 1888), and controls ($M = 7100$, SD = 2200), $F(2, 55) = .420$, $p = .659$. This means that all things considered, no group started with any a priori maths advantage.

Calendar calculation test

For accuracy scores, we conducted a 3×2 ANOVA contrasting group (autistic-savants, autistic-nonsavants, controls) and question type (primed vs. unprimed questions). As expected, we found a significant main effect of question type ($F(1, 55) = 26.82$, $p < .001$, ηp2 = .33) such that scores were higher for the easier primed questions ($M = 14.85$, SD = 5.15) compared to unprimed questions ($M = 12.97$, SD = 5.98). This suggests that participants were applying rules appropriately in our task and paying attention.

Table 2 Types of savant skills reported by the autistic-savant group in experiment 2, some participants reported having multiple savant skills

Skill types	Number of cases
Math	5
Calendar calculation	0
Musical instrument playing	2
Music reproduction	2
Absolute pitch	4
Art	2
Memory	5
Mechanical (building)	1
Fluency for different languages	1
Other	5

We also found a statistical trend for a main effect of group ($F(2, 55) = 2.56$, $p = .09$, ηp2 = .09), with controls ($M = 15.44$, SD = 6.04) tending to have overall higher accuracy scores compared to the autistic-nonsavants ($M = 11.60$, SD = 11.30; $p = .084$), but not compared to the autistic-savants ($M = 14.73$, SD = 9.92; $p = 1.00$). Finally, there was no significant interaction between group and question type ($F(2, 55) = 1.96$, $p = .15$, ηp2 = .07).

We also conducted a 3×2 ANOVA (again, group × question) looking at participants' response times. We again found a significant main effect of question type ($F(1, 55) = 16.78$, $p < .001$, ηp2 = .23) such that participants were significantly faster for the easier primed questions ($M = 12,351$, SD = 5703) compared to unprimed questions, as expected ($M = 13,994$, SD = 6241). Importantly, we found a significant main effect of group ($F(2, 55) = 4.55$, $p = .015$, ηp2 = .14) and a significant interaction between group and question type ($F(2, 55) = 5.12$, $p = .009$, ηp2 = .07). Detailed explorations revealed that autistic-savants ($M = 17,832$, SD = 7500) were significantly slower on the unprimed questions (Fig. 7) compared to both autistic-nonsavants ($M = 12,055$, SD = 6352; $p = .043$) and controls ($M = 12,094$, SD = 4129; $p = .006$), and autistic-savants ($M = 14,447$, SD = 7325) were significantly slower than controls even on the primed questions ($M = 10,371$, SD = 3148; $p = .043$).

Enjoyment/strategy questionnaire

A one-way ANOVA found no significant differences ($F(2, 53) = 1.41$, $p = .25$) in how much each group enjoyed learning to calendar calculate (i.e. collapsing questions Q7, Q8, Q9): for autistic-savants ($M = 3.44$, SD = .88), autistic-nonsavants ($M = 2.89$, SD = 1.17), or controls ($M = 3.42$, SD = .77).

In terms of strategy used, we conducted a 3×4 ANOVA crossing group (autistic-savant; autistic-nonsavant; control) and strategy question (Q1, Q2, Q3, Q4; relating respectively to picturing a mental calendar; using the on-screen timeline *Mon, Tues, Wed...*; using mental arithmetic; using rote memorisation of anchor dates). We found no main effect of group ($F(2, 51) = 1.77$, $p = .180$, ηp2 = .07) and no interaction ($F(6, 153) = .93$, $p = .476$, ηp2 = .35). But we found a significant effect of question ($F(3, 153) = 9.43$, $p < .001$, ηp2 = .16) in that the strategy of 'picturing a calendar in my head' was used least often compared to the other three strategies (all $p < .05$). No other comparisons were significant (all $p > .05$).

Discussion

The results for experiment 2 showed no clear a priori group advantages in being able to learn to perform calendar calculation skills. However, a significant pattern emerged for response times in that autistic-savants were slower than both autistic-nonsavants and controls, when

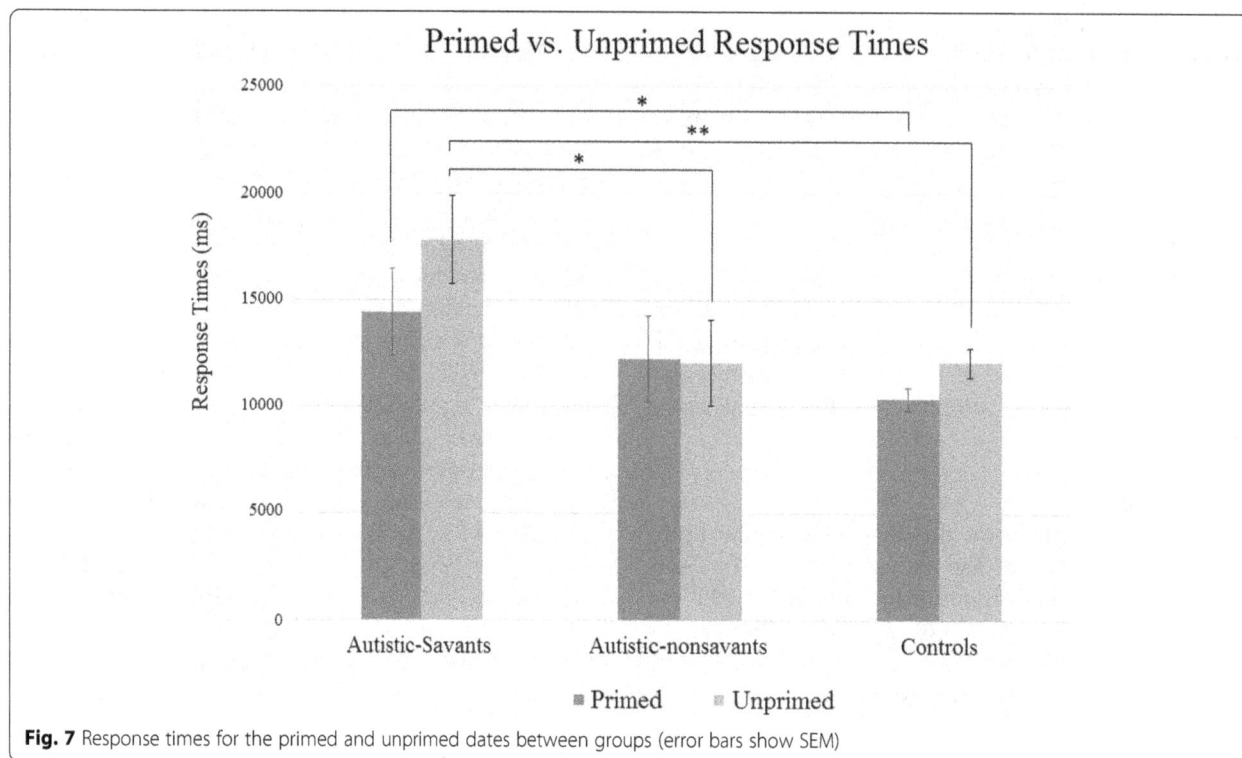

Fig. 7 Response times for the primed and unprimed dates between groups (error bars show SEM)

tackling the harder unprimed date questions. They were also slower than controls even in the simpler primed questions. This suggests that autistic-savants engaged with the task in a distinct way compared to the other groups in that they take longer to respond. We also found that the least-used strategy was 'picturing a calendar in my head' but that all groups reported similar strategies and enjoyed the task to a similar degree. The implications of these results are discussed below.

General discussion

The purpose of these studies was to profile the differences between autistic participants with and without a prodigious talent (autistic-savants and autistic-nonsavants, respectively). The third group was controls with neither autism nor a prodigious talent. Our findings present the first empirical evidence to adjudicate between different theoretical frameworks of savant syndrome in adults. Each of our results is discussed in turn below in terms of how they relate to previous models of the development of savant skills.

Experiment 1 investigated the profile of self-reported differences between autistic-savants, autistic-nonsavants, and controls. We asked all groups to complete self-report measures from six questionnaires: the Sussex Savant Questionnaire (SSQ), the Glasgow Sensory Questionnaire (GSQ) [30], the Leyton Obsessional Inventory—short form (LOI) [40], the Sussex Cognitive Styles Questionnaire (SCSQ) [41], the Systemising Quotient-Revised (SQ-R) [42], and

the Autism Spectrum Quotient (AQ) [43]. Our aim was to establish a general profile of individual differences that might distinguish between autistic individuals who develop talent and autistic individuals who do not. Our choice of questionnaires was motivated by previous theories and findings [3, 15, 16, 23, 24], and we focused on factors related to sensory sensitivity, obsessive behaviours, different aspects of cognitive style (e.g. local bias), and autism-related traits such as systemising and social awareness. We first briefly describe the (expected) pattern of results that distinguished all participants with autism from controls.

We found that both autism groups (autistic-savants and autistic-nonsavants) differed from controls on key measures, as predicted from previous literature [30, 43, 46] and theoretical accounts [3]. Both autistic-savants and autistic-nonsavants, relative to controls, reported more symptoms related to sensory sensitivity (known previously to be heightened in autism [30]) and obsessive behaviours (a common hallmark of autism [2]), increased systemising (previously shown in autism [46]), and a more locally oriented cognitive style (theorised as a feature of autism and savant syndrome and supported by findings [3, 25] but savant syndrome had not been separated from autism). Both autism groups also reported the expected generalised autism-related symptoms such as poor social, communication, and imagination skills, as well as poor attention switching and heightened attention-to-detail, which replicates previous findings using the same self-report measure in autism [43]. These findings are useful in confirming the validity of our autism classifications (autistic-savant and autistic-nonsavant) against controls and suggest that savant syndrome does indeed exist within or alongside autism based on our measures.

Our key findings relate to differences between autistic-savants and autistic-nonsavants. We found that these two groups differed in several ways. First, we considered two models that theorise why savants engage in many hours of practice [15, 16]. Happé and Vital's [15] mind-blindness theory suggests that autistic-savants practice as a result of re-dedicating cognitive resources to skill development that would otherwise be used to monitor social interactions. This predicts that autistic-savants may show poorer social skills compared to autistic-nonsavants. Our findings did not support this hypothesis: there were no differences between autistic-savants and autistic-nonsavants on social or communication skills in the AQ (and indeed no difference in any subscale of the AQ). Since it would have been expected that autistic-savants would score higher than autistic-nonsavants on generalised autism-related symptoms, we additionally showed that a Bayes factor analysis supported the null hypothesis of no differences between these groups for four out of the five AQ sub-scales (social skills, attention switching, communication, imagination). This does not necessarily rule out altogether the role of additional autism-related traits in the development of savant skills (e.g. a preference for solitary activities), but our current data suggests that differences on the above measures may not be strongly apparent when comparing autistic-savants and autistic-nonsavants.

Instead, we found support for an alternative model by Simner and colleagues [16] in which practice arises from increased obsessional traits in autistic-savants. The autistic-savant group showed higher obsessional traits compared to autistic-nonsavants, and this was specifically related to the 'worries/just right' factor. This factor relates to the inclination to take one's time about making sure things are 'just right' (e.g. 'I do not take a long time to dress in the morning' [reverse coded]). This factor could well be implicated in the development of talent, for example, when making sure the details of a painting are 'just right' or putting additional effort into learning a number list perfectly without error. The second feature of the 'worries/just right' factor (i.e. excessive worries about, e.g. bumping into people or the belief in unlucky numbers) raises an interesting possibility that obsessive rehearsal in savants might be driven by anxiety. If so, then savant skills may be guided by the same anxiety-laden motivations that drive, for example, repetitive OCD behaviour [19]. Indeed, seven autistic-savants (compared to two autistic-nonsavants and one control) scored above the threshold for OCD symptoms although our small numbers did not allow us to support this

statistically. We are therefore exploring in subsequent studies how anxiety may be implicated in the development of savant skills. Overall, the above results suggest that practice in savant skills is driven by obsessional (possibly anxiety-linked) behaviours in autistic-savants compared to autistic-nonsavants [16] rather than freed-up resources from mind-blindness [15].

We also investigated other areas of cognition/perception, drawn from several theoretical accounts [3, 23, 24]. We found that autistic-savants scored higher on the Systemising Quotient-Revised (SQ-R; although not on the shorter 'systemising' factor of the Cognitive Styles Questionnaire; SCSQ). We also found that autistic-savants scored higher on 'technical/ spatial' elements of the SCSQ which relates to technical interests, mathematical ability, and the use of spatial mental imagery—but also contains several questions which are systemising in nature (e.g. 'If I were buying a stereo, I would want to know about its precise technical features.'). Together, these findings of higher systemising and technical/spatial abilities of savants support the model by Baron-Cohen et al. [23] who proposed that savant skills emerge from increased systemising in autistic-savants. Where we found null results between all group comparisons, we additionally computed Bayes factors to assess whether our results truly reflected no differences. Here our analysis supported evidence for the null hypothesis of no differences between autistic-savants and autistic-nonsavants on the imagery ability and language and word forms sub-scales of the SCSQ; therefore, our current data suggest that these aspects of cognition may not be involved in the facilitation of savant skills.

Local processing has also been theorised as important in the development of savant skills, as suggested by the enhanced perceptual functioning model (EPF) [3]. However, we found no difference in self-reported local processing traits between autistic-savants and autistic-nonsavants, and so fail to support this proposal from the current data. Bennet and Heaton [22] found a similar pattern to us in savant children and adolescents based on parental reports (no local processing advantage for autistic-savants over autistic-nonsavants). Importantly, however, Pring et al. [26] show that enhanced local processing abilities in savants (relative to autistic-nonsavants) might only be revealed by a more engaging task. As such, the EPF model by Mottron et al. [3] has been supported by behavioural evidence in certain engaging tasks, but not by our self-report data here.

Finally, we investigated the theory that the development of savant skills might be tied to heightened sensory sensitivity [23]. Our autistic-savants reported significantly more symptoms related to sensory sensitivity lending support to the theory that sensory sensitivity could act as an initial catalyst in the emergence of savant talent. Baron-Cohen et al. also made claims that sensory sensitivity might increase attention-to-detail. However, although we found this trait to be heightened in our autism groups globally, there was no difference in attention-to-detail between our autistic-savants and autistic-nonsavants. Having said this, our Bayes analysis suggested that no firm conclusions could be drawn about group differences in attention to detail; therefore, future studies may wish to further investigate this. Interestingly, the finding of heightened sensory sensitivity in our savant group relates more broadly to another condition, synaesthesia, which also has a distinct sensory component. As noted in the Background, synaesthesia produces sensory experiences that are induced by unusual stimuli (e.g. letters or numbers might induce colour sensations). Synaesthesia has been linked to autism previously [48, 49], and Ward et al. [50] showed that both conditions share common links in their profile of sensory sensitivities. More recently, synaesthesia has been specifically tied to savant syndrome rather than autism per se [39]. So our current data combined with previous evidence further suggests that sensory components may be an important mediating link between autism and the development of savant skills, perhaps even via synaesthesia itself [16].

In experiment 2, we taught the three groups the novel skill of calendar calculation and tested their abilities after three tutorials. We aimed to examine whether autistic-savants would show advantages in learning this skill compared to autistic-nonsavants and controls, as predicted by the 'veridical mapping' model [24]. Veridical mapping links savant talent to an enhanced ability to detect regularities within and between systems. Calendar calculation requires this skill *par excellence* because weekdays can be mapped to dates by understanding the underlying regularities in the calendar—which we taught to the participants in our study. In contrast to veridical mapping, practice-based models of savant skills might not predict immediate advantages prior to prolonged training [15, 16]. We found no evidence to support the veridical mapping model since autistic-savants were no more accurate than autistic-nonsavants or even controls. It is possible that differences in accuracy may have been observed if participants were given a longer period of training, for instance, if autistic-savants were given more time to consolidate their learning. Indeed, calendar calculation is often assumed to develop as a result of periods of study which are far longer than our training session. However, we show that calendar calculation is surprisingly easy to acquire with around 75% accuracy after merely 35 min of training even in the control group.

Importantly, we did find that autistic-savants took significantly longer to answer our calendar calculation questions: they were slower than both autistic-nonsavants and controls for (difficult) unprimed questions and slower than controls even on (easier) primed questions. One interpretation of this is that our autistic-savant participants may have found the task more difficult compared to the other groups. But given that all subjects began with the same level of mental maths ability (as measure by our test in experiment 2), a more plausible interpretation is that, autistic-savants engaged with the task differently by adopting a more careful, effortful approach with increased checking. This would fall in line with the findings from experiment 1 that autistic-savants show more obsessional behaviours, specifically related to taking a long time to get things 'just right' (see results above for the Leyton Obsessional Inventory). Indeed, the magnitude of the differences between groups for response times (autistic-savants took more than 5 s longer on average than nonsavants) suggests again they may have taken longer to check and re-check their answers. Overall, experiment 2 lends support to practice-based models of savant skills rather than veridical mapping since autistic-savants did not show immediate advantages on this skill prior to extended training and they appear to display a more engaged, effortful approach to the task.

One limitation of the current study is that we validated savants with a detailed self-report questionnaire rather than by objective tests. This is largely because savant syndrome is an umbrella term for many different heterogeneous manifestations (e.g. calendar- calculation, drawing, music etc.). We did however validate our approach by showing a 'dose-like' effect of savant skills on one of our other measures: the number of savant skills reported in our questionnaire correlated positively with the strength of savants' technical-spatial abilities. In other words, although talents are described only in self-report (rather than objectively evaluated), this self-report appears to be a reliable metric since it correlates with a trait that particularly separates autistic-savants from autistic-nonsavants. Nevertheless, future investigations might focus on objectively verifying self-reported skills with a battery of tests designed to measure specific savant skills (e.g. absolute pitch, language skills), and we have embarked on this program of research in our own lab. A further limitation of our study was the fact that we had a high proportion of females in the control group compared to our two autism groups. Nonetheless, we conducted an additional analysis where we had found main effects (i.e. sensory sensitivity, obsessional traits, technical-spatial skills, and systemising) showing that our pattern of results was maintained across all groups even after controlling for gender.

Conclusions

Our results demonstrate a diverse range of attributes that distinguish autistic-savants from autistic-nonsavants in adults based on both self-report and an objective test. Our findings suggest that savant syndrome is defined by observable differences in aspects of cognition, perception, and behaviour that go beyond the mere presence of savant skills themselves. We found that areas of particular influence on savant talent relate specifically to higher sensory sensitivity (supporting Baron-Cohen et al. [23]), obsessive behaviour (supporting, e.g. Simner et al. [16]), and systemising and technical/spatial traits (supporting Baron-Cohen et al. [23]) along with a more careful and engaged learning style when presented with a novel savant skill (supporting practice models such as Simner et al. [16]). We did not find social skills [15], local processing [3], or increased pattern detection in calendar-calculation [24] to be distinguishing features between autistic-savants and autistic-nonsavants. Our study is novel in the savant literature by clarifying the role of different traits and behaviours in the development of prodigious talent, in order to distinguish between previous theories that suggested the developmental pathway of the emergence of talent in autism. Our preliminary findings should be used to guide further research in delineating the direction and relative contribution of the factors identified in our study. Exploring further how these factors might influence different abilities (e.g. maths, music, art etc.) could be an important next step in our understanding of savant skills. Our current findings are important in defining savant syndrome as a legitimate sub-group of autism.

Endnotes

[1]Calculation of a Bayes factor allows the evaluation of null results to determine whether the data supports evidence for the null against the alternative hypothesis [51]. Bayes factors are evaluated along a continuum although typically, a Bayes factor (BF) >.33 provides moderate support for the null hypothesis while a Bayes factor of > 3 provides moderate support for the alternative hypothesis, and values in between indicate no firm conclusions should be drawn.

[2]We note that there were gender imbalances in our participant samples across groups (see [46] for example gender effects in autism). Given this, we repeated all analyses where we had found main effects (i.e. sensory sensitivity, obsessional traits, technical-spatial skills, and systemising) but this time ran ANCOVAs with gender entered as a covariate. Even after controlling for gender, all of our main effects were maintained: for sensory sensitivity ($F(2, 111) = 28.06$, $p < .001$, ηp2 = .34), obsessional traits ($F(2, 111) = 7.74$, $p < .001$, ηp2 = .13), technical-spatial skills ($F(2, 111) = 6.36$, $p = .002$, ηp2 = .11), and systemising ($F(2, 91) = 22.09$, $p < .001$, ηp2 = .34). In addition, the pattern of results for all our post hoc comparisons were maintained with autistic-

savants scoring higher than both autistic-nonsavants and controls across all measures (all p's < 0.05) while autistic-nonsavants scored higher than controls across all measures (p's < .05) apart from obsessional traits and technical-spatial abilities ($p > .05$). In other words, gender had very little effect on our overall pattern of findings, and importantly, it had no effect whatsoever on our key findings comparing autistic-savants and autistic nonsavants.

Abbreviations
AQ: Autism Spectrum Quotient; CARD: Cambridge Autism Research Database; EPF: Enhanced perceptual functioning; LOI: Leyton Obsession Inventory; SCSQ: Sussex Cognitive Styles Questionnaire; SQ-R: Systemising Quotient-Revised; SSQ: Sussex Savant Questionnaire

Acknowledgements
We are grateful to Paula Smith for access to CARD.

Funding
JEAH, JS, and JW were supported by a grant from the Economic and Social Research Council (ESRC) (http://www.esrc.ac.uk/) grant ES/K006215/1. SBC was supported by the MRC and the Autism Research Trust during the period of this work.

Authors' contributions
JS and JW were responsible for the overall direction of the research. The data from the savant and autism samples were collected by JEAH, PS, and CA, and controls were collected by JEAH, PS, CA, and EG. JEAH, JS, JW, and EG conducted the analyses. The paper was written by JEAH, JS, JW, and SBC. All authors read and approved the final manuscript.

Competing interests
The authors declare that they have no competing interests.

Author details
[1]School of Psychology, Pevensey Building, University of Sussex, Brighton BN1 9QJ, UK. [2]Autism Research Centre, University of Cambridge, Cambridge CB2 8AH, UK.

References

1. Miller LK. The savant syndrome: intellectual impairment and exceptional skill. Psychol Bull. 1999;125:31–46. https://doi.org/10.1037/0033-2909.125.1.31.

2. American Psychiatric Association. Cautionary statement for forensic use of DSM-5. 5th edition. Arlington: American Psychiatric Publishing; 2013. https://doi.org/10.1176/appi.books.9780890425596.744053.

3. Mottron L, Dawson M, Soulières I, Hubert B, Burack J. Enhanced perceptual functioning in autism: an update, and eight principles of autistic perception. J Autism Dev Disord. 2006;36:27–43. https://doi.org/10.1007/s10803-005-0040-7.

4. Baron-Cohen. The extreme male brain theory of autism. Trends Cogn Sci. 2002;6:248–54. https://doi.org/10.1016/S1364-6613(02)01904-6.

5. O'Riordan M, Plaisted K. Enhanced discrimination in autism. Q J Exp Psychol Sect A Hum Exp Psychol. 2001;54:961–79. https://doi.org/10.1080/713756000.

6. Furniss GJ. Celebrating the artmaking of children with autism. Art Educ. 2008;61:2008.

7. Treffert DA. The savant syndrome: an extraordinary condition. A synopsis: past, present, future. Philos Trans R Soc B Biol Sci. 2009;364:1351–7. https://doi.org/10.1098/rstb.2008.0326.

8. Chia NKH. Autism enigma: the need to include savant and crypto-savant in the current definition. Acad Res Int 2012;2:234–240.

9. Henley DR. Review of bright splinters of the mind: a personal story of research with autistic savants. London: J. Kingsley; 2003. https://doi.org/10.1111/1469-7610.t01-1-00086.

10. Howlin P, Goode S, Hutton J, Rutter M. Savant skills in autism: psychometric approaches and parental reports. Philos Trans R Soc B Biol Sci. 2009;364:1359–67. https://doi.org/10.1098/rstb.2008.0328.

11. Bölte S, Poustka F. Comparing the intelligence profiles of savant and nonsavant individuals with autistic disorder. Intelligence. 2004;32:121–31. https://doi.org/10.1016/j.intell.2003.11.002.

12. Ericsson KA, Charness N. Expert performance: its structure and acquisition. Am Psychol. 1994;49:725–47. https://doi.org/10.1037/0003-066X.49.8.725.

13. Hu Y, Ericsson KA, Yang D, Lu C. Superior self-paced memorization of digits in spite of a normal digit span: the structure of a memorist's skill. J Exp Psychol Learn Mem Cogn. 2009;35:1426–42. https://doi.org/10.1037/a0017395.

14. Wilding JM, Valentine ER. Superior memory: Psychology Press; 1997. http://books.google.pl/books?id=IBHYHgpxDEkC. Accessed 12 Dec 2017

15. Happé F, Vital P. What aspects of autism predispose to talent? Philos Trans R Soc B Biol Sci. 2009;364:1369–75. https://doi.org/10.1098/rstb.2008.0332.

16. Simner J, Mayo N, Spiller M-J. A foundation for savantism? Visuo-spatial synaesthetes present with cognitive benefits. Cortex. 2009;45:1246–60. https://doi.org/10.1016/j.cortex.2009.07.007.

17. Baron-Cohen S. Mindblindness: an essay on autism and theory of mind: MIT Press; 1995. https://doi.org/10.1027//0269-8803.13.1.57.

18. Frith U. Mind blindness and the brain in autism. Neuron. 2001;32:969–79. https://doi.org/10.1016/S0896-6273(01)00552-9.

19. LePort AKR, Mattfeld AT, Dickinson-Anson H, Fallon JH, Stark CEL, Kruggel F, et al. Behavioral and neuroanatomical investigation of Highly Superior Autobiographical Memory (HSAM). Neurobiol Learn Mem. 2012;98:78–92. https://doi.org/10.1016/j.nlm.2012.05.002.

20. Parker ES, Cahill L, McGaugh JL. A case of unusual autobiographical remembering. Neurocase. 2006;12:35–49. https://doi.org/10.1080/13554790500473680.

21. O'Connor N, Hermelin B. Talents and preoccupations in idiots-savants. Psychol Med. 1991;21:959–64. https://doi.org/10.1017/S0033291700029949.

22. Bennett E, Heaton P. Is talent in autism spectrum disorders associated with a specific cognitive and behavioural phenotype? J Autism Dev Disord. 2012;42:2739–53. https://doi.org/10.1007/s10803-012-1533-9.

23. Baron-Cohen S, Ashwin E, Ashwin C, Tavassoli T, Chakrabarti B. Talent in autism: hyper-systemizing, hyper-attention to detail and sensory hypersensitivity. Philos Trans R Soc B Biol Sci. 2009;364:1377–83. https://doi.org/10.1098/rstb.2008.0337.

24. Mottron L, Bouvet L, Bonnel A, Samson F, Burack JA, Dawson M, et al. Veridical mapping in the development of exceptional autistic abilities. Neurosci Biobehav Rev. 2013;37:209–28. https://doi.org/10.1016/j.neubiorev.2012.11.016.

25. Bor D, Billington J, Baron-cohen S. Savant memory for digits in a case of synaesthesia and Asperger syndrome is related to hyperactivity in the lateral prefrontal cortex. Neurocase. 2007;13:311–9. https://doi.org/10.1080/13554790701844945.

26. Pring L, Ryder N, Crane L, Hermelin B. Local and global processing in savant artists with autism. Perception. 2010;39:1094–103. https://doi.org/10.1068/p6674.

27. Leekam SR, Nieto C, Libby SJ, Wing L, Gould J. Describing the sensory abnormalities of children and adults with autism. J Autism Dev Disord. 2007;37:894–910.

28. Kern JK, Trivedi MH, Garver CR, Grannemann BD, Andrews AA, Savla JS, et al. The pattern of sensory processing abnormalities in autism. Autism. 2006;10:480–94. https://doi.org/10.1177/1362361306066564.

29. Tomchek SD, Dunn W. Sensory processing in children with and without autism: a comparative study using the short sensory profile. 2007. http://sense-ability.co.za/article02.pdf. Accessed 1 Aug 2018.

30. McMahon C, Vismara L, Solomon M. Neural mechanisms of emotion regulation in autism spectrum disorder. J Autism Dev Disord. 2015;5:2–3. https://doi.org/10.1007/s10803.

31. Bertone A, Mottron L, Jelenic P, Faubert J. Motion perception in autism: a "complex" issue. J Cogn Neurosci. 2003;15:218–25. https://doi.org/10.1162/089892903321208150.

32. Mottron L, Burack JA, Stauder JEA, Robaey P. Perceptual processing among high-functioning persons with autism. J Child Psychol Psychiatry Allied Discip. 1999;40:203–11. https://doi.org/10.1017/S0021963098003333.

33. Bonnel A, Mottron L, Peretz I, Trudel M, Gallun E, Bonnel AM. Enhanced pitch sensitivity in individuals with autism: a signal detection analysis. J Cogn Neurosci. 2003;15:226–35. https://doi.org/10.1162/089892903321208169.

34. Heaton P, Davis RE, Happé FGE. Research note: exceptional absolute pitch perception for spoken words in an able adult with autism. Neuropsychologia. 2008;46:2095–8. https://doi.org/10.1016/j.neuropsychologia.2008.02.006.

35. Blakemore SJ, Tavassoli T, Calò S, Thomas RM, Catmur C, Frith U, et al. Tactile sensitivity in Asperger syndrome. Brain Cogn. 2006;61:5–13. https://doi.org/10.1016/j.bandc.2005.12.013.

36. Tommerdahl M, Tannan V, Cascio CJ, Baranek GT, Whitsel BL. Vibrotactile adaptation fails to enhance spatial localization in adults with autism. Brain Res. 2007;1154:116–23. https://doi.org/10.1016/j.brainres.2007.04.032.

37. Simner J. Defining synaesthesia. Br J Psychol. 2012;103:1–15. https://doi.org/10.1348/000712610X528305.

38. Ward J. Synesthesia. Annu Rev Psychol. 2013;64:49–75. https://doi.org/10.1146/annurev-psych-113011-143840.

39. Hughes JEA, Simner J, Baron-Cohen S, Treffert DA, Ward J. Is synaesthesia more prevalent in autism spectrum conditions? Only where there is prodigious talent. Multisens Res. 2017;30:391–408. https://doi.org/10.1163/22134808-00002558.

40. Mathews CA, Jang KL, Hami S, Stein MB. The structure of obsessionality among young adults. Depress Anxiety. 2004;20:77–85. https://doi.org/10.1002/da.20028.

41. Mealor AD, Simner J, Rothen N, Carmichael DA, Ward J. Different dimensions of cognitive style in typical and atypical cognition: new evidence and a new measurement tool. PLoS One. 2016;11:e0155483. https://doi.org/10.1371/journal.pone.0155483.

42. Wheelwright S, Baron-Cohen S, Goldenfeld N, Delaney J, Fine D, Smith R, et al. Predicting autism spectrum quotient (AQ) from the systemizing quotient-revised (SQ-R) and empathy quotient (EQ). Brain Res. 2006;1079:47–56. https://doi.org/10.1016/j.brainres.2006.01.012.

43. Baron-Cohen S, Wheelwright S, Skinner R, Martin J, Clubley E. The autism-spectrum quotient (AQ): evidence from Asperger syndrome/high-functioning autism, males and females, scientists and mathematicians. J Autism Dev Disord. 2001;31:5–17. https://doi.org/10.1023/A:1005653411471.

44. Mottron L, Lemmens K, Gagnon L, Seron X. Non-algorithmic access to calendar information in a calendar calculator with autism. J Autism Dev Disord. 2006;36:239–47. https://doi.org/10.1007/s10803-005-0059-9.

45. Boddaert N, Barthélémy C, Poline JB, Samson Y, Brunelle F, Zilbovicius M. Autism: functional brain mapping of exceptional calendar capacity. Br J Psychiatry. 2005;187:83–6. https://doi.org/10.1192/bjp.187.1.83.

46. Baron-Cohen S, Richler J, Bisarya D, Gurunathan N, Wheelwright S. The systemizing quotient: an investigation of adults with Asperger syndrome or high-functioning autism, and normal sex differences. Philos Trans R Soc B Biol Sci. 2003;358:361–74. https://doi.org/10.1098/rstb.2002.1206.

47. Hermelin B, O'connor N. Idiot savant calendrical calculators: rules and regularities. Psychol Med. 1986;16:885–93. https://doi.org/10.1017/S0033291700011892.

48. Neufeld J, Roy M, Zapf A, Sinke C, Emrich HM, Prox-Vagedes V, et al. Is synesthesia more common in patients with Asperger syndrome? Front Hum Neurosci. 2013;7:847. https://doi.org/10.3389/fnhum.2013.00847.

49. Baron-Cohen S, Johnson D, Asher J, Wheelwright S, Fisher SE, Gregersen PK, et al. Is synaesthesia more common in autism? 2013. https://doi.org/10.1186/2040-2392-4-40.

50. Ward J, Hoadley C, Hughes JEA, Smith P, Allison C, Baron-Cohen S, et al. Atypical sensory sensitivity as a shared feature between synaesthesia and autism OPEN 2017. doi:https://doi.org/10.1038/srep41155.

51. Dienes Z, Coulton S, Heather N. Using Bayes factors to evaluate evidence for no effect: examples from the SIPS project. Addiction. 2018;113:240–6. https://doi.org/10.1111/add.14002.

Permissions

List of Contributors

Lien Van Eylen and Jean Steyaert
Center for Developmental Psychiatry, Department of Neurosciences, KU Leuven, Kapucijnenvoer 7h, PB 7001, 3000 Leuven, Belgium
Leuven Autism Research (LAuRes), KU Leuven, 3000 Leuven, Belgium

Bart Boets
Center for Developmental Psychiatry, Department of Neurosciences, KU Leuven, Kapucijnenvoer 7h, PB 7001, 3000 Leuven, Belgium
Leuven Autism Research (LAuRes), KU Leuven, 3000 Leuven, Belgium
Department of Brain and Cognitive Sciences, Massachusetts Institute of Technology, Cambridge, MA 02139, USA

Johan Wagemans
Leuven Autism Research (LAuRes), KU Leuven, 3000 Leuven, Belgium
Laboratory of Experimental Psychology, KU Leuven, 3000 Leuven, Belgium

Kevin Sitek
Department of Brain and Cognitive Sciences, Massachusetts Institute of Technology, Cambridge, MA 02139, USA
Speech and Hearing Bioscience and Technology, Division of Medical Sciences, Harvard Medical School, Boston, MA 02115, USA

Pieter Moors
Laboratory of Experimental Psychology, KU Leuven, 3000 Leuven, Belgium

Ilse Noens
Parenting and Special Education Research Unit, KU Leuven, 3000 Leuven, Belgium

Stefan Sunaert
Translational MRI, KU Leuven, 3000 Leuven, Belgium

Matthew Benger and Nicholas D. Mazarakis
Gene Therapy, Centre for Neuroinflammation and Neurodegeneration, Division of Brain Sciences, Faculty of Medicine, Imperial College London, Hammersmith Hospital Campus, W12 0NN, London, UK

Maria Kinali
Present address: The Portland Hospital, 205-209 Great Portland Street, London W1W 5AH, UK

Chun-xue Liu, Chun-yang Li, Chun-chun Hu, Yi Wang and Xiu Xu
Division of Child Health Care, Children's Hospital of Fudan University, 399 Wanyuan Road, Shanghai 201102, China

Jia Lin and Qiang Li
Center for Translational Medicine, Institute of Pediatrics, Shanghai Key Laboratory of Birth Defect, Children's Hospital of Fudan University, 399 Wanyuan Road, Shanghai 201102, China

Yong-hui Jiang
Department of Pediatrics and Neurobiology, Duke University School of Medicine, Durham, NC 27614, USA

Quan Wang, Suzanne L. Macari and Katarzyna Chawarska
Child Study Center, Yale School of Medicine, 40 Temple St Suite 7D, New Haven, CT 06510, USA

Daniel J. Campbell
Vertex Pharmaceuticals Incorporated, 50 Northern Ave, Boston, MA 02210, USA

Frederick Shic
Center for Child Health, Behavior and Development, Seattle Children's Research Institute, 2001 8th Ave Suite 400, Seattle, WA 98121, USA
Department of Pediatrics, University of Washington, Seattle, WA, USA

Jean Golding, Steven Gregory, Genette Ellis, Alan Emond, Yasmin Iles-Caven and Caroline Taylor
Centre for Child and Adolescent Health, Bristol Medical School, University of Bristol, Oakfield House, Oakfield Grove, Bristol BS8 2BN, UK

Dheeraj Rai
Centre for Academic Mental Health, Bristol Medical School, University of Bristol, Oakfield House, Oakfield Grove, Bristol BS8 2BN, UK

Joseph Hibbeln
Section on Nutritional Neurosciences, LMBB, National Institute on Alcohol Abuse and Alcoholism, National Institutes of Health, 31 Center Drive 1B/58, Bethesda, MD 20892, USA

Dai-Hua Lu, Huang-Ju Tu, Houng-Chi Liou and Wen-Mei Fu
Pharmacological Institute, College of Medicine, National Taiwan University, Taipei, Taiwan

Hsiao-Mei Liao and Susan Shur-Fen Gau
Department of Psychiatry, National Taiwan University Hospital and College of Medicine, Taipei, Taiwan

Chia-Hsiang Chen
Department of Psychiatry, Chang Gung Memorial Hospital Linkou, Taoyuan, Taiwan
Department and Graduate Institute of Biomedical Sciences, Chang Gung University, Taoyuan, Taiwan

Sarah Cassidy
School of Psychology, University of Nottingham, University Park, Nottingham NG7 2RD, Uk
Centre for Innovative Research across the Life Course, Coventry University, Coventry, UK
Autism Research Centre, University of Cambridge, Cambridge, UK

Louise Bradley
Centre for Innovative Research across the Life Course, Coventry University, Coventry, UK

Rebecca Shaw
Centre for Innovative Research across the Life Course, Coventry University, Coventry, UK
Coventry and Warwickshire Partnership Trust, Coventry, UK

Simon Baron-Cohen
Autism Research Centre, University of Cambridge, Cambridge, UK
Cambridge Lifetime Asperger Syndrome Service (CLASS), Cambridgeshire and Peterborough NHS Foundation Trust, Cambridge, UK

Hanna den Bakker, Michael S. Sidorov and Benjamin D. Philpot
Department of Cell Biology and Physiology, University of North Carolina, Chapel Hill, NC 27599, USA
Carolina Institute for Developmental Disabilities, University of North Carolina, Chapel Hill, NC 27599, USA
Neuroscience Center, University of North Carolina, Chapel Hill, NC 27599, USA

Zheng Fan
Department of Neurology, University of North Carolina, Chapel Hill, NC 27599, USA

David J. Lee
Department of Neurosciences, University of California, San Diego, CA, USA

Lynne M. Bird
Department of Pediatrics, University of California, San Diego, CA, USA

Division of Dysmorphology/Genetics, Rady Children's Hospital, San Diego, CA, USA

Catherine J. Chu
Department of Neurology, Massachusetts General Hospital, Boston, MA 02114, USA
Harvard Medical School, Boston, MA 02215, USA

Hirokazu Kumazaki, Yuko Yoshimura, Takashi Ikeda, Chiaki Hasegawa, Daisuke N. Saito, Sara Tomiyama, Kyung-min An, Yoshio Minabe and Mitsuru Kikuchi
Research Center for Child Mental Development, Kanazawa University, 13-1, Takaramachi, Kanazawa, Ishikawa 920-8640, Japan

Yuichiro Yoshikawa, Jiro Shimaya and Hiroshi Ishiguro
Department of Systems Innovation, Graduate School of Engineering Science, Osaka University, 1-3, Machikaneryamachou, Toyonaka, Osaka 560-0043, Japan

Yoshio Matsumoto
Service Robotics Research Group, Intelligent Systems Institute, National Institute of Advanced Industrial Science and Technology, Ibaraki 305-8560, Japan

Orna Tzischinsky
Behavioral Science Department, Emek Yesreel College, Emek Yesreel, Israel

Gal Meiri and Orit Zivan
Pre-School Psychiatry Unit, Soroka University Medical Center, Beer Sheva, Israel

Liora Manelis, Asif Bar-Sinai and Michal Ilan
Pre-School Psychiatry Unit, Soroka University Medical Center, Beer Sheva, Israel
Psychology Department, Ben Gurion University, Beer Sheva, Israel

Ilan Dinstein
Psychology Department, Ben Gurion University, Beer Sheva, Israel
Cognitive and Brain Sciences Department, Ben Gurion University, Beer Sheva, Israel

Hagit Flusser, Analya Michaelovski and Michal Faroy
Zusman Child Development Center, Soroka University Medical Center, Beer Sheva, Israel

Idan Menashe
Public Health Department, Ben Gurion University, Beer Sheva, Israel

Katherine Kuhl-Meltzoff Stavropoulos
Riverside Graduate School of Education, University of California, 9500 University Avenue, Riverside, CA 92521, USA

Leslie J. Carver
University of California, San Diego, USA

Caroline Mann and Anke Bletsch
Department of Child and Adolescent Psychiatry, Psychosomatics and Psychotherapy, University Hospital, Goethe University Frankfurt am Main, Deutschordenstrasse 50, 60528 Frankfurt am Main, Germany

Christine Ecker
Department of Child and Adolescent Psychiatry, Psychosomatics and Psychotherapy, University Hospital, Goethe University Frankfurt am Main, Deutschordenstrasse 50, 60528 Frankfurt am Main, Germany
Department of Forensic and Neurodevelopmental Sciences, and the Sackler Institute for Translational Neurodevelopmental Sciences, Institute of Psychiatry, Psychology and Neuroscience (IoPPN), King's College London, London SE5 8AF, UK

Derek Andrews
Department of Psychiatry and Behavioural Sciences, The Medical Investigation of Neurodevelopmental Disorders (MIND) Institute, UC Davis School of Medicine, University of California Davis, Sacramento, CA, USA

Eileen Daly, Clodagh Murphy and Declan Murphy
Department of Forensic and Neurodevelopmental Sciences, and the Sackler Institute for Translational Neurodevelopmental Sciences, Institute of Psychiatry, Psychology and Neuroscience (IoPPN), King's College London, London SE5 8AF, UK

Jacob Ellegood
Mouse Imaging Centre (MICe), Hospital for Sick Children, 25 Orde Street, Toronto, Ontario M5T 3H7, Canada

Yohan Yee, R. Mark Henkelman and Jason P. Lerch
Mouse Imaging Centre (MICe), Hospital for Sick Children, 25 Orde Street, Toronto, Ontario M5T 3H7, Canada
Department of Medical Biophysics, University of Toronto, Toronto, ON M5S, Canada

Travis M. Kerr and Christopher L. Muller
Department of Psychiatry, Vanderbilt University, Nashville, TN 37235, USA

Randy D. Blakely
Department of Pharmacology, Vanderbilt University, Nashville, TN 37235, USA
Department of Psychiatry, Vanderbilt University, Nashville, TN 37235, USA
Department of Biomedical Science and Brain Institute, Florida Atlantic University, Jupiter, FL 33431, USA

Jeremy Veenstra-VanderWeele
Department of Pharmacology, Vanderbilt University, Nashville, TN 37235, USA
Department of Psychiatry, Columbia University, New York, NY 10027, USA

Federica Filice, Emanuel Lauber and Beat Schwaller
Anatomy Unit, Section of Medicine, University of Fribourg, Route Albert-Gockel 1, CH-1700 Fribourg, Switzerland

Karl Jakob Vörckel
Behavioral Neuroscience, Faculty of Psychology, Philipps-University of Marburg, Gutenbergstraße 18, 35032 Marburg, Germany

Markus Wöhr
Behavioral Neuroscience, Faculty of Psychology, Philipps-University of Marburg, Gutenbergstraße 18, 35032 Marburg, Germany
Marburg Center for Mind, Brain, and Behavior (MCMBB), Hans-Meerwein-Straße 6, 35032 Marburg, Germany

R. L. Moseley, R. Hitchiner and J. A. Kirkby
Department of Psychology, Bournemouth University, Fern Barrow, Poole, Dorset BH12 5BB, UK

Melanie Penner and Evdokia Anagnostou
Autism Research Centre, Bloorview Research Institute, Holland Bloorview Kids Rehabilitation Hospital, Toronto, Canada
Department of Paediatrics, University of Toronto, Toronto, Canada

Wendy J. Ungar
Technology Assessment at Sick Kids (TASK), Child Health Evaluative Sciences, The Hospital for Sick Children Research Institute, Toronto, Canada
Institute of Health Policy, Management and Evaluation, University of Toronto, Toronto, Canada

Danielle Smith
Research and Development Department, Cumbria Partnership NHS Foundation Trust, Carleton Clinic, Carlisle CA1 3SX, UK

Danielle Ropar and Harriet A Allen
School of Psychology, University of Nottingham, Nottingham NG7 2RD, UK

Nisim Perets
Sagol School of Neuroscience, Tel Aviv University, Tel Aviv, Israel

Daniel Offen
Sagol School of Neuroscience, Tel Aviv University, Tel Aviv, Israel
Sacklar School of Medicine, Department of Human Genetics and Biochemistry, Tel Aviv University, Tel Aviv, Israel

Stav Hertz and Michael London
Edmond and Lily Safra Center for Brain Sciences, Hebrew University, Jerusalem, Israel

James E A Hughes, Jamie Ward, Elin Gruffydd and Julia Simner
School of Psychology, Pevensey Building, University of Sussex, Brighton BN1 9QJ, UK

Simon Baron-Cohen, Paula Smith and Carrie Allison
Autism Research Centre, University of Cambridge, Cambridge CB2 8AH, UK

Index

A

Alpha Asymmetry, 115, 117-118, 121-123, 125-126

Angelman Syndrome, 21, 23-24, 67-68, 83, 87-89, 93-94

Anxiety, 20, 35, 56, 60-62, 65-69, 73, 75-79, 82, 106-107, 109, 112-113, 128, 144, 149, 153, 167, 175, 178, 199, 233, 236

Asperger's Syndrome, 49, 82, 97, 104, 128, 204, 206

Attentional Synchrony, 38

Autism, 1-3, 12-17, 19, 21-25, 36-41, 43-56, 65-76, 78-84, 91, 93-95, 97, 103-115, 117, 120-123, 127-132, 139-144, 150, 152-155, 166-180, 183, 185, 188-189, 191-197, 203-208, 215, 228-230

Autism Spectrum Disorder, 1-2, 12-13, 15, 21-25, 36-38, 40, 45-46, 54-56, 67-68, 81-82, 94, 97, 103-104, 113, 115, 117, 130, 140-144, 152-155, 167, 177-180, 191-193, 205-206, 219, 236

Autistic Symptomatology, 168-169, 176

Autistic Trait, 49-51, 53, 196, 222, 224

B

Brain Anatomy, 130, 141

Brain Serotonergic System, 143

C

Camouflaging Behaviour, 79

Caregiver Sensory Profile, 105-106, 111

Cerebral Cortex, 141, 166

D

Dental Amalgam, 47, 49-51

Depression, 18, 21, 56-58, 61-63, 66-70, 73, 75-82, 117, 128, 144, 153, 167

Depth Perception, 193-194, 203, 205

Diffusion-weighted Imaging, 1-2, 12

Dopamine, 18, 56-57, 59, 63-65, 67-68, 128, 166

Dorsal Raphe, 143-144, 146-147, 150-153

Dyspraxia, 73, 194, 206

E

Early Detection, 180

Empathy Problem, 79, 82

Epilepsy, 3, 15-16, 22-23, 68, 73, 83-84, 93, 131

Estradiol Treatment, 155-156

F

Factor Analysis, 176, 193, 196-198, 201, 205-207, 233

Fasciculus, 1, 4, 8-9, 12-13

Foveal Avascular Zone, 42

G

Gene Therapy, 15-23

Grey-white Matter Tissue, 130, 139-141

H

Hyperactivity Disorder, 3, 55, 73, 80, 117, 141, 179, 181, 206

Hypersensitivity, 105-112, 114-115, 153, 174, 236

I

Impaired Social Interaction, 15, 23, 56-57, 155

Inferior Longitudinal Fasciculus, 1, 4, 8, 12-13

Intellectual Disability, 15-16, 70, 80, 83-84, 176, 205

J

Joint Attention, 38, 40-43, 45-46, 95, 101, 103-104, 193

L

Learning Disability, 73

Lower Fractional Anisotropy, 2

M

Maternal Mercury, 50, 52

Mental Health, 55, 69-76, 78-80, 140, 152, 180-181

Mitochondria, 238-240, 247-248

Motor Skill, 193, 198, 201-204, 206

N

Neural Mechanism, 116

Neuroanatomical Difference, 140

Neurodevelopmental Disorder, 83

Neuroimaging, 2, 13, 18, 112, 130-132, 136, 141, 143, 151, 154, 218

Non-suicidal Self-injury, 69-70, 72-73, 80, 82

Norepinephrine, 56-57, 59, 63, 66-68, 128

O

Operationalizing Atypical Gaze, 38

Oscillatory Rhythm, 115

P

Paraformaldehyde, 57, 145, 152, 216

Path Analysis, 193, 201

Personality Disorder, 73

Pre-pulse Inhibition, 58, 63, 67

Prenatal Mercury, 47, 53, 55

Protein Parvalbumin, 155, 167

Psychological Profile, 220

R

Repetitive Behavior, 3, 6, 12-13, 31, 35, 43, 49-54, 81, 121, 153, 155-157, 163, 209-210, 217, 219

Reward Processing, 115-118, 120-123, 125, 127-128

S

Savant Syndrome, 220-223, 229, 232, 234-236

Sensory Processing, 2, 113-114, 127, 169, 179, 203, 219-220, 236

Sensory Sensitivity, 108-110, 112, 220, 222, 224, 229, 232-235, 237

Serotonin, 56-57, 59, 63, 66-68, 143-144, 147, 151-154, 218

Sleep Disturbance, 15-16, 105-107, 109-112

Sleep Dysfunction, 84

Social Behavior, 25, 45, 56-57, 65-66, 68, 118, 128, 141, 154-155, 158-160, 164-165, 167

Social Deficits, 56, 59, 66-67, 115-117, 125, 137, 177, 219

Social Motivation Hypothesis, 115-116, 125-126

Social Skills, 104, 118, 173, 193-194, 198, 201-204, 224-226, 235

Social Stimuli, 38, 46, 95, 103, 115-116, 118, 125, 127, 203

Stereoability, 193

Stereopsis, 193-195, 197-198, 201-207

Structural Connectivity, 1-2, 12-13, 91

Suicidality, 69-75, 77-81

Synaptic Dysfunction, 15, 22, 167

Synaptophysin, 25, 27, 32-33, 35-37

T

Theta, 83, 85, 87-89, 92, 115, 117-118, 121-123, 125-128

U

Ultrasonic Vocalization, 159

V

Viral Vector, 15, 18-20

Visual Processing, 1-3, 5-6, 9-13